Illustrated
Textbook of
Optics and
Refractive Anomalies

Illustrated

Textbook of
Optics and
Refractive Anomalies

AK Jain DNB, MNAMS

Assistant Professor
Department of Ophthalmology
Rama Medical College
Hapur, Uttar Pradesh

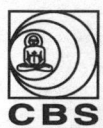

CBS

CBS Publishers & Distributors Pvt Ltd

New Delhi • Bengaluru • Chennai • Kochi • Kolkata • Mumbai
Hyderabad • Jharkhand • Nagpur • Patna • Pune • Uttarakhand

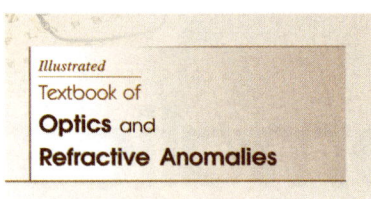

Illustrated
Textbook of
Optics and
Refractive Anomalies

ISBN: 978-93-86478-63-4

Copyright © Author and Publisher

First Edition: 2018

Published by Satish Kumar Jain and Produced by Varun Jain for

CBS Publishers & Distributors Pvt Ltd
4819/XI Prahlad Street, 24 Ansari Road, Daryaganj, New Delhi 110 002, India.
Ph: 23289259, 23266861, 23266867   Fax: 011-23243014   Website: www.cbspd.com
e-mail: delhi@cbspd.com; cbspubs@airtelmail.in.
Corporate Office: 204 FIE, Industrial Area, Patparganj, Delhi 110 092
Ph: 4934 4934   Fax: 4934 4935   e-mail: publishing@cbspd.com; publicity@cbspd.com

Branches

- **Bengaluru:** Seema House 2975, 17th Cross, K.R. Road,
  Banasankari 2nd Stage, Bengaluru 560 070, Karnataka
  Ph: +91-80-26771678/79   Fax: +91-80-26771680   e-mail: bangalore@cbspd.com
- **Chennai:** 7, Subbaraya Street, Shenoy Nagar, Chennai 600 030, Tamil Nadu
  Ph: +91-44-26680620, 26681266   Fax: +91-44-42032115   e-mail: chennai@cbspd.com
- **Kochi:** Ashana House, No. 39/1904, AM Thomas Road, Valanjambalam,
  Ernakulam 682 016, Kochi, Kerala
  Ph: +91-484-4059061-65   Fax: +91-484-4059065   e-mail: kochi@cbspd.com
- **Kolkata:** 6/B, Ground Floor, Rameswar Shaw Road, Kolkata-700 014, West Bengal
  Ph: +91-33-22891126, 22891127, 22891128   e-mail: kolkata@cbspd.com
- **Mumbai:** 83-C, Dr E Moses Road, Worli, Mumbai-400018, Maharashtra
  Ph: +91-22-24902340/41   Fax: +91-22-24902342   e-mail: mumbai@cbspd.com

Representatives

- **Hyderabad** 0-9885175004   • **Jharkhand** 0-9811541605   • **Nagpur** 0-9021734563
- **Patna** 0-9334159340   • **Pune** 0-9623451994   • **Uttarakhand** 0-9716462459

Printed at Goyal Offset Printers, GT Karnal Road, Industrial Area, Delhi, India

to

---

my beloved family members
for their support, encouragement and love

Foreword

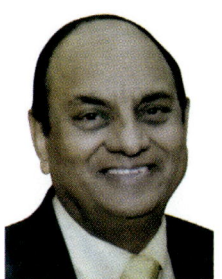

Optics and refraction is the foundation stone of ophthalmology and comprehensive knowledge of basics is essential in clinical practice. Majority of patients in ophthalmic practice have refractive errors, hence every ophthalmic personnel including ophthalmologist must be well trained to manage the refractive errors perfectly.

I am honoured and feel proud to write the Foreword to this book entitled *Illustrated Textbook of Optics and Refractive Anomalies*, as I had gone through the book and found it to be very useful for BSc and MSc optometry students and equally excellent for medical undergraduate and ophthalmology postgraduate students. This book is unique in the sense that it not only contains the basic concepts related to ocular optics and various refractive anomalies but also the live illustration of refraction methods. These illustrations of refraction give a clear image of real live reflexes seen during retinoscopy; hence students can understand the exact types of refractive error and can easily neutralize them when they perform retinoscopy on patients. The chapters on *refractive surgery* and *low vision* are very informative for ophthalmology postgraduate students. The language and text style is written in a very simple and crispy manner so that students can understand the basic concepts and reproduce them in examination. Section on problem-based learning is an exclusive representation in textbook of ophthalmology. Various footnotes and problem-based learning are the strengths of this book, which make the clear road for the clinical application of knowledge by the students in their daily practice. I congratulate the author for this unique endeavour on optics and refraction and wish him all the success for this book.

Prof DJ Pandey MS

Ex-Head, Department of Ophthalmology, and in-charge, Eye Bank and Cornea Clinic SN Medical College, Agra, Uttar Pradesh

Past President, UPSOS; Vice President, ACOIN Governor Awarded: Best Teacher Award

Preface

Refractive anomalies are one of the most common clinical problems encountered in the field of ophthalmology throughout the world and remain one of the difficult challenges to understand, hence a deep knowledge for correction of refractive anomalies is a prerequisite for the successful ophthalmic practice. *Illustrated Textbook of Optics and Refractive Anomalies* has been written to provide the basic information about optics and refractive errors. This book is written in a simple, concise and lucid manner with supportive illustrations in the form of ray diagrams, figures and tables so that the reader can acquire the profound knowledge about the subject with the help of diagrammatic representation of the respective topic.

This book comprises 5 sections including 18 chapters where each section contains the diagrammatic illustrations related to text for easy understanding of the students. Section I deals with the basic concepts of optics and lenses including light and its various properties, refraction and reflection through various surfaces and various types of lenses used in relation to the human eye. Basic knowledge of light and optics is essential to master the skill of refraction. This section serves as the foundation stone for correction of refractive anomalies of the human eye.

Section II covers various refractive anomalies associated with the human eye. This section consists of refractive status of the human eye in relation to not only the refractive errors but also with convergence and accommodation anomalies. This section also includes chapter on refractive errors seen with binocular vision anomalies and also the management of such refractive errors. Section III consists of chapters on vision and all the possible methods to evaluate the vision in the human eye. Visual status and the possibility in the amount of improvement in visual status form the basis for refraction. Evaluation of visual status is an art which requires the thorough knowledge of the examiner about the vision and cooperation of the patient, hence expressive examination techniques have been explained in this chapter to make it easy for readers. For mastering the art of refraction, optics of various kinds of retinoscopes and refraction tools is explained in great detail.

Section IV deals with the visual rehabilitation related to the management of different kinds of refractive anomalies. Detailed retinoscopy methods and various reflexes encountered during retinoscopy are also explained in simpler and illustrated manner. Chapter on retinoscopy contains the diagrams representing the actual reflexes seen in the patient's eye, hence the reader can master the technique of retinoscopy by reading this book. Section V at the end contains problem-based learning, where various problems related to refraction encountered during practice and the possible solutions have also been discussed in detail.

I hope this book will help teachers, residents, ophthalmologists and optometrists to widen their knowledge about optics and refraction. The knowledge and information gained from this book will assist the readers to comprehend the basic concepts of optics and various refraction anomalies of the human eye.

I believe that careful review and evaluation can create this book a better one and there is always scope of improvement. If there are mistakes and printing errors, please mail your feedback and suggestions to dramitjain75@gmail.com.

AK Jain

Acknowledgments

It is my great pleasure to express my gratitude to all those whose blessings and contribution have made this endeavour possible. First and foremost, I would like to thank God, the 'Almighty', who has provided me the strength to undertake this work and complete it successfully.

I would like to express my sincere thanks to Prof DJ Pandey for writing the Foreword to this book. I take pride in acknowledging the guidance of Prof AK Gupta (former Dean, Maulana Azad Medical College, New Delhi), ICARE Eye Hospital and Postgraduate Institute, Noida, who has been so helpful and cooperative in giving his support at all times to achieve my goal.

I also thank all my teachers, colleagues and students from Santosh Medical College; Narinder Mohan Hospital, Ghaziabad; Saraswati Medical College and Rama Medical College, Hapur; ICARE Hospital and Research Centre, Noida; and Sharp Sight Centre, Delhi; for their kind cooperation and valuable suggestions to complete this project. I am also thankful to Dr Sparsh Gupta, Dr Ashish Mehta, Dr Vivek Chhimpa, Dr Vikrant Sharma, Dr Vivek Jain, Dr Swati Gupta and Dr Amil A for their help and cooperation.

My acknowledgements would be incomplete without thanking all my family members for their indubitable support, love and encouragement in all my endeavours. I owe my special thanks to my wife Dr Seema and lovely sweet daughter Harshita Jain for her great patience, understanding and for giving me unlimited happiness and pleasure.

I would like to thank Mr Satish Kumar Jain (CMD), Mr Varun Jain (Director), CBS Publishers & Distributors, and their management team for the enthusiastic cooperation, professional skills, and suggestions and to finish this task in an impressive manner. I would like to take this opportunity to thank Mr YN Arjuna (Senior Vice-President—Publishing, Editorial and Publicity), Mrs Ritu Chawla (AGM Production), Mr Prasenjit Paul (copyeditor), Mr Ram Murti (graphic artist), Mr Neeraj Prasad (graphic artist) and Mr Vikrant Sharma (DTP operator) for preparing the book material in a press-ready form. My thanks go to artist Mr Sumit Sharma whose artistic representations created the magical illustrations.

Last but not the least I thank all my patients who make me knowledgeable enough to write this book on optics and refractive anomalies.

AK Jain

Contents

Optics and Ophthalmic Lenses

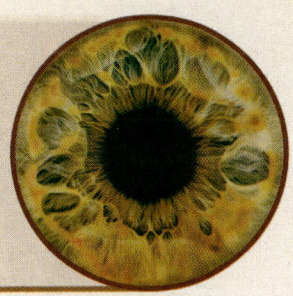

Elementary Optics

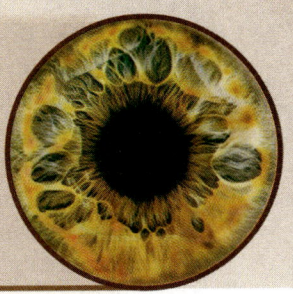

Learning Objectives

After studying this chapter the reader should be able to:
- Describe the various theories proposed for light.
- Describe the different properties of light.
- Explain the diffraction, polarization, interference, coherence, scattering, transmission and absorption phenomenon of light and their applications.
- Explain the fluorescence and photoelectric effect of light.
- Understand and explain various photometry and radiometry terms used for measurement of light.
- Understand the basic mechanism and basic properties of LASER.
- Explain the sensitivity of human eyes for various spectrum of light.

Chapter Outline

- Introduction
  - History of nature of light
- Properties of light
  - Physical properties
    - Character of light
    - Propagation of light
    - Intensity of light
  - Optical properties
    - Diffraction
    - Polarization
    - Interference and coherence
- Transmission and absorbance
- Scattering
- Illumination and brightness
  - Radiometry
  - Photometry
- Special properties
  - Fluorescence
  - Photoelectric effect
  - LASER
- Visible light versus human eye

INTRODUCTION

Light is an electromagnetic energy. The visible portion of the light which lies in between the ultraviolet and infrared wavelengths is the one which gives us the sensation of seeing the objects. This visible spectrum has seven colors represented as VIBGYOR, an acronym of Violet, Indigo, Blue, Green, Yellow, Orange and Red. To understand the light we need to look into the history of nature of light.

History of Nature of Light

- ***Particle theory of Newton:*** In the year 1675, Sir Isaac Newton postulated that light emits from a source in the stream form and is made up of minute particles called corpuscles. These corpuscles move in the air medium unaffected by gravity and give the feeling of sight when enters the eye. Newton's theory was able to describe the properties like propagation of light in vacuum, reflection and refraction, but was unable to describe the properties like diffraction, polarization and interference of light.

- *Wave theory of Huygens*: Subsequently, in the year 1678, Huygens tried to explain phenomenon such as diffraction and interference of light by proposing that light moves in the waveform after emitting from a source. According to this theory, the light wave has troughs and crests, which are circular in the shape for a given time. Wavefront is location of various points in the same phase at a given particular time of light wave. Various shapes of wavefront are dependent on the type of light source, e.g. point source produces spherical wave-fronts, whereas long slit source gives cylindrical wavefront.

- *Electromagnetic theory of Maxwell*: In the year 1873, Maxwell improvised the wave theory by proposing that light wave is not a mechanical wave but it is an electro-magnetic wave. Electromagnetic wave means that light wave has both electric and magnetic fields while travelling in vacuum. This theory could partially explain the scattering phenomenon of light but was unable to explain the photoelectric property of light.

- *Quantum theory of Einstein*: In the year 1905, Einstein came with a proposal that light with a given frequency consists of quanta (photon) with the same energy. It can be explained by equation

$$e = h\eta$$

Here e = energy, h = Planck's constant (6.626 × 10^{-34}), η = frequency of light

By this equation we can make out that energy (e) is directly proportional to the frequency of light but energy is inversely proportional to the wavelength of light; because frequency is inversely proportional to wavelength.

- *Dual-nature theory* is the recent concept about light and is accepted universally.

According to dual-nature theory, light behaves like both wave and photon (particle).

PROPERTIES OF LIGHT

To understand the principles of optics and refraction it is essential to know the various properties of the light. Table 1.1 summarizes the important and related properties of light so that readers can understand the various clinical applications of the light.

Physical Properties
Character of Light

Light is a dual natured form of energy, which acts like a wave in a medium and like a photon in the vacuum.

Different medium can be classified as

- Transparent
- Translucent
- Opaque

When light passes through a medium in unchanged form, that medium is called *transparent medium*. If only a part of light is disturbed when passing through medium, but still light can pass through a medium, then that medium is called *translucent medium*. If a medium does not allow any light to pass through it, then that medium is called *opaque medium*.

Light moves as an electromagnetic wave in a group and makes an energy spectrum of

Table 1.1: Different properties of light		
Physical properties	*Optical properties*	*Special properties*
• Character of light • Propagation of light • Intensity of light	• Diffraction • Polarization • Interference and coherence • Transmission and absorption • Scattering • Illumination and brightness	• Fluorescence • Photoelectric effect • LASER

Table 1.2: Types of rays with their respective wavelengths

Types of rays	Wavelength
Cosmic rays	1×10^{-5} nm
Gamma rays	1×10^{-3} nm
X-rays	0.14×10^{-1} nm
Ultraviolet rays	$13.6 \times 10^{+1}$ nm
Visible light (**VIBGYOR**)	
Violet ray	385–425 nm
Indigo ray	425–445 nm
Blue ray	445–490 nm
Green ray	490–555 nm
Yellow ray	555–585 nm
Orange ray	585–645 nm
Red ray	645–750 nm
Infrared ray	$750 - 1 \times 10^5$ nm
Electromagnetic ray	More than 3×10^{13} nm

different wavelengths and types of rays. Summary of types of rays and wavelength is shown in Table 1.2.

Propagation of Light

Wave theory: Wave theory is the most popular and widely accepted theory for the propagation of light. According to wave theory, once light is emitted from a luminous body and passes through a homogeneous medium, it propagates in all the directions. Although light propagate in all the directions but it moves only in a straight line in the form of a wave as shown in Fig. 1.1.

'I' shows a light wave at particular instance.

'II' shows a second light wave after a short interval.

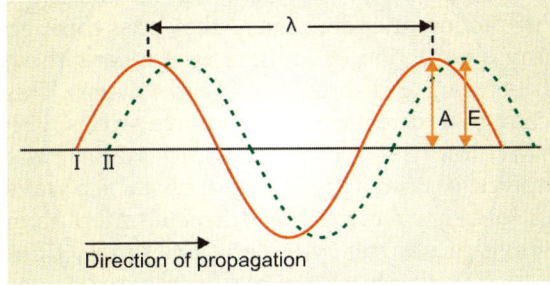

Fig. 1.1: Motion of light in waveform

'λ' is the distance between two consecutive crest of light waves and represents wavelength. At any given instance of time the crest (or trough) of light wave is circular in shape.

'E' represents the electric field of the light wave at a defined point and this electric field always remains perpendicular to the direction of propagation of light wave.

'A' indicates the maximum value of electric field and it represents amplitude of wave, which determines the intensity of the wave.

During propagation of light wave there is no movement of matter rather with the passage of wave the electric field increases, decreases and reverses in its direction at each point.

Another important characteristic of a wave is its frequency, which is defined as number of crests that pass a fixed point in duration of one second.

In addition to electric field, light wave has a magnetic field which decreases and increases in relation of the electric field. This magnetic field is a three-dimensional representation which lie perpendicular to the direction of propagation in one plane and electric field of wave in another plane.

Propagation of light in a wave form explains various properties of light such as

- Diffraction
- Polarization
- Interference
- Illumination
- Reflection
- Refraction

Photon theory: Interaction of light with matter results in either emission or absorption of individual quanta of energy (photon). Photon is also a form of light because some consider that light is a stream of particles moving together. Amount of energy (*e*) per photon is calculated by formula

$$e = h\eta$$

where η represents frequency of light wave and *h* is Planck's constant

As it is clear from the formula that photon energy and frequency of light wave are directly proportional to each other, whereas frequency of light wave is inversely proportional to the wavelength of light. So, energy of a photon is also inversely proportional to wavelength of light, hence photon of wavelength 400 nm will have double energy than 800 nm photon. Thus, a red light with 800 nm wavelength is less harmful than ultraviolet light (< 400 nm) or X-ray (< 350 nm) which can burn or can severely damage the tissues.

To explain the photon theory we can consider the phenomenon of fluorescence as shown by fluorescein molecule during fundus angiography. A single molecule of fluorescein absorbs a single photon of blue light. When this fluorescein molecule emits light, photon with lower energy is emitted which lies in the yellow green spectrum and the remaining energy of photon is used for heat production or chemical reaction with fluorescein molecule.

Various properties of light can be explained by the phenomenon of photon theory such as

- Scattering of light
- Fluorescence
- Photoelectric effect

Intensity of Light

As we all know that light travels in all the directions. When light moves from one point to other, its intensity rapidly decreases as the distance increases from the point of source of light. In other words, the intensity of light is inversely proportional to the distance of light source. Light obeys the law of inverse square (Fig. 1.2) means intensity will be more (brighter) near the light source and it will decrease (dim) far from the light source.

Suppose L_1 and L_2 are amounts of light falling per second per unit area on two spheres A and B having radius r_1 and r_2, respectively (Fig. 1.2). As we know that area of a sphere is $4\pi r^2$, hence the amount of light falling on spheres A and B is $L_1 4\pi r_1^2$ and $L_2 4\pi r_2^2$,

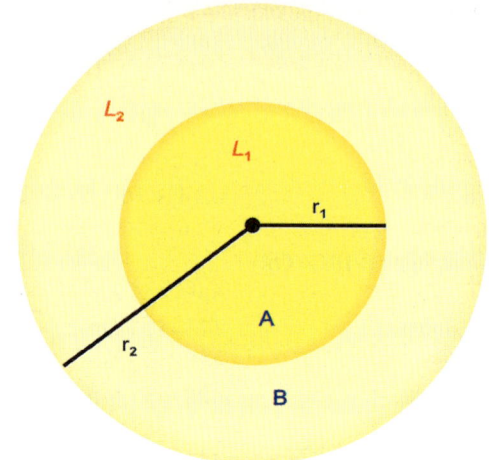

Fig. 1.2: Law of inverse square

respectively. Since the light is equally distributed on both the spheres, hence

$$L_1 4\pi r_1^2 = L_2 4\pi r_2^2$$

$$\frac{L_1}{L_2} = \frac{4\pi r_2^2}{4\pi r_1^2}$$

$$= \frac{r_2^2}{r_1^2}$$

So to simplify light intensity at any given point on a surface and square of distance from the light source are inversely proportional to each other.

Optical Properties

Diffraction

All types of waves when pass through an obstacle, an aperture or through any form of irregularities in the medium get diffracted. It means there is a change in the direction of the waves. Similarly, the light waves also show diffraction phenomenon as they pass through any obstruction or an aperture, means there is bending and spreading of light waves. This change in direction of light wave varies with wavelength of the light and size of the aperture. With a given size of obstacle a wave of longer wavelength is diffracted more than wave of shorter wavelength. Hence, light wave with shorter wavelength produces minimal amount of appreciable change of direction. Furthermore, the diffraction is much more evident when the size of the obstacle/ aperture is small.

Types of diffraction: Two types of diffraction may occur depending on the distance between the source and the screen.

- **Fresnel diffraction:** This type of diffraction will occur when source of light or screen or both are present at a fixed distance from the diffracting material (obstruction or aperture), i.e. source of light and screen are not far away from each other. As shown in Fig. 1.3 that incident wavefront is spherical in nature because point light source is situated at finite distance. Similarly, wavefronts emitting after getting diffracted from obstacle or aperture are also spherical in nature. Because of the spherical nature of wavefronts, a definite diffraction pattern can be produced on screen, without any additional lens.

- **Fraunhofer diffraction:** It occurs when the light source and screen, or either of them, are present at infinite distance from the obstruction or aperture, means source of light and screen are far away from each other. As shown in Fig. 1.4, in this type of diffraction the incident wavefronts are plane or straight because light source is situated at infinity. Similarly, wavefronts leaving the obstruction or aperture are also plane or straight in nature. Because of straight wavefronts there is need of a convex lens to converge these wavefronts so that a definite diffraction pattern can be produced on the screen.

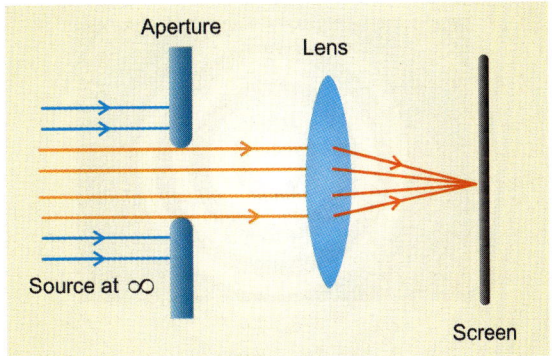

Fig. 1.4: Fraunhofer diffraction

Many other optical effects of light like interference or refraction may also combine with diffraction and may be seen in various forms. Suppose many optical effects are present together and diffraction becomes dominant among them; then we observe the specific pattern of diffraction only. For example, if we see the specific pattern of a distant light through a fine woven curtain or through a windshield (which is repeatedly rubbed by the windshield wipers over a car glass), then in these cases the bending of light ray will be perpendicular to the incidence ray, hence a diffraction perpendicular to light ray will be seen. However, in the case of a cross woven curtain, an array of bright spots of two dimensions is seen because in this case the interference is getting mixed with the diffraction, and both together are producing bright spots of light. If only diffraction could have occurred, then a continuous streak of light would have seen rather than spots of light.

Effect of diffraction on visual acuity: Let us see the effect of diffraction on visual acuity. In emmetrope having pupil size of 2.5 mm or less, the limit of visual acuity is determined by diffraction. A distant light source forms an image on retina of the eye. This image has concentric dark and light rings which are surrounding a bright central disc of light. This central bright disc is called airy disc (Fig. 1.5).

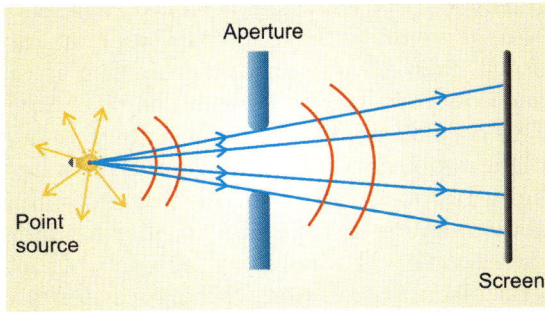

Fig. 1.3: Fresnel diffraction

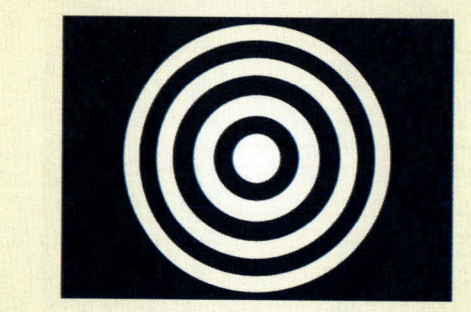

Fig. 1.5: Airy disc

This can be represented by an equation:

$$D = 2.44\,f\,\frac{\lambda}{d}$$

Here D = diameter of disc

    f = focal length of optical system, i.e. eye

    λ = wavelength

    d = diameter of aperture, i.e. pupil

When light waves of different wavelengths pass through pupil of the same size, then light wave of longer wavelength (red) will diffract

Optical Applications

- Various studies concluded that amount of best resolution produced by an optical instrument or eye is restricted by the phenomenon of diffraction. The radius of airy disc is approximately equivalent to the minimal resolvable distance. For example, resolution of telescopes can be increased by increasing the aperture of its objective lens.
- Aspherical irregularities of the cornea and crystalline lens rarely allow the formation of an airy disc, even if we are looking at a small source of light through a very small pupil.
- For any optical system diffraction decides the limit of its finest resolution. Because of this in fabrication of optical components a degree of precision is present, after this there will be no improvement in the image quality, even if we change the resolution.
- Rayleigh criterion sets limit of resolution that can be produced by an optical system. This criterion states that *"no further improvement will be seen in the resolution of an optical system, if the optical system produces a wave front that lies within one quarter wavelength limit of being perfect"*.

Clinical Applications

Rayleigh criterion is used to set standards in the fabrication of optical components in optical devices.

more than the shorter wavelength (blue). Hence, it is clear from the above equation that an airy disc of larger diameter will be formed by a wave having longer wavelength (red light) as compared to a wave with shorter wavelength (blue light). Diameter of disc (D) is inversely proportional to size of pupil (d) so if the size of pupil decreases, the diameter of central disc increases and vice versa.

Polarization

Usually, human eye is not sensitive to perceive polarized light except in case of the Haidinger's brushes phenomenon where polarized light is perceived as a yellowish bar in the center of visual field. In ophthalmology there are several clinical applications of polarized light.

Normally visible light has vast number of waves emitted by molecules of light source, because each molecule produces a wave oriented in its own specific plane. These light waves which are propagating in all the directions and oriented in different planes are termed as unpolarized light.

Hence, an unpolarized light is a haphazard mixture of polarized beams of light directed in various planes. Mixture of unpolarized light and polarized light (plane, circular or elliptical) is termed partially polarized light.

To understand polarization in simpler way, consider a rope which has been tied at one end. Now if we move free end of the rope up and down, then a wave of rope propagate as up and down oscillations along the length of rope. This oscillation of wave up and down in one plane represents a linear or plane polarized light. Suppose if we rotate the free end of this abovementioned rope in a circular manner, then a wave will travel along the length of rope in a circular manner which represents a circularly polarized light.

Partially polarized light can be produced from a plane reflecting surface by phenomenon of specular reflection. Naturally occurring plane surfaces like water and snow cause polarization of light on incidence, although a polarized light will be produced only when the angle of reflection from these surfaces is equal to polarizing angle (Brewster angle φ) of medium or surface (Fig. 1.6).

When visible light faces an edge situated between surfaces of two refracting media having different refractive indices, some part of the light is usually reflected. The part or fraction of the visible light which gets reflected can be expressed by the help of Fresnel equations. These expressions are dependent upon the polarization of incident light beam and its angle of incidence. For example, consider a light ray is reflecting from a glass medium (refractive index ≈ 1.5) into the air medium (refractive index ≈ 1), then the polarization angle is approximately 56°, whereas when light ray is reflecting from an air–water interface (refractive index ≈ 1.33), then the Brewster's angle (φ) to produce polarization is approximately 53°. By these examples we can make out that Brewster's angle (φ) or polarizing angle is not only dependent on the angle of incidence but also dependent on the refractive index of a given medium.

As discussed the degree of polarizing angle of incident light ray varies according to the refractive index of the medium; certain materials show differential refractive index which decides the polarization and direction of propagation of light. These materials are known as birefringent (birefractive) material and exhibit an optical property called as birefringence. This birefringence property of a material is responsible for the phenomenon of double refraction, where an incident light ray when falls on a birefractive material, polarization takes place and single incident ray split into two rays, out of them one ray is fully polarized. These two light rays after polarization do not propagate in the same direction rather moves into slightly different paths. Crystal having non-cubic structures like calcite crystal, and plastic under mechanical stress are examples of a birefringent material.

Unpolarized light can be transformed into plane polarized light by passing an unpolarized light beam through a polarizing material like plastic sheet or certain crystals like tourmaline or calcite crystals. These polarized materials or filters allow passing of light wave which is propagating in one particular plane and prevent passing of remaining light waves, which are propagating in other planes. So the resultant light wave coming out through these polarized filters propagate in one particular plane only. As we can see in Fig. 1.7, a tourmaline crystal C_1 (whose axis is cut parallel to unpolarized light) has been placed in the path of light wave. This will produce a polarized light in the same direction of light beam.

Now, if we place another crystal C_2 (whose axis is also cut parallel to unpolarized light) after C_1, the resultant light wave will also be a polarized light in the same direction as before (Fig. 1.8). Now, suppose we keep the axis of crystal C_1 fixed and rotate the axis of crystal C_2, then the light emerging from C_2 becomes dimmer and dimmer in proportionate with amount of rotation of crystal C_2. When the axis of crystal C_2 becomes perpendicular to axis of C_1, no light will come out of C_2 as shown in Fig. 1.9.

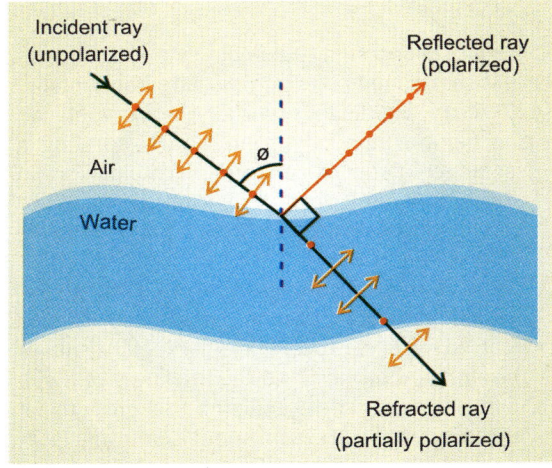

Incident ray
(unpolarized)

Reflected ray
(polarized)

Air

Ø

Water

Refracted ray
(partially polarized)

Fig. 1.6: Brewster's angle (φ)

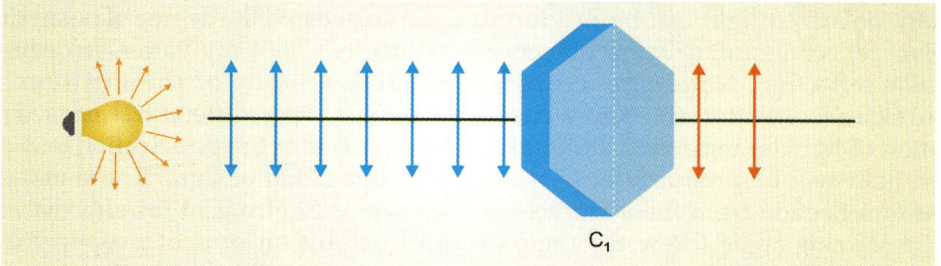

Fig. 1.7: Phenomenon of polarization, transverse wave passing through crystal C_1

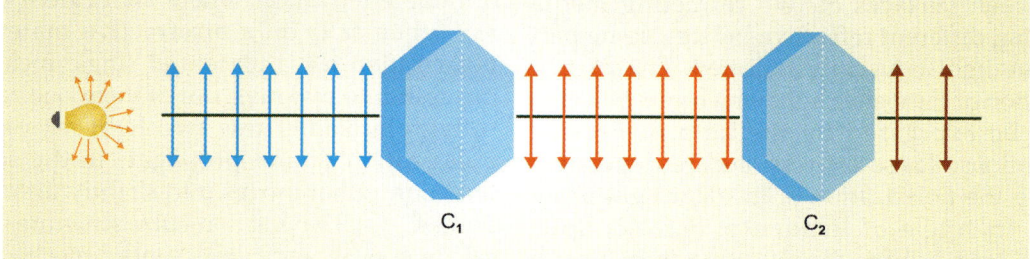

Fig. 1.8: No change occurs after placing another crystal C_2, which is rotating in same direction

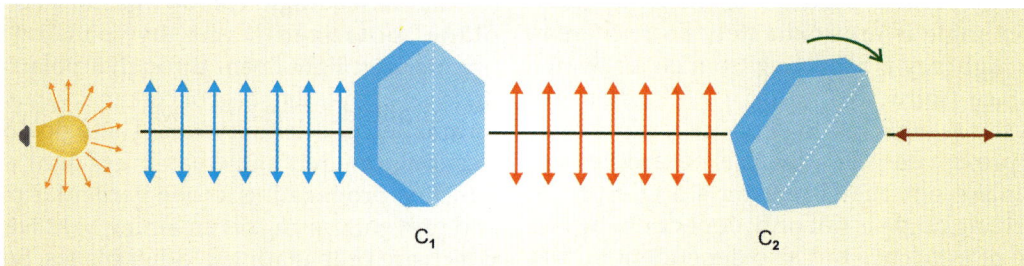

Fig. 1.9: First crystal (C_1) kept fixed second crystal (C_2) rotate; polarized light vanishes when C_2 becomes perpendicular to C_1

Clinical Application

- The phenomenon of polarization has been incorporated in number of ophthalmic instruments like slit lamp, ophthalmoscope, mainly to eliminate unwanted strong reflex from cornea.
- Polarizing sunglasses are very useful in reducing glare produced due to reflected sunlight from natural surfaces like water surface (during boating) or snow surface (during skiing). Since the predominant polarization in natural surfaces occurs horizontally, these sunglasses are designed in such a way that only vertically polarized light can pass through them. Similarly, light reflected from surface of roads or glass surface of oncoming automobiles (during driving) is also partially polarized, usually horizontally.
- Clinically Haidinger's brushes phenomenon can be demonstrated by continuously rotating a polarizer in front of a uniform blue field. Normal individual will observe a rotating structure having double ended brush or a propeller. This phenomenon can be used in localization of fovea during sensory testing or to evaluate the retinal nerve fiber layer at macula.
- Retinal nerve fiber layer (RNFL) shows birefringent property, so the thickness of RNFL can be measured by utilizing this property of birefringence. An instrument scanning laser polarimetry (e.g. GDx-VCC) uses polarized light

and measures the thickness of RNFL by calculating the amount of retardation in laser beam.

- Polarizing projection charts are clinically very useful because after wearing of specialized polarizing glasses it is possible to test only single eye while the patient is seeing polarizing projection chart binocularly. This test is successfully applied on malingering patients to detect the status of visual acuity. For example, alternate letters on Snellen's chart can be polarized at 90 degree to each other. When a patient wearing polarized glasses is asked to see these letters, the letters are seen separately through each of the eye. Suppose if a patient complains that he/she is blind uniocularly, but after wearing polarized glasses he/she reads all letters from 6/6 line correctly on Snellen's chart, it indicates that this patient is malingering the blindness.
- Similarly, several other charts based on the principal of polarization have been designed, which provide sensitivity tests for binocular functions or abnormalities. For example, Titmus fly test for streopsis, Mallett card test for fixation disparity and stereo projector method for aniseikonia.

Interference and Coherence

When two light waves arising from the same source are bring together, the phenomenon of interference occurs. This phenomenon of interference is better appreciated when the light wave is either monochromatic or its wavelength lies within narrow bandwidth, although a white light under favorable conditions can also produce an interference.

As shown in Fig. 1.10, waves produced from a single light source are made to pass through a small aperture. This produces a wavefront of light moving in defined direction. The curved lines in Fig. 1.10 are representing crests of waves at a particular instance. Now let us see what happens when this wavefront of light is made to pass through two small apertures. These light waves superimpose with each other and produces interference. Two types of interference can occur, depending on the way by which these waves superimpose with each other.

Constructive interference: When the crests (maxima) or trough (minima) of two waves coincide with each other, the energy of electromagnetic fields is added together and a wave of maximum intensity is produced. The amplitude of resulting wave will be equal to the sum of the amplitude of two waves which were superimposing. Hence, they produce constructive interference represented as light bands in Fig. 1.10(A). As shown in Fig. 1.11, when two light waves travelling in

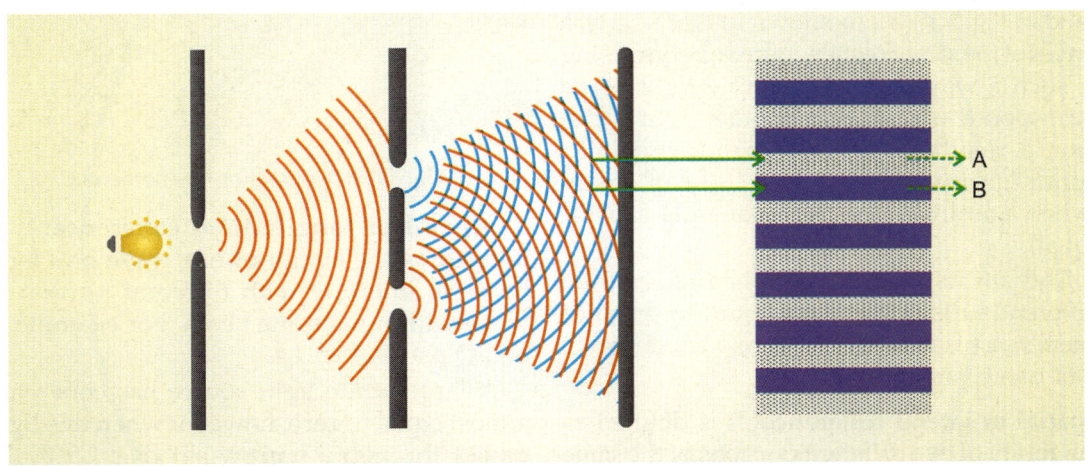

Fig. 1.10: Interference pattern. A: Light band (constructive interference); B: Dark band (destructive interference)

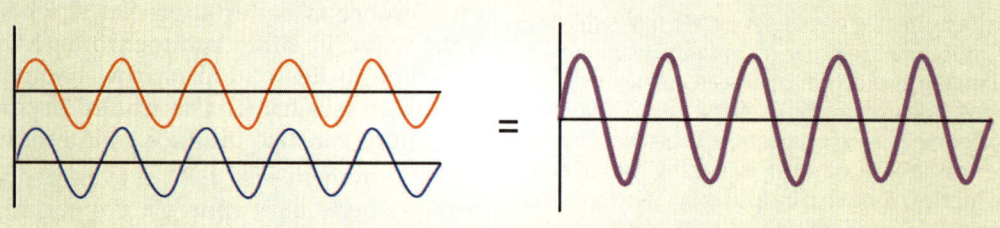

Fig. 1.11: Constructive interference

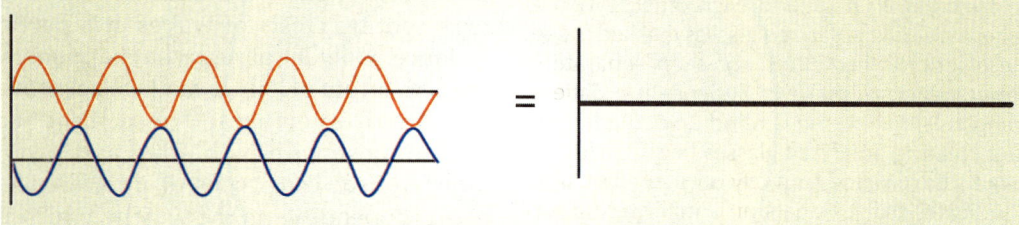

Fig. 1.12: Destructive interference

same direction having the same frequency gets merged in such a way that their crests coincide with each other then they produce a resultant wave of maximum intensity.

Destructive interference: When the crest (maxima) of one wave coincides with the trough (minima) of other wave, then a wave of minimum intensity is produced because energy of two electromagnetic fields is cancelled by each other. Hence, they produce destructive interference represented as dark band in Fig. 1.10(B). As shown in Fig. 1.12, two waves of the same frequency are superimposing in such a way that crest of one light wave corresponds with trough of other light wave, then a resultant wave is produced with minimum intensity or zero light intensity (when amplitude of two waves is exactly equal).

The ability of two light beams, or two different parts of the same beam to produce interference is termed coherence. The coherence is of two types:

Spatial or lateral coherence: It is defined as the ability of two different portions of the same light wave to generate interference. For example, O and P part in Fig. 1.13.

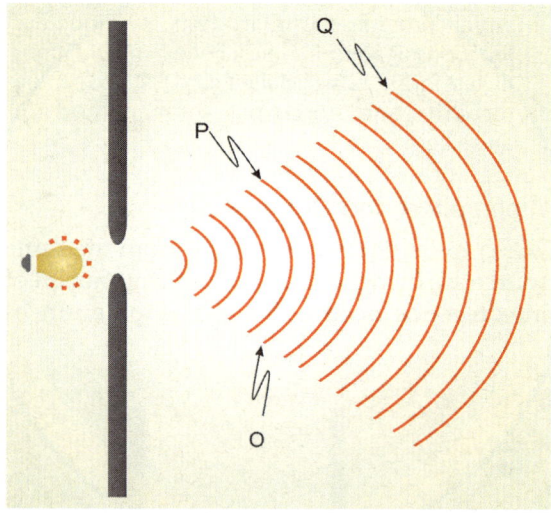

Fig. 1.13: Coherence phenomenon

Temporal or longitudinal coherence: It is defined as the ability of one wave of a light beam to interfere with different portion of wave within the same beam. For example, P and Q part in Fig. 1.13.

A large white light source has coherence almost equal to zero, however when this light passes through a narrow slit (Fig. 1.13), the spatial coherence between O and P improves and it may approach unity as slit width

Clinical Applications

- The LASER interferometry technique is based on phenomenon of interference of laser beams. This laser interferometry is used to evaluate the retinal function; hence potential vision can be assessed in patients having media opacities due to cataract.
- 3D images in holography are produced by phenomenon of interference.
- During fluorescein angiography excitation and barrier filters of fundus camera are based on interference. Excitation filter used in fundus camera transmits short wavelengths (below 500 nm), which cause fluorescein to fluoresce. The barrier filter used in fundus camera transmits only long wavelengths (above 500 nm), hence only fluorescent emission is received by film, whereas remaining excitation light is blocked.
- Based on interference filters, the cold mirrors are coated in multiple layers. These multilayers are designed in such a manner that they allow infrared waves to transmit, whereas visible light gets reflected.
- Spectacles glasses having anti-reflection coating works on the principle of destructive interference.
- OCT (optical coherence topography) is based on principles of interference and uses infrared rays as light source.

approaches to zero. Temporal coherence can be improved by using filters, which selects only a narrow band of wavelength. Laser light is an example of highly coherent beam.

Transmission and Absorption

Passing of radiant energy through a medium or space is termed transmission. This is measured as transmittance which is defined as percentage of the light energy that can pass through a particular medium or substance. For example, if the intensity of the incident light falling on a semi-transparent material is I', and the intensity of transmitted light is I, then transmittance (T) would be

$$T = \frac{I}{I'}$$

Transmittance is expressed as unitless number between 0 and 1.

When it is represented as a percentage, then it is called the percentage transmittance (%T).

$$\%T = I \times \frac{100}{I'}$$

Absorbance measures the amount of an incident light that is absorbed by molecules of material when it travels through a material. As a result of absorbance the intensity of light will decreases exponentially with distance as the light passes through the material. In other words, absorbance increases as path length of light increases. Absorbance is usually expressed in terms of optical density (OD) and is measured by using an absorption spectrophotometer. It is based on the principle that every substance or medium can absorb or transmits certain wavelengths of radiant energy but not other wavelengths. The absorption of a sample or material can be calculated from value of transmittance. It is defines as the negative logarithm of the transmittance.

$$\text{Absorbance (OD)} = \log \frac{1}{T} \text{ or } \frac{100}{\%T}$$

As clear from formula if transmittance of light is 10%, then absorbance (OD) will be 1. Similarly, if transmittance is 1% and 100%, then absorbance (OD) will be 2 and 0 (zero), respectively.

Scattering

When parallel light beam passes via a substance or gas medium, a few rays move in directions other than the direction of its initial

Clinical Applications

- Absorbed light can excite an electron into a higher level as seen in fluorescence phenomenon.
- Several optical devices like light filters and sunglasses utilizes the phenomenon of absorption to produce effects like polarization. Birefringent crystals like tourmaline or calcite completely absorbs the specific wavelengths of light, which are not in alignment with their molecular structures; hence they transmit only a single ray of linearly polarized light.

Applications of Scattering

- Amount of scattering is dependent on two factors, i.e. wavelength of the light and size of particles in atmosphere.
  - Light having shorter wavelengths (blue) will scatter more as compared to longer wavelengths (red light). Hence, blue light scatters more as compared to red light. Due to this fact the color of sky appears blue. Similarly, red color is used to indicate danger in signals because it can be seen from a longer distance as there is no significant loss of red color due to scattering of light.
  - Rayleigh phenomenon occurs due to scattering of light by smaller size particles in air and is dependent on wavelength of incident light, whereas larger particles like dust particles scatter light irrespective of the wavelength of incident light. For example, sky appears blue in mid-day light and appears reddish during sunset time, because blue light (shorter wavelength) scatters strongly by small particles in mid-day time and during sunset time only longer wavelengths (red) remain (because they scatter less during daytime).
- Scattering of light affects vision in two ways, one by phenomenon of glare and second by reduction in the amount of light.
  - Glare: Bright sources of light like sunlight or vehicle headlights when fall on an eye, a fraction of light get scattered inside the ocular media and then it reaches the retina. As a result, the contrast of fovea decreases due to this scattered light and objects look blur.
  - Reduction in amount of light: A few ocular pathologies like cataract, anterior chamber flare and corneal edema cause more scattering of light. Large molecules in nucleus of lens in the early stages of cataract are responsible for scattering of light and hence multiple images of very distinct object like moon are seen in intumescent cataract. Similarly, proteins molecules in anterior chamber and fluid in cornea will scatter the light and person complaints of diminished vision.

incidence. In other words, the light emerges from medium in a different direction from the incident light. This movement of light rays in different directions is called scattering of light. Phenomenon of scattering takes place at molecular and atomic level, i.e. gas atoms or molecules present in the medium when get stroked by the incident light rays, electrons of these molecules absorb energy from the light and then release or re-radiate this absorbed energy into various directions as shown in Fig. 1.14. Due to this reradiation the light appears as if scattered in the various directions.

Scattering due to very small molecules or particles present in the atmosphere produces a phenomenon called Rayleigh phenomenon (Fig. 1.14). Usually this Rayleigh phenomenon is very weak in nature and it may vary according to the wavelength of the incident light; means *shorter is the wavelength, greater will be the scattering*. For example, sky appears blue because the blue light (shortest wavelength) from the sun is scattered more as

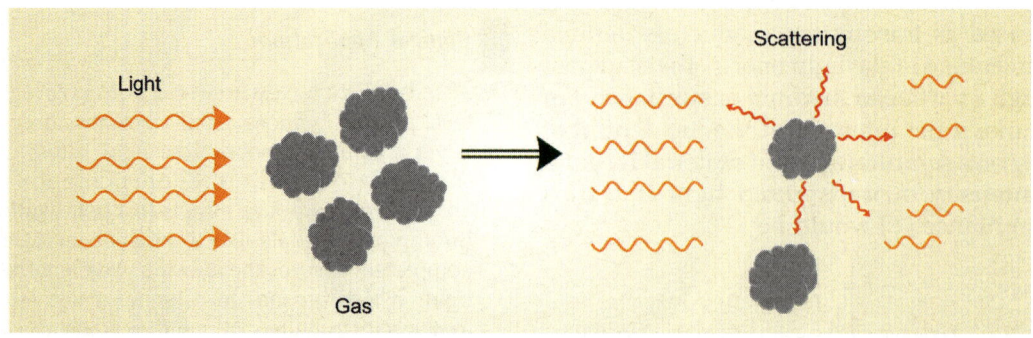

Fig. 1.14: Scattering phenomenon of light

compared to other wavelengths present in the sunlight. Larger particles such as dust particles in the atmosphere will scatter the light more intensely and is less dependent on the wavelength of incident light ray.

Illumination and Brightness

In normal physiological state, human eyes respond only to visible light, whereas identification of other spectrum waves require very sophisticated and advance scientific instruments like radio receivers or scintillation counters. For better understanding of illumination and brightness, we should be well aware of methods and terminologies required for measurement of light. Visible light can be measured by means of

- Radiometry
- Photometry

Radiometry: In broader terms radiometry is referred as measurement of light in terms of power, however, practically radiometry is used to measure the infrared, visible and ultraviolet lights with the help of optical instruments.

Following terms are used for the understanding of radiometric measurements:

- Radiant energy
- Radiant flux (radiant power)
- Radiant flux density

Radiant energy: Light as such is a form of radiant energy and electromagnetic radiation cause transport of this radiant energy through the space. These electromagnetic radiations can be considered as either wave or particle which is dependent on the fact that in which form we are measuring these electromagnetic radiations. Light energy is converted into another form of energy after getting absorbed by an object. Radiant energy of visible light which is a part of electromagnetic radiations is transferred into electrons of matter in the form of kinetic energy. This kinetic or motion energy causes the movement of electrons in the form of an electric current to flow in a photographic light meter. Thus in simpler words, radiant energy is the energy transferred,

received or emitted from source in the form of electromagnetic radiations and it is represented by symbol Q and is measured in unit as joules.

Note: Spectral radiant energy is nothing but the amount of radiant energy per unit wavelength interval and its unit of measurement is joules per nanometer.

Radiant flux (Radiant power): Radiant energy measured for each unit time is referred as Radiant power. It means that the energy transferred, received or emitted per unit time in the form of electromagnetic radiation is radiant power and is measured as joules per second or *watts*. As we know that light flows through the space so in simpler words, the flow of radiant energy per unit time can be termed radiant power or radiant flux. Radiant flux is denoted as ω and is measured in watts.

Note: Spectral radiant flux is nothing but radiant flux per unit wavelength interval and its unit of measurement is watts per nanometer.

Radiant flux density: It measures the amount of the radiant flux arriving or leaving at or from unit area of a real or unreal surface in unit time. The amount of radiant flux which is falling on or leaving from the given surface in unit time is known as *Irradiance and Radiant exitance, respectively.*

Irradiance (I_R) and *Radiant exitance* (R_E) can be calculated as

$$I_R \text{ or } R_E = \frac{d\omega}{dA}$$

where 'ω' denotes radiant flux received or released at or from a point on the given surface

d = differential derivative

A = area surrounding the point.

Unit of measurement for both *Irradiance* (I_R) and *Radiant exitance* (R_E) is watts per square meter.

Radiance: Radiance is the amount of radiant flux incorporated in the light ray arriving at or leaving a point on a surface in a given direction and its unit of measurement is watts per square meter per steradian (steradian is measurement of solid angle of an area).

Radiant intensity: Radiant intensity is referred as the amount of intensity of light emitted by a given source of light and its unit of measurement is watts per steradian.

Photometry: Photometry is the measurement of visible light in terms of units which can be adjusted to a representative value depending on the sensitivity of the visual system. The visual system of humans is very complex and is capable to detect the electromagnetic radiation in the wavelengths ranging from 360 nm to 760 nm (commonly referred as visible light).

Human eye show variable sensitivity level for different wavelengths of light; for example, a source of light having radiance of one watt per square meter steradian of yellow wavelength will appear brighter as compared to a source of light having equal radiance with red wavelength. In photometry watts of radiant energy is not measured, rather the subjective impressions are measured which are obtained when human eye visual system is stimulated with radiant energy.

Thus, subjective measurement of light is very complex and variable because along with wavelength, several other physical and physiological factors can also influence these impressions. Various factors like radiant flux, lightening conditions (whether constant or flickering), adjustment of the iris diaphragm and retina, psychological condition of viewer plays an important role in the measurement of light during photometry.

Light can be measured as monochromatic form or in combination form or even as continuum of wavelengths. In the year 1924, the Commission Internationale de l'eclairage (CIE) performed a study, in which under controlled conditions they studied the response of more than 100 observers who visually matched the brightness of various monochromatic light sources having different wavelengths. Statistical results of study were plotted as CIE photometric curve, which provided weighing functions to convert radiometric measurement into photometric measurements.

Various terms used in photometric measurements are

- Luminous intensity
- Luminous flux
- Luminous flux density

Luminous intensity: Luminous intensity is defined as light emitted by a given source of light in a specific direction per unit solid angle and its unit of measurement is candela (Cd). Measurement of luminous intensity does not depend on the distance of light source; rather it will depend on the amount of light released in a given angular span. This angular span is represented as steradian. For example, in Fig. 1.15 the amount of light (intensity) received on screen A will be equal to screen A′ (considering that screen A is not obstructing the fall of light on screen A′) because both the screens covers the same angle at light source.

Luminous intensity of one candela means that source of light is releasing monochromatic radiation of 540×10^{12} Hertz frequency (or

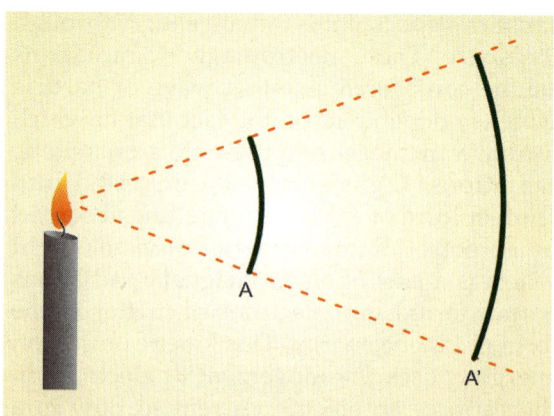

Fig. 1.15: Luminous intensity on screen A and A′ is equal

nearly 555 nm wavelength which corresponds to maximum photopic luminous efficiency). It is equivalent to the radiant intensity of 1/683 watts per steradian.

One steradian represents the solid angle (s) of one meter square surface area taken from a sphere having radius of one meter as shown in Fig. 1.16.

> **Note:** Two-dimensional measurement of an angle is usually done in units like degree and radian. However, a three-dimensional measurement of an angle is expressed in steradian.

Radiometric measurements can be converted into photometric measurements by the use of candela along with CIE photometric curve.

Luminous flux (Luminous power): Luminous flux is equivalent expression for radiant flux (watt) measured photometrically and its unit of measurement is *lumen* (*lm*). One lumen is equivalent to 1/683 watts of radiant power at a frequency of 540×10^{12} Hertz. Thus luminous power is total flow of light in all possible directions after getting emitted from a light source.

Lumen can be represented as $\Phi = E\,\sigma$

where, Φ = lumen

E = intensity of light

σ = angular span in steradian

As clear from the above equation, a point source of light having intensity of one candela will be emitting one lumen of luminous flux for each unit solid angle. Hence by simple mathematic calculations a point light source having intensity of one candela will emit a total of 4π lumens (because area of a sphere is equal to 4π).

Luminous flux density: Luminous flux density is equivalent expression for radiant flux density measured photometrically and its unit of measurement is *lumen* per square meter. Similarly, photometric equivalent of irradiance is *illuminance*, and that of radiant exitance is called *luminous exitance*.

Illumination: Illumination is also referred as illuminance, which in turn is equivalent to irradiance. As we know that irradiance is the amount of radiant flux arrived at a surface, similarly, illumination is amount of light arrived at a given surface and is expressed as number of lumens per square meter (lumen/m²). Earlier illumination was also expressed in units, meter-candle and lux.

Lux (l_x): Illumination of a given surface can be measured as lux. The major difference between lux and candela is that lux simply represents the illumination of a given surface, whereas candela actually measures illumination in terms of angular span. So illumination at a given surface in terms of lux will depend on the distance between the light source and surface; whereas in candela unit, as discussed above, the distance has no relevance.

As shown in Fig. 1.17, screen A and A' are equal in size but screen A' is less illuminated as compared to screen A; because farther the screen from the light source, poorer it will be illuminated. As we know that sphere of one meter diameter gives a one meter square area, which is expressed as one steradian. So if measuring distance is one meter, then values of one candela (lumen per steradian) will be equal to one lux (lumen per meter square).

Luminance: Photometrically weighted radiance is referred as luminance. It is defined as total amount of light falling or leaving at

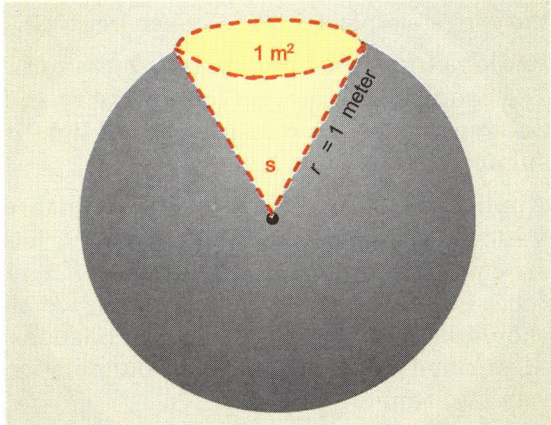

Fig. 1.16: Steradian measurement

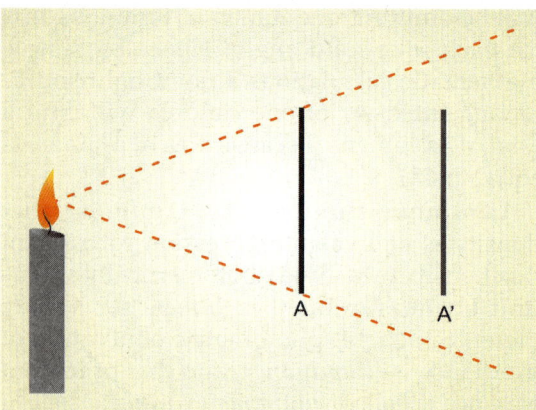

Fig. 1.17: Illumination at screen A and A' is different

or from a given surface in a specific direction. It simply means that brightness (viewed from a specified direction) of a given surface is referred in terms of luminance.

Luminance is commonly represented in Candela per square meter (Cd/m^2). Various other units used to measure luminance are

- Lambert
- Foot lambert
- Apostilb
- Bril
- Nit
- Skot

Among these abovementioned units the most commonly used units for measurement of luminance are lambert, foot lambert and Apostilb.

Lambert: This unit was coined by renowned scientist Johann Heinrich Lambert. He defined lambert as the brightness of a Lambertian surface (means a perfectly diffusing surface) that reflects or emits one lumen per square centimeter ($lumen/cm^2$).

Foot Lambert: It is defined as the luminance of a surface radiating or emitting one lumen per square foot and is more routinely used as compared to Lambert.

> **Note:** Lambertian surface are the perfectly diffusing surface which either reflect or emit constant amount of luminance (radiance) irrespective of the angle of viewing.

The luminance of a perfect diffuse reflecting surface (Lambertian surface) is equal to the incident illuminance in foot candles.

Luminance (foot lambert) = Illuminance (foot candles).

Apostilb: It is an older unit of luminance and now it is expressed in terms of stilb. One stilb is equivalent to one candela per square centimeter or 10^4 candelas per square meter (1 stilb = 10^4 cd/m^2). As one apostilb is equal to $1/\pi\ 10^{-4}$ stilb, so one candela per square meter is equal to 3.14 apostilb. An apostilb is defined as luminance of a Lambertian surface radiating or emitting one lumen per square meter.

Lighting efficiency: A surface or a room can be illuminated by ample number of ways such as incandescent lamps, fluorescent tubes, electroluminescent sheets, halogen bulbs, etc. All these appliances are compared with each other in their effectiveness of altering electrical energy into luminous energy. This conversion efficiency of an appliance is termed lighting efficiency and is called luminous efficacy of a source. Luminous efficacy is measured in lumen per watt (lm/W). In simpler words, suppose the power of a light source output in watt is known to us, then we can calculate light source output in lumen.

Lighting efficiency is defined in terms of percentage which depends on a hypothetical maximum value of 683 lm/W, at a wavelength of 555 nm. It simply means at a wavelength of 555 nm the conversion factor is 683 lumen per watt.

Radiometric versus photometric measures

The equivalent term used in radiometry and photometry for the measurement of light is summarized in Table 1.3.

Applications of illuminance and luminance

Various illumination recommendation levels are employed by engineers to utilize different types of appliances in routine life, so we all should be aware of these recommendations. Most commonly recommended illumination standards are

- Foot lambert is used in motion picture industry to measure the luminance of image

Table 1.3: Equivalent terms in radiometry and photometry

Light measurements	Radiometric terms		Photometric terms	
	Term	Unit	Term	Unit
Per unit time rate of flow of radiant energy	Radiant flux	Watt	Luminous flux	Lumen (one Candela = 4π Lumen)
Quantity of light arriving per unit area at a point on a given surface	Irradiance	Watt per square meter	Illuminance	Lumens per square meter or foot candle
Quantity of light leaving per unit area at a point on a given surface	Radiant exitance	Watt per square meter	Luminous exitance	Lumens per square meter
Intensity of light emitted per differential solid angle	Radiant intensity	Watt per steradian	Luminous intensity	Candela
Total amount of light emitted or reflected per unit area per unit solid angle	Radiance	Watt per steradian per square meter	Luminance	Candela per square meter

on a projection screen. A screen luminance of 16 foot lamberts is recommended for commercial movie theatres.

- Flight simulation industry also utilizes foot lambert to measure highlight brightness of display systems. Generally 3–6 foot lamberts are recommended for simulation devices in aviation industries.
- Various panels, switches and displays used in military require illumination even in daylight. Luminance levels ranges from 100 foot lamberts in daylight to a few foot lamberts in nighttime.
- Full unobstructed sunlight has an illumination of approximately 10,000 foot candle. Normal illumination standards recommendations in foot candles (fc) for various places are
  - Classroom   50–60 fc
  - Lecture hall   100 fc
  - Nursing station   30 fc
  - Hospital corridors   10 fc
  - Operating table   3000 fc
  - Reading   80 fc
  - Fine job   100–300 fc
  - Room   30 fc
  - Toilets   10 fc

- Apostilb unit is used to decide the luminance of background as well as targets in perimetry instruments.

Special Properties

Fluorescence

When short wavelength light is absorbed by an electron (excited electron) present in specific types of substances, they move to an excited state from their ground state. This excited electron can come to a lower level under special conditions. Suppose this excited electron comes to a lower level, which is still a level higher than original ground state of electrons; then this electron will emit energy. This energy is emitted in the form of a photon. However, this emitted photon will have less energy as compared to the photon which had absorbed the light energy. Hence the emitted photon will be of longer wavelength. This process of emission of photon with longer wavelength is known as fluorescence. The chemical fluorescein used in fundus angiography works on this phenomenon.

Fluorescein dye when exposed to light by fundus camera, then unbound fluorescein absorbs light of a wavelength in the range of 465–490 nm, which is in bluish green region.

Clinical Applications

Fluorescence property is used in performing fundus angiography and various other angiographies done for diagnosing ocular, cardiac, cerebral and liver conditions.

Subsequently, the molecules of dye fluoresce and excited fluorescein molecule re-radiates and emits the light with longer wavelength (520–530 nm), which lies in greenish yellow region. Hence, a blue light is emitted as green light due to fluorescence and details of fundus can be studied easily. Some other chemicals like Indocyanine green dye (absorbs 790 nm and emits 835 nm) shows similar properties.

Photoelectric Effect

Several studies had concluded that when some metals are illuminated by specific type of lights (ultraviolet) or wavelengths, these metals emit electrons. This process of emission of energy after illumination is termed photoelectric effect.

Similar to metals some specific tissues like retinal cells when absorb the light, a chemical phenomenon happens inside retinal cells. This chemical phenomenon generates an electric impulse. This electric impulse transmits the signals to brain and hence one can see the objects. This entire phenomenon of absorption of light, formation of chemical substance and conversion of chemical substance into an electrical signal is known as photoelectric effect.

LASER

LASER is all acronyms for **Light Amplification by Stimulated Emission of Radiation** and represents a very useful and special property of light. Laser has several unique properties which can be used for diagnostic and therapeutic purposes in medical science.

Elements of a laser

All lasers used in ophthalmology consist of the following basic elements (Fig. 1.18).
- An active medium
- Energy input (pumping)
- Optical amplifier
- Release of laser

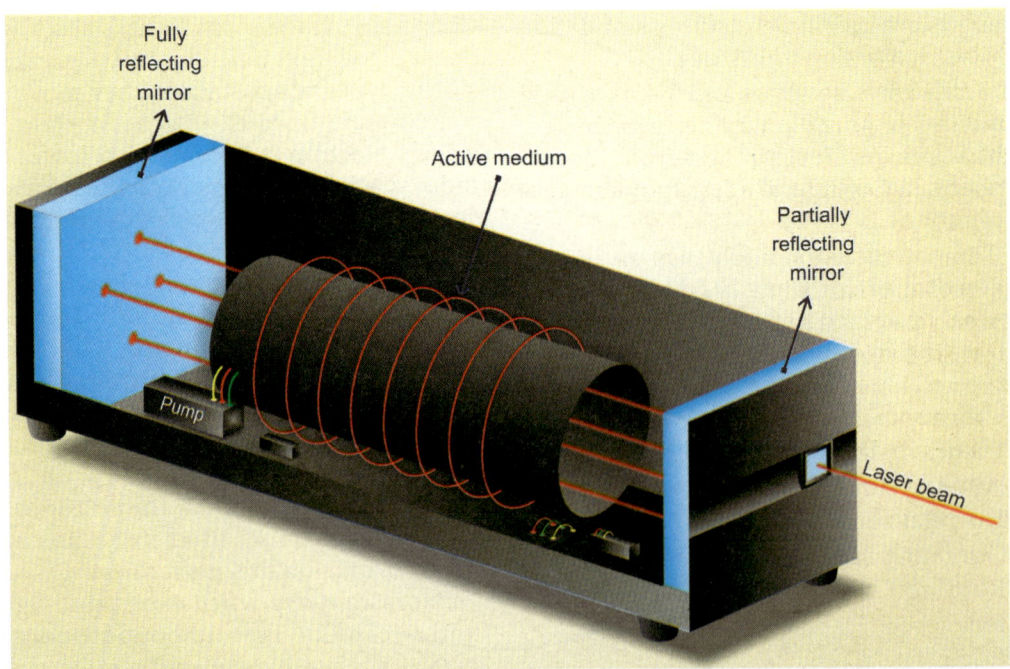

Fig. 1.18: Laser system

Active medium: An *active medium* in laser provides an atomic or molecular environment. Due to presence of this medium, a large number of atoms in the active medium (solid, liquid or gas) get energized above their original ground state on stimulation by a photon of light followed by stimulated emission. It means a photon of the same wavelength is emitted when the atom comes back to its lower energy state. In ophthalmology, various active mediums are used to produce laser beam and are named on the basis of active medium. Some commonly used active mediums are:

- Gas mediums having gases such as argon (Ar), krypton (Kr), carbon dioxide, argon fluoride (ArF).
- Liquid mediums used in dye lasers having dyes such as Rhodamine, Fluorescein and Coumarin.
- Solid mediums have crystal which is activated by an active element, for example, neodymium activating a crystal yttrium-aluminum-garnet (Nd: YAG) and erbium activating an yttrium-lanthanum-fluoride (Er: YLF). Semiconductors like diode also are solid state active medium which produces laser.

Energy input (pumping): Laser system also requires a source of energy (energy input) to keep majority of atoms in an energy state higher than their original ground state in the active medium. This state is termed *population inversion* as it is opposite of normal situation where majority of atoms remain in their ground energy state. This energy input in the form of optical or electrical energy, which keeps the electrons in population inversion state is termed *pumping*. For example, in gas lasers electrical discharge between electrodes in gas are source of energy input while in liquid dye laser energy input is given by other solid or gas laser. Similarly, solid crystal lasers are pumped by an incoherent light source like Xenon arc flash lamp.

Optical amplifier: Third requirement for a laser system is optical amplification where light is amplified by an optical feedback system. The main function of it is to promote stimulated emissions in the active medium where population inversion had been already achieved. To achieve this, entire laser cavity acts like an optical resonator which means at each end of cavity mirrors are placed to reflect the light beam to and fro through the active medium so that coherence of light beam is increased and total coherent energy increased through stimulated emission. Therefore, stimulated emission is coherent. Spontaneous emission may also occur from stimulated atoms in active medium. However, this spontaneous emission occurs randomly in all the directions, but usually do not strike on reflecting mirror; so there is no optical amplification of spontaneous emission.

Release of laser: Laser system also contains mechanism to release laser beam from the laser cavity. Releasing of laser is achieved by making one mirror fully reflective and another mirror partially reflective. Those amplified stimulated light waves which strike the partially reflecting mirror gets emitted from the laser cavity as laser beam (**Fig. 1.18**).

Properties of laser: Laser can also be considered as a type of light energy but has certain unique properties compared to ordinary light, like
- Monochromaticity
- Coherence
- Polarization
- Directionality
- Intensity

Laser systems usually emit light (photons) having same energy and thus one particular wavelength as per requirement. As discussed ordinary visible light is a mixture of seven colors having a range of wavelengths, however, a laser light has a only single color because laser is produced by the transition of only one atom with a single particular wavelength. So the laser light is normally very pure (not a mixture) in wavelength or has monochromatic property. However, sometimes these laser systems can emit light which is combination of multiple wavelengths. These light beams having multiple wavelengths can be easily separated using specially designed instruments. As a result, monochromatic or pure form of light beam consisting of single wavelength of light is produced. Another advantage with laser light is that being monochromatic in nature it can be focused even to a smaller spot as compared to white light. In addition, it is also not affected by chromatic aberration in lens system.

In case of ordinary light the emitted photons have no phase relationship with each other and are not coherent. Coherence is another important property of laser light. It means the photons emitted from the laser source are "in step" and "in phase" which means that the maxima (crest) or minima (trough) of the wave of one photon will occur at same time as on the wave associated with the other photon. It may be temporal coherence or spatial coherence and both are utilize to produce the interference which is used to produce three-dimensional images (holograms).

Polarization is another important characteristic of laser light. Many lasers emit linearly polarized light, it means the electric field of coherent light beam oscillates in a particular stable direction.

Directionality is another important property of laser means the laser beams are very narrow and moves together in a beam (highly directional) and does not spread out or diverge. Lasers cause amplification of only those light rays (photons) which travel along a very narrow path between two mirrors of laser system. It is because of directional property of laser beam that laser light can be focused on a small spot as it is easy to collect all the energy in a simple lens system.

Intensity or brightness of laser beam is the most important property as it determines the effect of laser on target tissue. Intensity of laser beam can be defined as the power emitted per unit surface area per unit solid angle.

Types of laser

Laser beam are of two types

- Continuous wave (CW) laser: This means that the laser energy stored in a laser material (like ruby crystal) is released as a steady continuous wave.
- Pulsed laser: This means that the laser energy stored in a laser material is released as pulses of light energy.

For continuous wave type laser we need to determine the minimum and maximum power of wavelength for assessment of laser strength. Wavelength powers can be measured by the use of a *photodiode* or *thermocouple* type sensor.

For pulsed type of laser a *pyroelectric sensor* is used. This sensor is designed to measure the laser energy at every pulse and is able to convert joules into an average power of laser beam in watts. Repetition of pulse frequency can be measured by combining this sensor with display units. Stability of laser output on every pulse basis can be measured by use of silicon joule meter probe (type of pyroelectric probe).

In case where only laser output measurement is required for optical adjustment purposes, a simpler and cheaper device like *thermopile* (series of thermocouples) power meter can be used instead of a pyroelectric sensor.

In clinical practice effect of laser beam on target tissue is represented by focal point size or spot size (for example, 100 µm)

Laser types like Argon, krypton delivers continuous laser wave and hence the power is displayed on a panel in unit watt. Whereas laser type like Nd: YAG is expressed as energy per pulse in unit joules on display panel; because Nd: YAG delivers a pulse of laser not a continuous wave of laser. Representation of energy in joules for pulsed laser type is easier because energy of light beam varies with the settings of pulse shutter. For example, a laser beam of power 50 mW pulsed at time interval of 0.1 second will deliver energy of 5 mjoules per pulse; whereas same laser beam with 50 mW power pulse for 0.2 second interval will deliver energy of 10 mjoule per pulse.

Tissue interactions of laser

Light energy had been used therapeutically to heat and to alter the target tissue permanently much before the invention of laser; however, laser does these tissue interactions in more controlled and precise way. Various tissue effects seen by laser beam are

- Photocoagulation
- Photodisruption
- Photoablation

Selective absorption of light energy and then conversion of this light energy into heat, which subsequently produces permanent structural changes in target tissue, is termed *photocoagulation*. The process of photocoagulation and its therapeutic results are dependent on laser wavelength and laser pulse duration. At present several lasers clinically used for photocoagulation are blue–green (488–514 nm), argon, krypton red (647 nm), dye, diode infrared (810 nm), holmium and gallium arsenide.

The process where high peak powered pulsed lasers are used to ionize the target and rupture the surrounding tissue, is termed *photodisruption*. In clinical practice photodisruptive laser is utilized like a virtual microsurgical scissor, cutting through ocular tissues such as lens capsule, iris, vitreous strands and inflammatory membranes; without disturbing the surrounding tissue. Currently Nd: YAG (1024 nm) laser is used as photodisruptive laser in ophthalmology practice.

A laser tissue interaction process where high powered ultraviolet laser pulse precisely engraves the cornea is termed *photoablation*. During photoablation the energy state of only a single photon of ultraviolet light having wavelength 193 nm will exceed the covalent bond strength of corneal protein. A submicron layer of cornea is removed precisely by absorption of these laser pulses;

without opacifying the adjacent corneal tissue because of the relative absence of thermal injury. Commonly used lasers for photoablation in ophthalmology are excimer ultraviolet (193 nm), holmium: yttrium-aluminum-garnet (Ho: YAG) infrared laser (2060 nm), erbium: yttrium-aluminum-garnet (Er: YAG) infrared laser (2940 nm) and CO_2 (10,600 nm) infrared laser.

Note: Pulsed Nd: YLF (1053) infrared laser is used in plasma ablation of tissue.

Clinical Applications

Lasers are used extensively in various ophthalmic conditions, for both diagnostic and therapeutic purposes.

VISIBLE LIGHT VERSUS HUMAN EYE

Light sensitivity of human eye

- Human eye is very sensitive to a wide range of light and can see light energy from a few photons (5–9) per milliseconds up to bright sunlight; means a difference of 10^{15} in sensitivity.

- Visible light is appreciated by human eye in the form of pulses or images. These images or light pulses repeatedly appear and/or disappear in front of the eyes. Consider a situation when the repetition frequency of these pulses crosses a specific threshold level; then the eye cannot feel two pulses as separate, rather feel them as single. The phenomenon where eye feel of the pulses of light as single is termed persistence of eye for light or image. Persistence of fovea for red light is 0.0209 second; for yellow light 0.0179 second; for blue–violet light is 0.0349 second. Hence on average light persistence time (time interval between two successive light pulses) is between 0.02 and 0.04 second.

- Daylight vision also called photopic vision, requires surrounding light levels in high range (luminance more than 3 cd/m^2); vice versa night time vision also called scotopic vision, requires surrounding light levels in low range (luminance less than 0.003 cd/m²). Vision level in between photopic and scotopic vision is called mesopic vision, needs surrounding light levels in an average range (luminance in a range of 3 to 0.003 cd/m²); hence it is most commonly used for routine activities.

- In human eye light sensitive retina has visually sensitive elements: Rod cells and cone cells. Rods are more sensitive than cones; where rods are responsible for scotopic vision, whereas photopic vision is related to cones. In human eye the photopic sensitivity has maximum sensitivity to wavelength 555 nm (spectral range of green and yellow); whereas peak scotopic sensitivity occurs at range of 507 nm. Similarly a maximum luminous efficacy (lm /W) of 683 is also seen at 555 nm range (Fig. 1.19).

- Weber's law: This law is useful to assess several sensory functions like brightness, loudness, mass, etc. Weber's law simply correlates that the just noticeable difference in luminance of stimulus upon luminance of original stimulus is a constant value. Suppose original luminance is L and minimal noticeable difference in luminance is ΔL, then as per Weber's law

$$\frac{\Delta L}{L} = K \text{ (where } K \text{ is a constant)}$$

For example, two spotlights have intensity of light 100 units each, and intensity of one light increases till observer sees just noticeable difference in light intensity (say at 110 units). Then difference threshold is 10 units (110–100) and Weber's fraction will be 0.1 (10/100). Now by applying Weber's law the value of the viewer's difference in the threshold for a light spot having any other intensity value (say 1000 units) can be calculated. As per formula change in stimulus brightness is constant proportion equal to Weber's fraction (0.1 in our example) for spotlight having intensity of 1000 unit just noticeable difference would be 100 (0.1 × 1000). Weber's constant for rods and cones is 0.14 and 0.02 to 0.03 respectively (lower values of Weber's constant indicates high sensitivity to increments).

- Fechner's law: Weber's law was explained in detail by statements given in Fechner's law. The initial statement is that only a visual response which exceeds some amount of threshold is capable of discriminating two stimuli. The other statement is that logarithmic power for a given intensity (say E) is equal to visual response (say V) and is represented by equation V = log (E). To simplify the Fechner's law, it means a subjective sensation is proportional to logarithm of stimulus sensitivity.

Light transmittance of human eye

- Normally human eye appreciates electromagnetic spectrum present in natural environment in a range of 400 to 600 nm. While considering the ultraviolet light this UV spectrum is divided as UV-C rays (100–280 nm), UV-B (280–320 nm) and UV-A (320–400 nm). UV rays are harmful for eyes, but majority of these rays are filtered or absorbed by ocular structures.

- Our natural atmosphere usually gives us protection from UV rays below 280 nm. Human eye cornea absorbs 100% of UVC, 90% of UVB and 60% of UVA rays. Remaining majority of UVA rays are absorbed by crystalline lens, hence only a very small fraction of UVA rays reaches retina.

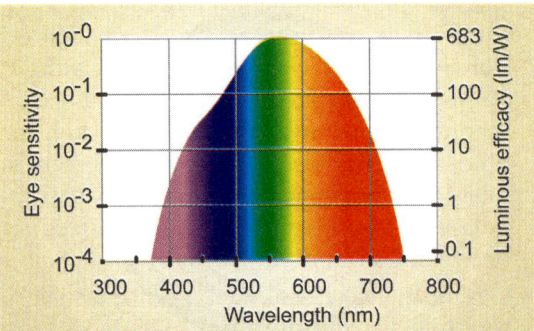

Fig. 1.19: Eye sensitivity in relation to wavelengths of light and luminous efficacy

- In normal circumstances majority of high energy visible (HEV) light wavelength between 380 and 450 nm (blue light spectrum) are absorbed by crystalline lens in human eye. After surgical removal of crystalline lens (aphakia), HEV light wavelengths can pass the eye and will reach retina. So these aphakic patients usually complain that they are seeing the objects much bluer than before the surgery.

- UV radiations can damage anterior portion of eye, whereas blue light portion (HEV light) can damage retinal structures. This damaging process could be in terms of photothermal, photomechanical or photo-chemical. Photothermal damage is mainly caused by longer wavelengths in the visible spectrum and also in near infra red region. Photochemical damage is caused by exposure of retinal structure to HEV spectrum and also UV spectrum.

Reflection and Refraction

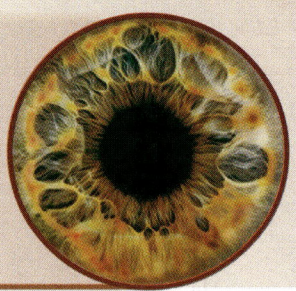

REFLECTION

When a light ray strikes on a surface or medium, three possibilities may occur with it. A certain part of it will be absorbed, a part of ray will be refracted and a part will be reflected. The amount of reflection depends on the smoothness and polishing of the surface; smoother or well polished surface will reflect the light completely. Basic principles of reflections of light enable us to understand the laws of reflections from plane and curved surfaces and prisms.

On the basis of nature of surface, reflection is of two types:

Specular reflection: This type of reflection occurs from smooth or regular surfaces, e.g. plane or curved mirrors. The angle of incident and angle of reflection for a set of parallel rays remains same after reflection so there is no scattering of rays.

Diffuse reflection: This type of reflection occur from rough or irregular surfaces, e.g. paper, clothing, etc. The rays get scatter in different directions because the angle of incident and angle of reflection for a set of parallel rays are different.

Laws of Reflection

- The incident light ray (i), the reflected light ray (r) and the normal (perpendicular line drawn from the surface point, where incident ray is meeting at the surface), all these elements lie in the same plane as shown in Fig. 2.1.

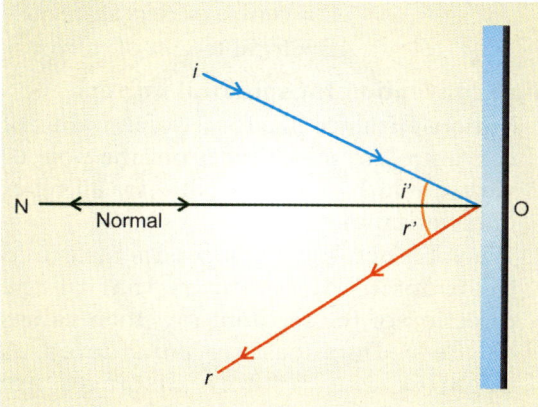

Fig. 2.1: Laws of reflection

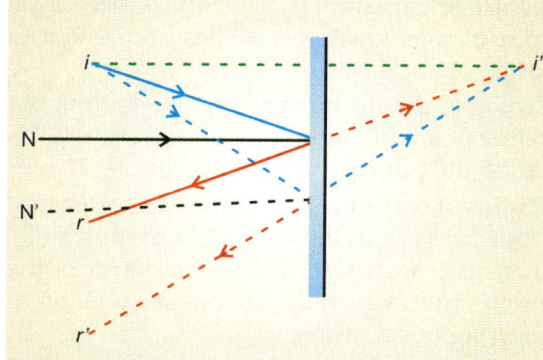

Fig. 2.2: Reflection in plane mirror and image formation

- The incident light ray and reflected light ray both lie opposite to each other on either side to the normal.
- Angle between incident light ray and normal (i') is always equal to angle between reflected light ray and normal (r').

Reflection Through Mirrors

Usually surfaces or mirrors used in various optical devices are plane, convex or concave. Let us see the reflection through these various types of mirrors.

Plane Mirror

Plane mirror is a type of mirror having plane or flat reflecting surface. Reflected rays from plane mirror are divergent in nature. Because these rays are divergent they do not meet with each other and real image is not formed. However, after drawing imaginary lines in opposite direction, a virtual image is formed behind the mirror (Fig. 2.2).

This virtual image formed behind the mirror is equal in size and is situated at the same distance as that of the object from mirror as shown in Fig. 2.3. The size of image can be calculated by the formula:

$$I = \frac{v}{u}$$

Here, I = size of image
v = distance between the image and mirror
u = distance between the object and mirror

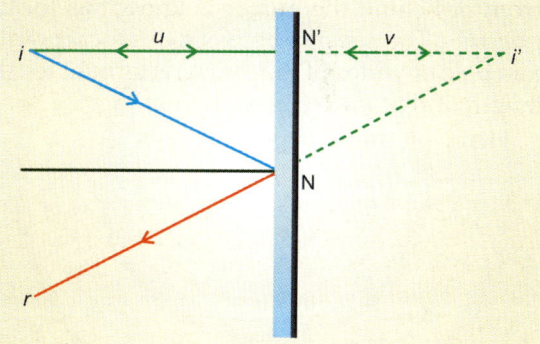

Fig. 2.3: Reflection in plane mirror proving that i' is image of i.

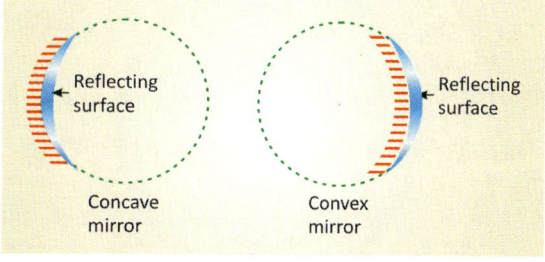

Fig. 2.4: Spherical mirrors

Spherical Mirrors

The portion of a sphere, in the form of an arc is called a spherical mirror. These mirror can be convex or concave (Fig. 2.4), depending on the side of surface which is polished.

Important cardinal points related to spherical mirror:

Vertex or pole (Fig. 2.5) of a mirror is nothing but the centre of arc (A).

Centre of curvature (C): It is the centre of the sphere from which the arc has been taken to form spherical mirror.

Principal axis of mirror: The line joining the centre of arc (A) and centre of curvature (C) is called the principal axis of mirror.

Radius of curvature (r) of mirror is the distance from pole (A) to the centre of curvature (C). In simpler words, it is the radius value of the sphere from which the arc has been taken to form spherical mirror (Fig. 2.6).

Focal point: The point where two reflected parallel rays meet on principle axis, either in front or behind the mirror is known as focal point (F). The distance between this focal point and pole or vertex of mirror (A) is termed focal length of that mirror as shown in Fig. 2.7.

Here, r_1 and r_2 = parallel rays
 F = focal point

C = centre of curvature
AF = focal length of mirror

Sign convention for spherical mirrors

1. Various distance like focal point, radius of curvature are measured from the pole or vertex, which is a fixed point for all types of spherical mirrors.

2. When all of these distances are measured in opposite direction as that of the direction of the incident ray, then values of these distances are considered as **negative** and if these distances are measured in the same direction as that of the incident ray, then values of these distances are considered as **positive** as shown in Fig. 2.8.

3. All those distances which are measured perpendicular and above the principal axis are taken as positive (as for erect image),

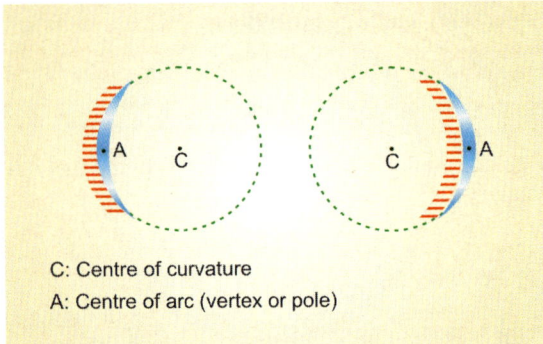

C: Centre of curvature
A: Centre of arc (vertex or pole)

Fig. 2.5: Spherical mirror showing vertex or pole

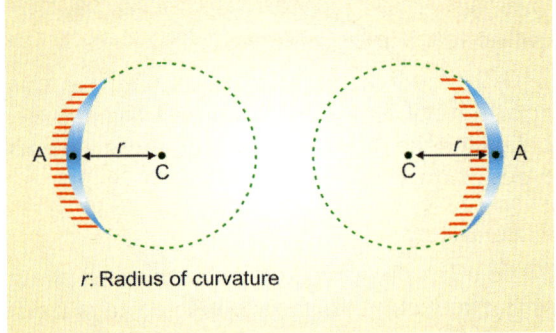

r: Radius of curvature

Fig. 2.6: Radius of curvature in spherical mirrors

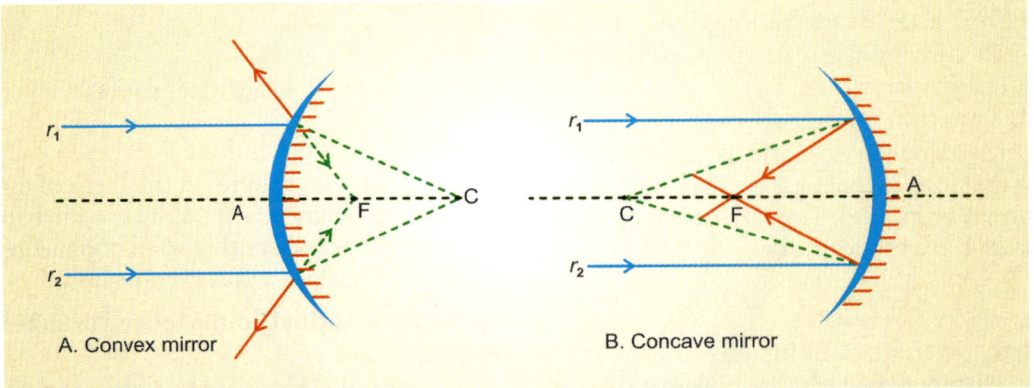

A. Convex mirror

B. Concave mirror

Fig. 2.7: Focal length of the spherical mirrors

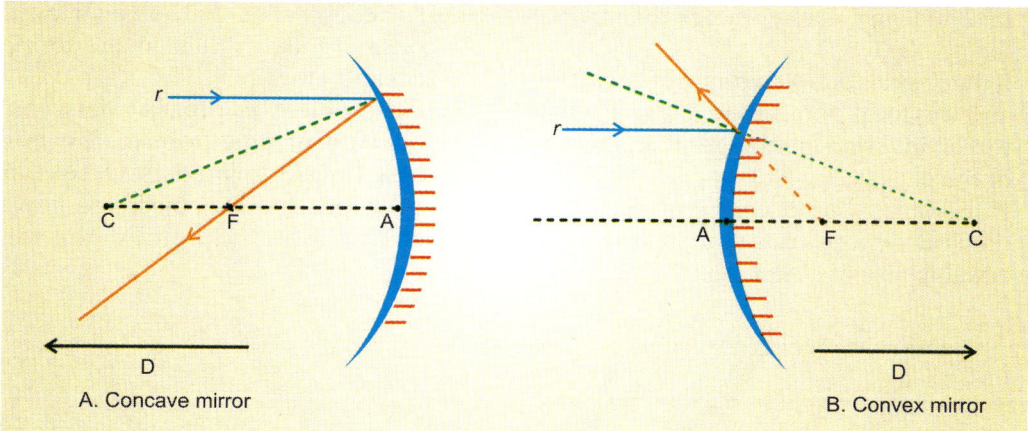

Fig. 2.8: Measurement of various distances in spherical mirrors. D = direction of measurement of various distances from pole or vertex

while the distances which are measured perpendicular and below the principal axis are taken as negative (as for inverted image).

Convex mirror When polished **(reflecting)** surface of the arc is away from the centre of curvature it becomes convex mirror. The focal point of convex mirror is behind the polished surface of the arc. Both the focal point and radius of curvature of a convex mirror are represented in positive values. The image formed in a convex mirror varies in size, distance and location depending upon the position of object in relation to the focal length of convex mirror. However, the images formed in a convex mirror are always virtual and erect. Size of image is always smaller than the object's size as shown in Fig. 2.9.

Concave mirror When polished **(reflecting)** surface of the arc of sphere faces towards the centre of curvature it behaves as a concave mirror. The focal point of concave mirror lies in front (towards object) of the polished surface of arc. Both the focal point and radius of curvature of a concave mirror are represented in negative values. The images formed in a concave mirror are dependent on the relative position of the object (Fig. 2.10).

Let us see the various types of images seen in a concave mirror considering that the object is situated at various positions from pole.

- If the object is at infinity then real and pinpoint image is formed at the focal point of mirror (Fig. 2.11).
- If the object is between infinity and centre of curvature, then image formed is real,

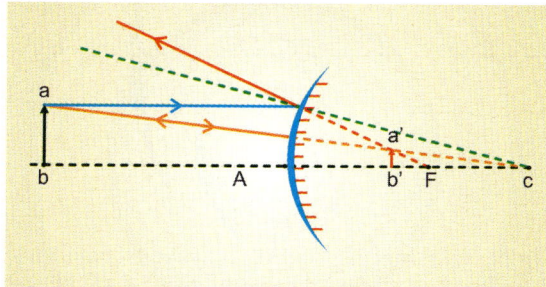

Fig. 2.9: Image in convex mirror (virtual, erect and smaller) ab = object; a'b' = image

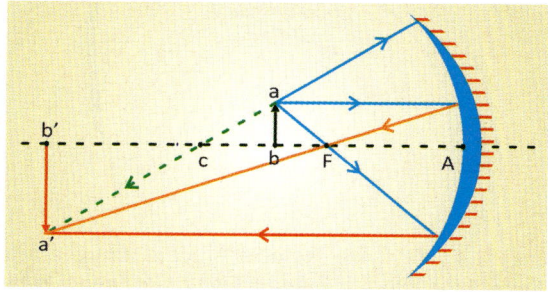

Fig. 2.10: Image in concave mirror (real, inverted, larger) ab = object; a'b' = image

inverted, and smaller in size than that of the object (Fig. 2.12).

- If the object is between centre of curvature and the focal point, then image formed is real, inverted and bigger than the size of the object (Fig. 2.13).
- If the object lies at centre of curvature then image formed is real, inverted and equal in size of object (Fig. 2.14).

- If the object is at the focal point of concave mirror, then image formed is real and at infinity (Fig. 2.15).
- If the object is present between the focal point and pole of the mirror, then image formed is virtual, erect and larger than the object size, however, will be situated behind the mirror (Fig 2.16).

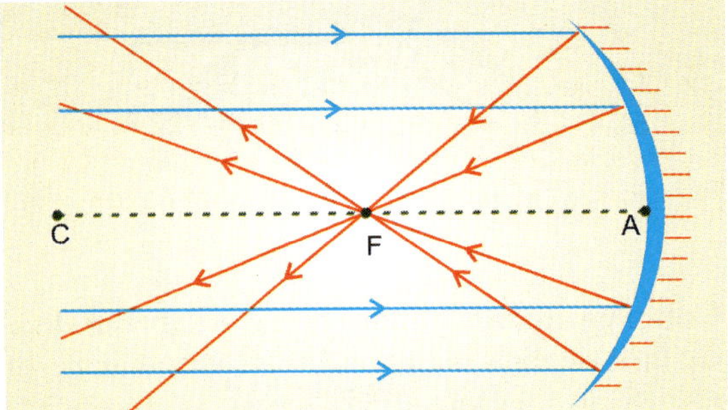

Fig. 2.11

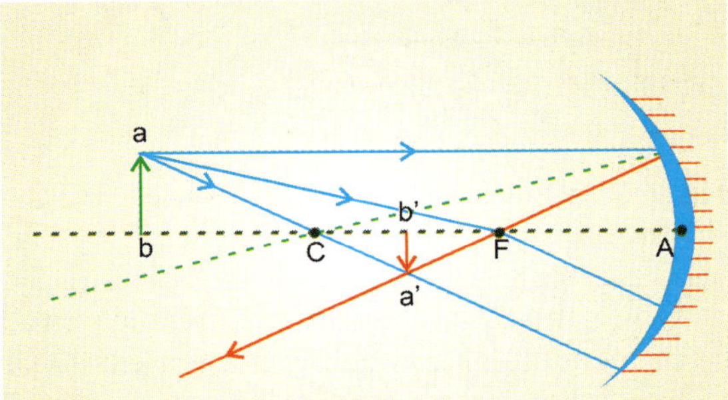

Fig. 2.12

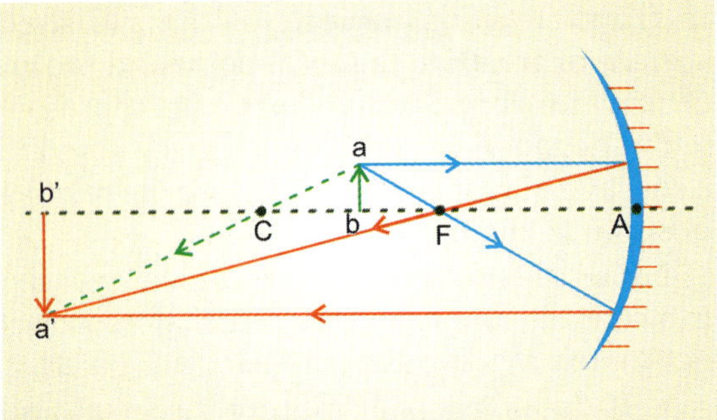

Fig. 2.13

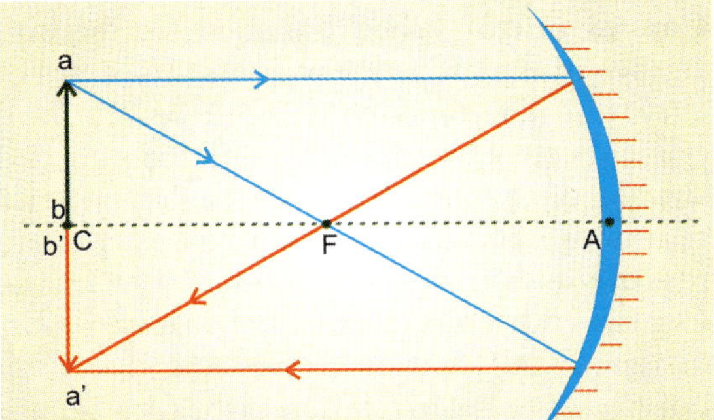

Fig. 2.14

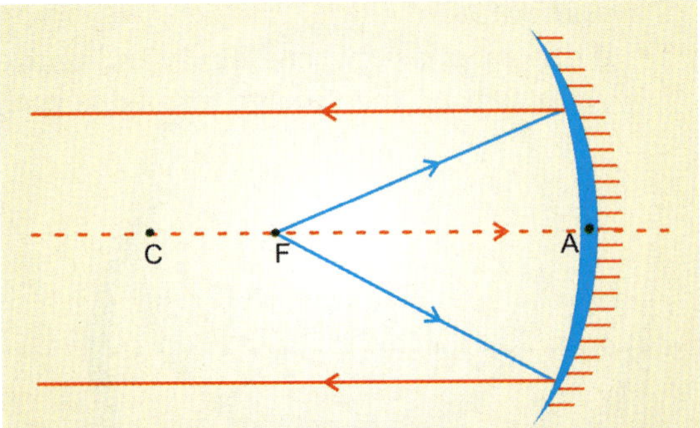

Fig. 2.15

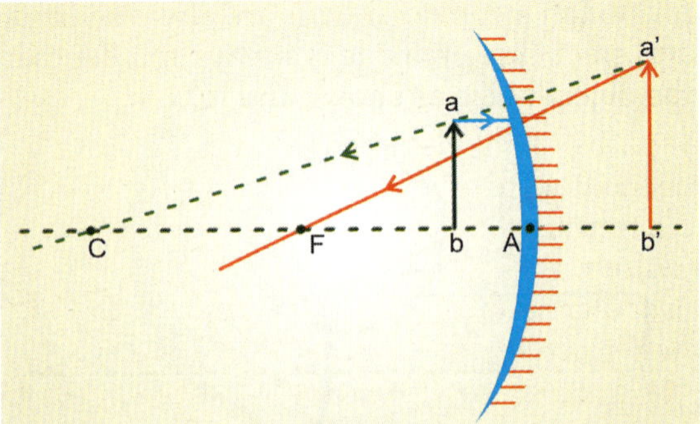

Fig. 2.16

Figs 2.11 to 2.16: Relationship of images and object, considering object at various positions; **Fig. 2.11:** Object at infinity; **Fig. 2.12:** Object between infinity and centre of curvature; **Fig. 2.13:** Object between centre of curvature and focal point; **Fig. 2.14:** Object at centre of curvature; **Fig. 2.15:** Object at focal point; **Fig. 2.16:** Object between focal point and pole

Note: In concave mirror all images are formed in front of the mirror except in Fig. 2.16 where object is situated in between the focal point and pole (vertex) of concave mirror.

Clinical Applications

Plane mirrors and concave mirrors are used in various ophthalmic instruments to magnify the images. However, convex mirrors are not routinely used in ophthalmic devices except for analysis of images formed by corneal reflections and to understand principles of Retinoscopy and Keratometry.

REFRACTION

Introduction

Light rays once emitted from a light source, travel in all the directions. For all practical purposes we consider that the light travels in a straight line when moving in the space. This straight line movement of light ray helps in better way to understand various optical systems and its related problems. As explained earlier that when light ray meets to various substances while travelling in the space, it gets absorbed completely or partially in opaque or translucent substances, respectively or may pass unabsorbed through a transparent substance.

Theoretically, if we consider that there is no resistance in the path of light then it travels with an approximate speed of 3×10^9 miles/sec in the space but practically every substance gives some resistance, hence speed of light is retarded when it travels through various substances. Due to change in the speed of light, the path of light also changes as it passes from one medium to other. The change in speed will be determined by the refractive index of the medium. If the speed of light is higher in a particular medium than in the air, it indicates low refractive index of that medium.

To understand the phenomenon of refraction we should consider the movement of light rays through a transparent medium.

1. When light rays enter a transparent medium exactly perpendicular to the surface, then speed of light gets retarded inside the medium as shown in Fig. 2.17. However, once it comes out of the medium, the speed of the emerging light ray remains same as before.

2. When light ray enters the substance/medium at an oblique angle, then the retardation in the speed at one edge of the light beam will be different as compared to the other edge of the beam. This is due to the fact that one edge of the beam strikes the surface earlier as compared to the other edge. The beam of light which strikes earlier will retard before, as compare to the other beam which enters later in the medium. The light ray which entered first will losses its speed first, but will still comes out first. Similarly the ray which enters last will also losses its speed in same proportion and comes out last. In between these two rays there will be several rays which will enter and comes out as per there angle of incidence. The resultant light beam will have various speeds as the rays will be coming out at different time intervals. (Fig. 2.18)

This emergent light beam will be not in same plane as before. The direction of this emerging beam will be changed due to retardation of rays having different speeds. The change in the direction of light ray or the bending of light beam when it passes through a transparent medium is termed as refraction.

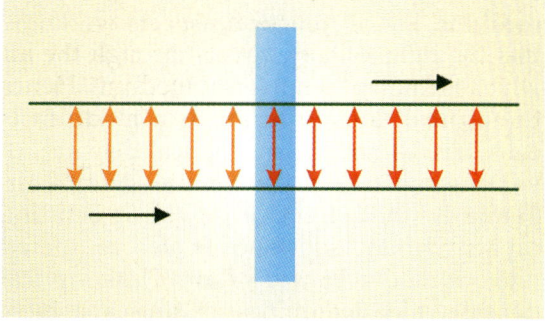

Fig. 2.17: Light wave moving perpendicular to medium

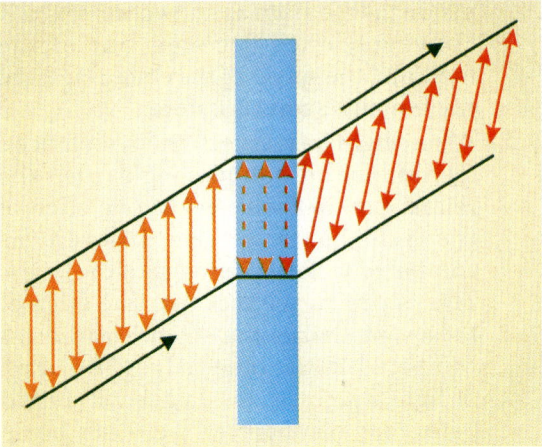

Fig. 2.18: Light wave moving oblique to medium

Refractive Index

As light travels through a medium it gets resistance from that medium also. The retardation of speed of light ray will depend on amount of resistance exerted by medium. More is the resistance exerted by medium, more will be decrease in the speed of light. This retardation of speed in turn is directly proportional to the amount of bending of light ray, means if there is more reduction in the speed of light ray, then emerging light ray will bend more acutely.

Property of any substance by which resistance is given to the light ray is called optical density of that substance. In simpler terms, if the density of the medium is more, then this medium will exert more resistance on the light ray as compared to less dense medium. For all practical aspects we know that the light usually travels through the air which is known as universal medium. Hence the optical density of air as a medium is considered standard and optical densities of various substances are compared with air. Similarly, the refractive power or bending capacity of any substance is also compared with refractive power of air. Thus, optical density which determines bending capacity of a substance is called refractive index of that substance. In other way, refractive index of

substance indicates the measure of the bending of light beam when these light rays passes across one medium to another medium.

For all practical purposes the refractive index of air is taken as 1.00 and other substances are compared with air. For example, water has refractive index of 1.33, crown glass of 1.5, cornea of 1.376 and crystalline lens has refractive index of 1.41.

Laws of Refraction

- The incident light ray, the refracted light ray and the normal all are situated in the same plane.
- Incident light ray and refracted light ray lie opposite of the normal.
- **Snell's law** states that ratio of sin i (means sine of incidence angle) and sin r (means sine of refraction angle) is always a constant for all angles of incidence. Therefore,

$$\text{Constant (K)} = \frac{\sin i}{\sin r}$$

Here i = angle of incidence

            r = angle of refraction

or $\dfrac{\sin i}{\sin r} = \dfrac{\mu'}{\mu} = \text{Constant (K)}$

Where, μ is the refractive index of medium 1 and μ' is the refractive index of medium 2.

When one of these mediums is air (say μ), then this constant (K) becomes the refractive index of second medium (μ'); since refractive index of air is 1.00.

There are three factors which can influence the amount of refraction or degree of bending of light beam:

- *Refractive index of the medium:* Through which the light ray is travelling.
- *Angle of incidence of ray (i):* Higher is the value of incidence angle (i), greater will be the refraction or bending of the light ray. It means more obliquely the rays strike, more will be bending.
- *Wavelength of light ray:* Shorter is the wavelength of light ray, more will be the degree of its bending. For example, blue

ray will bend more than red ray in any medium because blue light has shorter wavelength (380 nm) as compared to red light (780 nm).

Refraction of light ray occurs at every interface present between two mediums. For example, when light passes through a glass plate from air, it gets deviate at first interface of air and glass, then deviates at second interface of glass and air. We know that incident ray bends towards perpendicular while passing from rarer (air) to denser (glass) medium and away from perpendicular when passes from denser to rarer medium; hence the incident ray A will emerges out as refracted ray A' as shown in Fig. 2.19.

Here, i and i' are angle of the incidence at the air–glass interface, whereas r and r' are angle of the refraction at the glass–air interface.

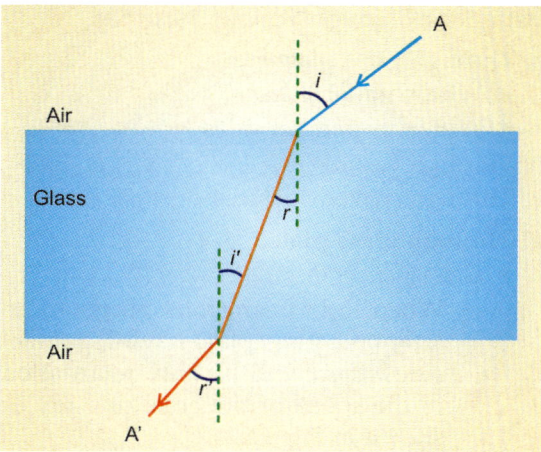

Fig. 2.19: Refraction of light

Total Internal Reflection

As discussed above when light travels from denser (glass) medium to rarer (air) medium, then the angle of refraction (r') is always more than the angle of incidence (i'). The angle of incidence (i') and the angle of refraction (r') are inversely proportional to each other. There is a particular angle of incidence at which the angle of refraction will become 90° and at this angle the refracted light ray will just graze at the interface of two mediums. This particular angle of incidence at which angle of refraction is 90° is termed as the ***critical angle*** (c) of that denser medium (Fig 2.20).

Suppose the angle of incidence gradually increases and becomes more than that of the critical angle (c), then the refracted ray of light will not enter into other medium, rather it will reflect back into the same medium. This phenomenon is known as ***total internal reflection*** (Fig. 2.21). Because of this total internal reflection phenomenon, we cannot visualize the angle of the eye directly so we require gonioscope to visualize the angle of eye.

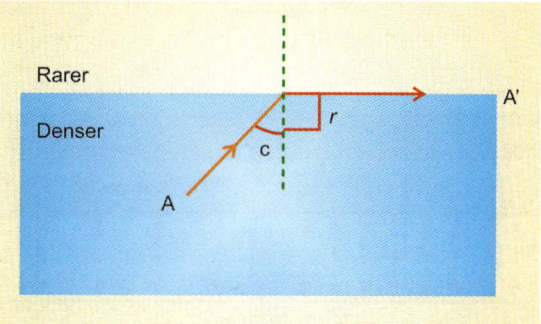

Fig. 2.20: Critical angle

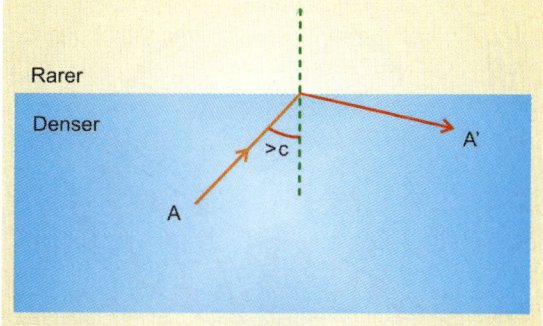

Fig. 2.21: Total internal reflection

Clinical Applications

Principle of total internal reflection is used in many optical appliances such as fiber optic lights, applanation tonometer.

Refraction Through Various Surfaces

a. Through glass plate
  - With parallel sides
  - With non-parallel sides
b. Through prisms
c. Through curved surfaces

a. **Through glass plate:**
  - *Glass plate with parallel side:*
    - When light beam falls perpendicularly on a glass plate having parallel sides, there will be only retardation in the speed of the emerging ray as shown in Fig. 2.22.
    - When light beam falls obliquely on a glass plate having parallel sides, then there will be both retardation and bending of light beam as shown in Fig. 2.23.

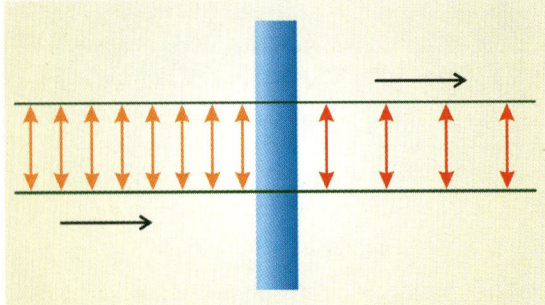

Fig. 2.22: Retardation of speed, when light beam is perpendicular to medium

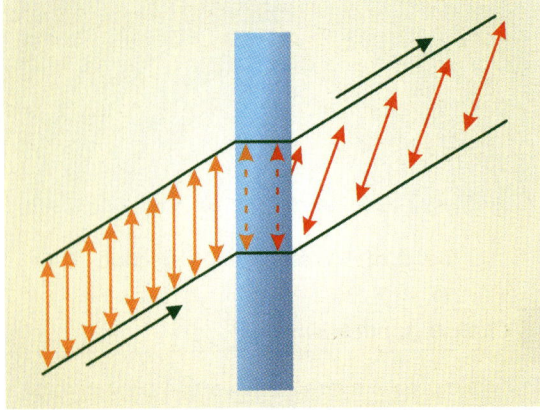

Fig. 2.23: Retardation of speed and bending of light, when light beam is oblique to medium

Note: In both these situations, the emerging beam of light will be parallel to the incident beam; though the path may be changed, if it falls obliquely.

  - *Glass plate with non-parallel sides:* When light falls perpendicularly or obliquely on a glass plate having non-parallel sides, then there will be both retardation of speed and bending of emerging beam. However, here the path of the emerging light beam is not parallel to the incident light beam rather it is in all different direction as shown in Fig. 2.24.

b. **Through prism:** As discussed above, when a light beam is passed through a glass plate with non-parallel sides, its speed get retarded and the direction of bending beam is also different from that of incident beam. Now let us see what will happen when a light ray is passed through a prism.

Prism consists of two unparallel plane refracting sides, meeting at a point called apex (N) of the prism. These two inclined refracting sides are connected at the bottom through a plane surface, called base (LM) of the prism. The angle between two refracting surface is called angle of refraction (*r*). (Fig. 2.25 A). As per basics of physics when light ray enters from rarer to denser medium, it bends towards the perpendicular and vice versa occurs when light ray enters from the denser medium to the rarer medium, i.e. light ray bends away from the perpendicular. Correspondingly

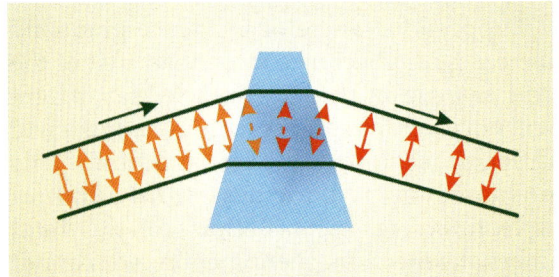

Fig. 2.24: Refraction through unparallel surfaces showing both retardation of speed and bending of light.

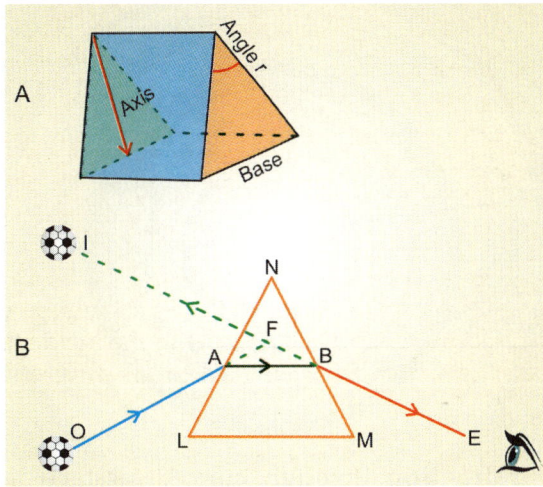

Fig. 2.25: Refraction through prism

in case of prism, when a ray (OA) enters from air (rarer) to glass (denser) medium, it bends towards perpendicular and when ray (BE) comes out of prism, i.e. from glass (denser) medium to air (rarer), medium ray bends away from the perpendicular (Fig 2.25 B).

Thus, the entire path of incident ray will become OABE, because the incident ray (OA) will bend towards perpendicular and emerging ray (BE) further bends away from the perpendicular means bending again toward base (LM) of the prism. Hence, the final outcome of an incident ray falling on a prism is that it bends towards the base of the prism.

The total amount of deviation between incident ray (OA) and emergent ray (BE) is called the angle of deviation.

Now, we presume that we are observing the object (O) through the prism from position E of emerging ray (BE). The object will be seen at position 'I' towards the apex (N) of the prism, though in reality, the object is situated at position 'O' near the base of the prism.

Refractive status of prisms
The refractive status of a prism depends upon three factors:
• Refractive index of the material by which prism is made.

• Angle at which the light beam falls on the prism, i.e. angle of incidence.
• Amount of refracting angle of prism.

Usually the ophthalmic prisms are made using crown glass and the angle of incidence of light ray is usually kept symmetrical. Suppose if these two factors, i.e. refractive index of the material and the angle of incidence (which influence the deviation of light ray through prism) are

Clinical Applications

Prisms can be used for various diagnostic and therapeutic purposes in ophthalmology practice.

I. **Diagnostic uses**
   • Incorporated in ophthalmic instruments such as gonioscope, applanation tonometer to diagnose glaucoma.
   • Used as beam splitter in many ophthalmic devices like interferometers, surgical microscope, slit lamp and keratometer.
   • Can be used as unmounted loose prisms or in combination with other prisms (prism bar) for either subjective measurement (with Maddox rod) or objective measurement (Prism bar test, Krimsky's test), of angle of deviation.
   • Clinical evaluation of microtropia (4D prism test) and suppression scotoma (induced prism test) is done with the help of prisms.
   • Diagnosis of malingering is done by performing simulated blindness test using high power prisms.

II. **Therapeutic uses**
   • In visually impaired patients to enhance the visual field special types of prisms called Fresnel prisms are used.
   • Prisms are incorporated in bifocal glasses (having high refractive power) to increase the comfort of wear.
   • In cases of strabismus to correct small degree deviations, prisms are added in spectacle corrections.
   • In cases of convergence insufficiency various convergence exercises are performed with the help of prisms.

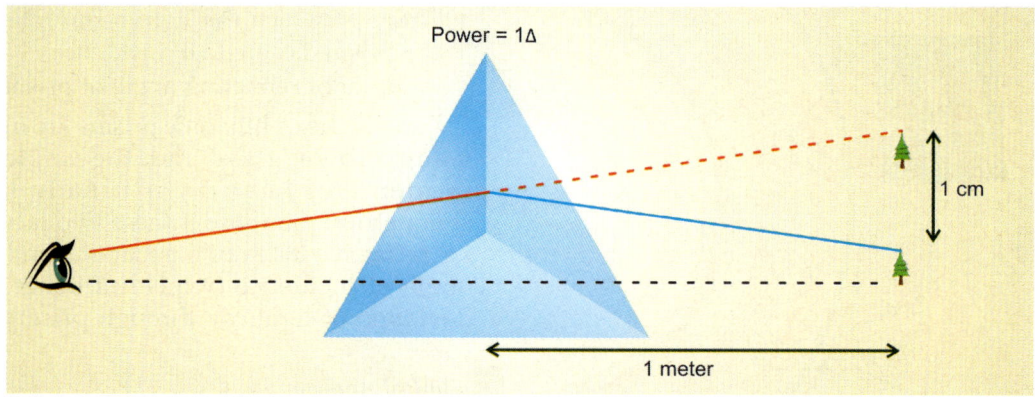

Fig. 2.26: Prism dioptre

kept constant, then it is only the angle of refraction of the prism which will decide the amount of deviation of light ray.

Various methods had been tried in the past to standardize the refractive status of the prism but no conclusive way is derived. Most commonly used terminology to express the refractive power of the prism is called prism dioptre. One (1) prism dioptre means prism will cause displacement of an object by 1 cm which is kept 1 meter away from the prism (Fig. 2.26).

However, in the case of large prisms, the measurement of the prism dioptre gives a significant error because measurement is done on a tangent scale. To minimize this error use of a *centrad prism unit* has been recommended where displacement of 1 cm of the object is measured on an arc instead of a tangent at one meter distance. However, prism dioptre is still used normally in our routine clinical practice. The relationship between degree of arc and prism dioptre is expressed as: One degree of arc ~ Two prism dioptres.

To conclude refraction through prism, the light ray gets deviated towards the base and image of the object is displaced towards the apex when we see through a prism.

c. **Through curved surfaces:** Cornea, being a curved surface is most powerful refracting surface in human eye, hence knowledge of refraction through curved surface is practically important in ophthalmology.

Let us study Fig. 2.27, where a curved transparent refracting surface is represented as XY. Centre of curvature of this curved surface is denoted as 'C' and radius of curvature as 'r' (where r is the distance between C and N). Light ray falling at point 'O' follows the Snell's law of refraction, hence bend towards the normal. In Fig. 2.27 the light ray is travelling from air (rarer) to glass (denser) medium, as a result the incident ray (OA) is bending towards normal and emerging as OB. Amount of refraction is dependent on the degree of the angle of incidence and refractive index of the medium. On the basis of this fact, anterior and posterior focus of curved

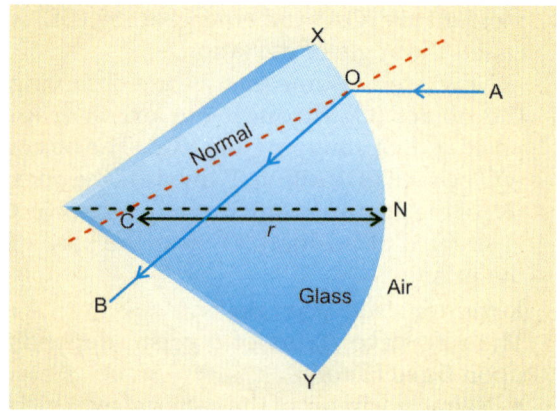

Fig. 2.27: Refraction through curved surfaces

Note: Knowledge of anterior and posterior focus will help us to understand various terminologies like vergence, dioptric power and focal length in upcoming chapters.

surface can be calculated by these simple formulas.

$$F_1 = \frac{\mu r}{\mu' - \mu} \text{ and } F_2 = \frac{\mu' r}{\mu' - \mu}$$

where

F_1 is anterior focus

F_2 is posterior focus

μ = refractive index of medium of incident ray (air in our example)

μ' = refractive index of medium of emerging ray (glass in our example)

r = radius of curvature of curved surface (in meter)

Ophthalmic Lenses

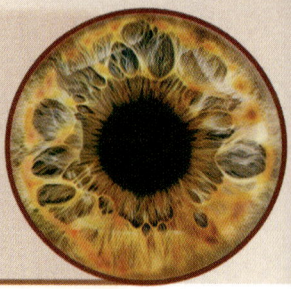

INTRODUCTION

When a bundle of light rays fall on a spherically curved surface, the individual ray will bend at different angles. These all bend rays will meet at a point called focus. The distance of focus will depend on the curvature of surface, optical density of the medium and also on the wavelength of the light falling on this spherical surface.

Convergence and divergence: When a ray strikes on a curved refracting surface, it gets deviated from its path. This phenomenon of deviation or bending of ray is called vergence, which is of two types.

Convergence: When two parallel rays strike a curved refracting surface and both rays bend towards each other after striking. This phenomenon is termed as convergence (Fig. 3.1A).

Divergence: If two parallel rays after striking a refractive surface get deviated from its path and move away from each other. This phenomenon is termed as divergence (Fig. 3.1B).

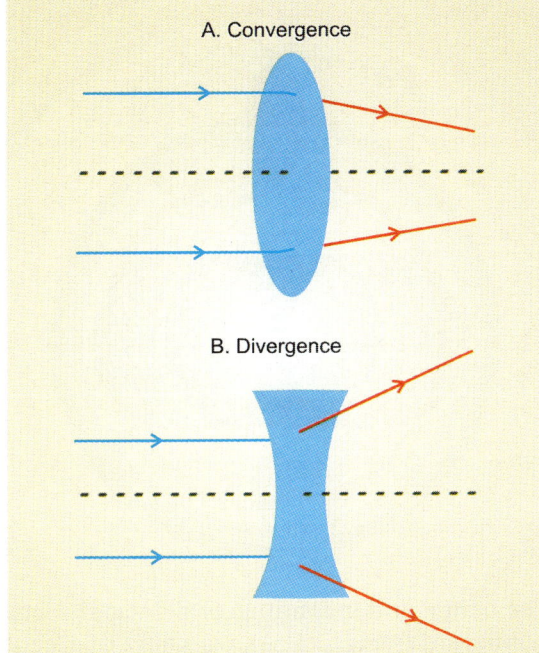

A. Convergence

B. Divergence

Fig. 3.1A and B: Phenomenon of vergence of light rays

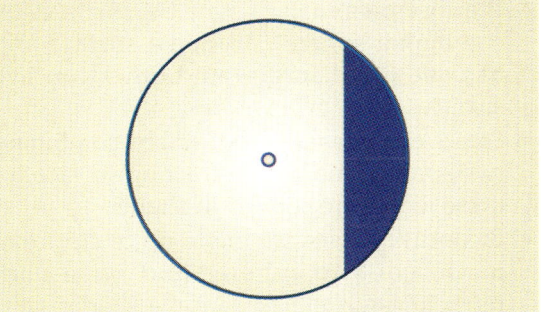

Fig. 3.2: Plano convex lens

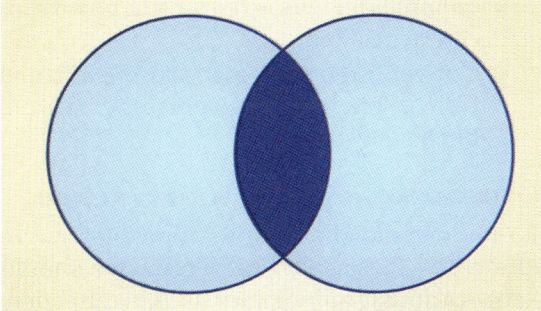

Fig. 3.3: Biconvex lens

These two terminologies, convergence and divergence, will be used commonly in upcoming chapters.

Spherical Lenses

Sphere when cut at certain side can become a lens; hence the name spherical lens came into nomenclature. Thus, these lenses have their (one or both) surfaces curved in the form of sphere.

As shown in Fig. 3.2 when a part of sphere is cut, it forms a plano convex lens. Similarly, if two spheres are combined and a portion is cut, it will form a biconvex lens (Fig. 3.3).

Types of Spherical Lenses

Various types of lenses can be created from solid sphere alone or by combining sphere with various refractive surfaces as shown in Fig. 3.4.

Common types of lenses are

- Plano convex lens can be formed by cutting the part of the sphere and it has one plane surface and the other convex surface.

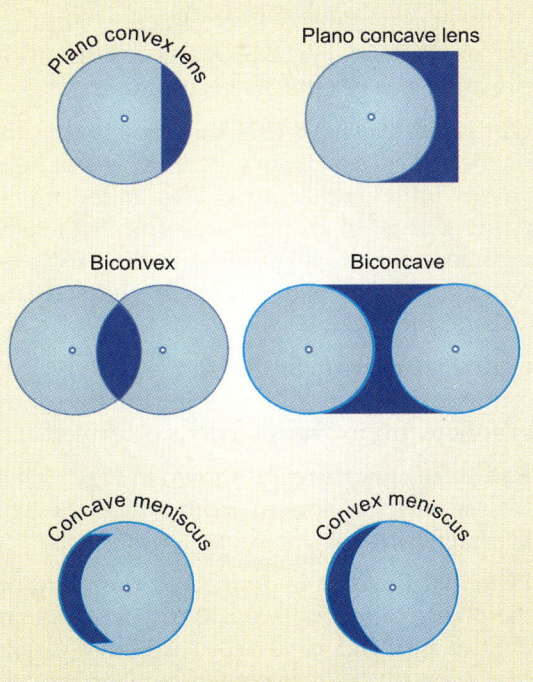

Fig. 3.4: Various types of spherical lenses

- Plano concave lens can be formed by combining sphere and plane surface and has one plane surface and other concave surface.
- Biconvex lenses are produced by combining two spheres and both refracting surfaces of these lenses are convex in shape.
- Biconcave lenses are made up by approximation of two spheres and have both refracting surfaces of concave shape.
- Meniscus lenses are of two types
  - Concave meniscus can be formed from a sphere and has greater curvature of concave shape.
  - Convex meniscus also can be formed from a sphere and has greater curvature of convex shape.

Terminologies Related to Spherical Lenses

To understand the various types of images formed by these spherical lenses, we should know various terminologies used in refraction.

Principal axis or optical axis: It is defined as the common axis represented by the line joining centre of curvatures of two refracting surfaces. For example in **Fig. 3.5**, *XY* is representing principal axis or optical axis of the lens.

Optical centre (O): It is the principal point on the optical axis from where the ray of light passes undeviated and is also called nodal point of lens. In all types of spherical lenses optical point is situated inside the lens, however, in case of meniscus lens it lies outside the lens.

Centre of curvature: As shown in **Fig. 3.5**, centre of curvature 'C' is nothing but the centre of sphere, from which the lens is formed.

Radius of curvature: As shown in **Fig. 3.5** it is the radius (*r*) of sphere, from which the lens has been formed.

Principal focus: It is defined as the point on the principal (optical) axis of the lens, where all the parallel rays from infinity either converges (in case of a convex lens) or appears to be diverge (in case of a concave lens).

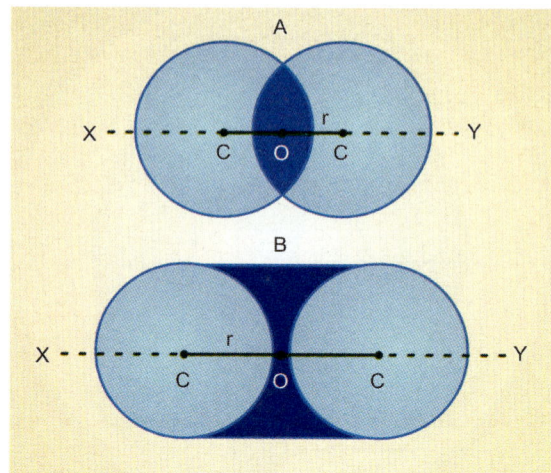

Fig. 3.5: Terminologies in lenses
XY: Principal/optical axis
O: Optical centre and C: Centre of curvature

For better understanding of principal focus points, study **Fig. 3.6**. As we know that light ray can pass through lens from either side of it, hence lens has two principal foci; one on each side of the lens.

- First principal focus (F_1) is a point situated on the optical axis of lens. Light ray originating from this point become parallel to optical axis, after getting refracted by the lens (**Fig. 3.6A**).
- Second principal focus (F_2) is a point situated on the optical axis of lens, where all the light rays travelling parallel to optical axis either converge (in case of convex lens) or appear to be diverge (in case of concave lens) after getting refracted by the lens (**Fig 3.6B**).

Focal length: It is defined as the distance between optical centre (*O*) and principal focus point, measured along the principal axis of lens. Two focal lengths f_1 and f_2 are seen for each lens, because every lens has two principal foci on either side.

- First focal length (f_1) is the distance between optical axis of the lens and first principal focus (F_1) (**Fig. 3.6A**).

Note: When lens is situated in air or medium on both the sides of a lens is air, then $f_1 = f_2$.

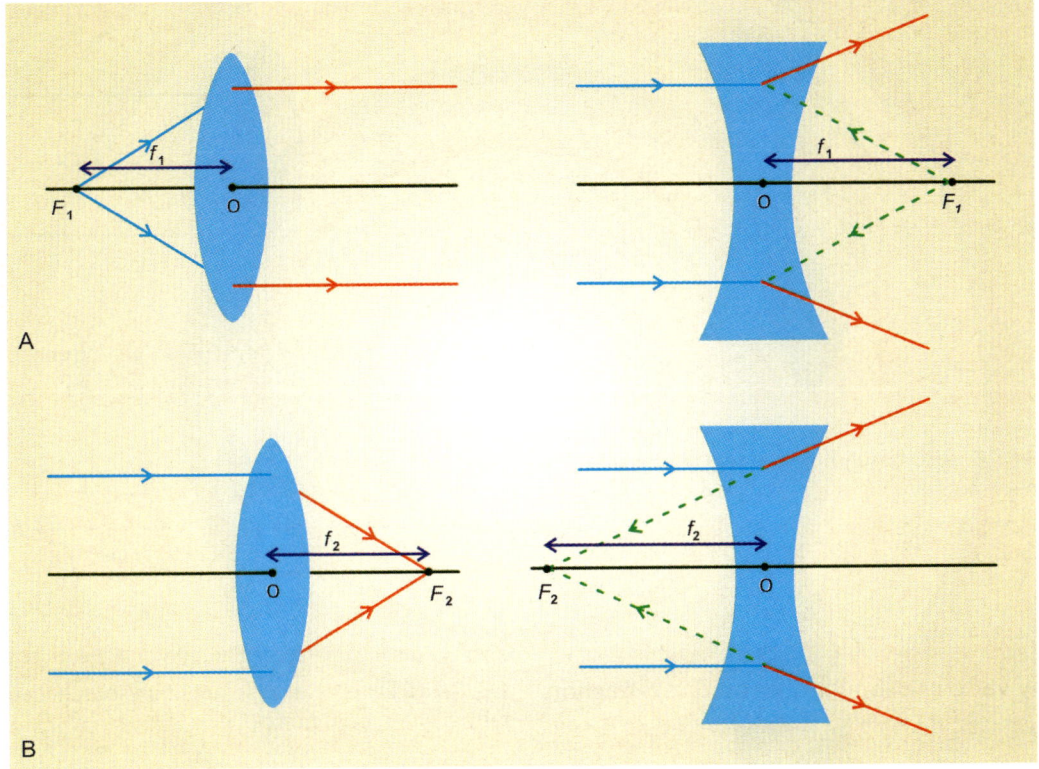

Fig. 3.6: Principal focus points in convex and concave lenses

- Second focal length (f_2) is the distance between optical axis of the lens and second principal focus (F_2) (Fig. 3.6B).

Refraction through Spherical Lenses

To understand refraction through spherical lenses, we should recall the basics physics where we learnt the refraction of light ray through prism in Chapter 2. As we can see in Fig. 3.7 that an incident ray falling on the prism will bend towards its base. On the basis of this simple fact we can explain the refraction through various types of lenses.

Convex lens: Convex lenses can also be considered as combination of two prisms attached base to base as shown in Fig. 3.8.

As discussed above the light rays will bend towards base of the prism and when both the rays bend towards the base of prism, they will meet at certain point; this meeting point of bent rays becomes the focal point of the convex lens

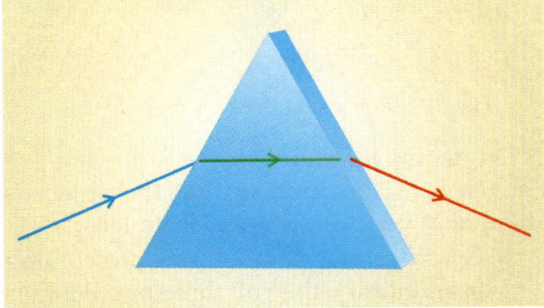

Fig 3.7: Refraction through prism

(Fig. 3.9). As it is clear from Fig. 3.9 that the parallel rays after falling on a convex lens are getting converge at focal point, so these types of lenses are also known as convergent lenses. Here we also noticed that a central ray of light passes through the lens without any deviation and goes straight through the lens. The line in which this unaffected ray moves is called the principal axis of the lens.

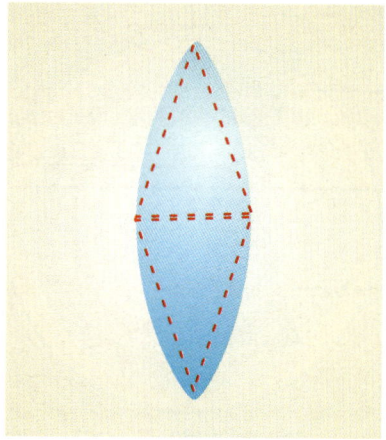

Fig. 3.8: Base to base joining of two prisms, making a convex lens

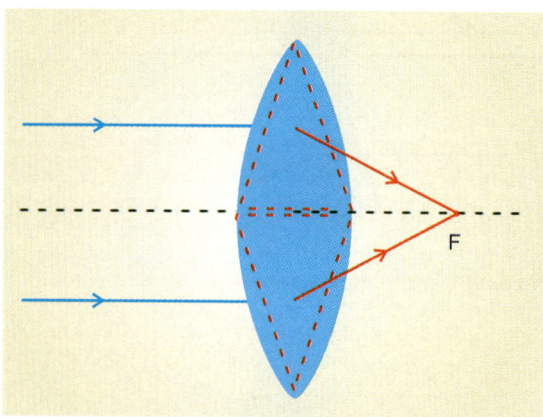

Fig. 3.9: Refraction through convex lens

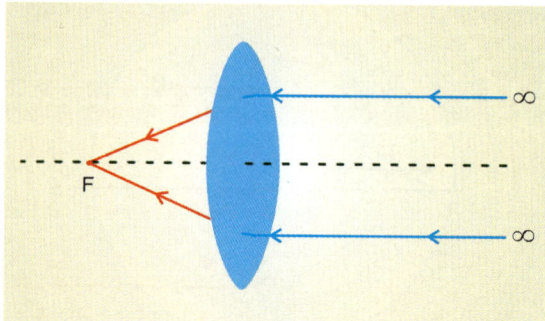

Fig. 3.10: Parallel rays from infinity getting converged

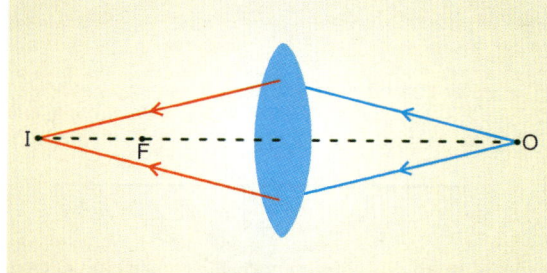

Fig. 3.11: Divergent rays from point source focusing farther than focal point

Let us study various images formed by the convex lens considering that the object is situated at various distances from lens:

- Consider that parallel rays are coming from infinity; then all these parallel rays will converge and focus on a single point. This point is called principal focus (F) of convex lens. The distance between the convex lens and the principal focus is termed focal distance or focal length (Fig. 3.10).
- Now consider that rays are coming from a point source (O) which is nearer than the infinity. These rays are divergent in nature and when they strike the lens surface, they get focused at a

point (I) farther than the principal focus (F) (Fig. 3.11).

Figures 3.12 to 3.15: Images formed by convex lenses considering objects at various distances.

- Suppose the point source of light (O) is between the focal point (F) and convex lens, then the image will form behind the source of light (O) and will be virtual in nature (Fig. 3.12).
- When an object (AB) is present beyond the principal focus (F) at finite distance, then a real, inverted and larger size image (A′B′) will form on the other side of a convex lens (Fig. 3.13).
- An object (CD) present between principal focus (F) and lens will form a virtual, erect and larger image (C′D′) on the same side of the lens (Fig. 3.14).
- An object (AB) present at the centre of curvature will form a real, inverted and equal size image (A′B′) at centre of curvature on the other side of lens (Fig. 3.15).

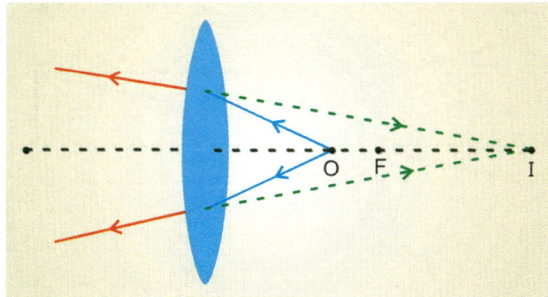

Fig. 3.12: Point light source between focal point and convex lens

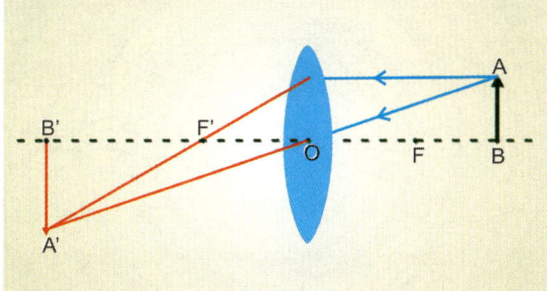

Fig. 3.13: Object AB between centre of curvature and focal point

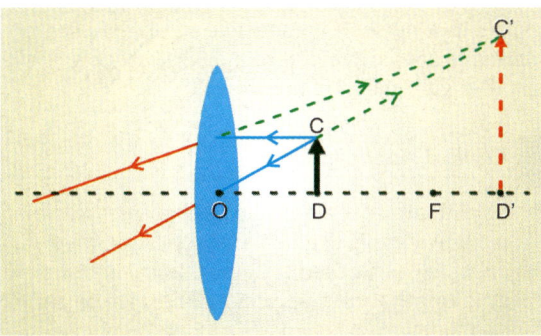

Fig. 3.14: Object CD between focal point and convex lens

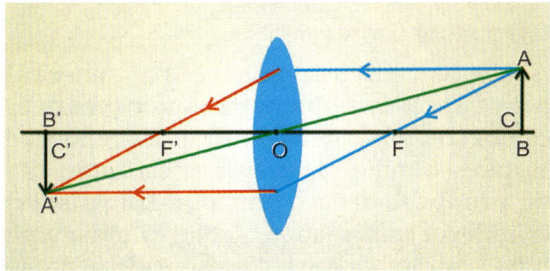

Fig. 3.15: Object AB at centre of curvature

Concave lens: Concave lenses can be considered as combination of two prisms, which are joined apex to apex as shown in Fig. 3.16.

Again by the rule of refraction through a prism the light ray bends towards base of the prism, so in case of a concave lens both the incident rays bend towards the base of prism or diverge from each other as shown in Fig. 3.17.

As we can see in Fig. 3.17, that the parallel rays falling on a concave lens are getting diverged from each other, thus these lenses are also called as divergent lenses. Similar to convex lens a central ray of light also passes through the concave lens unaffected and goes straight through the lens. The line in which this unaffected ray moves is called the

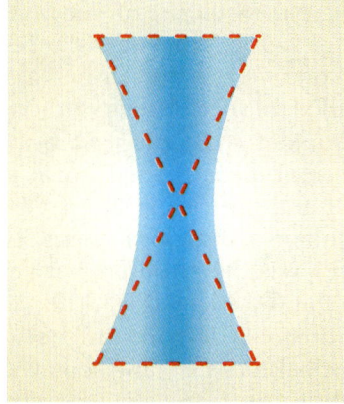

Fig. 3.16: Apex to apex joining of two prisms, making a concave lens

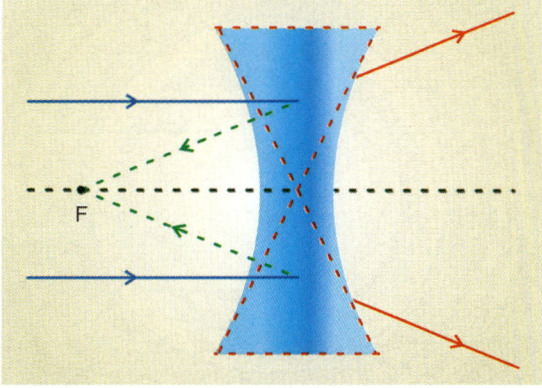

Fig. 3.17: Refraction through concave lens

principal axis of the lens. By drawing an imaginary line in the backward direction of emerging divergent rays, these rays meet on the principal axis of lens at a point *F*. This point (*F*) is the focal point of concave lens.

Let us study various images formed by the concave lens considering the object is situated at various distances from lens.

Figures 3.18–3.20: Images formed by concave lenses considering objects at various distances.

- Consider that parallel rays are coming from infinity, then the rays will diverge and do not meet at one point. But if we move along these divergent rays in backward direction, then these rays appears to meet at single point on the principal axis of lens on the same side of source of light. This point is called the principal focus (*F*) of concave lens as shown in Fig. 3.18. The distance between the concave lens and principal focus (*F*) is called the focal distance or focal length.
- An object (*AB*) present beyond the principal focus (*F*) will form a virtual, erect and smaller image (*A'B'*) on the same side of the concave lens. The image (*A'B'*) will be situated between focal point and the lens (Fig. 3.19).
- An object (*CD*) present between the principal focus (*F*) and lens will form a virtual, erect and smaller size image (*C'D'*) on the same side of the lens and this image will be situated between the object (*CD*) and the lens (Fig. 3.20).

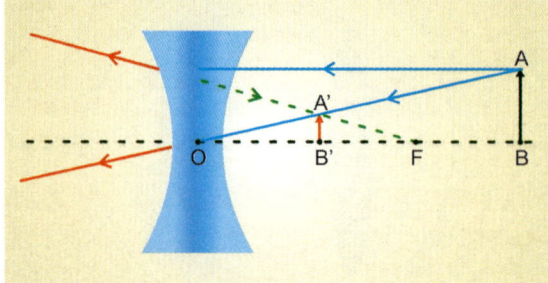

Fig. 3.19: Object between infinity and focal point

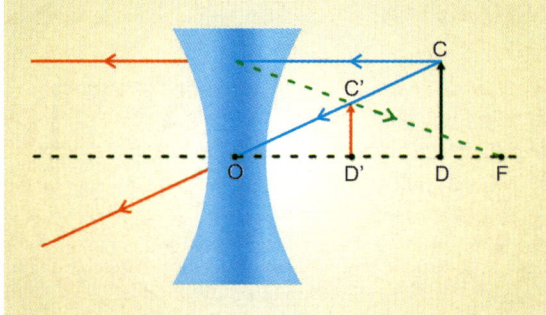

Fig. 3.20: Object between focal point and lens

Note: In a nutshell irrespective of object position concave lens always forms a virtual, erect and smaller size image of an object.

Clinical Applications

- Spherical lenses are used to correct various refractive errors like hypermetropia and myopia.
- These lenses are used in various optical instruments and ophthalmic devices, either alone or in combination.
- Spherical lenses are also used in various low visual aid devices for improvement in vision.

Cylindrical Lenses

As we had discussed above that spherical lenses are formed by portion of a sphere or combination of sphere with other refractive surfaces. Similarly, the cylindrical lenses can be produced from a cut portion of solid cylinder or combination of solid cylinder with other refractive surfaces; hence the name cylindrical lenses came in nomenclature.

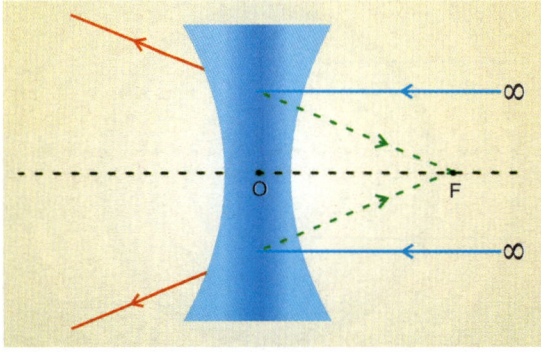

Fig. 3.18: Object at infinity

Types of Cylindrical Lens

Similar to spherical lenses cylindrical lenses are also classified according to their refracting status as

• Convex cylinder
• Concave cylinder

Convex cylinder: To form a convex cylindrical lens a solid glass cylinder having its axis of rotation as *XY* is cut vertically via a surface *ABCD* along *XY* axis as shown in Fig. 3.21. Now when this cut portion is separated from the solid cylinder, it will work as a convex cylindrical lens.

Concave cylinder lens: Similarly to form a concave cylindrical lens a solid glass cylinder having its axis of rotation as *XY* is combined with a rectangular plate as shown in Fig. 3.22. Now when a portion is cut along *XY* axis and separated, then this separated portion will work as a concave cylindrical lens.

Cylindrical lenses have only one axis of refraction, i.e. either convex or concave. Rest of the area of these lenses is non-refracting in nature and thus rays falling in these areas will pass unaffected.

Refraction Through Cylindrical Lenses

Refraction through cylindrical lenses is not as simple as it occurs through spherical lenses. In spherical lenses all the rays strike on a

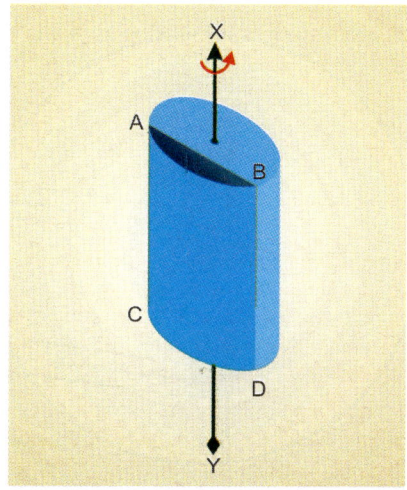

Fig. 3.21: Convex cylinder formation

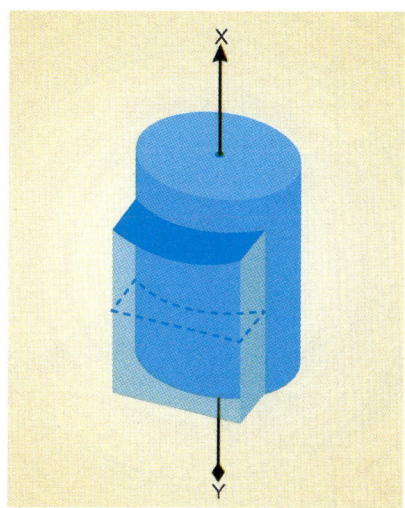

Fig. 3.22: Concave cylinder formation

regular curved surface either convex or concave and gets converge or diverge, respectively. Whereas in cylindrical lenses, one meridian is curved while the meridian perpendicular to it is plane in nature, hence the rays will bend only at one meridian, i.e. on curved one while the rays will pass unaffected through the meridian perpendicular to it.

Convex cylindrical lens: As represented in Fig. 3.23 portion of the solid glass cylinder is cut via a surface *ABCD*. This cut portion behaves as a convex cylindrical lens. The axis *XY* along which the portion was cut is termed as refractive axis of cylindrical lens. There are two perpendicular planes (meridians) of this cylindrical lens, namely *LMNO* and *PQ*. As we can see in Fig. 3.23 plane *LMNO* is not a curved surface (rather it is plane surface), so this surface will not refract the light rays. Whereas a plane perpendicular to it, i.e. *PQ* is having a convex surface; hence the ray falling on *PQ* plane will converge at the focal point of lens. In this convex cylindrical lens the effective power will be perpendicular to its axis *XY*.

Concave cylindrical lens: As represented in Fig. 3.24, solid glass cylinder *ABCD* is combined with a solid glass plate *LMNO*. The portion cut from these combined surfaces will

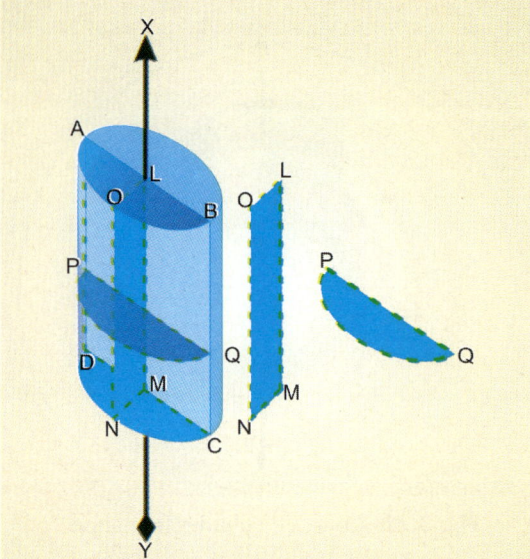

Fig. 3.23: Convex cylindrical lens

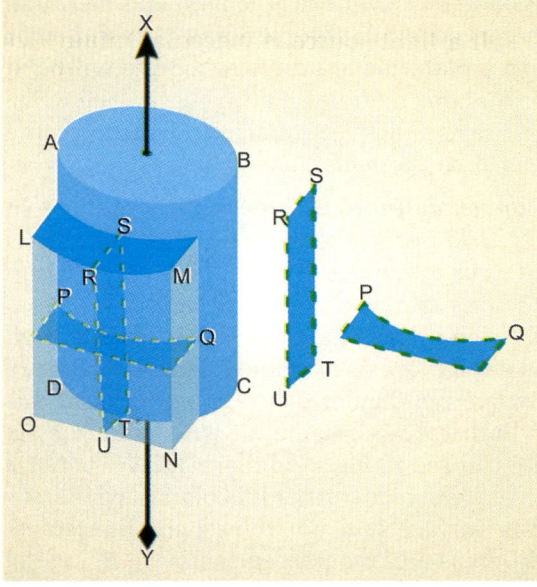

Fig. 3.24: Concave cylindrical lens

form a concave cylindrical lens. The axis *XY* along which the portion was cut is termed as refractive axis of cylindrical lens. As shown in Fig. 3.24 *RSTU* and *PQ* indicate two perpendicular planes of this concave cylindrical lens. The plane *RSTU* is not curved so it will not refract the light ray. Whereas a

plane perpendicular to it, i.e. *PQ* is having a concave surface, hence the ray falling on this plane will get diverged. In this concave cylindrical lens the effective power will be perpendicular to its axis *XY*.

Refraction Through Convex Cylindrical Lens

A convex cylindrical lens having its axis *XY* in vertical direction will focus the divergent rays coming from a point source '*O*' as a vertical line (*I*) as shown in Fig. 3.25.

Similarly, when light rays perpendicular to axis *XY*, passes through a convex cylindrical lens, these rays get focus at focal plane *FF'*. However, the rays which travel in the same plane as that of axis *XY* will pass undeviated as shown in Fig. 3.26.

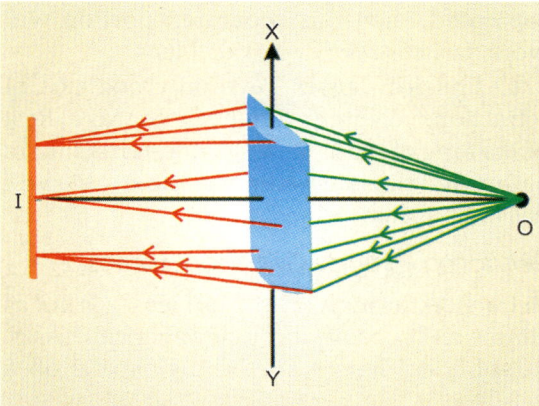

Fig. 3.25: Point source is focusing as line in convex cylindrical lens

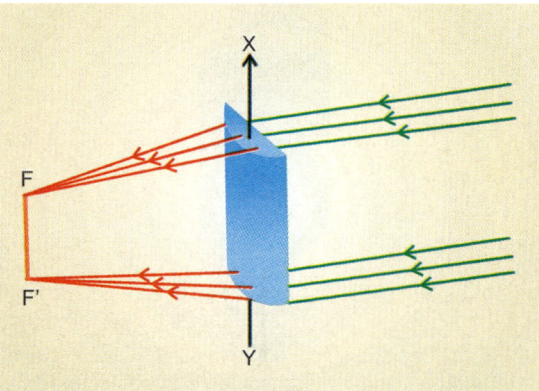

Fig. 3.26: Refraction through convex cylinder

Refraction Through Concave Cylinder Lens

As shown in Fig. 3.27 when light rays perpendicular to cylindrical axis *XY* passes through a concave cylindrical lens, they focus at a virtual focal plane *FF'*; because these rays get diverged when they strike the concave surface of cylindrical lens. However, the rays which are travelling in the same plane as that of cylindrical axis *XY* will pass undeviated.

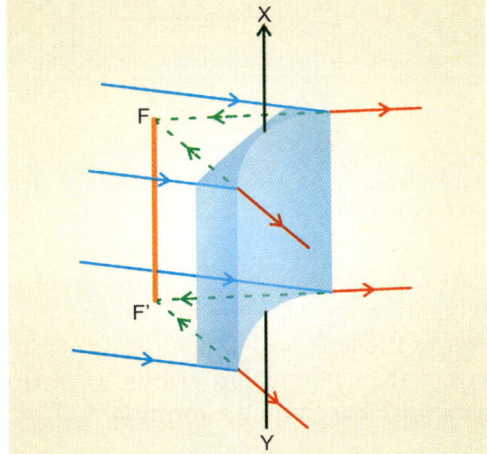

Fig. 3.27: Refraction through concave cylinder

Note: So to simplify and understand refraction through cylindrical lenses; in both types of cylindrical lenses the rays which strike perpendicular to the axis XY of cylinder will deviate and rays which strike the lens at same plane as axis XY of cylinder will pass undeviated.

Clinical Applications

- Cylindrical lenses are used for correction of refractive error like astigmatism.
- Cylindrical lenses are also used in various muscular imbalance conditions like heterophoria and heterotropia.
- These cylindrical lenses are also used in various low visual aid devices for improvement in visual fields.

REFRACTIVE STATUS OF LENSES

As we know that any natural light source (usually and almost always) emits rays of diverging nature. These emitted rays move in such a manner that radius of curvature (vergence) of the wavefront gradually increases as waves move away from the light source (Fig. 3.28A). This phenomenon of increasing vergence of wavefront is known as negative vergence.

Now if these diverging rays emitting from a natural light source are merged with the help of a convex lens, then the radius of curvature of the wavefront will gradually decrease as the wave moves away from the light source (Fig. 3.28B). This phenomenon of decreasing vergence of wavefront is termed as positive vergence.

In a nutshell curvature of wavefront is dependent on its radius and on the distance of wavefront from its source of origin. More is the distance of wavefront from the light source, lesser will be the curvature of wave front. In other words, curvature of the wave front is inversely proportional to the distance from the light source.

If a light source is placed at infinity then the curvature of a wave front originating from this light source will be so flat that the rays coming out of source are almost parallel to each other. This phenomenon where waves in a wavefront are parallel to each other is termed a zero (plano) vergence (Fig. 3.28C).

In simpler words, refraction means bending of light rays or we can say that refraction alters the vergence of light rays. If the light rays pass straight via a medium, then their vergence is unchanged and it indicates that no refraction has taken place. When light rays while passing through a medium gets bend or refracted, then it indicates that the vergence of light ray has changed. Lens is such medium that cause change in the vergence of light rays.

Refractive status of a lens determines
- Its power to deviate the image of a given object and
- Its power to either magnify or minify the image of a given object.

Note: More powerful lens will refract the light ray to a higher degree, whereas image size of an object is also more differentiated as compared to the object.

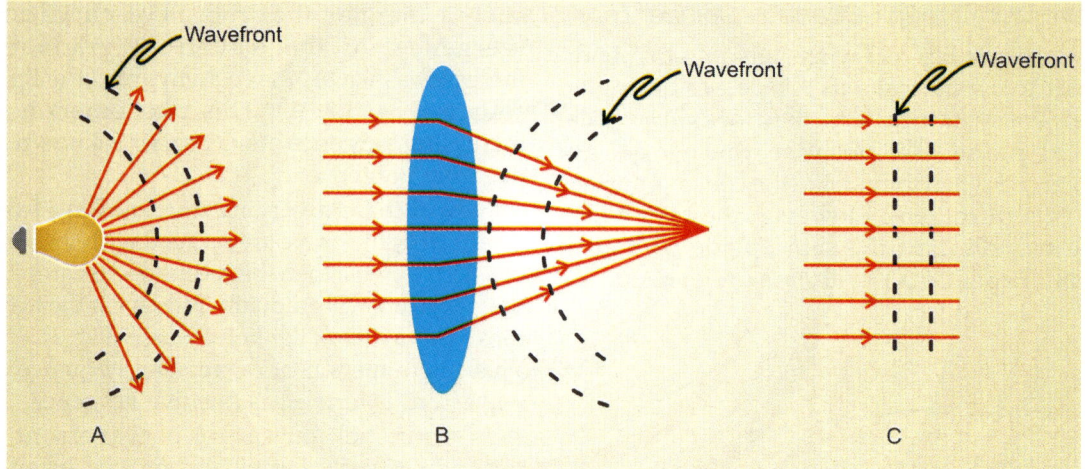

Fig. 3.28: Curvature of the wavefront depends on vergence of rays. A. Negative vergence (divergence); B. Positive vergence (convergence); C. Zero vergence (source at infinity)

The refractive power (vergence power or dioptric power) of lens indicate its ability to converge or diverge light. Refractive power of a lens is expressed as dioptre (D).

In clinical practice the refractive power of the lens is represented in terms of its focal length and is equal to the reciprocal of the focal length of the lens

$$p = \frac{1}{F}$$

where p = power of the lens
and F = focal length of the lens

Refractive power of lens depends upon three factors:

- Curvature of the lens surfaces
- Distance between two surfaces or thickness of the lens
- Refractive index of the lens material

Note: For all practical purposes lens material is standard and practically the thickness of lens is very less, hence primarily refractive power of a lens is decided by the curvature of the lens surface.

As we can see in **Fig. 3.29A, B,** when parallel rays meet at the focal point which is situated at 1 meter distance from the optical centre of the lens, then the power of such a lens is termed 1 Dioptre (D) power. Focal point distance (focal length) is a convenient and practically adoptable method to decide the power of the lens.

For a thin lens calculations of various distance are based on the formula

$$\frac{1}{F} = \frac{1}{V} - \frac{1}{U}$$

Here F = focal length of lens
          V = distance between the lens and image
          U = distance between the object and lens

Focal point distance is inversely proportional to the refractive power of the lens; means when power of the lens is more, then the distance of the focal point will be less.

- 1 D powerful lens will have a focal point distance of 1 meter
- 2 D power lens will have a focal point distance of 0.5 meter
- 0.5 D power lens will have a focal point distance of 2 meters

Role of Dioptre

Dioptre plays an important role in determining various properties of the lenses and helps us to calculate several data in relation of the lenses.

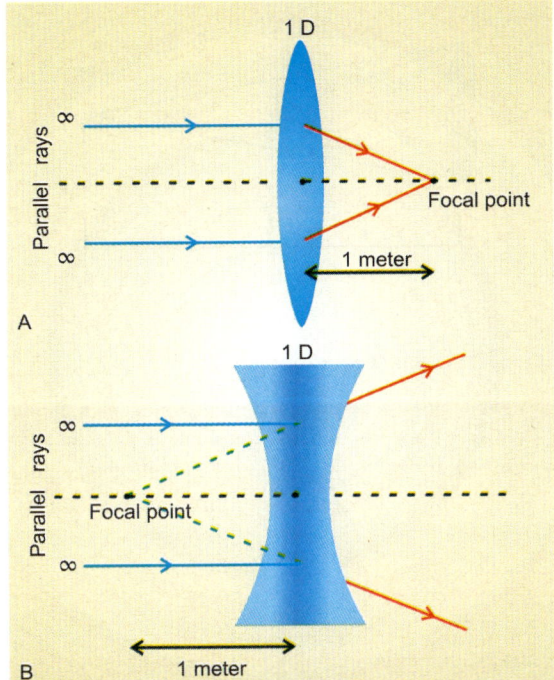

Fig. 3.29: Dioptric power of lens. A. Converging lens; B. Diverging lens

Measurement of vergence: Curvature of a refracting surface determines the vergence of rays and we measure the curvature of refracting surface in terms of dioptres (D). Curvature of refracting surface (wavefront) and simultaneously the vergence of light rays both vary inversely with the distance from the light source means when shorter is the distance from source, greater will be the vergence of ray.

As vergence is inversely proportional to the distance from the light source and as we know that dioptres can be used to measure the focal point distance so on the basis of this we can correlate the vergence of wavefront in terms of dioptres.

For example, a wavefront present at 1 meter distance from its source of origin will have a vergence of 1 dioptre (1 D). Accordingly vergence at 1/2 meter distance will be of 2 D and vergence at 2 meters distance will be of 0.5 D. For all practical purposes vergence at 6 meters distance is calculated as zero or nil, considering that wavefront distance from the light source is infinite.

Measurement of distance: As discussed above, we can describe the vergence as either positive or negative. Similarly, dioptres are also prefixed with signs of either plus or minus. Plus dioptres express the convergence (positive vergence) and minus dioptres express the divergence (negative vergence).

As shown in Fig. 3.30A when light rays are diverging from a point source, then they produce a negative vergence of one dioptre (–1 D) at 1 meter distance. Now if we decrease the distance to half from the source, then vergence gets doubled, i.e. –2 D (because vergence is inversely proportional to distance from the light source) and when the distance from the source remains one-fourth of a meter, then the vergence become four times, i.e. –4 D.

Similarly, when parallel rays from infinity are made to converge as a point focus at a distance of one meter by using convex lens, means a positive vergence of +1 D is produced. Similarly, when parallel rays are made to focus at one-fourth of a meter distance from converging lens, means a four dioptres (+4 D) positive vergence is produced as shown in Fig. 3.30B.

Note: In simpler words, a distance from point of vergence can be represented either as one-fourth of a meter or four dioptre.

Measurement of lens power: Along with measurement of vergence and distance, dioptre also helps in measurement of power of lens. In other words, dioptre indicates the ability of any lens in terms of its light bending capacity. The power of a lens can be described in terms of dioptric distance (meters) of the focal point.

For example, + 1 D power convex lens will converge parallel rays from infinity to a point located at the distance of 1 meter from the lens (Fig. 3.31A). Similarly, a – 1 D power concave lens will diverge the parallel rays from infinity

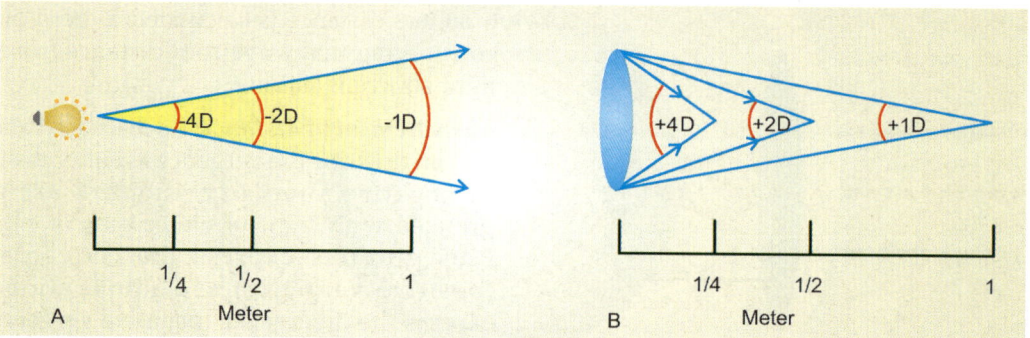

Fig. 3.30: Measurement of vergence and distance in dioptres

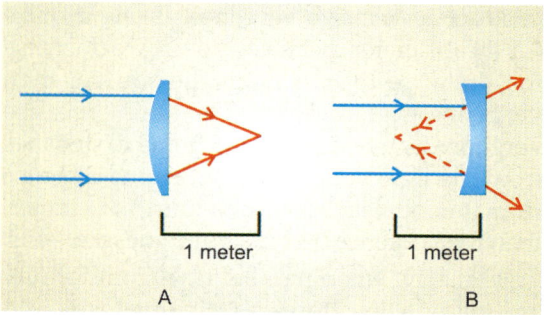

Fig. 3.31: Effect of one dioptre power lenses on vergence
A: +1 D power convex lens converges parallel rays at a point situated one meter distance from the lens
B: –1 D power concave lens diverges parallel rays, as if they are coming from a point (focal point) 1 meter distance from the lens

Table 3.1: Equivalent dioptric distances	
Dioptric power	*Focal distance*
Nil	Infinity or 6 meters
0.5 D	2 meters
1.0 D	1 meter
2.0 D	50 cm
3.0 D	33 cm
4.0 D	25 cm
5.0 D	20 cm
10.0 D	10 cm

which when joined backward will meet at 1 meter distance (Fig. 3.31B).

As discussed above the dioptric power of a lens is reciprocal to the focal distance (in meters) means shorter is the distance more will be the number of dioptres. For example, lens of +4 D will converge the parallel rays at a focus distance of 0.25 meter (25 cm); similarly a –5 D lens will diverge parallel rays and the form a virtual image at focus distance of 0.20 meter (20 cm). Equivalent focal distances for routinely used dioptric powers are summarized in Table 3.1.

Measurement of curvatures: The light ray bending capability of a lens is primarily correlated to the curvatures of lens surfaces, predominantly at air–lens interface. As the curvature of lens surface increases, the degree or amount of refraction also increases proportionately; means the lens having a steeper curved surface or a shorter radius of curvature will refract incident light rays more as compared to the lens having flatter curved surface or longer radius of curvature.

Note: The total power of a lens is decided by the power of its both refracting surfaces (front and back curves), but practically it is sufficient to remember that front surface of the cornea (convex shape) will produce a positive vergence (plus power) on light rays passing through it.

In relation to refraction, the primary role of the eye is to focus all the incident rays of light on the retina. To achieve this eye must exert a substantial amount of positive vergence on incident parallel rays to converge them; so that these parallel rays get focused on fovea situated about 23 mm away from the cornea. Normally total amount of plus power exerted by both the cornea and crystalline lens is equal to nearly 60 D.

Lens Representations

The spherical lenses and cylindrical lenses can be represented in the following way:

A symbol of S/sph for sphere and symbol of C/cyl for cylinder are post-fixed the power, however, the axis of cylinder is also written after the expression of power separated by a '*x*' sign.

- *For example:* Spherical (converging) lens and cylindrical lens of 1 D can be represented as + 1 DS (+ 1 Dsph) and + 1 DC (+1 Dcyl) × axis of power (e.g. 90° or 180°), respectively. While spherical (diverging) lens of 1 D can be represented as – 1 DS (– 1 Dsph) and cylindrical lens as – 1 DC (– 1 Dcyl)) × axis of power (say 90° or 180°).

Cylinder orientation: This is a universal way to represent the axis of a cylindrical lens. The examiner sees the patient's right and left eyes as shown in Fig. 3.32. When the examiner is facing the patient, the right eye of the patient will be towards his left side and thus from examiner's left side the axis representation is started.

Vertically the scale will be read as 90° and horizontally as 180° starting from the left of examiner. Similarly, 45° and 135° are represented at right angle to each other. The axis of the cylinders recorded by this universal representation is written after the dioptric power of cylinders as described above.

Refraction Through Combination of Lenses

The practical advantage of dioptre system and signs of plus/minus is that when two lenses are used in combination, it became easy to

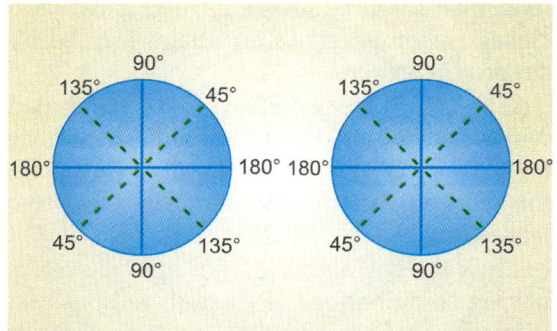

Fig. 3.32: Representation of cylindrical orientation

calculate the effective outcome easily by using the specific formula.

1. If a + 2 Dsph lens is converging the parallel rays, and before these rays reach to the focal point, another diverging lens of – 4 Dsph is placed in the path of these converging rays; then the effective outcome is calculated as explained below.

   To calculate the equivalent power we mathematically combine the powers of these two spherical lenses:

   + 2 Dsph + (–4 Dsph) = –2 Dsph

   For better understanding we use universal representation method of lens power values in the form of a cross as shown in Fig. 3.33.

   The final image formed with combination of these two spherical lenses will be that as if a minus 2 Dsph lens is placed, means a virtual, erect image will be formed at 0.5 meter distance from the lenses.

2. Similarly, when two cylindrical lenses whose axis are perpendicular to each other are placed in contact, then their effective power will be as that of a sphere. For example, if + 1 Dcyl with 90° axis (vertical axis) is combined with another +1 Dcyl having 180° axis (horizontal axis), then the final effective power will be of + 1 Dsph. This can also be represented as shown in Fig. 3.34.

Note: Effective power of a cylindrical lens is actually perpendicular to the represented axis.

3. Similarly, we can also combine spherical lenses with cylindrical lenses in various combinations, so that we can get different types of images with these combinations. Suppose if a +2 Dsph is combined with – 2 Dcyl having axis at 90°, then the resultant effective power will be of +2 Dcyl at 180° or horizontal meridian as shown in Fig. 3.35.

4. If a converging spherical lens is combined with the plus cylindrical lens, then in the axis of cylinder the effective power will be combination of both but in the remaining area of the lens the power will be equal to spherical lens power. For example, when

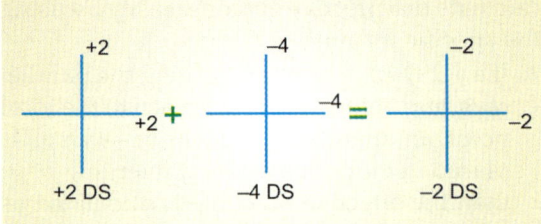

Fig. 3.33: Representation of combination of spherical lenses

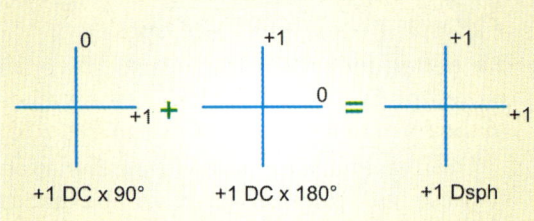

Fig. 3.34: Formation of an equivalent spherical lens by combination of two cylindrical lenses

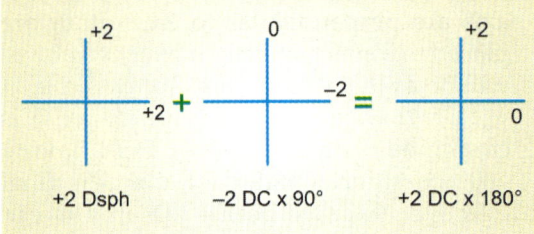

Fig. 3.35: Combination of plus spherical lens and minus cylindrical lens forms a plus cylinder of opposite axis

+2 Dsph is combined with + 1 Dcyl at the axis 90°, then the resultant effective refractive power at 90° meridian (axis) will be of +3 D, whereas in all other meridians it will be of +2 D only.

These all calculations which have been discussed above to find out the power of an effective lens holds good only when the two lenses are very thin and/or are placed in contact with each other. However, entire calculations to find out the effective power of lenses will change if either the lenses are thick and/or are placed at a distance from each other.

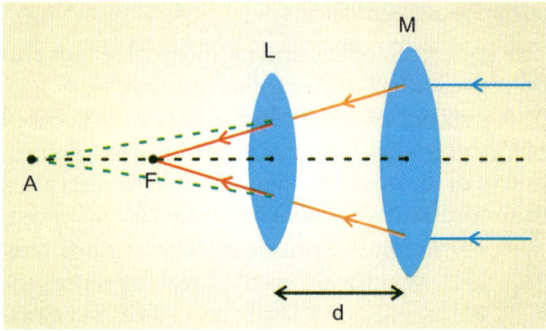

Fig. 3.36: Image formation after combination of two convex lenses

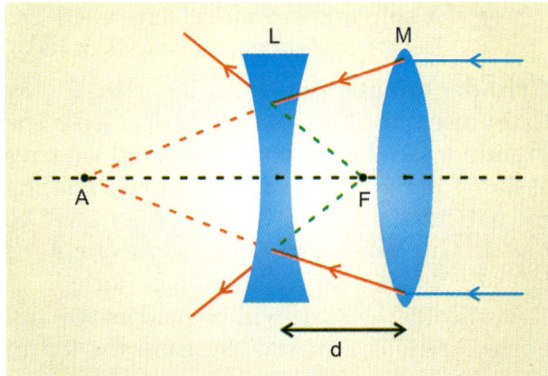

Fig. 3.37: Image formation after combination of concave and convex lens

For example, as shown in Fig. 3.36, a convex lens (L) will form image at point A, but when this lens is combined with another convex lens (M) placed at a distance (d) from the convex lens (L), then the effective image will be formed at focus F. We can also notice that if a convex lens is combined with another convex lens, then the final image formed is real and closer as compared to an image formed by single convex lens.

Likewise, if a convex lens (M) is combined with a concave lens (L) and placed at a distance (d) from each other, then the final image (F) formed is virtual and situated in between two lenses (Fig. 3.37).

Thus the calculations from optical system having combinations of lenses is tedious and difficult, however, this can be done easily if only a few lenses or refractive surfaces are

Clinical Applications

Combination of lenses leads to discovery of various telescopes and forms the optical principle for both Astronomical and Galilean telescopes.

present and they all lie on the same optical axis. Scientist Gauss and Listing worked a lot on mathematics of these combinations, and made the calculations easy for various optical systems.

Refraction Through Special Lenses

Thick Lenses

Till now we studied all calculations considering the lens to be very thin (thickness of lens is negligible) and contain a single refracting surface. As compared to thin lens, thick lens have two refracting surfaces separated by a glass medium and not by the air medium as seen in thin lens. Thickness of thin lenses has no influence on light rays, hence they pass through thin lens unaffected. However, in case of thick lenses it is important to know a few additional parameters to understand refraction through thick lens.

In Fig. 3.38, we can see that in thick lens when parallel light ray strikes the refracting surface, i.e. R_1 it get converge and then light ray further strikes the second refracting surface, i.e. R_2 and finally focused at focal point (F_2). Suppose, if this light ray had not met at the second surface, i.e. R_2 then it could

have been focused at point F_1 (as seen in the case of a thin lens). However, in the case of a thick lens the final effective focus became F_2 in place of F_1.

Total power of a thick lens cannot be obtained by simple addition of the powers of the two refractive surfaces (i.e. R_1 and R_2 in our example). The formula used to calculate the total power of a thick lens is:

$$\text{Total power } (\theta) = r_1 + r_2 - \left(\frac{t}{\mu}\right) \times r_1 r_2$$

Here r_1 = power of first refracting surface of the lens (R_1) in dioptre

r_2 = power of second refracting surface of the lens (R_2) in dioptre

t = thickness of the lens in meters

μ = refractive index of the lens material

For example, consider a 2 cm (0.02 meter) thick lens having refractive powers +6 D (r_1) and +8 D (r_2) is made up of crown glass with refractive index (μ) of 1.5, then the power of this lens will not be just simple addition, i.e. $6 + 8 = +14$ D, rather it will have total refractive power of +13.36 D (calculated by above mentioned formula). This difference of 0.64 dioptre power is due to the change in the vergence happened in light ray while travelling from front to back refracting surface inside the lens. Knowing the calculation for the final refractive power of a thick lens is very useful in many practical situations.

Clinical Significance

Contact lenses and intra ocular lenses are considered as thick lenses, although they practically appear very much thinner than routine spectacle lenses.

Astigmatic or Cylindrical Lenses

In spherical lenses all the meridians have the same curvature, hence the rays coming from a point source will focus as a point at focal length of the spherical lens. But in cylindrical lenses one meridian is curved (either convex or concave) and the other meridian (perpendicular to first meridian) is not curved (i.e. plane), hence the

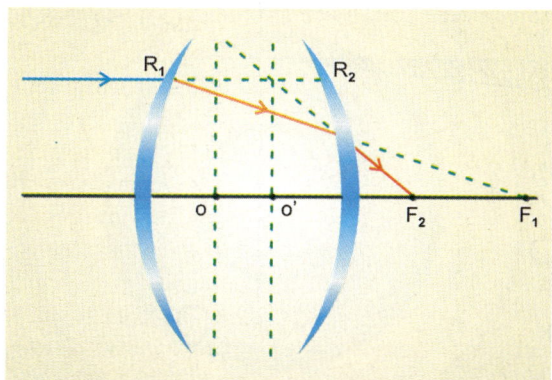

Fig. 3.38: Refraction through thick lens

rays coming from a point source will focus as a straight line at focal length of the cylindrical lens. This type of cylindrical lens which has only one curved meridian is called simple cylindrical or astigmatic lens (planocylindrical lens). Another type of astigmatic lens which is termed compound or spherocylinder astigmatic or cylindrical lens has both the meridian curved at different degrees. This type of lens will never form a point image or a line image of a point light source. For example, a spoon which has a steeper curvature from side to side (VV') as compared to the curvature from tip to handle (HH') (Fig. 3.39).

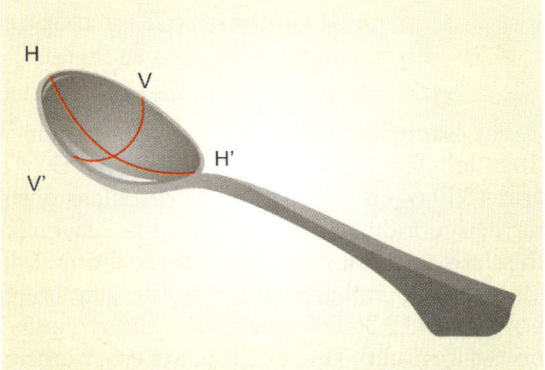

Fig. 3.39: Spoon representing two different curved meridians

Sturm's Conoid

Refraction through a compound astigmatic lens having two meridians can be understood by Sturm's conoid. As seen in Fig. 3.40 lens has two meridians with different curvatures, namely LL' (vertical) and MM' (horizontal). If vertical meridian (LL') of the lens is more curved (steeper) as compared to horizontal meridian MM' of the lens as seen in Fig. 3.40, then the rays from LL' meridian will focus nearer as compared to rays from MM', while rays from horizontal meridian (MM') will focus at far point, thus there will be two foci and the distance between these two foci is known as focal interval (**sturm conoid interval**). There is overlapping of light rays in between these two focal points so that a series of images of various shapes of the object or source of light is formed at different intervals. These images represent the images of object seen by an astigmatic eye.

If sections are made at different intervals (points a, b, c, d, e, f and g in Fig. 3.40) in sturm's conoid, then the shape of images or shape of bundle of light rays at these sections will be as follows

- Section at point a = both vertical and horizontal rays are converging at this

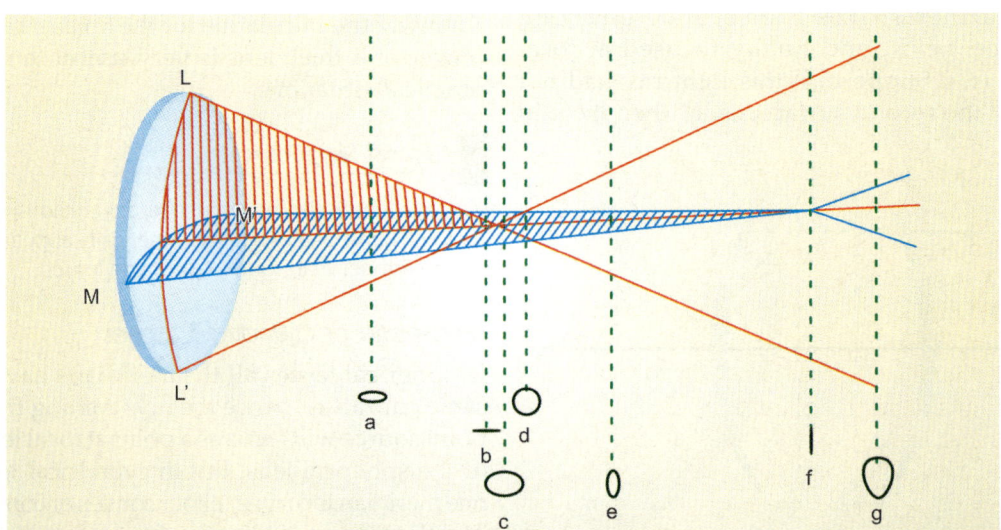

Fig. 3.40: Sturm's conoid

point but vertical rays are converging more rapidly than horizontal rays. Hence, section of light bundle here will be a horizontally oval-shaped ellipse having more horizontal diameter

- Section at point *b* = all vertical rays meet at this point (first focus), while horizontal rays are still converging, hence a horizontal line is seen at this section.
- Section at point *c* = the horizontal rays are converging but divergence of vertical rays has started, hence a horizontal oval ellipse is formed at this section.
- Section at point *d* = horizontal rays are converging and vertical rays are also diverging in almost same proportion, hence a circle is formed at this section. This is the point where least distorted image is formed and this circle is called ***circle of least diffusion or confusion*** which is situated near the middle of interval.
- Section at point *e* = degree of divergence of vertical rays is more than convergence of horizontal rays, hence a vertically oval ellipse with large vertical diameter is formed at this section.
- Section at point *f* = all horizontal rays meet here (second focus), hence a vertical line is seen at this point, whereas vertical rays are still diverging.
- Section at point *g* = both vertical and horizontal rays are diverging, hence vertical oval ellipse is formed.

When in an astigmatic lens the two meridians are at right angles to each other, then they produce the regular astigmatism and if meridians are not at right angle to each other, then they produce an irregular astigmatism. The details about astigmatism and their management will be dealt in Chapter 5.

Note: Distance between vertical focal point 'b' and horizontal focal point 'f' is known as **focal interval of Sturm**.

Practical Evaluation of Lenses

The parameters of lenses can also be evaluated without any instrument. We can asses not only the type of lens but also their approximate power to a near accuracy.

Different types of lenses and their approximate power can be assessed as follows.

Convex Lens

Hold a convex lens in front of the eye and a distant object is observed through it. Now, if we move the lens side by side, the object image will move in opposite direction of the movement of lens (Fig. 3.41). This phenomenon is due to the fact that the image formed by convex lens is inverted.

To know the power of this convex lens under examination, we can hold a concave lens of known power in close contact with convex lens and now observe the movement of the same object. The opposite directional movement of object image will decrease after addition of concave lens of known power. Now gradually change the power of concave lens until no movement of image is observed through both the lenses. At this point of no movement of object the unknown power of convex lens is same as that of the known power of concave lens; although with a plus sign.

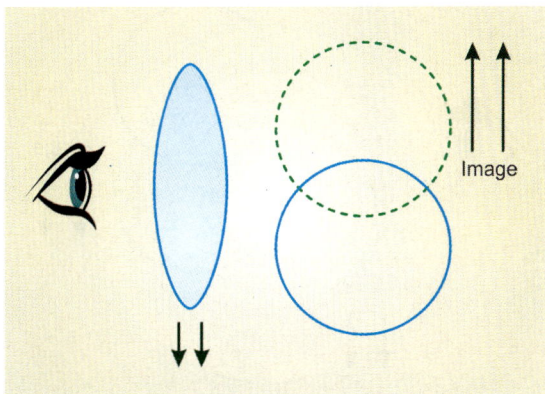

Fig. 3.41: Opposite movement of an object image when viewed through convex lens

Concave Lens

Similarly, a concave lens is held in front of the eye and a distant object is observed through it. Now by moving the concave lens side by side the object image also moves in the same direction of the movement of lens (Fig. 3.42). This phenomenon is due to the fact that the image formed by concave lens is erect.

To know the power of this concave lens under examination, we can hold a convex lens of known power in close contact with this concave lens and now observe the movement of object image. The same directional movement of image will decrease by adding convex lens of known power. Continue to change the power of convex lens till there is no further movement of image in any direction. At this point of no image movement the power of concave lens is the same as that of convex lens; although with a minus sign.

Cylindrical Lens

When we hold a cylindrical lens in front of the eye and view a linear object like tube light through this cylindrical lens, the object image appears as if it is unequally displaced or elongated in one direction (Fig. 3.43). This phenomenon happens because of the fact that cylindrical lenses have power only in one meridian.

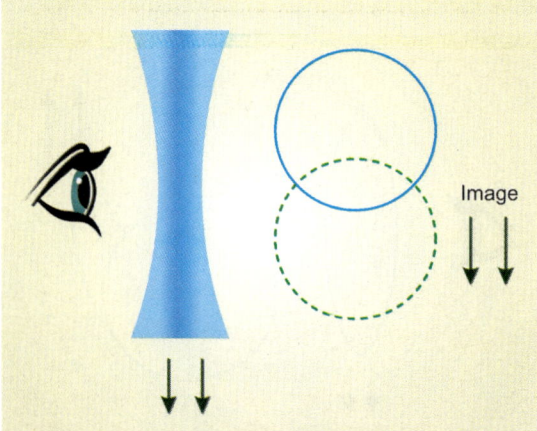

Fig. 3.42: Same directional movement of object image when viewed through concave lens

Test procedure

- Hold the cylindrical lens in front of the eye and observe the illuminated tube light of the examination room.
- Rotate the cylindrical lens in either vertical or horizontal meridian; while simultaneously observe the movement of tube light.
- We will observe movement of tube light in any one of these two meridians. Now note the meridian of cylindrical lens where there is no movement of object (tube light); this is the axis of cylindrical lens because when we move the cylindrical lens in the line of its axis, no movement of object is seen.
- Now slowly rotate the cylindrical lens in any other plane, there will be displacement of object either with or against the movement of the cylindrical lens.
- By this rotational movement of object, we can make out whether it is convex (if against movement, Fig. 3.43A) or concave (if with movement is seen, Fig. 3.43B) cylindrical lens.
- Now slowly keep rotating the cylindrical lens in the same plane of examination until the movement of the object becomes maximum, this will be the perpendicular axis to the axis of the cylindrical lens.
- Now we can hold another cylindrical lens of known power having opposite sign in front of the lens in question; so that we can neutralize the rotational movement of image.
- Keep changing the power of additional cylindrical lens having opposite sign, until there is no rotational movement of the object is seen, this will give the power of cylinder in question.

In a nutshell remember these points during evaluation of a given lens

- When we see an object through a lens and object moves with the movement of lens, then it is a concave lens and if the object moves against the movement of lens then it is a convex lens.

Note: At axis of the cylindrical lens there was no movement of the object.

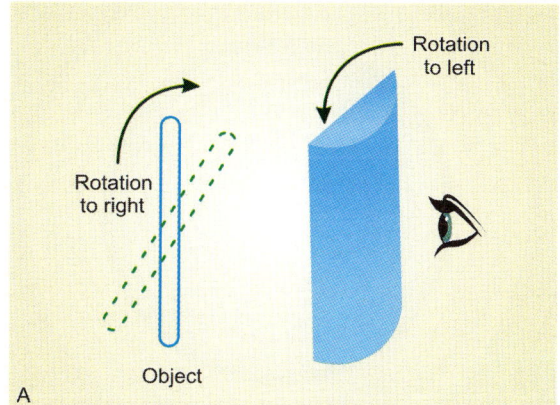 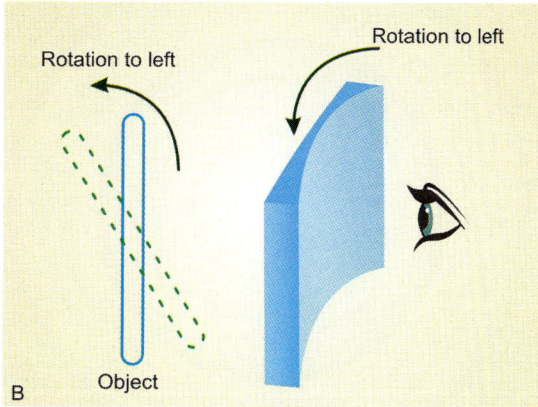

Fig. 3.43: Movement of object image when viewed through cylindrical lens. A. Convex cylinder; B. Concave cylinder

- When image movement is only in one plane along with the rotation of linear object, then the lens is cylindrical lens.
- When rotation of linear object is with the movement of lens, then it is the concave cylinder and if rotation of linear object is against the movement of lens, then it is the convex cylinder.

- Power of cylindrical lens is determined by using opposite sign spherical lens or cylindrical lens of known power, until there is no movement of linear object.
- For neutralization of lenses hold the known power lens in close contact with unknown power lens keeping their optical axes in the single line.

Ocular and Refractive Anomalies

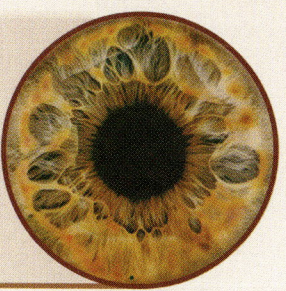

CHAPTER 4

Optical System and Optical Defects of Human Eye

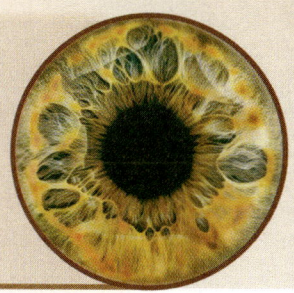

After studying this chapter the reader should be able to:
- Understand the refraction through various surfaces in human eye.
- Enlist the main factors affecting refraction through cornea and lens in human eye.
- Describe various theoretical eye models and their comparison in terms of cardinal points.
- Define and understand the visual axes and visual angles of the eye.
- Describe various physiological and pathological optical defects of human eye.

Chapter Outline

- Introduction
  - Refraction through cornea and lens
  - Theorem of Gauss
  - Gullstrand's schematic eye
  - Listing's reduced eye
  - Donder's simplified eye
  - Retinal image size
- Refractive Status of Eye
  - Visual axes and angles of eye
  - Image formation due to reflection from surfaces
- Optical Defects of Human Eye
  - Physiological optical defects of eye
    - Diffraction of light
    - Spherical aberration
    - Chromatic aberration
    - Oblique aberration
    - Coma
    - Decentring
    - Distortion
- Pathological Optical Defects of Eye
  - Refractive surface anomalies
  - Refractive index anomalies
  - Disposition of optical elements
  - Obliquity of optical elements
  - Absence of optical element of eye

INTRODUCTION

Human eye is the most sophisticated optical device created by the nature. The eye has various refracting surfaces and various medium through which light rays travel to ultimately reach at neurological tissue called retina, which sends signals to the brain about the perceived light ray's information. This forms the basis of image formation in the brain. Let us see the structures coming in the pathway of a light ray while passing through the human eye. Various refracting surfaces coming across the light pathways as shown in Fig. 4.1 are

- Anterior surface of cornea (C1)
- Cornea substance (C)
- Posterior surface of cornea (C2)
- Aqueous humor (A)
- Anterior surface of lens (L1)
- Lens substance (L)
- Posterior surface of lens (L2)
- Vitreous humor (V)

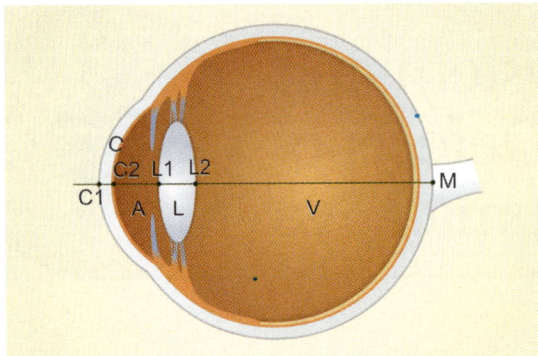

Fig. 4.1: Human eye showing various refracting surfaces

This looks very complicated that a light ray gets refracted at numerous ocular structures but in reality only the anterior corneal surface and crystalline lens act as the effective refractive surfaces of the eye, rest of the structures contribute very little in refraction because the difference in their refractive indices (RI) is negligible.

To understand this better it is important to know the RI of air and various ocular surfaces as summarized in Table 4.1.

As we can see that the RI of various ocular structures are more or less similar but there is a significant difference in the RI of air and cornea.

Another important factor which affects the refraction in the eye is radii of curvature of the cornea and crystalline lens. The values of radius of curvatures of different ocular surfaces are:

- Anterior surface of cornea: 7.7 mm
- Posterior surface of cornea: 6.8 mm
- Anterior surface of lens: 10.0 mm
- Posterior surface of lens: 6.0 mm

Table 4.1: Ocular structures and refractive indices

Structure	Refractive index
Cornea	1.376
Aqueous humor	1.336
Vitreous humor	1.336
Crystalline lens	1.41
Air	*1.00*

As per various hypotheses crystalline lens plays a major role in accommodation of the eye by changing its curvature. During maximum accommodative state the anterior and posterior lens curvatures become +5.33 and –5.33, respectively.

Refraction Through Cornea and Lens

Both cornea and crystalline lens cause convergence of light rays as both have convex surfaces. The cornea plays a major role in ocular refraction with power of about 40–45 D, because there is a huge difference in refractive indices of air (1.0) and cornea (1.376). Whereas crystalline lens in the eye lies between aqueous and vitreous humor (having same RI), hence refractive power of crystalline lens is about half compared to refractive power of cornea, i.e. nearly 18–20 D.

In the eye, cornea mainly works as single refracting surface. Cornea has homogeneous material with very less thickness; hence cornea work as single unit. In contrast, lens is thick and its material is also not homogeneous in nature. Hence, lens simply does not work as two refractive surfaces (anterior and posterior) rather it works as multiple refracting surfaces. Crystalline lens consists of several layers with different refractive indices. For example, central nuclear portion of the lens has higher refractive index than peripheral cortical layers. The curvatures of different layers of the lens are also different.

As it is clear from Fig. 4.2 that layers of the crystalline lens are not concentric as well as the curvature of inner layer is greater than the consecutive outer layers. The curvature of the peripheral cortical layer is much less than that of central nuclear layer. Hence, the refractive status at different places varies significantly in the crystalline lens. The refractive index of peripheral cortical matter of the lens is approximately 1.386 and refractive index of the central nucleus of lens is about 1.42, with an average RI of 1.41.

Greater RI of central nuclear portion of the lens as compared to peripheral cortical matter

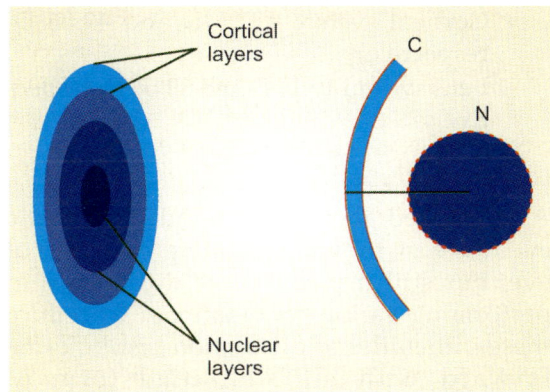

Fig. 4.2: Layers of crystalline lens

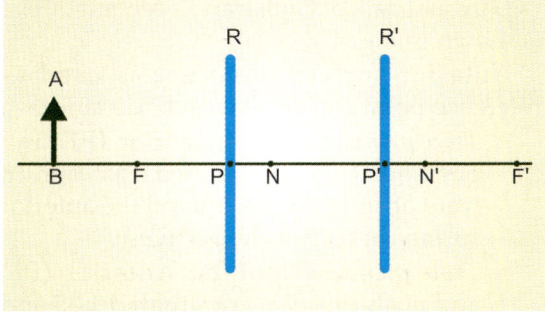

Fig. 4.3: Cardinal points with two refracting surfaces

has a great importance biologically; because variation in the refractive indices helps the crystalline lens to converge the light rays over the retina. The cortical and nuclear pattern of crystalline lens also declines the chances of various optical errors like spherical and chromatic aberrations; these patterns of crystalline lens also help in accommodation.

Furthermore, the anterior and posterior surface curvatures of crystalline lens are also unequal. Anterior surface of lens is more flat than posterior surface. Thus, the anterior surface curvature has the power of 10.0 D and posterior surface curvature has the power of 6.0 D only. This difference in power of curvatures is also responsible for an unequal refractive status of lens.

Thus optical system of human eye is complex and behaves like a combination of lenses or as a thick lens system which makes mathematical calculation tedious. Gauss proposed a simple concept and suggested that homocentric system of lenses could be treated as a whole rather than in various parts. Any complicated optical system can be reduced to a simple system by the application of theorem of Gauss, which simplify the refraction in eye and makes the mathematical calculations easy.

Theorem of Gauss

Each optical system has its own cardinal points, i.e. focal point, principle point and nodal point. The focal points and principle points are associated with focal planes and principle planes, respectively.

Single optical system has one pair of each cardinal point and two optical systems will have six pairs of cardinal points. If these points lie on a single plane and we know the value of any two cardinal points pairs, then we can calculate the remaining values easily. Similarly the effective outcome of the ray can be calculated in two optical systems by reducing these cardinal points to a single cardinal point system by using calculations of great mathematician Gauss.

In Fig. 4.3, AB is an object, F and F′ are focal points, P and P′ are principal points and N and N′ are nodal points for two refracting surfaces R and R′ respectively.

Based on the Gauss theorem many models of human eye were proposed. All of these following schematic eye models tried to explain the optics of human eye in as simple manner as possible.

Gullstrand's Schematic Eye

As discussed above, the scientist Gauss put forward the three pairs of cardinal points, all lying on the principal axis of optical system to understand the multiple optical devices in an easy way. Further, Tscherning and Helmholtz contributed a lot to understand the optics of human eye. Ultimately, it was Gullstrand who presented the most authentic model of schematic eye for better understanding of optics of the eye.

Cardinal data of Gullstrand's schematic eye is shown in Fig. 4.4.

Anterior surface of cornea is used as reference point for calculation of distance.

- *Two principal foci:* Anterior (F1) and posterior (F2) are situated 15.7 mm in front of and 24.4 mm behind the anterior surface of cornea, respectively.
- *Two principal points:* Anterior (P1) and posterior (P2) are situated 1.35 and 1.60 mm away from the anterior surface of cornea, respectively
- *Two nodal points:* First (N1) and second (N2) are located 7.08 and 7.33 mm behind the anterior surface of cornea, respectively.

Refractive indices of various refracting surfaces when accommodation is relaxed are

- Cornea—1.376
- Aqueous humor and vitreous humor—1.336
- Crystalline lens cortex—1.386
- Crystalline lens nucleus—1.406

Dioptric power or refracting power of the eye while accommodation is minimum and maximum is

- Complete eye 58.64 D and 70.57 D, respectively.
- Corneal system 43.05 D and 43.05 D, respectively.
- Lens system 19.11 D and 33.06 D, respectively.

Listing's Reduced Eye

As discussed above Gullstrand's schematic eye was easy for understanding the optics of eye; but still it poses some difficulties in performing various calculations. To reduce these difficulties of calculation Listing came forward with his simplified form of schematic eye, which is popularly called as reduced eye.

In Listing's reduced eye (Fig 4.5) also, all the distances of various cardinal points are calculated from anterior surface of cornea as reference point.

- Anterior focal point F1 and posterior focal point F2 are situated at 15.7 mm in front and 24.4 mm behind the anterior surface of cornea, respectively.
- Principal point P is located 1.5 mm behind the reference plane (anterior surface of cornea).
- Nodal points N is placed 7.2 mm behind the reference plane.
- Anterior focal length of the eye is 17.2 mm and posterior focal length is 22.9 mm.

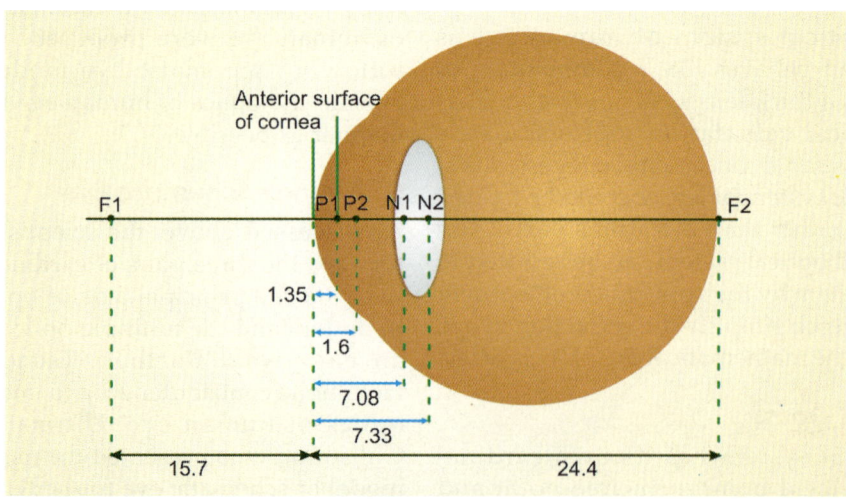

Fig. 4.4: Gullstrand's schematic eye

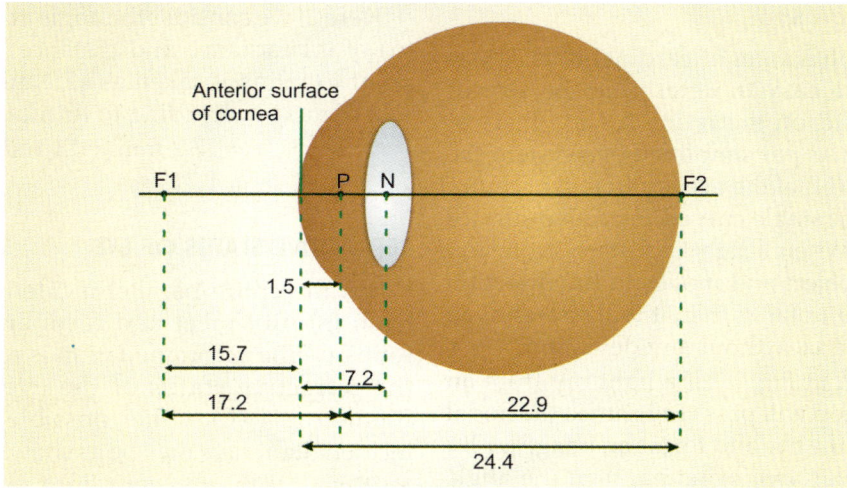

Fig. 4.5: Listing's reduced eye

- Uniform refractive index of ocular structures is 1.336.
- Total dioptric power of the eye is 58.2 D

The total refractive power of the eye is calculated by formula

$$F = \frac{\text{Refractive index}}{\text{Focal length (meters)}}$$

Hence, by using anterior focal length 17.2 mm

$$F = \frac{\text{Refractive index of air}}{\text{Anterior focal length (meters)}}$$

$$= 1 \times \frac{1000}{17.2}$$

$$= 58.2$$

Similarly, by using posterior focal length 22.9 mm

$$F = \frac{\text{Refractive index of vitreous}}{\text{Posterior focal length (meters)}}$$

$$= 1.336 \times \frac{1000}{22.9}$$

$$= 58.2$$

Donders' Simplified Eye

Scientist Franciscus Cornelis Donders further simplified the cardinal point data of Listing's reduced eye by converting them into round figures. He oversimplified the data so that readers can remember them easily. He considered the eye as single curved refracting surface and reduced the cardinal data as shown in Fig. 4.6.

Reference plane in Donder's simplified eye model is situated 2 mm behind the anterior corneal surface of the eye.

- Nodal point N is situated 5 mm behind the reference plane
- Anterior focal length is 15 mm
- Posterior focal length is 20 mm
- Uniform refractive index of ocular structures is 1.336
- Total dioptric power of the eye is 60 D

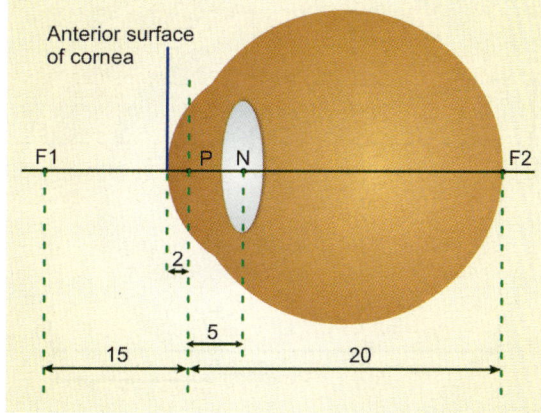

Fig. 4.6: Donders' simplified eye

Retinal Image Size

Due to simplification of cardinal data, it has now become easy to determine the size of image formed on the retina by an object of known size. As per simplified eye system the nodal point (N) of the eye is situated at centre of an anterior single curved refractive surface of the eye. When a light ray starts from top edge of an object and moves in the direction of nodal point of eye, then it will straightway reach the retina without any deviation.

As shown in Fig. 4.7 if a light ray from an object (AB) top will pass straight via the nodal point (N) of the eye and forms an image (A′B′) in the macular area of retina, then the angle (α) formed between the object (AB) and image (A′B′) at nodal point will be equal. The distance between the nodal point (N) and image (A′B′) is 17.2 mm, i.e. equal to that of anterior focal length.

Angle (α) is measured in radians and can be calculated by simplified formula

$$\tan \alpha = \frac{\text{Object size}}{\substack{\text{Distance between the} \\ \text{object and nodal point}}}$$

The size of retinal image (A′B′) can be calculated by the following formula =
Distance between nodal point (N) and retina (mm) × Angle of image (α) at the nodal point (radians)

Here, if we consider the angle at nodal point (α) of 0.1 radiance and distance from nodal point to retina is taken as 17.2 mm, then the size of image according to formula will be

= 17.2 mm × 0.1 radiance

= 1.72 mm

REFRACTIVE STATUS OF EYE

When the entire parallel incident light rays from infinity meet and form an image on retina (while accommodation is at rest), then the refractive status of the eye is termed Emmetropia (E). Other possible destiny of incident light rays may be as shown in Fig. 4.8.

- When all the incident light rays focus in front of the retina, then it is termed myopic state of the eye (M).
- When all the incident light rays focus behind the retina, then it is called hypermetropic state of the eye (H).
- When a few light rays meet in front of the retina, a few rays meet on the retina or a few rays meet behind the retina, then this condition is termed astigmatic state of the eye.

Visual Axes and Angles of Eye

Visual axes of eye (Fig. 4.9)

- *Optical axis:* A straight line which passes through the centre of cornea (C), then through centre of crystalline lens (L) and then reach the retina at point R is called optical axis (OR) of the eye. Optical axis lies nasally to fovea of the retina.

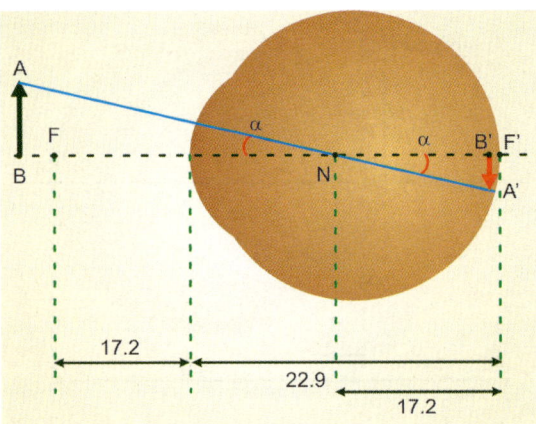

Fig. 4.7: Retinal image size

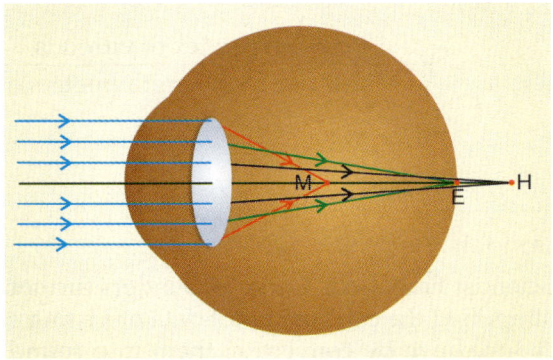

Fig. 4.8: Various refracting status of eye

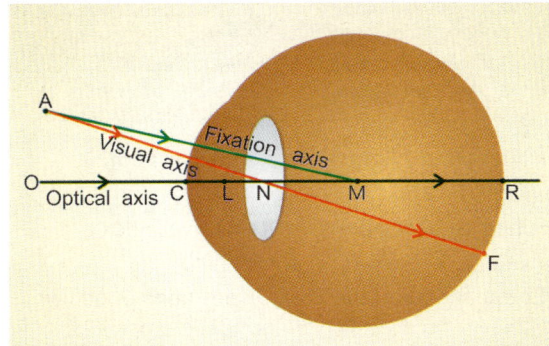

Fig. 4.9: Visual axes of eye

- *Visual axis:* A straight line which passes through fixation point from object (A) via nodal point (N) and meets the retina at its fovea (F) is called visual axis (AF) of the eye.
- *Fixation axis:* A straight line which passes through fixation point on object (A) and meets at centre of rotation of the eye (M) is termed fixation axis (AM) of the eye.

Visual angles of eye (Fig. 4.10)

- Angle alpha (α): The angle (ONA) formed between the visual axis (AF) and the optical axis (OR) at the nodal point (N) of the eye is called angle alpha. Normally, it is 5°. This small degree of deviation between the visual axis and the optical axis plays an important role in correcting the chromatic aberrations of eye.
- Angle gamma (γ): The angle (OMA) formed between the optical axis (OR) and fixation

Note: For all practical purposes center of cornea (C) is considered corresponding to the center of pupil.

axis (AM) at centre of rotation of eye (M) is termed angle gamma (γ).
- Angle kappa (κ): The angle (OCA) formed between an imaginary pupillary line (AC) corresponding to center of the pupil and the optical axis (OR) is called angle kappa.

Image Formation due to Reflection from Surfaces

Purkinje Images

In the year 1823, physiologist Purkinje discovered that images of a candle gets reflected from anterior and posterior surfaces of cornea and that of crystalline lens, which he named them Purkinje's images. Basically four principal images **(Purkinje I, II, III, IV)** are seen one each from anterior and posterior surfaces of cornea **(I, II)** and also one each

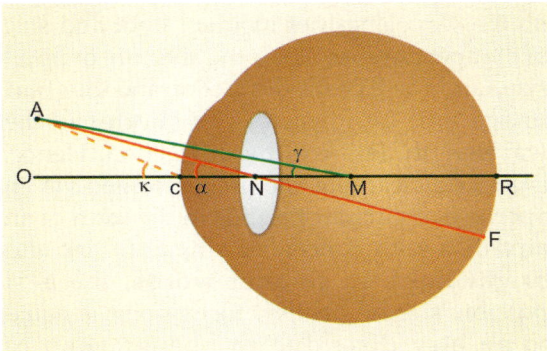

Fig. 4.10: Visual angles of eye

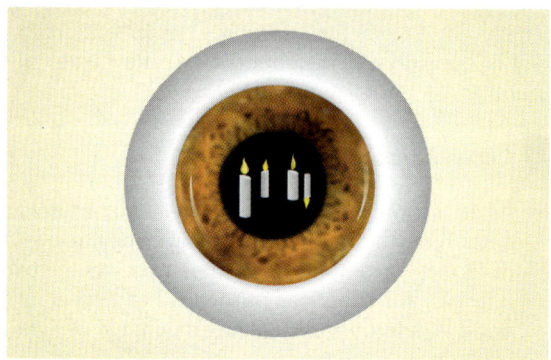

Fig. 4.11: Purkinje images

from anterior and posterior surfaces of crystalline lens (III, IV). All images formed were upright except the one formed from posterior surface of crystalline lens. Images I, II, and III were virtual and erect, whereas image (IV) from posterior surface of lens was real and inverted as shown in Fig. 4.11. Among these four images the anterior corneal surface image was largest in size and brightest in nature.

OPTICAL DEFECTS OF HUMAN EYE

Above mentioned various cardinal data and parameters of the eye help us to understand various optical defects of the eye. Optical defects of the human eye can be physiological or pathological.

Various types of physiological and pathological optical defects of the eye are summarized in Table 4.2.

Physiological Optical Defects of Eye

Diffraction of Light

Sir George Airy, an eminent scientist, reported that when light rays pass through an aperture, the light ray gets diffracted by the edge of this aperture (pupillary margins or rim of crystalline lens in human eye). The pattern which is formed due to diffracted images contains series of concentric rings which have alternative dark and bright bands along with a bright central disc. This central disc is known as *Airy disc* (Fig 4.12).

Table 4.2: Various types of physiological and pathological optical defects of the eye

Physiological optical defects of the eye	Pathological optical defects of the eye
Diffraction of light	Refractive surface anomalies
Spherical aberrations	Refractive index anomalies
Chromatic aberrations	Dispositions of ocular optical elements
Oblique aberrations	Obliquity of the ocular optical elements
Coma	Absence of optical element of the eye
Decentring	
Distortion	

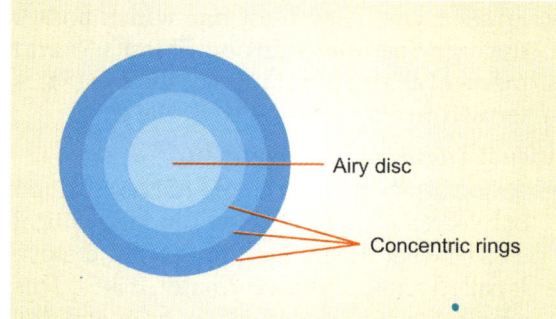

Fig. 4.12: Airy disc

Because of diffraction of light even a perfect lens (aberration free) will not form a sharp point image of a point source of light. Instead the image of a point light source is formed as an airy disc. The size of the airy disc depends on the wavelength of incident light and size of the aperture. Smaller is the aperture or pupil size, larger will be the diffraction and thus blur image will be formed. The shorter is the wavelength, less will be diffraction. Hence, even by a clear lens the image formed via an aperture or circular pupil is in the form of an airy disc with concentric rings of dark and bright light. In simpler words, the best possible size of smallest focus point is equal to an airy disc, due to phenomenon of diffraction.

Spherical Aberrations

As we know that refraction of light depends on many factors, among them curvature of the refracting surface is an important factor for refraction. Crystalline lens of eye has more curvature at the periphery than the center. Due to this difference in curvatures of lens the refraction of the peripheral rays of light is stronger than the rays falling in the center of lens. As a result, the central rays bend less and focus away from lens while peripheral rays focus near the lens. It means the central and peripheral rays do not focus at a single point after refraction, thus the image formed is not sharp rather it is blur at the edges as shown in Fig. 4.13.

Human eye has a dioptric power of about +60 D which is primarily due to cornea and crystalline lens. Theoretically, because of this high dioptric power human eye should produce a great amount of spherical aberrations, but practically when these aberrations of the eye were measured by a technique called aberrometry, it was found that majority of these aberrations were coma type aberrations, not the spherical type aberrations.

There are various ocular structural factors which help in decreasing the spherical aberrations of the eye

- Distinctive curvature of the cornea, i.e. it is more curved in the center and flatter at its periphery. Hence, at periphery there is less bending of light rays than

center and rays from center bend more because it is more curved, hence rays from both the portions will meet almost at the same point.

- Crystalline lens of eye has more refractive index in the center than peripheral cortex and also the central layers are more curved than peripheral layers. Because of this peculiar arrangement of lens layers and density of material, the rays are refracted more from central portion as compared to the peripheral portion of crystalline lens; hence decreases the spherical aberrations.

- Finally, iris behaves like a diaphragm and block the entry of majority of peripheral rays into the eye, so that only axial and paraxial rays can enter the eye.

Chromatic Aberration

Light rays when passes through a transparent medium the amount of its refraction is decided by the wavelength of incident light ray. As discussed before white light is actually a representation of VIBGYOR, where violet color ray has shortest wavelength and red color ray has longest wavelength. As per the law of refraction blue ray will refract more as compared to red ray of the light. So when white light passes through the eye, blue light deviates more strongly and will focus in front of the red light while the red light being of longer wavelength will focus at a longer distance than the blue light. In between these two color rays other colors of the spectrum are focused at different distances according to their wavelengths. In normal circumstances emmetropic eye is slightly myopic for blue light (blue rays focusing in front of retina) and hypermetropic for red light (red rays focusing behind the retina) as shown in Fig. 4.14.

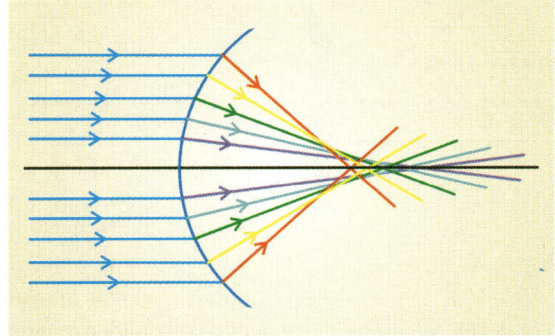

Fig. 4.13: Spherical aberration

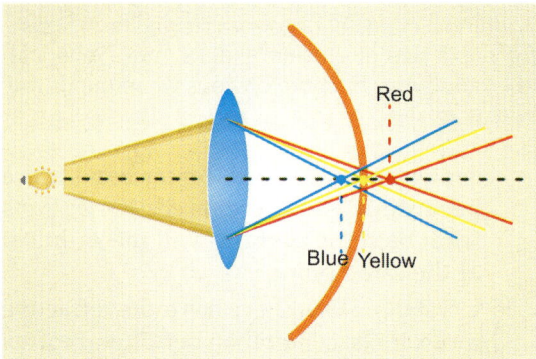

Fig. 4.14: Chromatic aberration

As shown in Fig. 4.14, it is mainly the yellow light of spectrum which falls on the retina as compared to the blue or red light. Various ocular factors that help to decrease these chromatic aberrations of the eye are:

- Fovea of retina is having very less number of blue cones, so blue light is not much appreciated by fovea.
- Long wavelength and medium wavelength cones in eye have very narrow band of spectrum of sensitivity. So the fovea is less sensitive for blue or red color rays.
- During normal focusing process of the eye the rays having more intensity (i.e. yellow color) gets well focused and forms a sharp image on the retina. Whereas, blue light rays of shorter wavelength and red light rays of longer wavelength form lower intensity circles as compared to the yellow rays; hence the images formed by blue and red colors are not sharp on the retina, so get neglected by the brain.

Oblique Aberrations

An object present in the peripheral visual field of eye does not focus like central visual field objects; rather object image is seen as a thin form of pencil ray due to improper focusing of the oblique rays.

As shown in Fig. 4.15, a sturm's conoid is formed at peripheral portion of spherical lens. Due to this conoid two line foci Fa and Fb will be formed in any of the peripheral oblique axis of eye. So the emergent rays from the peripheral portion of retina get affected due to oblique astigmatism of eye. This oblique astigmatism is more pronounced when either biconvex or biconcave lenses are used, on contrary, meniscus lenses or periscopic lenses show less oblique astigmatism as shown in Fig. 4.16.

Factor which mainly reduces this oblique astigmatism is the curvature of retina, which is adapted to the optical system of eye in such a manner that the peripheral visual field of eye is not affected in practicality. Pupil also reduces the amount of pencil rays to reach the retina of eye and helps in reduction of oblique astigmatism.

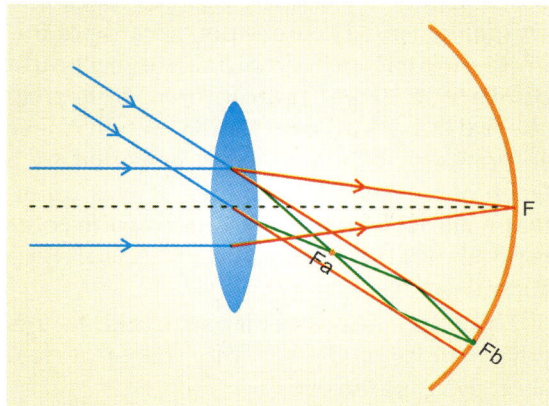

Fig. 4.15: Oblique aberration

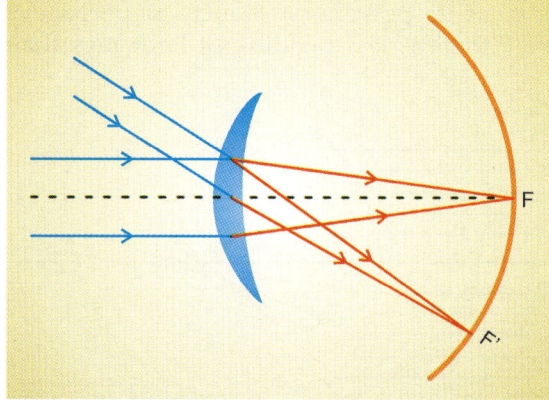

Fig. 4.16: Meniscus lenses decreasing oblique aberrations

Coma

This is again a type of peripheral aberration because the light rays after getting refracted from different areas of crystalline lens form different planes of foci. The peripheral rays from an object form an image having bright central portion and a tail having reduced brightness (similar to a comet). It means point source of light forms the chief focus along with an imaginary plane of multiple foci; this effect is termed coma (Fig. 4.17). This optical aberration (coma) can be reduced by preventing the entry of peripheral rays refracting from the ocular surfaces.

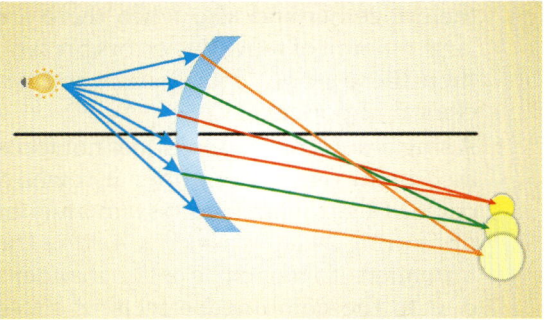

Fig. 4.17: Coma aberration

Decentring

Normally incident light rays initially fall on cornea and then pass through the crystalline lens to get focus at retina; because practically cornea and lens are two main refracting surfaces of the eye. Center of these two major refracting surfaces do not have a common axis, rather the crystalline lens of eye is slightly decentred as compared to the cornea. Axis OA of crystalline lens L is situated approximately 0.25 mm above the center of curvature of cornea C, which in turn is positioned in common with that of visual axis as shown in Fig. 4.18. This small decentring of lens does not functionally affect the vision and hence usually gets neglected.

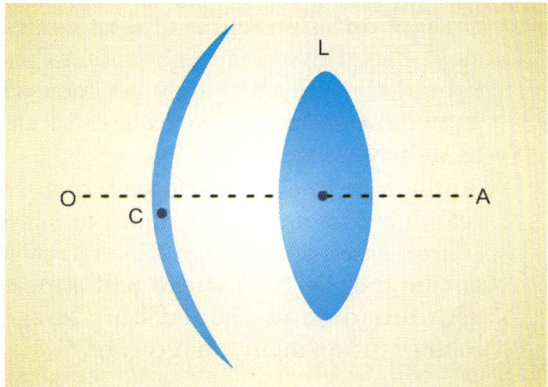

Fig. 4.18: Decentration phenomenon of crystalline lens

Distortion

As discussed above the image size on retina varies in accordance with change in image angle at nodal point. This image angle is in turn varies with change in distance between optical axis and object height. In simpler terms magnification of object is dependent on relative position of object and optical axis of eye.

Suppose peripheral portion of an object is magnified more than the central portion of an object; then pincushion type of distortion in image is seen. Whereas, if central portion is more magnified than peripheral portion of an object, then barrel type of distortion in image will occur (Fig. 4.19). For example, in aphakic

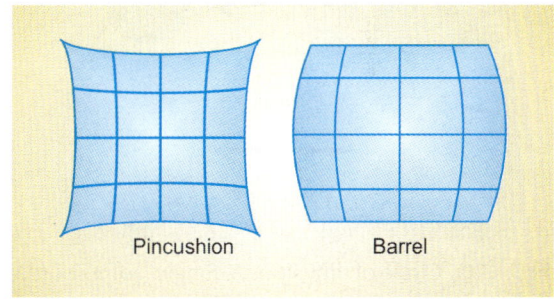

Pincushion   Barrel

Fig. 4.19: Distortion of images pincushion and Barrel type

patients or patients wearing high plus power lenses, a significant pincushion image effect is a matter of concern.

Practical aspects of physiological optical defects of eye

- In our today's life these physiological optical defects occur normally but they do not produce any problem and are not noticed by us. However, when we see them together and also when there are large amount of refractive errors present; then these unnoticed aberrations get clinical importance.

- A single-point light source does not focus as a point on retina; rather it forms a circle of light which has certain amount of blurring as shown in Fig. 4.20A. The formation of a blur circle of light happens due to the combined effects of these physiological optical defects in normal eyes. This blur circle of light is called circle of diffusion (circle of least confusion). When two-point light sources are kept at close distance they get focused as two overlapping blur circles of light as shown in Fig. 4.20B.

- Similarly a line light source which in reality is combination of multiple point sources will form an image of overlapping circles and the final image will appear as a broad band shaped blur image instead of a linear image (Fig. 4.21).

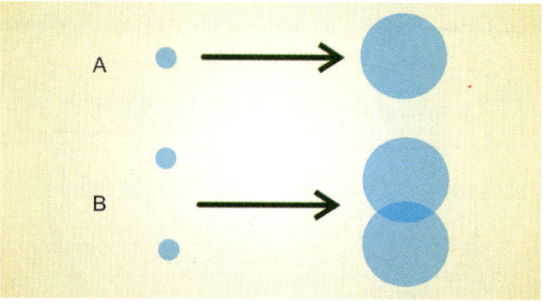

Fig. 4.20: Circle of diffusion. A. Single-point source; B: Two-point sources

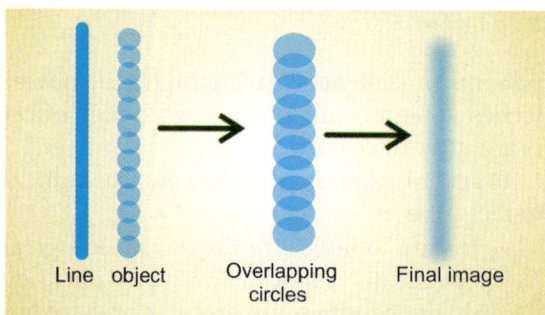

Fig. 4.21: Line of diffusion

However, smaller circles of light will produce clearer image and in turn a good vision. Thus, human eye tries to produce these circles of least diffusion to get a clear and sharp image of an object.

Pathological Optical Defects (Refractive Errors) of Eye

Parallel rays from infinity when falls on a physiologically normal eye they get refracted and converge to focus on the retina to form a circle of least confusion. When this happens in an eye with the accommodation at rest, it is termed emmetrope state of eye (Fig. 4.22).

This state of emmetropia is a theoretical assumption and is difficult to attain in realism because to attain emmetropic state various ocular elements must be perfect in their dimensions. For example, to attain emmetropic state in an eye the axial length, corneal curvature and curvature of the crystalline lens must poses such an accurate dimensions that there is no difference of even fraction of mm in size. Hence emmetropia is not a common clinical presentation rather more commonly small optical errors are seen.

So in other words, a condition where all the parallel rays of light do not focus on the retina becomes more common state of eye than emmetropia. These conditions where all the parallel rays from infinity do not focus on the retina and do not form circle of least confusion, while the accommodation is at rest are termed ametropia. This ametropic state of eye is

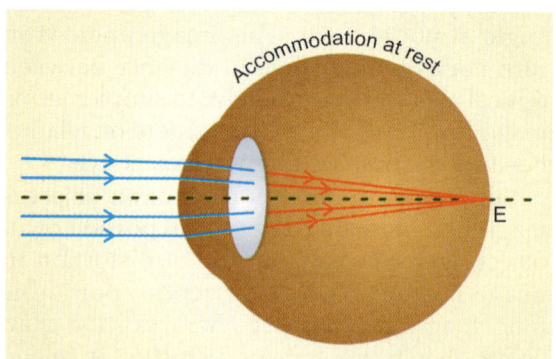

Fig. 4.22: Emmetropic state of eye

commonly called refractive errors of the eye. Usually the refractive errors of both the eyes are of equal degree (isometropia), however, when the refractive errors of both the eyes are unequal in amount, it is called Anisometropia.

Refractive errors of eye are broadly classified as

- Hypermetropia (hyperopia or long sightedness)
- Myopia (short sightedness)
- Astigmatism

Hypermetropia: In emmetropic eye the principal focus of the eye is formed on the retina. However, when the parallel light rays from infinity get focused behind the retina (i.e. principle focus is formed behind the retina), while the accommodation is at rest; this state of eye is termed hypermetropic state of the eye as shown in Fig. 4.23.

Myopia: When all the parallel light rays from infinity get focused in front of the retina (or principal focus of the eye is located in front of the retina), when accommodation is at rest then this form of the eye is termed myopic state of the eye as shown in Fig. 4.24.

Astigmatism: This is the refractive state of eye wherein the parallel light rays from infinity are not focused at a single focus while the accommodation is at rest. This state of eye is termed astigmatic state of the eye (Fig. 4.25). In astigmatism the refraction of rays varies in

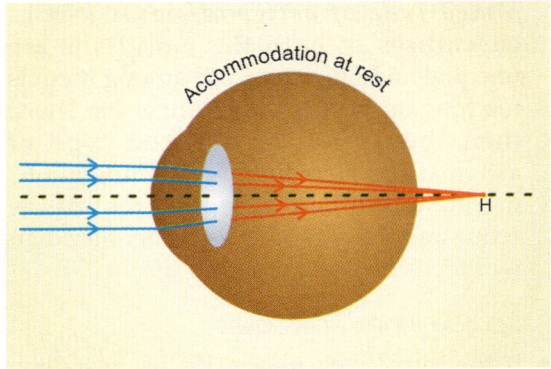

Fig. 4.23: Hypermetropic state of eye

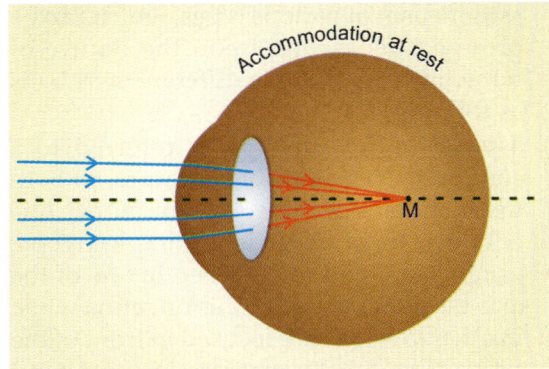

Fig. 4.24: Myopic state of eye

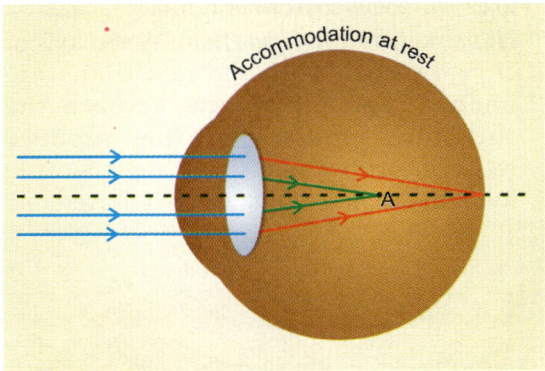

Fig. 4.25: Astigmatic state of eye

different meridians so a few rays will get focus in front of the retina, a few on the retina and a few behind the retina that is why no single focus is formed.

Several pathological conditions may lead to refractive errors like hypermetropia, myopia or astigmatism of eye. Pathology may be seen in dimensions of ocular structures or position of ocular elements.

Refractive Surface Anomalies

- Curvatural refractive errors may occur because of too steep or too flat curvature of either cornea or crystalline lens. These too flat or too steep curvatures of the refracting surfaces can lead to curvatural hypermetropia or myopia, respectively.
- Similarly, irregular or different curvatures of cornea, crystalline lens or retina in different meridians will give rise to

astigmatism of various types, which can be grouped depending upon the nature of refracting curvatures in different meridians as follows:

Myopic astigmatism: It is referred to a condition where axes of curvatures of both the meridians are unequal and either one or both of them are too long. Simple myopic astigmatism will result when in one of the axis the light rays will focus on retina while in other axis rays are focused in front of the retina (Fig. 4.26A), whereas in compound myopic astigmatism light rays in both the axes will focus in front of retina (Fig. 4.26B).

Hypermetropic astigmatism: When axis of curvatures of both the meridians are unequal and either one or both the curvatures are too short they produce hypermetropic astigmatism. Simple hypermetropic astigmatism is referred to a

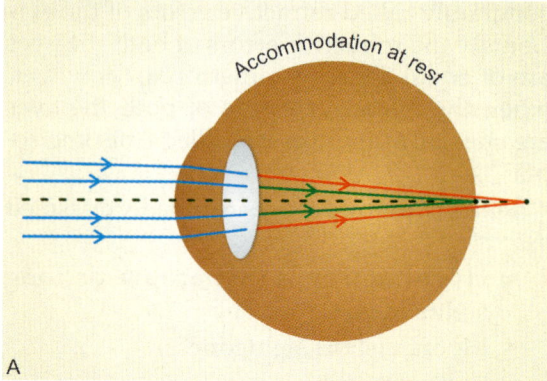

A

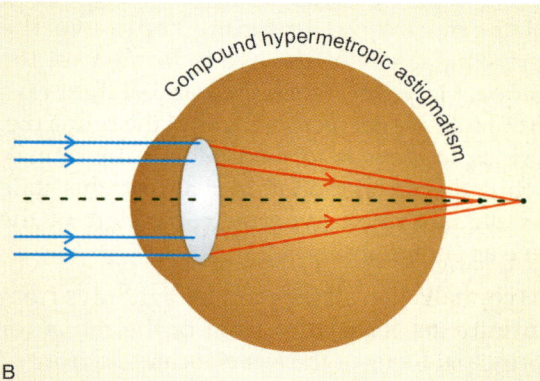

B

Fig. 4.27: Hypermetropic astigmatism. A. Simple hypermetropic astigmatism; B. Compound hypermetropic astigmatism

condition when rays in one meridian will focus on retina and in other meridian rays will focus beyond retina (Fig. 4.27A). In compound hypermetropic astigmatism rays in both the meridians will focus behind the retina as shown in Fig. 4.27B.

Mixed type of astigmatism: If axis of curvatures of both the meridians are unequal and one curvature among them is too long and other curvature is too short, then they produce a mixed type of astigmatism. Here light rays falling in one meridian will be focused in front of the retina and the rays falling in other meridian will focus behind the retina (Fig. 4.28).

Refractive Index Anomalies

- If the refractive indices (RI) of crystalline lens, aqueous humor and vitreous humor

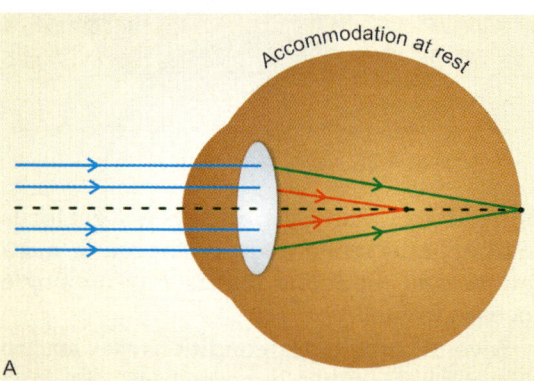

A

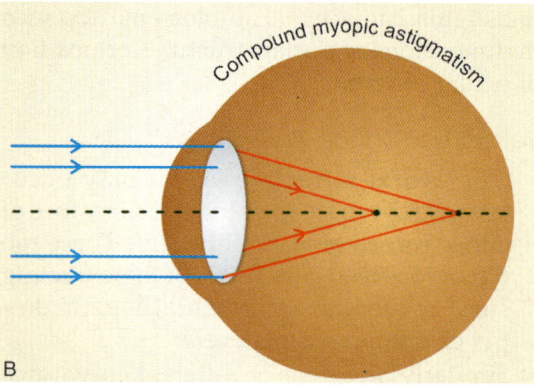

B

Fig. 4.26: Myopic astigmatism. A. Simple myopic astigmatism; B. Compound myopic astigmatism

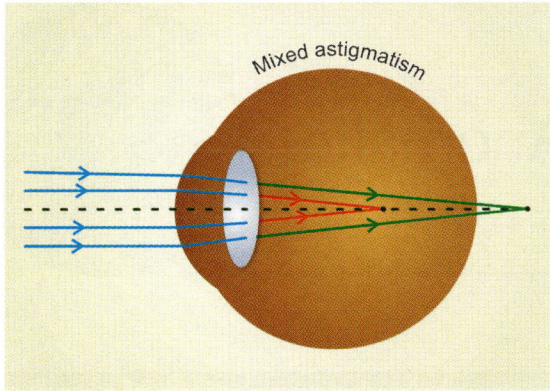

Fig. 4.28: Mixed astigmatism

becomes too low (as in diabetes), then it produces index type hypermetropia.

- When the refractive indices of crystalline lens, aqueous humor and vitreous humor becomes too high (as in nuclear sclerosis of lens), then also it will cause index type myopia.
- Change in the values of refractive index of crystalline lens in different meridians can cause astigmatism.

> **Note:** These index errors are difficult to notice in clinical practice and a small change in refractive index of either aqueous humor or vitreous humor will not produce much change in the refractive status of ocular system.

Dispositions of Optical Elements of Eye

The relative position of optical elements like cornea, crystalline lens and the retina within the eyeball serves an important role in maintenance of refractive status of the eye.

- If anterio-posterior diameter of eye is too long and the retina is situated far away from refracting optical elements like cornea and crystalline lens; then the incident light rays will focus in front of the retina. This type of refractive anomaly is termed as axial myopia.
- If anterio-posterior diameter of the eye is too short and the retina is situated very near to refracting optical elements like cornea and crystalline lens, then the incident light rays will focus behind the retina. This type of refractive anomaly is called as axial hypermetropia.
- In several congenital anomalies crystalline lens gets dislocate and move forwards near to cornea, then this condition will cause myopia; Whereas, if crystalline lens is dislocated backward towards the retina, then it will cause hypermetropia.

Obliquity of Optical Elements of Eye

- **Lenticular obliquity:** A condition where crystalline lens is placed either oblique or subluxated from its original axis. It will cause an astigmatic type of refractive error.
- **Retinal obliquity:** If posterior pole of the eye is obliquely placed then it may cause refractive errors. For example, in staphyloma the posterior pole of eye bulges backward and will cause high degree of myopia. If its summit is not in alignment with the fovea, then rays will fall obliquely in this region of posterior pole and will cause high astigmatic error.

Absence of Optical Element of Eye

A condition where crystalline lens is absent is termed aphakia. Common causes of aphakic are congenital disorders or post-surgical removal of crystalline lens. Aphakia causes a refractive error in terms of high degree hypermetropia.

Refractive Anomalies

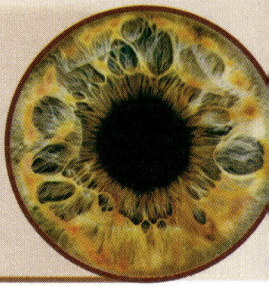

Chapter Outline

HYPERMETROPIA

Introduction

Hypermetropia is a refractive state of the eye where the incident parallel rays of light from infinity get focus behind the retina while the accommodation is at rest (Fig. 5.1). Commonly, it is also known as long sightedness or hyperopia. In hypermetropia the principal focal point (F) is behind the retina so the image formed on the retina will be a blurred image.

Classification of Hypermetropia

Depending upon various factors hypermetropia can be classified in to different types as shown in Table 5.1.

Based on Etiology

a. **Axial hypermetropia:** It is commonest etiological type of hypermetropia. Shortening of the axial length (anterio-posterior

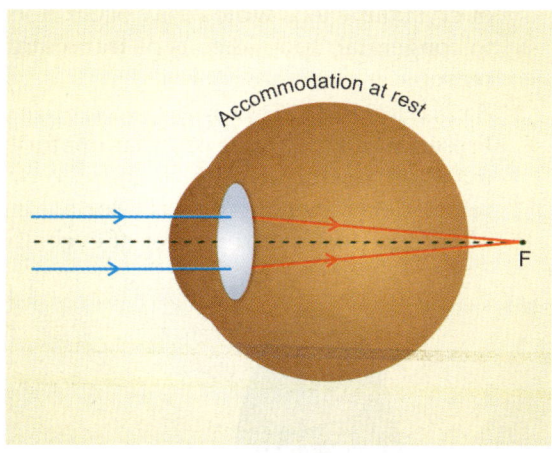

Fig. 5.1: Hypermetropia

Note: Normal axial length of eye is approximately 24 mm.

diameter of the eye) of the eyeball is most common cause of hypermetropia. Although there is decrease in total length of the eyeball but the total refractive power of eye remains normal, hence the principal focus is formed behind the retina. About 1 mm shortening of the axial length causes hypermetropia of nearly 3 D.

b. **Curvatural hypermetropia:** This type of hypermetropia develops when either the curvature of cornea or crystalline lens or both becomes more flat (i.e. corneal plana or lens plana) as compared to the normal emmetropic eye. It may be congenital or acquired. As a result, the refractive power of the eye gets reduced. Generally, a 1 mm flattening of the curvature (or 1 mm increase in radius of curvature) produces hypermetropia of about 6 D.

Note: Normal radius of curvature of the cornea is 7.8 mm anteriorly and 6.8 mm posteriorly. Normal radius of curvature of lens is 10 mm anteriorly and 6 mm posteriorly.

c. **Index hypermetropia:** Reduction in refractive index of aqueous humor, crystalline lens material or vitreous humor may cause index type hypermetropia. For example, hypermetropia in old age (physiological) or in diabetic patients (pathological) is mainly due to decrease in the refractive power of crystalline lens.

Table 5.1: Classification of hypermetropia		
Based on etiology	*Based on clinical presentation*	*Based on the degree of hypermetropia*
a. Axial hypermetropia	a. Simple hypermetropia	a. Mild hypermetropia: Having low degree error (+0.25 to +2 D)
b. Curvatural hypermetropia	b. Pathological hypermetropia	b. Moderate hypermetropia: Having medium degree error (+2.25 to +5 D)
c. Index hypermetropia	c. Functional hypermetropia	
d. Displacement hypermetropia		c. Severe hypermetropia: Having high degree error (> +5 D).
e. Aphakic hypermetropia		

d. **Displacement (positional) hypermetropia:** Displacement or positional hypermetropia occurs due to backward displacement of crystalline lens in vitreous cavity towards the retina. For example, in buphthalmos.

e. **Aphakic hypermetropia:** Congenital disorders, surgical removal or traumatic posterior dislocation of crystalline lens cause a condition known as aphakia (i.e. absence of crystalline lens). Aphakia leads to high degree of hypermetropia.

Note: About 1 mm of change in the axial length usually cause 3 D change in the refractive error and 1 mm change of the curvature usually cause change of 6 D in refractive error.

Based on Clinical Presentation

a. **Simple hypermetropia:** This is the most common clinical type of hypermetropia. Normal biological variations of ocular structures occurring at the time of development, e.g. axial and curvatural hypermetropia may occur due to underdevelopment of eye. Hence, the axial and curvatural types of hypermetropia are included in simple type of hypermetropia.

b. **Pathological hypermetropia:** Abnormal variations other than normal biologic variations of the refractive components of the eye during development may result in either congenital or acquired problems of ocular structures. These pathological variations will lead to the pathological hypermetropia.

   • *Senile or acquired hypermetropia:* Occur in advancing age due to change in the curvature or in index of an ageing crystalline lens.

      1. *Curvatural pathological hypermetropia:* Outer lens fibers develop at later age, hence they have less curvature as compared to inner younger lens fibers. This difference in curvatures leads to hypermetropia in old age.

      2. *Index pathological hypermetropia:* In younger age group, the refractive index of the cortex of crystalline lens is usually much less than the refractive index of the lens nucleus. It is because of this difference in refractive index, a meniscus type lens is formed inside the lens and the total refractive power of crystalline lens remains more (Fig. 5.2). While with advancing age the cortex of lens undergoes sclerosis and its refractive index increases. Therefore, the lens turned into more homogenous in terms of index and meniscus lens now act as a single lens. Hence, the total converging power of crystalline lens is decreased as a whole due to sclerosis of lens cortex. This decrease in converging power of an ageing crystalline lens leads to an index type hypermetropia.

   • *Positional pathological hypermetropia:* May occur due to posterior displacement of crystalline lens which may occur due to congenital, spontaneous or traumatic reasons.

   • *Axial pathological hypermetropia:* Presence of any tumor or inflammatory mass on posterior pole of the eye or retinal detachment may cause shortening of anterio-posterior diameter of eyeball.

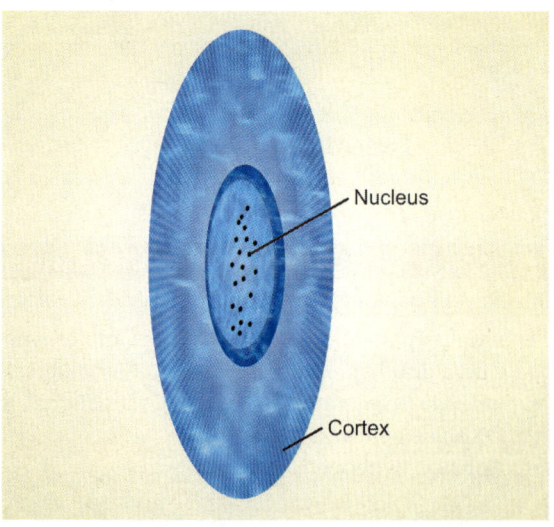

Fig. 5.2: Layers of crystalline lens

- *Aphakia:* means crystalline lens is absent, may be due to congenital or acquired causes. This will give a high degree of hypermetropia.
- *Consecutive pathological hypermetropia:* This type of hypermetropia occurs as a consequence of either surgical aphakia or overcorrected myopia or under-corrected pseudophakia.

c. **Functional hypermetropia:** Functional hypermetropia occurs due to paralysis of accommodation. For example, as seen in patients of oculomotor nerve (III rd nerve) paralysis or internal ophthalmoplegia.

Based on the Degree of Hypermetropia

a. **Mild degree hypermetropia:** When the degree of hypermetropia or amount of refractive error is in the range of +2.00 D or less. In mild hypermetropia the asthenopic symptoms are generally more pronounced than visual symptoms because accommodation in younger age tries to compensate for visual difficulties.

b. **Moderate degree hypermetropia:** When the degree of hypermetropia or amount of refractive error is in the range of +2.25 to +5.00D. Patients having moderate hyperopia usually present with difficulty in vision (mainly in near vision).

c. **Severe or high degree hypermetropia:** When the degree of hypermetropia or amount of refractive error is more than +5 D. Patients having severe hyperopia present with difficulty in vision (both distance and near vision) along with significant asthenopic symptoms.

Normal Age Variations in Hypermetropia

Normally, the status of human eyes at birth is of hypermetropia (approximately 2–3 D), which may increase a little degree in first year of infant life. In majority of individuals this refractive status gradually decreases and by the age of 5–7 years eye status starts to shift towards emmetropia.

Note: However, if there is marked nuclear sclerosis of lens as seen in early cataract there will be a refractive error of myopia type instead of hypermetropia, because there is an increase in the optical density of nucleus also along with cortex of lens.

This emmetrope refractive status of the eye remains stationary after puberty till the old age (approximately 50 years) and will again shift towards hypermetrope in old age due to sclerosis of lens fibers. An eye which was emmetropic at an age of 30 years may have 0.25 D hypermetropia at an age of 55 years and 0.75 D at an age of 60 years. Similarly, at an age of 70 years person may have hypermetropia of 1 D and at 80 years may have even 2.5 D hypermetropia. This is called acquired hypermetropia which is mainly due to continuous growth of the outer layers of cortex of crystalline lens and also due to the change in the refractive index of lens material. In old age the hypermetropia is mainly of index type and occasionally of curvatural type.

Relationship in Accommodation and Hypermetropia

Hypermetropia either caused by decrease in the length of eyeball or decrease in the curvatures of refracting surfaces or change in the refractive index of eye, with all reasons the outcome remains same, i.e. the parallel rays from infinity will focus behind the retina. The diffusion circles formed at retina will produce blur and indistinct images.

Since the eyeball in hypermetropia is short in anterio-posterior diameter, the retina lies nearer to the nodal point of eye as compared to the emmetropic eye. Due to this reason the image formed in hypermetropic eyes will be smaller in size as compared to that formed in emmetropic eyes.

In emmetropic eyes the rays coming from a point on retina (R) will leave the eye in parallel way, whereas the rays from hypermetropic eyes will leave as divergent rays. Hence, in the case of emmetropia the rays

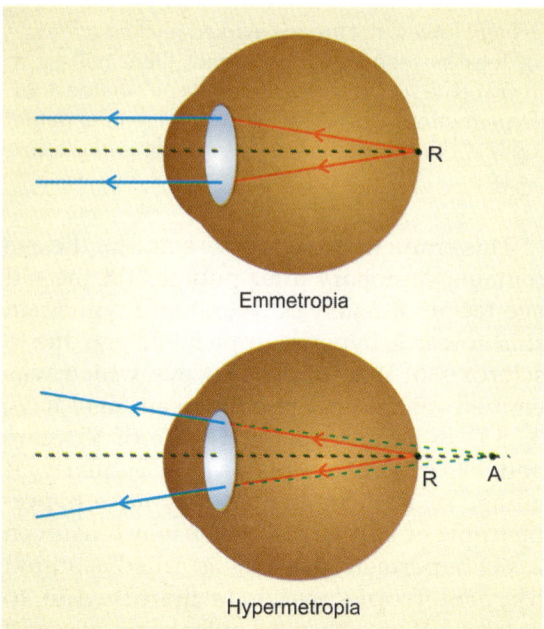

Fig. 5.3: Emmetropic and hypermetropic eye

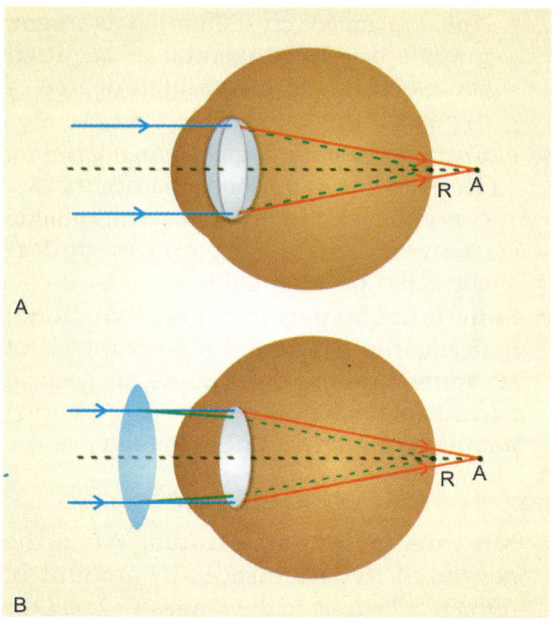

Fig. 5.4: Correction of hypermetropia. A. Accommodation of eye; B. Convex lens

will meet at infinity while in hypermetropia they meet behind the retina at a point (A) as shown in Fig. 5.3.

So, theoretically any object present at infinity or practically at any distance of more than 6 meters will form a sharp and clear image on the retina in case of emmetropic eyes, whereas in hypermetropic eye a clear image will not form on the retina at any distance of object, keeping accommodation at rest. So, in case of hypermetropia the refractive (converging) power of optical system should be increased to receive a clear image of object. Converging power of the optical system can be increased either by efforts of eye (accommodation) or by artificially supporting the eye (using convex lens).

As shown in Fig. 5.4A during accommodation of eye there is change in the curvature of crystalline lens. This change will increase the converging power of the eye and make rays to focus on the retina. On the other hand, a convex lens can be used in spectacles so that convergence is increased and rays get focus on the retina (Fig. 5.4B).

Accommodation is an act where eye tries to adjust its focal length through the contraction of ciliary muscle, which is attached to the lens capsule. This contraction of ciliary muscle will increase the refractive power of lens by changing its curvature (making more convex) and hence certain amount of hypermetropia gets corrected due to accommodation and person remains asymptomatic. It is known that normally physiological tone of ciliary muscle can cause correction of an appreciable amount of hypermetropia, hence to know the total degree of hypermetropic refractive error, it becomes essential to relax the tone of ciliary muscle by using cycloplegic drugs, e.g. atropine.

Thus, accommodation has a significant influence on hypermetropia and on the basis of the action of accommodation hypermetropia can be represented into various components like:

- Latent hypermetropia
- Manifest hypermetropia
  - Facultative hypermetropia
  - Absolute hypermetropia
- Total hypermetropia

Latent Hypermetropia

This is the amount of hypermetropia which normally gets corrected by the physiological tone of ciliary muscle. Usually, it is in the range of about 1 D, but in the children the range of latent hypermetropia is more than adults and it progressively decreases with advancement of age. Latent hypermetropia can be revealed clinically only by testing refraction after abolishing the tone of ciliary muscle (by use of atropine). It means that if analysis of refraction is done in the absence of cycloplegics, then latent hypermetropia can be overcome by accommodation of patient and remains nondetectable.

Manifest Hypermetropia

This is the remaining amount of refractive error from the total refractive error which is not corrected by the normal tone of ciliary muscle. It has two components:

a. **Facultative hypermetropia:** This portion of manifest hypermetropia can be corrected by the efforts of accommodation exerted by patient.

b. **Absolute hypermetropia:** This is the remaining portion of manifest hypermetropia which cannot be corrected by efforts of accommodation exerted by the patient.

Total Hypermetropia

It is the total amount of refractive error of eye, which is measured after using cycloplegics like atropine which abolishes the tone of ciliary muscles. The sum of latent hypermetropia and manifest hypermetropia indicates total magnitude of hypermetropia.

Total hypermetropia = Latent hypermetropia + Manifest hypermetropia (Facultative hypermetropia + Absolute hypermetropia)

Clinical Tests to Find out Accommodation Based Hypermetropia

Absolute Hypermetropia

Assume a hypermetrope person who is unable to see the distant objects clearly (vision is not 6/6) and to correct this we have to place a convex (or plus) lens in front of his eyes. Now, we will increase the power of this convex lens gradually till the person just sees the distant object clearly with weakest convex lens. At this point of correction, the power of convex lens and accommodation of that person are working together and he/she is able to see the object clearly. So, the convex lens used externally is compensating for only that portion of hypermetropia which is not corrected by efforts of person's accommodation, hence it is equal to absolute hypermetropia. This absolute hypermetropia is represented by the weakest convex lens which is giving the maximum visual acuity.

Manifest Hypermetropia

Now keep on increasing the power of convex lens till that person sees the distant object clearly with the strongest convex lens or we can say note down that power of convex lens at which blurring of distant object starts. This power of stronger convex lens is also compensating for the accommodation of that hypermetrope. Thus, the strongest convex lens is the measure of manifest hypermetropia by which the visual acuity of a person is recorded as maximum.

Facultative Hypermetropia

The above described process of testing had also measured that amount of hypermetropia which is corrected by accommodation efforts of a person. The difference in the power of strongest and weakest convex lens indicates the amount of facultative hypermetropia.

Total and Latent Hypermetropia

Now instill a drop of atropine in the eyes of hypermetrope and correct the refractive error of patient by using stronger convex lens than before by which maximum visual acuity can be obtained. The power of this strongest convex lens represents the total hypermetropia, which will be usually a little more than the power of that convex lens which represented the manifest hypermetropia.

Note: An apparent increase in hypermetropia is also seen in advancing age after 40 years due to failure of accommodation. With decrease in the tone of ciliary muscle, the greater part of latent hypermetropia will become manifest hypermetropia. This decreases the range of accommodation and with decreased possibility of correction more of facultative hypermetropia will become absolute hypermetropia. In younger age accommodative power can correct most of hypermetropia and hypermetropia is absolute only when hypermetropia is of very large degree. But after an age of 65 years practically all manifest hypermetropia will become absolute hypermetropia because with age there will be gradual weakening of ciliary muscles (decrease inherent tone of muscle) followed by total failure of accommodative efforts. As a result both facultative and latent hypermetropia becomes nonfunctional.

Difference between the powers of two strongest convex lenses (representing total hypermetropia and manifest hypermetropia, respectively) will give the amount of latent hypermetropia.

As we can see that whether a person has high degree or low degree of total hypermetropia, he will not be able to see the distant objects clearly without using accommodation. However, if a person has low degree of hypermetropia within limits of facultative hypermetropia, this person can see the distant objects clearly by using his/her accommodation power. In one way it is advantageous that accommodation is compensating the hypermetropia but constant use of accommodation for a long period will lead to stress and various convergence anomalies.

Clinical Features of Hypermetropia

Symptoms

As discussed above active accommodation tries to compensate the adverse effects of hypermetropia on vision. This impact of accommodation on vision may vary according to age, degree of refractive error and demand placed on the visual system.

Asymptomatic hypermetropia: In younger patients a small degree of hypermetropia (i.e. latent hypermetropia) remains corrected by the action of accommodation of patients and hence they usually remain asymptomatic. However, symptoms may appear later on as there is increase in the visual stress and accommodation fails to overcome the increased visual stress.

Symptomatic hypermetropia

Symptoms due to eye strain (asthenopia): Sometimes hypermetropia gets fully corrected by the efforts of accommodation hence no visual symptoms are produced. But in long term due to continuous overuse of accommodation (over action of ciliary muscles) to see distant objects clearly, the patient may develop symptoms of accommodative asthenopia (eye strain). The common symptoms of asthenopia are watering of eyes, heaviness or dull pain of eyes, general fatigue, frontal or frontotemporal headache, mild photophobia or light sensitivity.

Usually, patients complaint of worsening of asthenopic symptoms as the day progresses and more pronounced with prolonged use of near vision. These symptoms get relieved by giving rest to eyes.

Diminution of vision with asthenopia: When hypermetropia becomes of moderate to severe degree, then it is not fully corrected by effort of accommodation. So, the patient will complain of visual symptoms along with asthenopia. There is more diminution of vision for near than distance because of continuous use of accommodation.

Diminution of vision: In high degree of hypermetropia (usually > 4 D), accommodative efforts fail to compensate for high degree of hypermetropia. Patient develops diminution of vision for near as well as for distance. Diminished vision for distance and near is more commonly seen in older individuals who have high degree of hyperopia with more visual demanding needs, but have decrease amplitude of accommodation.

Intermittent sudden blurring of vision:
Sometimes there may be spasm of accommodation in hypermetropes which can shift vision towards myopia (a state of pseudo myopia) leading to sudden intermittent blurring of vision. Accommodative spasm can be detected by performing cycloplegic refraction which discloses underlying hypermetropia.

Accommodative convergent squint or "Crossed-eyes" sensation without diplopia:
Excessive accommodation in some patients can give a feeling that their eyes are getting crossed (esotropia or inward deviation of the eyes or convergent squint) without producing any diplopia. The eyes cross due to extra-ocular muscle imbalance which happens in an attempt to focus near objects requiring the excessive convergence.

Clinical Signs

- Effect of hypermetropia on visual acuity depends on degree of hypermetropia, accommodation power and age of the patients. Low degree of hypermetropia is usually gets corrected by accommodation and patient has normal visual acuity. Approximate estimation of visual acuity can be obtained on the basis of degree of absolute hypermetropia as shown in Table 5.2. As the absolute hypermetropia increases, the visual acuity decreases proportionally.
- On ocular examination hypermetropic eyeball is usually small in size. It is not only that anterio-posterior diameter is smaller

than normal, but also eyeball as a whole is small in all directions. Rare developmental conditions such as coloboma, microphthalmos, etc. may be associated with small eyeball and hence predispose hypermetropia.

- Size or diameter of the cornea is also small as compared to the normal emmetropic eyes. However, the crystalline lens varies very little in size even in hypermetropia so in comparison to size of cornea it is relatively larger. Thus, the anterior chamber of eye appears shallower in hypermetropic as compared to an emmetropic eye.
- Anterior chamber of eye seems relatively shallow in hypermetropia and angle of anterior chamber is also narrow as compared to the normal eye. Due to narrow anterior chamber chances of development of primary angle closure glaucoma are relatively high.
- On fundoscopy, fundus shows a characteristic appearance of optic disc and retinal reflex. Optic disc appears of dark grayish red color with blur and irregular margins, which can be sometimes confused with optic neuritis (papillitis). Since there is no true swelling of optic disc in hypermetropia, hence hypermetropic condition is also referred as *pseudopapillitis*. Haziness of the disc is sometimes accentuated by a grayish areola or by grey striations emerging from it. Occasionally on examination, an inferior crescent may be seen around optic disc. Disc vessels may be tortuous and more branching in appearance. Retina shows a peculiar bright reflex effect resembling a water silk or shot silk appearance. Retinal blood vessels appear accentuated because of shiny retinal reflexes. These all changes are accentuated largely due to disturbances in the reflexes of fundus. Macular reflex is seen more eccentric to optic disc and is darker than normal.
- In hypermetropic eyes, macula is situated further away from the optic disc as compared to emmetropic eyes and cornea is more decentred than usual. Due to these two factors the visual axis cuts the cornea

Table 5.2: Visual acuity relationship with absolute hypermetropia	
Absolute hyperopia (D)	*Visual acuity*
+ 0.5	6/9
+ 1.0	612 to 6/18
+ 1.5	6/24
+ 2.0	6/36
+ 3.0	5/60
+ 4.5	3/60

Note: Drugs which cause dilatation of pupil (mydriatics) should be administered carefully in hypermetrope because dilation of pupil sometimes can precipitate an attack of angle closure glaucoma in hypermetrope.

markedly inside towards the optical axis of the eye. This gives a large positive angle alpha and subsequently an apparent divergent squint.

Sequel of Hypermetropia

Uncorrected hypermetropia for prolonged duration can lead to various complications

- Recurrent problems related to eyelids like blepharitis, stye or chalazion are common with uncorrected hypermetropia. Probable reason for occurrence of these problems is recurrent infections that occur as a result of repetitive stroking of eyelids, which is done by patient to get clear vision and to get relief from fatigue and exhaustion.
- In some children amblyopia may develop. For example: Uncorrected binocular high hypermetropia, unequal high uniocular hypermetropia or an accommodative squint can produce ametropic, anisometropic or strabismic amblyopia, respectively.
- In very young children (about 2–3 years) an excessive use of accommodation can produce an accommodative convergent strabismus.
- Development of primary narrow angle glaucoma can be seen in hypermetropes. As we know that overall eyeball size is small, with a comparative shallow anterior chamber and lens size is relatively large in hypermetropes so these patients are at risk for an acute attack of angle closure glaucoma. A precaution has to be taken while using mydriatics in these patients.

Management of Hypermetropia

Investigations

- **Ultrasonography or A-scan biometry** can be done to know the axial length of eyeball. It may be smaller or normal in length.

- **Gonioscopy** may reveal the mild narrowing of angles in hypermetropic eyes as compared to emmetropic eyes.
- **Ultrasound biomicroscopy (UBM) or anterior segment Optical Coherence Tomography** can detect a shallow anterior chamber in hypermetropic eye.

Treatment

1. **Asymptomatic patients:** There is no need of any treatment in asymptomatic patients having
   - Good general health
   - Younger age group with good accommodation
   - Small degree of hypermetropia
   - Not complaining about accommodative asthenopia.
   - Having no muscle imbalance or squint.
2. **Symptomatic patients:** In symptomatic patients, hypermetropia should be treated by optical and/or surgical correction.

Optical Correction

The optical correction is done by prescribing the convex or plus lenses, which enables the rays to get focus on the retina by increasing the total converging power of optical system (Fig. 5.5). These lenses either can be fit in spectacles or can be given in form of contact lens.

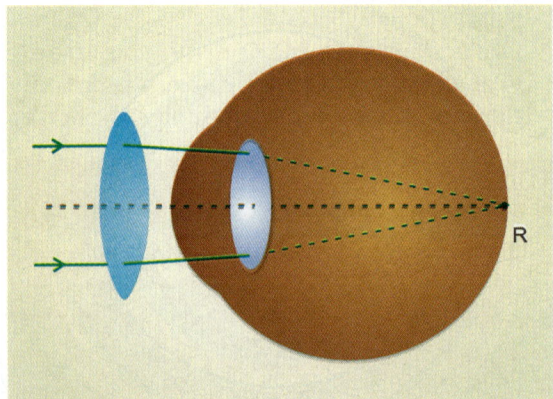

Fig. 5.5: Optical correction of hypermetropia by convex lens

Basic rules to remember while prescribing convex lens for hypermetropic patients are as follows:

- Cycloplegic refraction (using atropine for children <6 years and cyclopentolate or homatropine for older children and adults) should be done in all the cases to know the total amount of hypermetropic error.
- Young children (<6–7 years) have some amount of physiological hypermetropia and need glasses only when the hypermetropia is of high degree or a small degree of squint is present along with it.
- Suppose, if total manifest hypermetropia is of 1 D or lesser degree and the patient is asymptomatic, then there is no need of correction.
- Younger children (<5 years) if require any amount of hypermetropic correction, then the full amount of cycloplegic refraction should be prescribed in this age group because they will accept this full correction. However, at school going age, the amount of refraction may be reduced to a degree of one-third of total refraction, keeping in mind that child should not use accommodation of more than 2.5 D power for his/her distant vision.
- School going children (6–16 years) if having accommodative squint and/or definitive symptoms of ocular fatigue or decreased visual acuity, then even a small amount of hypermetropia needs correction.
- Older children will not accept full amount of cycloplegic refraction, hence initially they are always undercorrected up to that amount of refraction which they accept comfortably. After this at every 6 months interval the amount of spherical correction should be increased gradually till it reaches to the full amount of cycloplegic refraction.
- Hypermetropia in children usually decreases with the growth of child, hence it is mandatory to repeat the refraction in children at an interval of 6 months so that overcorrection is not prescribed and if required, amount of correction can be reduced accordingly.
- Children who are presenting with symptoms of eye strain (headache, early tiring, dislike to work, itching or rubbing of eyes or any combinations of these) and having refractive error of more than 3 D, it is advised them to wear correcting glasses constantly however, if refractive error is less than 3 D, then glasses can be worn only at the time of near work.
- Full cycloplegic correction has to be given in all cases of accommodative convergent squint at all age group.
- An undercorrection of about 1–2 D should be given in those cases where exophoria is associated with hypermetropia.
- Full cycloplegic correction along with occlusion therapy should be done in cases where amblyopia is associated with hypermetropia.
- Young adult (aged 25 years) may be asymptomatic even with 3 D of hypermetropia but will complaint of difficulty in reading at an age of 35 years. This is because accommodation declines with age and an additional power of accommodation is required in performing near work. In these kind of cases if spectacles are not influencing distant vision, then glasses should be worn only for near work. As the age advances, accommodation declines completely and whole refractive error becomes absolute hypermetropia so the person will need glasses even for distant vision, thus should wear glasses constantly.
- For older people glasses are prescribed according to their symptoms and amount of vision. Manifest hypermetropia should be corrected completely and glasses are advised to be worn regularly.
- Optical treatment can be given in the form of spectacles or contact lenses. Spectacles with convex lenses are most

acceptable, safe and simple method for hypermetropic correction. Contact lenses are often prescribed in unilateral hypermetropia (anisometropia) to avoid diplopia or amblyopia.

Surgical Correction

Various refractive procedures have been recommended for the correction of hypermetropia though the outcomes are not as encouraging and reliable as in the case of myopia. Various surgical modalities for the correction of hypermetropia are:

- Hyperopic LASIK
- Photorefractive keratectomy
- Conductive keratoplasty
- Thermal laser keratoplasty
- Refractive lens exchange
- Phakic intraocular lenses

  These refractive procedures are described in detail in Chapter 15.

MYOPIA

Introduction

Myopia is the refractive state of the eye where parallel rays of light from infinity get focus in front of the retina while accommodation is at rest (Fig. 5.6). Commonly, it is also known as short sightedness. In myopic eye, the principal focal point (F) is in front of the retina so the image formed on the retina is blurred.

The prevalence of myopia alters with age and other associated factors. The prevalence of myopia is more in premature infants than normal and it increases in school-age group and young adult and declines somewhat in the population above the age 45 years, being about 20% in age 60–65 years and 14% in 70 years of age. Some studies indicate more chances of myopia in females than in males. The chances are also more in those persons who work in occupations requiring lots of near work. The prevalence is high (35–60%) in those children whose both parents have myopia than who have one parent with myopia (25–40%).

Optics of myopia

- Myopic eyes have very powerful optical system in relation to the axial length of the eyeball. The focusing power of the cornea and the lens is too great with respect to the length of the eyeball so that the parallel rays of the light focus in front of the retina and after focusing these light rays start getting diverge and eventually fall on the retina forming a blur image due to circles of diffusion (Fig. 5.7).
- In myopic eye, nodal point is situated far away from the retina as compared to the emmetropic eye. As a result, the image formed in myopes will be relatively larger as compared to emmetrope (Fig. 5.8A). The

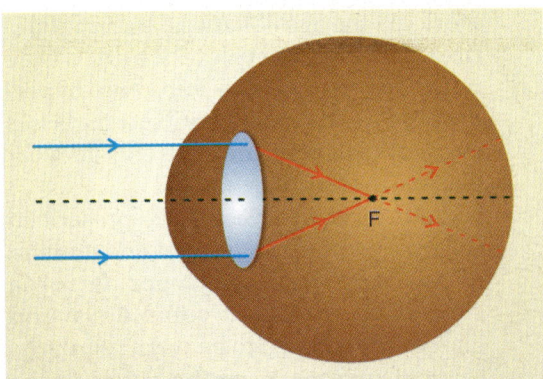

Fig. 5.6: Parallel rays from infinity focusing in front of retina in myopia

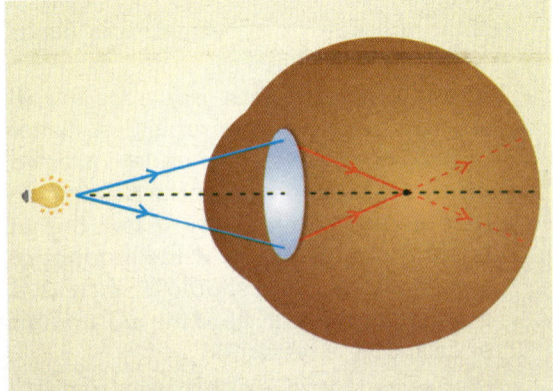

Fig. 5.7: Point light source beyond far point is focusing in front of retina in myopia

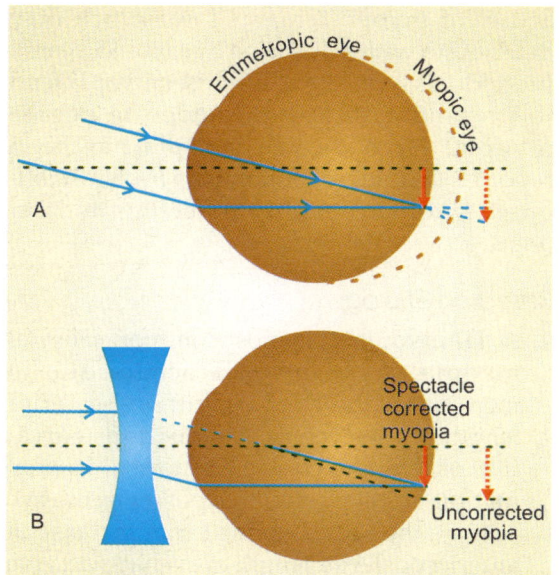

Fig. 5.8: Relative positions of retinal images in myopes. A. Retinal image before correction; B. Retinal image after correction with lens

phenomenon of enlargement of image is also seen in myopic eyes which are corrected by the spectacles (Fig. 5.8B). This enlargement of image provides some amount of compensation for the decreased visual acuity in myopes.

- In myopes the far point of the eye is situated in front of the eye at a finite distance. Any near object at far point of myopic eye will be focused without any effort of accommodation and will be seen easily. Thus, use of accommodation in myopes has

no or a little value because it may accentuate his/her visual problems. Thus, generally in an uncorrected myope accommodation remains underdeveloped. As we know that there is a direct relationship between the effort of accommodation and the effort of convergence. In myopes this relationship between accommodation and convergence is broken. Hence, this disparity may cause convergence insufficiency, exophoria, ultimately exotropia and development of presbyopia at early age.

- In myopes the macula lies slightly nearer to optic disc than normal eye, leading to some change in visual axis. As a result the angle alpha (angle between optical axis and visual axis) is slightly negative which gives sense of an apparent convergent strabismus.

Classification of Myopia

Depending upon the cause, age of onset, degree or clinical presentations, myopia can be classified as summarized in Table 5.3.

Based on Age of Onset

a. **Congenital or infantile myopia:** Congenital myopia may be present where eye is myopic (instead of hypermetropic) since birth, however, this type of myopic refractive error does not progress and myopic error remains static throughout whole life. Congenital myopia is usually associated with systemic disorders or premature birth.

Table 5.3: Classification of myopia			
Based on age of onset	Based on etiology	Based on degree of error	Based on clinical presentation

a. Congenital
b. Youth onset
c. Adult onset myopia
  • Early adult onset
  • Late adult onset
	a. Axial myopia
	b. Curvatural myopia
	c. Index myopia
	d. Positional myopia
	e. Excessive accommo-
	   dative myopia
		a. Low degree error
		  < –3 D
		b. Medium degree:
		  3 D to < –6 D
		c. High degree myopia:
		  > –6 D
			• Congenital myopia
			• Simple myopia
			• Pathological myopia
			• Acquired myopia
			• Nocturnal myopia
			• Space myopia
			• Pseudomyopia
			• Drug induced myopia

b. **Youth onset (childhood or early or school myopia):** This type of myopia develops during the period of childhood to early teenage years (8–14 years). As discussed previously, eye is usually hypermetropic at birth and slowly with the advancement of age the eye becomes emmetropic (mainly due to growth and enlargement of the eyeball). During this change of refractive status from hypermetropia to emmetropia sometimes eye overshoots the emmetropic point and becomes myopic in a few percentage of population. This is termed simple myopia which generally remains asymptomatic till early teenage. However, in subsequent years the myopic refractive error usually progress and may reach up to 5–6 D. This progression of refractive error usually stops at age of about 18–20 years and this type of myopic refractive error gets stabilized nearly at the age of 20–21 years.

c. **Adult onset myopia:** This type of myopia starts usually after 18–20 years of age and can be grouped as
   - *Early adult onset:* Starts between 20–40 years of age.
   - *Late adult onset:* Develops after 40 years of age.

The prevalence of adult-onset myopia may vary significantly depending on the demographics of the sample population being studied. Development of myopia after 18–20 years is very uncommon, however, if it occurs, it indicates either the refractive error was neglected for long duration in the previous years or we have to look carefully for some other causes of myopia.

Early adult onset myopia is less likely to be stationary, rather it progresses very fast and sometimes amount of refractive error may reach up to 25–30 D. It is usually associated with degenerative changes in posterior segment of the eye. However, there will be some amount of progression in myopia till old age. Due to this high degree of myopia, degenerative changes in ocular structures will be seen and in later decades of life visual acuity of myope remains low, which may deteriorate with advancing age (60–65 years). Individuals with late adult-onset myopia tend to present with low to moderate degree myopia. High degree myopia has been reported to be less common than in childhood-onset myopia, possibly reflecting its later onset.

Based on Etiology

a. **Axial myopia:** It is most common cause of myopia. Axial myopia occurs due to increase in the axial or anterio-posterior length of the eyeball. Although the curvature of lens and cornea are normal in axial myopia so total refractive power of the eye may be the same. About 1 mm increase in anterio-posterior length of eyeball will give rise to myopia of nearly 3 D.

b. **Curvatural myopia:** Curvatural myopia occurs when eye has normal axial length but either the curvature of the cornea or crystalline lens or both becomes steeper, as a result the refractive power of eye is increased. Increase in the curvature of cornea is seen in conditions like ectasias or in conical cornea (i.e. keratoconus or keratoglobus). Although, spherical refractive errors due to increase in the corneal curvature are less common than astigmatic errors. Increase in curvature of crystalline lens is seen in rare conditions like anterior or posterior lenticonus. About 1 mm decrease in the radius of curvature of the eye is associated with myopia of nearly 6 D.

c. **Index myopia:** Change in the refractive index of the lens will cause index myopia. For example, an increase in the refractive index of crystalline lens due to nuclear sclerosis in advancing age causes myopia. In contrary, decrease in the refractive index of lens cortex (as seen in diabetes) may also lead to index myopia.

d. **Positional or displacement myopia:** This type of myopia occurs due to forward displacement of crystalline lens towards the anterior chamber in eye. Probable mechanism is weakening of zonules which lead to displacement of crystalline lens, as occur in Ehlers-Danlos syndrome or Homocystinuria. Displacement of lens is also seen after glaucoma surgery.

e. **Excessive accommodative myopia:** Excessive accommodation (spasm of ciliary muscle) will relax the suspensory ligaments of crystalline lens capsule and will change the curvature of lens surface. Patients having spasm of accommodation develop myopia due to this mechanism and presents with an artificial myopic state of eye (pseudomyopia).

Based on Degree of Error

a. Low degree myopia: Have myopia of –3.00 D or less.
b. Medium degree myopia: Having myopia between –3.00 and –6.00 D.
c. High degree myopia: Usually myopia of –6.00 D or more. Persons with high myopia usually may have retinal detachments and primary open angle glaucoma.

Based on Clinical Presentation

Congenital myopia

• Congenital myopia is present since birth and usually manifest at an age of 2–3 years.
• It is more common in those children who had history of premature births or having various systemic disorders like Marfan's syndrome, Bardet-Biedl syndrome, Homocystinuria, Alport syndrome, etc.
• Congenital myopia may be associated with other ocular diseases also like congenital cataract, microphthalmos, megalocornea, aniridia, posterior staphyloma and congenital separation of retina.

Clinical features
• Congenital myopia most commonly presents as unilateral high degree of myopia (anisometropia) rarely, it may present as bilateral myopia.
• Degree of myopia is usually very high (8–10 D) and it generally remains stationary without any improvement.

• In cases of bilateral myopia, the child will have great difficulty in seeing the distant objects so child tries to hold the object very near to the eyes. This typical symptom usually gives a clue to the parents about problem in the vision of child and myopia gets diagnosed.
• In case of unilateral myopia as child is having some useful vision in one eye, myopia is detected only during routine school eye examinations or when child has developed strabismus because of anisometropic amblyopia.
• Timely diagnosis and early treatment of congenital myopia is very important to restore good distant vision in child. Cycloplegic refraction should be performed and full correction of myopia with associated astigmatism (if present) is done by prescribing spectacles. It is advised to use glasses constantly to prevent any visual deficit; however, it is very difficult to achieve a visual acuity of 6/6 in majority of cases of congenital myopia.

Simple myopia

It is also termed developmental myopia, physiological myopia or school myopia. This type of myopia is not associated with any systemic disease, hence termed developmental or physiological myopia. It is much more common than the other types of myopia and myopic error seldom goes beyond 6 D. Simple myopia usually develops during the developmental growth of the child. Normally it starts at an age of 5–6 years and progresses slowly up to an age of 16–18 years. Usually simple myopia starts with a small degree of refractive error 1–2 D and with the growth of child may reach up to a degree of 4–5 D (rarely> 6 D). In majority of cases, it becomes stationary up to the age of 18–20 years. Degree of myopia may vary from low to moderate. About 30% population have low degree of myopia (< 2 D), whereas, nearly 6% population have moderate degree (2–5 D) of myopia error.

Causes of simple myopia: Normal biological variations taking place during the development of eyeball will cause simple myopia. These variations may or may not be genetically determined and may have an autosomal dominant type or autosomal recessive type of inheritance. Simple myopia may occur due to various factors:

- Due to physiological variation in the anterio-posterior diameter of eyeball during development: As a result axial length of eyeball is increased leading to axial type of simple myopia. It means eye is an otherwise normal eye but is too long for its optical power.
- Due to underdevelopment of eyeball during childhood so that eye is too optically powerful for its axial length. It causes curvatural type of simple myopia.
- Near work hypothesis or "use abuse theory": It states that risk of simple myopia is increased by doing excessive near work, watching television too long or not using corrective glasses. However, this hypothesis is supported by only some studies.
- Some advocated that supplementation of diet with vitamins and minerals have a role in reducing myopia or slowdown the progress of myopia. But this thought has not been concluded by any confirmative study.
- Genetics also play an important role. It has been found that prevalence of myopia is increased in those children whom both parents are myopic as compared to children having one parent myopic, being 20% and 10%, respectively.

Clinical features
Symptoms
- *Near or short-sightedness:* The most common symptom associated with uncorrected myopia at any age group is diminished vision for distant objects and it is usually constant. An approximate estimate of amount of distance vision and degree of refractive error is shown in **Table 5.4**.

Table 5.4: Relationship of myopic error with distance vision

Myopic error (D)	Visual acuity
−0.5	6/9
−1.0	6/18
−2.0	6/36
−3.0	6/60
−4.0	5/60
−5.0	3/60
−6.0	2/60

- *Ocular asthenopic symptoms:* These are not characteristic of myopia, however, myopes with small degree of refractive error may compliant of these symptoms. These symptoms develop due to break in the relationship of convergence and accommodation. Asthenopic symptoms produced by either of accommodation or convergence problem are as follows:
  a. Myopic patients use less accommodation to see the near objects clearly, hence they also use less convergence, leading to convergence insufficiency and eventually exophoria. There may be suppression of vision in one eye due to exophoria.
  b. Sometimes, to see near objects myopes may converge and to keep pace with the convergence there is overuse of accommodation (ciliary spasm), leading to spasm of accommodation which may further results in artificial increase in the degree of myopia.
- Parents of uncorrected myopic children sometimes report of developing psychosocial symptoms in the child. These children may be reported as very academic with shy nature and not interested in outdoor activities. Most of these children think that maximum distance vision is what they see, so they mainly concentrate on activities where distant vision is not much needed.

Note: Usual presentation in myopes is the poor convergence due to insufficient use of accommodation; rather than the excessive accommodation.

Signs:
- Poor visual acuity for distance.
- Slit lamp examination of anterior segment will show
  - Eyes look large and prominent because of large diameter (increase axial length) of eyeball.
  - Cornea may be larger and steeper than normal.
  - Anterior chamber of eye appears deep as compared to emmetrope.
  - The size of crystalline lens is normal as compared to larger eyeball, hence space in anterior chamber increases and it appears deep.
- Pupil is large in size as compared to emmetropes and pupillary reaction is slightly sluggish. There is increase in ciliary tone which probably keeps the pupil size larger than normal.
- Fundus examination is grossly normal though mild tessellations of retina and/or a temporal crescent at optic disc may be seen.
- Intraocular pressure is normal; sometimes because of thin cornea and/or eyeball coats false raised IOP may be seen.

Pathological myopia

Pathological myopia is also known as progressive or degenerative or high myopia. Pathological myopia is a rapidly progressing type of refractive error, usually responsible for high degree of myopia along with degenerative changes in eyeball especially, in retina and choroid. This type of myopia generally starts in adolescent age (10–12 years) and then rapidly progress till adulthood, may reach up to 25–30 D.

Clinicopathology: In pathological myopia during the process of development the eye gets elongate. This elongation of eye is mainly confined to its posterior half of eyeball while the anterior half relatively remains normal in the size as shown in Fig. 5.9.

However, due to this elongation the entire eyeball becomes larger in pathological myopic eyes as compare to the emmetropic eyes.

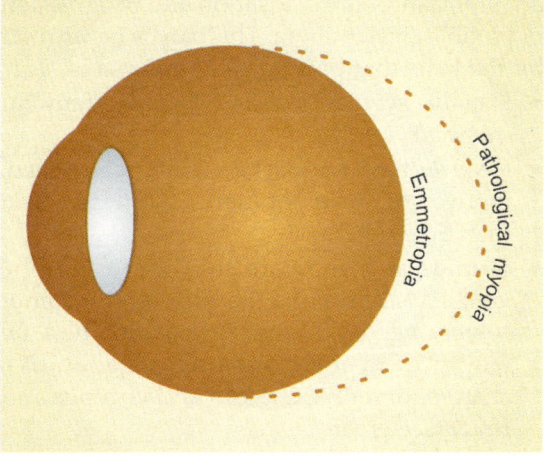

Fig. 5.9: Pathological myopia showing elongation of posterior half of eyeball

When the posterior pole of eyeball moves inward, then the equatorial part of eyeball comes out of palpebral fissure line and the flatness of curvature of eyeball becomes prominent.

Anterior chamber of the eye is relatively deep and the pupillary reaction is sluggish as compare to emmetropes. As we know that myopic patients do not need to use accommodation to see the near objects clearly, the ciliary muscle undergoes disuse atrophy (especially circular fibers). This will keep the pupil a little larger in size with poor light reaction.

Posterior half of sclera also becomes thin due to mechanical stretching of the eyeball and sometimes in severe cases sclera may be as thin as ¼th of normal scleral thickness.

Fundus examination reveals generalized atrophic changes in retina as well as in choroid.

Etiology: Several hypotheses have been postulated to explain the cause of pathological myopia but till now, no single hypothesis could explain the exact cause of these degenerative changes in choroid or retina. However, the common factors explained in many theories show that the pathological myopia has a definite connection with either genetic factors or environmental factors.

Genetic factors: Several recent studies had concluded that genetic basis or inheritance play

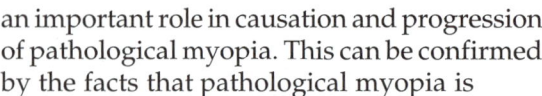

an important role in causation and progression of pathological myopia. This can be confirmed by the facts that pathological myopia is

- Usually seen as familial disease (familial myopia)
- Geographical and racial variation also seen, more common in population with East Asia than South Asia.
- Studies also indicate that there may be genetic variation in the different chromosomes or genes that are linked with the axial length of eyeball, various degenerative changes of retina, choroid and vitreous and refractive error.

Environmental factors: During growth period there is expansion of eyeball to the proper length. Posterior pole of eyeball elongates specifically during the period of active growth process and various factors like endocrine disorders, diet and presence of disease by affecting the growth may cause change in axial length of eyeball, leading to myopia.

Clinical features

Symptoms:

- Decreased vision: A profound diminution of visual acuity is found in these patients. In many cases, because of very high refractive error as well as due to associated retinal degenerative changes, the visual acuity is not correctable to normal by using myopic corrective methods.
- Symptoms due to vitreous degeneration: Patients with high myopia may complaints of seeing black spots or vitreous floaters or Muscae volitantes in the field of vision, specifically during bright light. The degenerated vitreous gel gets liquefy and the shadows of these liquefied portions of gelatinous vitreous body are appreciated by patients as floaters in front of the eye. These floaters move with the movement of eyeball.
- Diminished night vision (Night blindness): Myopes with high degree of refractive error often complain of blurred distance vision in dim illumination or night. More common in pathological myopes having chorioretinal

and pigment epithelium degenerations and amount of nocturnal myopia is in correlation with severity of chorioretinal degeneration.

Signs:

- **Visual acuity:** Visual acuity for distance is severely affected and error is of high degree than simple myopia. Refractive error increases gradually every year with an average of 3–4 D and goes very high up to 25–30 D till the age of 20–25 years. Sometimes the errors may increase progressively for life time.
- **Anterior segment:**
  – The eyes appear large and prominent and may be confused with exophthalmos or proptosis.
  – Cornea usually appears larger than normal.
  – Anterior chamber appears deep as compared to emmetrope eyes.
  – Pupils are larger in size and poorly reactive to light.

  Fundus examination (Fig. 5.10) will show tilted optic disc with marked degenerative changes in retina and choroid layers and vitreous of eyeball. It is important to note that degenerative changes observed on examination are not necessarily related to degree of myopia.

  – **Tilted optic disc:** The optic disc appears large, pale with prominent cups. Tilted disc appearance is due to oblique insertion of the optic nerves into the elongated globe. The tilt is usually located inferionasal or inferiotemporal.
  – **Myopic or temporal crescent:** On temporal side of disc a white sharp defined area can be seen, which is formed as a result of stretching of eyeball. Backward bulging of posterior pole causes separation of retina as well as choroid for some distance from the temporal margin of optic disc so that sclera present behind these layers can be seen directly as a crescent.
  – **Peri-papillary atrophy:** Hypopigmented finding seen on fundus examination when RPE attenuation surrounds the optic disc.

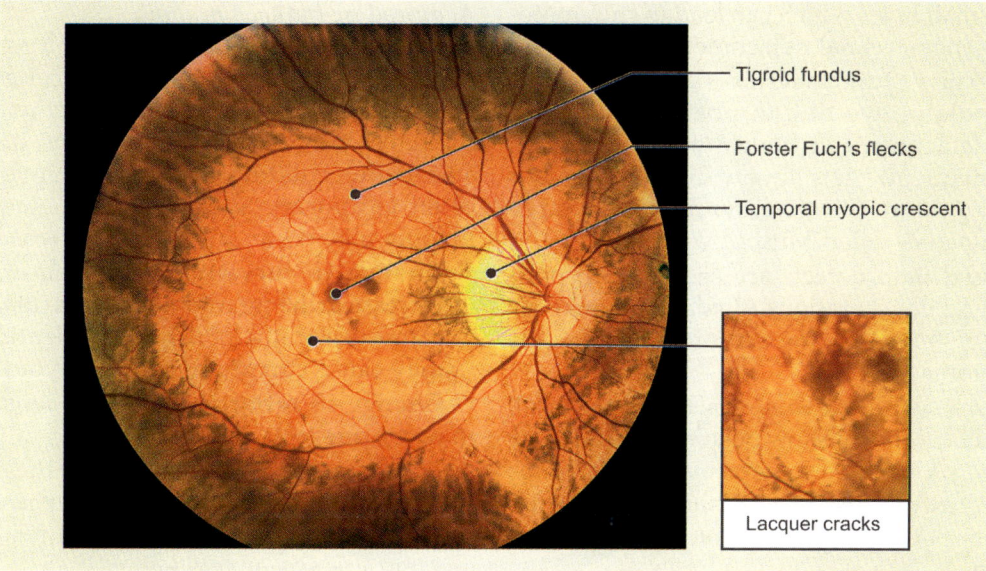

Tigroid fundus

Forster Fuch's flecks

Temporal myopic crescent

Lacquer cracks

Fig. 5.10: Myopic fundus

- **Choroidal crescent:** Can be seen on temporal side of myopic crescent. It is formed due to atrophy of retinal pigment epithelium so that choroidal vessels can be seen in form of crescent. However, with progression of disease, the choroid itself get atrophied and the choroidal vessels become less visible. This appearance of fundus is also called as Tigroid Fundus or tesselated fundus.
- **Supertraction crescent:** May be seen on nasal side of optic disc due to extension of retina over disc margin, thus blurring disc margins on its nasal side.
- **Choroidal atrophic patches** are present in posterior pole. These white patches are surrounded by pigments and sometimes haemorrhages. Such white patches at macula are very common and are main cause of diminished central vision in high myopes. Once these white patches with spots of pigments get accumulated they get spread widely all over the posterior pole of fundus.
- *Lacquer cracks* are formed due to microscopic separation in Bruch's membrane, which occurred as a result of overstretching

of eyeball. They appear as yellowish linear lesions and may be associated with subretinal haemorrhages.
- *Forster Fuch's flecks* are uncommon presentation and can occur spontaneously. They appear as dark red spots in macular region probably appear due to proliferation of retinal pigment epithelium along with intra-choroidal haemorrhages or thrombosis of choroidal vessels.
- **Posterior staphyloma** may be seen in high degree of myopia and occurs due to outpouching of scleral tissue while other layers are pushed backwards at posterior pole of eye. This condition is identified on indirect ophthalmoscopic examination as sudden kinking of retinal blood vessels where they dip at optic disc edge. Staphyloma in the long run can lead to atrophy and loss of vision.
- **Cystoid degenerations** at periphery of retina near ora serrata is a very common presentation in high myopes.
- **Lattice degenerations** may also be seen at the periphery of fundus. They are also called snail track lesions and may have

small holes which can lead to rhugmato-genous retinal detachments.

- **Weiss's fundus reflex** is seen at posterior pole of eye due to posterior vitreous detachment in high myopes. Vitreous frequently gets liquefy due to degeneration and will give symptoms of large floaters called Muscae volitantes.

- Visual field defects are seen due to peripheral degenerations. Visual field analysis may show the ring scotomas or discrete scotomas.

- A- scan will show large axial length of eyeball and B- scan will show posterior staphyloma along with posterior vitreous detachments.

- Electroretinogram will show subnormal wave pattern due to chorioretinal degeneration.

Sequelae of pathological myopia

- **Changes in lens:** Lens in high myopes shows changes due to nuclear sclerosis. These sclerotic changes will further increase the amount of refractive error.

- **Development of glaucoma:** Primary open angle glaucoma is commonly associated with myopia probably due to large eyeball.

- **Development of secondary or complicated cataract:** It may occur due to deprivation of nutrients to the posterior surface of lens as a result of overstretching of ocular structures.

- **Damage to retina:** Retinal tears can occur due to lattice degenerations, which may lead to retinal detachment. Retinal haemorrhages, if occur will give severe vision related complications.

- **Choroidal and vitreous haemorrhage:** Choroidal haemorrhage and choroidal thrombosis is a common complication of high myopes and can give rise to a significant loss of visual acuity if it involves the foveal or macula area. Vitreous haemorrhage may occur along with retinal tear or choroidal haemorrhage. In cases of choroidal haemorrhage the blood may leak into the vitreous and can fill the vitreous cavity.

Acquired or induced myopia

This type of myopia may occur as a result of exposure to various pharmaceutical agents, variation in blood sugar levels, changes in refractive index and position of lens, or other anomalous conditions. Acquired myopia is often temporary and reversible. Acquired myopia may occur due to various reasons

- **Change in curvature of cornea or lens:** Increase in the curvature of cornea (in keratoconus or keratoglobus) or lens (lenticonus) may cause curvatural type of myopia.

- **Change in refractive index of lens:** May occur due to
  - opalescent nuclear sclerosis of the central zone of the lens will increase the refractive index of lens and results in progressive myopia
  - In diabetics, refractive index of lens cortex is decreased probably because of change in carbohydrate metabolism of lens, causing myopia.

- **Change in position of cornea or lens:** Forward displacement (subluxation) of lens as seen in Homocystinuria and Ehlers-Danlos syndrome lead to positional myopia.

- **Consecutive myopia:** May develop due to:
  - Refractive surgical overcorrection of hypermetropia
  - The intraocular lens (IOL) implanted for pseudophakia overcorrects the refraction of eye means power of implanted IOL is more than required.

- **Conditional myopia:** Various atmospheric situations may induce myopic state for emmetropic persons. Some causes are as follows.

Nocturnal myopia (night or twilight myopia)

Some persons may complaints of greater difficulty seeing at low level of illumination, i.e. become symptomatic from increasing myopia at night, although, their daytime vision is normal. This myopia occurs because of increased sensitivity of eye for shorter wavelength of light at low illumination (i.e. modification in spectral sensitivity or Purkinje

Note: Purkinje shift means change in peak sensitivity to light under different illumination condition, from wavelengths close to 555 nanometers (green-yellow) in photopic vision to 507 nanometers (blue-green) in scotopic vision.

shift). Younger people are more likely to be affected by night myopia than the elderly. Such person especially myopic night drivers may require increased correction for clear vision at night.

Space myopia

As we know that when eye receives any visual stimulation from an object situated at some distance, it will adjust its focus accordingly. Although in the absence of any object in the visual field (e.g. when looking into empty space), there is no stimulus for eye for distance fixation. In this situation accommodative mechanism of eye adopts a position that corresponds to certain amount of accommodation (0.5–1.0 D) so that eye becomes more powerful and its focal point is displaced towards lens, leading to myopic state of eye. This type of myopia is experienced by fighter pilots or aviators when flying in cloud or fog.

Pseudomyopia (false nearsightedness or artificial myopia)

Excessive accommodation or spasm of accommodation may cause intermittent and temporary shift of refraction towards myopia. Pseudomyopia is usually seen after doing near work for prolonged time, where ciliary muscle goes into spasm leading to increase in the power of lens. Occasionally, full correction of hypermetropia in young children can produce a state of artificial myopia.

Drug induced myopia

Chronic use of many drugs can produce myopia of various degrees by allergic reaction. Drugs can increase the refractive power of eye by various mechanisms like:

- By causing sustained spasm of ciliary muscles
- By increasing refractive power of lens through water imbibitions

Note: Instrument myopia may occur due to over-use of accommodation when looking into an instrument like microscope.

- By causing swelling of ciliary process and its rotation which cause forward displacement of lens.
- Use of various drugs like sulfonamide derived drugs, steroids, cholinergic drugs, topiramate, etc. can precipitate myopia.

Management of Myopia

Myopia can be corrected by:
- Optical correction
- Surgical correction
- Supportive and prophylactic measures

Optical Correction

Corrective lens are prescribed in the form of eyeglasses and contact lenses.

The optical correction is done by prescribing the concave or minus lenses, which enables the rays to get focus on the retina by altering the total converging power of optical system (Fig. 5.11). Concave lenses will diverge the parallel incident rays and helps in focusing of these rays on retina.

These lenses either can be fitted in spectacles or can be given in contact lens form. Basic rules to remember when prescribing the concave lenses for myopia are as follows

- Unlike hypermetropia, in myopia minimal accepted power, which gives maximum visual acuity should be prescribed.

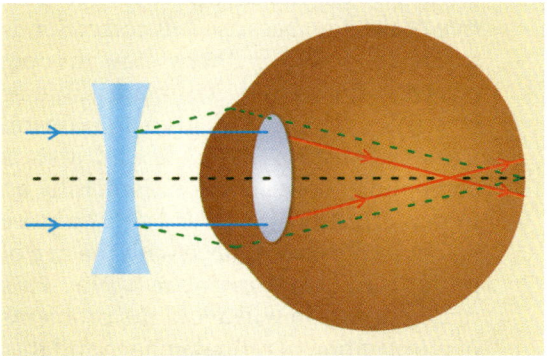

Fig. 5.11: Optical correction of myopia

- Young children below the age of 6–7 years should be given full correction and a constant use of glasses both for distant and near work is advised. This constant use will help in preventing the deviation of eyes as well as will develop a normal accommodation convergence reflex. Constant use of glasses for near work is advised not to improve the near vision but to improve the reading distance and to maintain the normal eye relationship.
- In adolescent myopic patients never overcorrect or fully correct the refractive error. These patients usually wants more minus power than best corrected visual acuity power, because this additional minus power will increase the contrast sensitivity of letters in the vision chart. To avoid overcorrection always ask the patient that whether the letters are more clearer or became small or large in size after adding a little more minus power than before.
- Young adults less than 30 years of age usually accept full optical correction. The patients older than 30 years of age who were never given a myopic correction before, having a refractive error of more than 3–4 D, usually do not accept full correction in first sitting. Hence these patients are undercorrected initially and advised to step up the correction in further sittings.
- In high myopes (more than 8–10 D) always do an under correction irrespective of the age, because full correction is rarely tolerated by these high myopic patients. Try to undercorrect as little as possible, which will give maximum visual acuity for distance and also is compatible for near vision. Generally an undercorrection of power 1–2 D or more is required in accordance with the age of patient and amount of myopia. This undercorrection will avoid the problems of minification of retinal images and that of related to near vision.

Surgical Correction

Various refractive procedures are done for the correction of myopia. The outcome of these procedures are very encouraging and reliable in cases of myopia, hence various newer procedure has also been introduced for high myopic patients.

These refractive procedures have been described in Chapter 15.

Supportive and prophylactic treatment

Various other measures are also advised to decrease the incidence or progression of myopia:

- **Intake of balanced diet:** Deficiency of certain vitamins and minerals (calcium, magnesium, vitamin A, vitamin D, etc.) and proteins are also associated with progression of myopia. Intake of these nutrients can slow the progression of myopia in children. Though this hypothesis has no evidential proof, but still many believe this theory.
- **Visual hygiene:** To decrease the development of myopia, it is advised that intensive visual near task like reading, computer work, etc. should be done with certain visual hygiene measures like maintaining proper distance and posture during reading and writing, keeping sufficient illumination and taking break frequently when doing near work. Research also indicates that children who spent more time outdoors are less prone to the development of myopia than those who spent less time.
- Low vision aids can be prescribed for very high myopes to provide some useful vision as they are not getting corrected by spectacles or contact lenses. They also have very poor visual acuity due to degenerative changes of retina and choroid and hence need low vision aids. Details of low vision aids are described in Chapter 16.
- As genetic has a role in pathological myopia, it is recommended that genetic counseling should be done before marriage. Persons having pathological myopia are advised to avoid the marriage with another pathological myope.

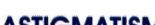
ASTIGMATISM

Introduction

The word astigmatism is derived from Greek where "a" means absent and "stigma" means point. Astigmatism is a refractive state of the eye wherein the parallel rays of the light from infinity get focused differently in different meridians while accommodation is at rest (Fig. 5.12). In astigmatism, the power of refraction varies in different meridians and hence the light rays entering in the eye undergo unequal refraction so that they are not focused at a single focal point rather they are focused as focal lines (formation of sturm's conoid).

It is a common refractive error accounting for about 13% of all refractive errors and occurs with equal frequency in males and females. Prevalence is very high in first year of life as the curvature of cornea is very steep. Nearly 50% of infants have astigmatism of about 1D in their first year of life. The degree and percentage of astigmatism gradually decrease with age as the cornea flattens. Almost half of the population has at least 0.5 D of astigmatism, while an astigmatism of >1 D is seen in nearly 10–15% of adults whereas, only 2% adults have an astigmatic error of <3 D. Ethnic variations also exist. For

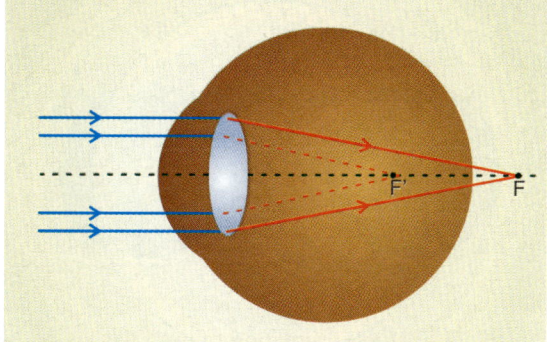

Fig. 5.12: Astigmatic state of eye

example, high prevalence is seen in East Asian people, probably due to narrower palpebral apertures and greater tightness of the eyelids.

Classification of Astigmatism

Astigmatism can be classified in various ways as shown in Table 5.5.

Before we discuss the types of astigmatism, it is important to know about **meridians** of eyes. Normally these **meridians** are defined for both eyes in the degrees from 1 to 180 as shown in Fig. 5.13. There is no "zero" meridian, nor any angle larger than 180°.

Generally, astigmatism is of two types:
- Regular astigmatism
- Irregular astigmatism

Table 5.5: Classification of astigmatism				
Regular astigmatism				*Irregular astigmatism*
On the basis of etiology	*On the basis of positions of meridians*	*On the basis of principal focus*		*On the basis of etiology*
Corneal astigmatism	With the rule astigmatism	Simple astigmatism	Simple myopic astigmatism	Corneal irregular astigmatism
Lenticular astigmatism	Against the rule astigmatism		Simple hypermetropic astigmatism	Lenticular irregular astigmatism
• Curvatural astigmatism	Oblique astigmatism	Compound astigmatism	Compound myopic astigmatism	Retinal irregular astigmatism
• Positional astigmatism	Bi-oblique astigmatism		Compound hyperopic astigmatism	
• Index astigmatism				
Retinal astigmatism		Mixed astigmatism		

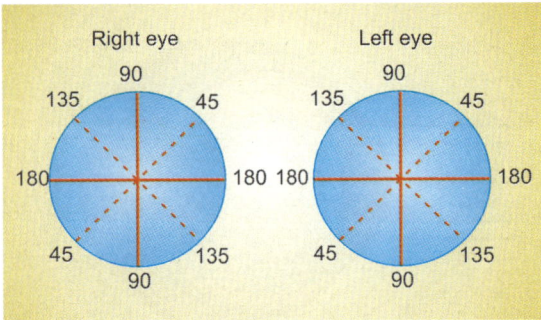

Fig. 5.13: Orientation of meridians

Regular Astigmatism

In this type of astigmatism only two principal meridians (horizontal and vertical) are present having different refractive power and there is uniform change in refractive power from one meridian to another meridian.

Classification

Regular astigmatism on the basis of etiology can be classified into:

- **Corneal astigmatism:** It is one of the most common causes of regular astigmatism. Change in the curvature of the cornea in different meridians leads to corneal astigmatism. Most of regular astigmatism is corneal in origin. Change in curvature may be congenital or acquired like after ocular surgery (cataract surgery or excimer laser), trauma to cornea, keratoconus, abnormal growth of tissue on the cornea (Pterygium), etc. Change in curvature of cornea due to acquired factors usually produces irregular astigmatism.

- **Lenticular astigmatism:** It is less common cause of astigmatism. Lenticular astigmatism may occur due to error in the curvature, position or refractive index of crystalline lens:
    - Due to congenital abnormality in the curvature or shape (spherical or oval shape) of lens. For example, lenticonus anterior and lenticonus posterior can produce a significant degree of astigmatism.

- Lens may be congenitally tilted or obliquely placed or there may be congenital or traumatic subluxation of lens producing a varying degree of astigmatism.
    - Refractive index of either cortex or nucleus of lens may change in diabetic or cataract patients leading to astigmatism.

- **Retinal astigmatism** is a rare type of astigmatism. It may occur due to an oblique placement of macula or due to different curvatures of retina in different meridians.

Regular astigmatism on the basis of position of meridians can be classified into:

Regular astigmatism can also be classified on the basis of position of its two principal meridians (horizontal and vertical). On the basis of axis, nature of curvature and angle between these two principal meridians, regular astigmatism is classified as follows:

- **With the rule astigmatism (direct astigmatism):** When two principal meridians (horizontal and vertical) are present at right angle to each other and the vertical meridian is more curved (steeper) than the horizontal meridian. This type of astigmatism is termed "with the rule" astigmatism (Fig. 5.14) because it is like physiological type of astigmatism seen in normal eye.

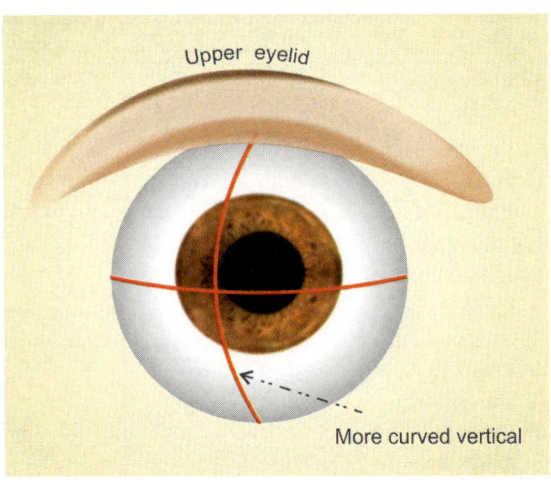

Fig. 5.14: With the rule astigmatism

In normal eye a small degree of physiological astigmatic error (0.12 D) exists because the vertical meridian of cornea is more curved (steeper) than horizontal meridian due to pressure of eyelids on anterior corneal surface. In other words, horizontal meridian of cornea is more flat as compared to vertical meridian. That is why this type of regular astigmatism is named "with the rule astigmatism". The vertical meridian being steeper in nature also has more refractive power than horizontal meridian. A concave cylinder at horizontal axis, i.e. 180 ± 10° or convex cylinder at vertical axis, i.e. 90 ± 10° will correct this type of astigmatism because cylinders have their principal meridians perpendicular to each other and power of the cylindrical lens is perpendicular to its axis.

- **Against the rule astigmatism (indirect astigmatism):** When two principal meridians (horizontal and vertical) are present at right angle to each other but horizontal meridian is more curved (steep) than vertical meridian, then this type of astigmatism is termed "against the rule" astigmatism. (Fig. 5.15). Here the curvature of meridians are not like of normal eye (where vertical meridian is more curved), hence named "Against the rule" astigmatism.

As horizontal meridian is steeper than vertical meridian so the refractive power at 180° will be more as compared to 90°. A convex cylinder at 180 ± 10° or concave cylinder at 90 ±10° will correct this type of astigmatism because power of a cylindrical lens is acting perpendicular to its axis.

- **Oblique astigmatism:** When two principal meridians are present at right angle to each other but they are not horizontal or vertical in nature (i.e. tilted). It means two principal meridians are not present at usual 90°/180° configuration. For example, two principal meridians present at 45° and 135° or at 30° and 120° (difference in both is still 90°) will cause oblique astigmatism (Fig. 5.16) Curvatures of these oblique meridians may be equal or unequal. Oblique astigmatism may be further sub-classified as

  - *Symmetrical oblique astigmatism:* When cylindrical correction required in both the eyes is at symmetrical axis, e.g. at 20° in both the eyes.
  - *Complimentary oblique astigmatism:* When cylindrical correction required in one eye is at complimentary axis to other eye. For example, 45° in one eye and 135° in the other eye.

- **Bi-oblique astigmatism:** When two principal meridians are not at right angle to each other and also are not horizontal or

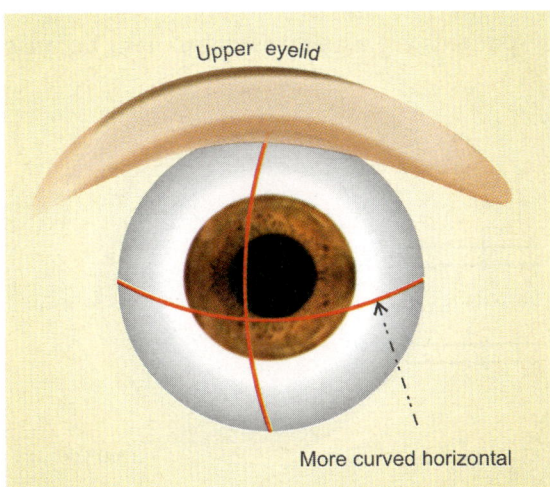

Fig. 5.15: Against the rule astigmatism

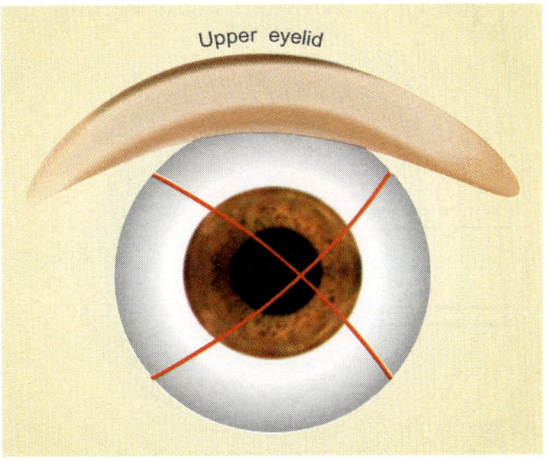

Fig. 5.16: Oblique astigmatism

vertical in nature, this type of astigmatism is called bi-oblique astigmatism. For example, two principal meridians at 20° and 140°.

Regular astigmatism on the basis of position of focal lines or type of refractive error in two meridians:

On the basis of position of the two principal focal lines in relation to retina and type of refractive error in meridian, regular astigmatism is classified as follows:

- **Simple astigmatism:** When the light rays from one principal meridian are focused on the retina while rays from other principal meridian focused either in front or behind the retina. Hence, one meridian is emmetropic while other meridian has refractive error (myopic or hypermetropic). Depending upon the refractive error present in meridian, simple astigmatism can be further subclassified as follows (Fig. 5.17A and B)
  - *Simple myopic astigmatism:* When rays from one meridian focus on the retina while rays from other principal meridian focus in front of the retina. For example, a plano cylinder –1.75 DC × 180° (here vertical meridian rays are focusing in front of the retina)
  - *Simple hypermetropic astigmatism:* When rays from one principal meridian focus on the retina while rays from other principal meridian focus behind the retina. For example, a plano cylinder + 1.5 DC × 90° (here horizontal meridian rays are focusing behind the retina)
- **Compound astigmatism:** In compound astigmatism both meridians have same type of refractive error with different refractive power and none of the meridians is focused on the retina. Hence, when the light rays from both the principal meridians are either focused in front or behind the retina, it is called compound astigmatism. It is of two types (Fig. 5.18A and B):
  - Compound myopic astigmatism: When rays from both the principal meridians focus in front of the retina. For example, –2.5 DS × –1.5 DC × 90° (here horizontal meridian is more steeper)
  - Compound hypermetropic astigmatism: When rays from both the principal meridians focus behind the retina. For example, +2.75 DS × + 1 DC × 180° (here vertical meridian is more flat)
- **Mixed astigmatism:** In mixed astigmatism both principal meridians have different types of refractive errors, i.e. the light rays from one principal meridian focus in front of the retina while rays from other principal meridian focus behind the retina. In other words, eye is myopic in one principal meridian and hypermetropic in other principal meridian (Fig. 5.19). These patients are usually asymptomatic because

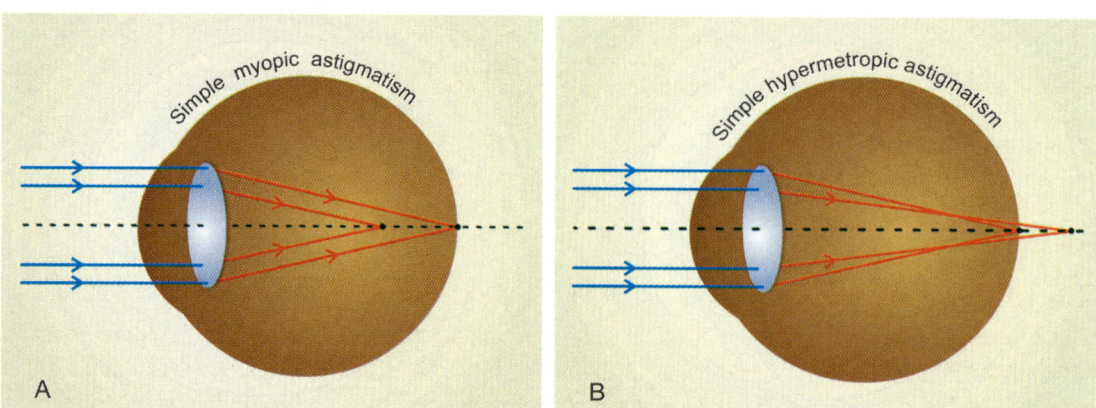

Fig. 5.17: Simple astigmatism. A. Simple myopic astigmatism; B. Simple hypermetropic astigmatism

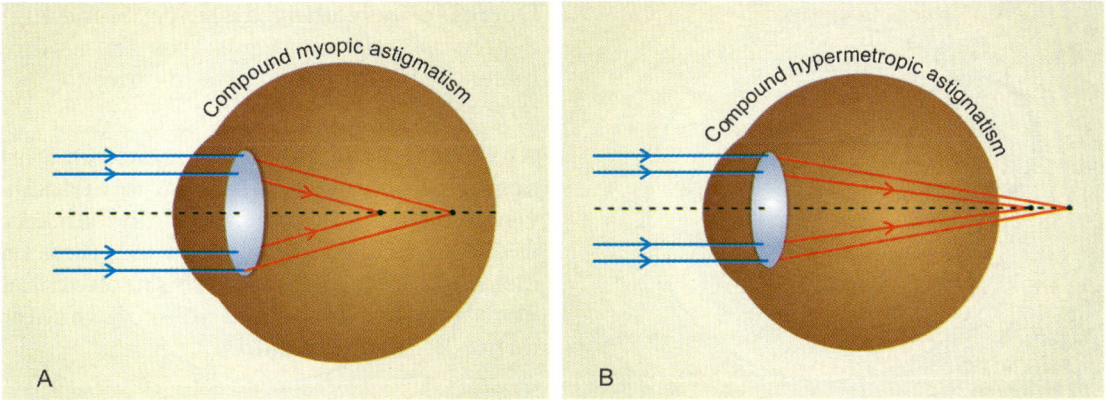

Fig. 5.18: Compound astigmatism. A. Compound myopic astigmatism; B. Compound hypermetropic astigmatism

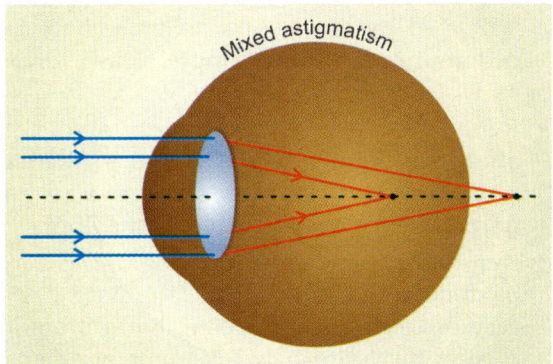

Fig. 5.19: Mixed astigmatism

Note: Simple, compound and mixed astigmatism may be with the rule or against the rule. Remember to get a mixed astigmatism cylindrical error is always more than spherical error with opposite sign.

the circle of least diffusion falls usually on the retina. For example, –2.5 DS × + 3.5 DC × 180°.

Clinical Features

Symptoms: Severity of symptoms mainly depends on the type and degree of astigmatic error.

Asthenopia (eye strain): Astigmatic patients may compliant of tiredness of eyes, mild brow ache or frontal headache or sometimes severe cephalgia with reflex neurological turbulence such as irritability, giddiness, light intolerance, fatigue or lethargy. These symptoms occur due to an excessive effort of accommodation to see the objects clearer. Asthenopic symptoms are relatively more common in astigmatic error as compared to spherical refractive error. These asthenopic symptoms are more pronounced in case of

- Small degree astigmatism
- With the rule astigmatism
- Hypermetropic astigmatism

Diminution of vision: Person with astigmatism may compliant of blurring of vision specially when doing work for distant fixation. Blurring gets increased with increase in the degree of astigmatism. Transient blurring of vision get relieved by closing or rubbing of eyes. To see the object clearly these patients try to focus in one meridian clearly which is nearest to emmetrope. Usually these patients prefer the vertical meridian for clear focus. Depending upon the type and degree of astigmatism, objects may appear proportionately elongated in astigmatic patients as follows

- Circular objects appears as an elongated oval images (Fig. 5.20)
- Line appears as fused elongated blurred oval images, in succession to each other as shown in Fig. 5.21. These oval images of a line object are seen in both the parallel and perpendicular axis of principal meridian in

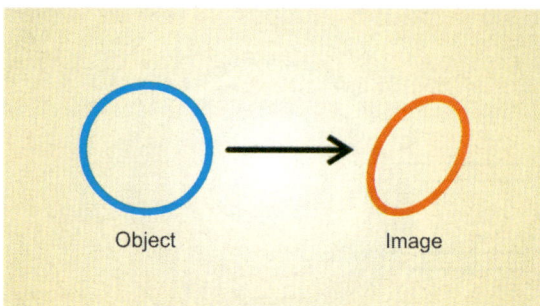

Fig. 5.20: Blur vision, circle appearing as oval

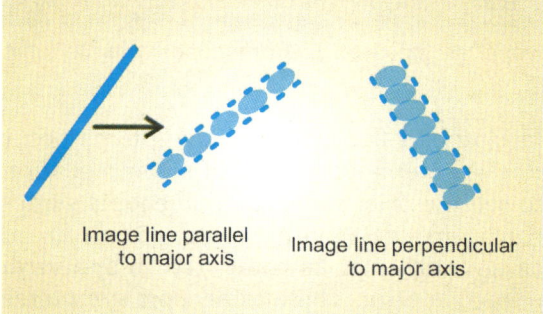

Fig. 5.21: Blur vision, line appearing as elongated oval images

astigmatic errors, depending upon the type of astigmatism.

- Point light source appears as blurred point image with a tail (point of light begins to tail off).

Recurrent ocular infection: Patients having low degree of astigmatism usually develop a habit of constant rubbing of eyes, probably because of itching or burning sensations in eye. This constant rubbing may result in falling of eyelashes, hyperemia of lid margins and frequent stye or chalazion formation.

Half closure of eyes: Like myopes, patients having high degree of astigmatism develop the habit of squeezing or forcefully closing the eyes partially. By doing this they make a stenopic slit of eyelids and avoid the rays in one meridian. This helps them to see the object clearer and distinct, but will also produce significant amount of brow pain; probably because of constant use of eyelid muscles.

Decrease in reading distance: Some high degree astigmatic patients keep the reading material closer to their eyes in order to see a larger image.

Abnormal head posture: In case of high degree of oblique astigmatism to make the visual axis straight, patient may tilt their head to one particular side, in order to reduce the distortion of blurred image. This habit of tilted head posture may lead to scoliosis and torticollis in some children.

Signs
- Visual acuity is diminished in direct proportionate with the amount of astigmatism. Because of distortion of images the patient will read the letters in Snellen's chart as different letter. For example, E as F or Y as T.
- Retinoscopy or autorefractometry: Will tell about different powers in two principal meridians and their axis. They may be perpendicular to each other or may not.
- Keratometry and corneal topography: Can be done to rule out corneal astigmatism. In case of corneal astigmatism, two different corneal curvature in two different meridians will be seen.
- Jackson cross cylinder test is an important method to check the power and axis of astigmatic error.
- Astigmatic fan test or Maddox V test is an older method but is an effective method to estimate the amount and type of astigmatic error.
- Stenopic slit or pinhole: Gives information about the refraction and principle axis in astigmatism. The slit aperture of stenopic slit allows the entry of light rays only in the axis of the slit. Suppose the astigmatic axis and slit axis are not in alignment, then the

Note: Total astigmatism comprises both of these factors, i.e. corneal astigmatism (due to anterior surface of cornea) and supplementary astigmatism (astigmatism of lens and posterior surface of the cornea).

visual acuity will decrease, hence we can confirm the correct astigmatic axis by use of stenopic slit.

- Anterior and posterior segments of eye are usually normal in low astigmatic error. However, some changes in shape of lens can be seen in lenticular type high astigmatic error cases.
- On fundus examination oval or tilted optic disc may be seen in patients with high degree of astigmatism.

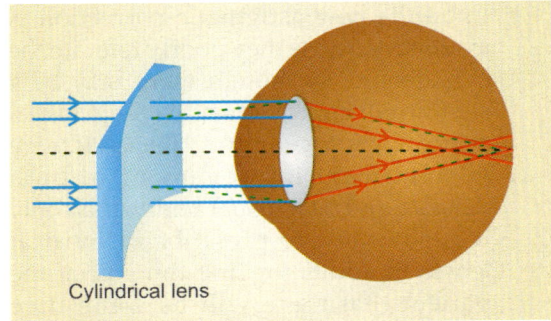

Cylindrical lens

Fig. 5.22: Optical correction of astigmatism

Javal's rule and its subsequent modifications, Grosvenor rule, etc. are used to estimate the magnitude of total astigmatism from Keratometry reading

Javal's rule formula: $A_t = p(A_c) + K$

Here, A_t = total refractive astigmatism, A_c = corneal astigmatism; p = about 1.25, K = 0.50 D against the rule

Or $A_t = 1.25(A_c) - 0.50 \times 90°$

Grosvenor rule: $A_t = 1.00(A_c) - 0.50 \times 90°$. It has no fudge factor value of 1.25.

Astigmatic fan test and Jackson cross cylinder test are explained in details in Chapter 11.

Treatment of Regular Astigmatism

Similar to other refractive errors regular astigmatism is treated by means of either optical correction or surgical procedures.

Optical correction: The optical correction in regular astigmatism is done by prescribing the appropriate cylindrical lenses. These may be minus or plus cylinders identified after an accurate retinoscopy (Fig. 5.22).

Cylindrical lenses with appropriate axis can be prescribed in form of spectacles or contact lenses. Hard contact lenses may be prescribed for correction of low degree (2–3 D) astigmatism while toric contact lenses (truncated or ballistic to maintain their correct axis) are prescribed for higher degree of astigmatism.

Basic rules to remember in prescribing the cylindrical lenses in cases of astigmatism are as follows

- Low degree of astigmatism (0.5–1 D) needs optical correction only when patient is symptomatic, i.e. there is eye strain symptoms and deterioration of vision. It is essential to do a thorough estimation of refraction in these patients before prescribing the cylindrical lenses. If some amount of astigmatic error remained uncorrected, then patient will try to correct it by own efforts and symptoms of eye strain may exaggerate.
- High degree astigmatism (>3 D) needs full correction irrespective of symptoms. However, full correction in form of cylindrical lenses in first instance may cause distress and discomfort to patient as object appears distorted and make the floor appear to tilt. It is advised that when prescribing for first time the error should be undercorrected so that the patient gets habituated to the cylinder. Gradually, at regular interval the cylindrical power can be increased until the full correction is tolerable in these patients.
- A change in axis of cylindrical power, especially in adult patients accustomed to their older axis, is to be done with great precautions. This change in cylindrical axis is usually poorly tolerated by older patients and they may develop asthenopic symptoms. Even if it is absolutely necessary to change the older axis, then the patient is advised to wear the newer cylinders in a trial frame and walk around in examination room for a few minutes. If no symptoms develop, then the newer axis can be prescribed.

- In adults new astigmatic correction is avoided, because they poorly tolerate the cylinders, even though there may be a significant improvement in their visual acuity by these cylindrical lenses. If there is significant improvement in both distance and near visual acuity, then only it is advisable to prescribe cylindrical lenses in adults for first time. Brief the patient that there will be some time period requires to get adjusted to these cylindrical lenses.
- Contact lens is a better option than spectacles to treat bi-oblique astigmatism, mixed astigmatism or high degree astigmatism.
- In mixed astigmatism or compound astigmatism the spherical lenses are prescribed as per the guidelines of myopia or hypermetropia correction in various age group patients.

Surgical correction: Refractive surgical procedure are very effective in correcting astigmatism.

These refractive procedures are described in detail in Chapter 15.

Irregular Astigmatism

Irregular astigmatism is the refractive state of eye where refractive power of eye changes irregularly in different ocular meridians. In irregular astigmatism the principal meridians are not at right angles and each meridian in the cornea show separate type of refraction.

Causes of Irregular Astigmatism

- Corneal irregular astigmatism: A condition where the refractive power of corneal meridians is different in different meridians due to irregular corneal surface. Irregular corneal astigmatism may occur due to keratoconus or widespread corneal scarring.
- Lenticular irregular astigmatism: During maturation of cataract the crystalline lens develops variable refractive index in different portions of cortex and nucleus. Thus the refractive status of lens varies in different layers, so a cataractous lens may produce an irregular astigmatism
- Retinal irregular astigmatism: Various conditions like retinal scarring, tumors of retina or choroid pushes the macular area and may cause the distortion of macular area. Thus, the light rays get refracted at different planes due to this distortion of macula. Hence, the astigmatism produced is of high degree and irregular in nature with poor visual acuity.

Clinical Features

Irregular astigmatism produces symptoms such as

- Diminution of vision
- Distorted images of objects
- Multiple images or polyopia

Treatment

- Optical correction: Irregular astigmatism cannot be corrected by spectacles. It is done by prescribing contact lenses (hard or semisoft), where contact lens will replace the anterior surface of cornea and helps in restoration of useful vision.
- Surgical correction is needed in cases where corneal scaring is extensive or optical correction has failed to improve the vision. Penetrating keratoplasty is usually required in severely damaged cornea. Alternatively, excision of scar and its replacement with graft can be done. Lenticular irregular astigmatism caused by cataract can be corrected satisfactorily by performing cataract surgeries and intraocular lens implantation.

Note: Optical correction of retinal irregular astigmatism is not successful, however, surgical correction of various retinal pathologies had been tried with variable results.

Binocular Vision and its Anomalies

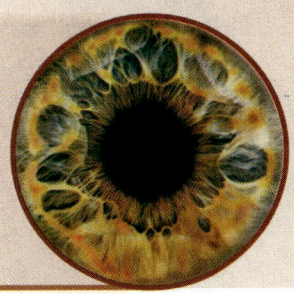

Chapter Outline

BINOCULAR VISION

Introduction

Binocular vision can be defined as "the vision obtained by the synchronized use of both the eyes, so that the images formed in each eye separately are appreciated as a single image in the visual cortex of the brain".

Binocular single vision (BSV) is simply not an inborn characteristic feature, rather it is an acquired phenomenon developed during the first few years of life as a gradual developmental process.

Various mechanisms involved in the development of binocular vision and which enable the eyes to function in a coordinated manner are described below.

A. Sensory Mechanism

Factors which constitute sensory mechanisms in the development of BSV can be grouped as

- *Visual acuity value of retinal receptors of each eye:* Foveal and macular area of the retina which mediate central vision has high visual acuity value as compared to rest of the retina which has a low visual acuity value. Integrity of fovea and macula in each eye is important because there must be adequate degree of central vision for development of binocular vision. Difference in the size of two retinal images should not be too great to prevent the fusion of images. Peripheral visual acuity also contributes in development of binocular vision.

- *Normal correspondence of retinal receptors of two eyes:* Extreme temporal part of peripheral visual field is uniocular, but rest of the visual field is binocular. It means the visual fields of both the eyes overlap in majority of portion. Retinal correspondence is a functional rather than an anatomical phenomenon. Two fovea of each eye may be regarded as corresponding retinal points and there are numerous other pairs of corresponding retinal points in temporal retina.

- *Hemi-decussation of optic nerve fibers at optic chiasma along with integrity of visual pathway:* Afferent optic nerve fibers arising from retina hemi-dessucate at optic chaisma, which enables these fibers from corresponding retinal area of two eyes to associate with one another in visual cortex. This implies that fibers from corresponding retinal points, i.e. temporal retina of one eye and nasal retina of other eye, travel in same optic tract and terminate in same lateral geniculate body where they relay in optic radiation and then to visual cortex.

- *Proprioceptive impulses from extrinsic ocular muscles:* Extrinsic ocular muscles give sensory information to the brain in a proprioceptive nature and this information is essential in establishment of binocular vision.

B. Motor Mechanisms

Motor factors contributing in development of binocular vision can be grouped as:

- *Anatomical factors:* Anatomical factors are the one, which determine the position of eyes and are concerned with structure of bony orbit and its content. These structures are important to ensure that eyes lie in bony orbit in such a way that their visual axis are aligned correctly with each other at rest and even during movement of eyes.

- *Physiological factors:* Physiological factors which determines the position of eyes are of three types:

Postural reflex: These are independent of visual stimuli and concerned with maintenance of two eyes in their correct relative positions within the orbit. Hence visual axes of two eyes are aligned to each other despite the change in head posture relative to body or body to space. Two groups of postural reflex are:

Static reflex: These reflexes are initiated by movement of head relative to body and are controlled by labyrinth and proprioceptive impulses from neck muscles.

Stato-kinetic reflex: These reflexes are initiated by movement of head relative to space.

Psycho-optical reflexes: These reflexes are dependent on visual stimuli. Maintenance of correct position of two eyes within the orbit is done by the help of the psycho-visual reflexes. In spite of movement of head relative to body or space the alignment of visual axis of two eyes remain in position because of visual stimuli which reach the visual cortex via afferent visual pathway. Various components of this reflex are:

Fixation reflex: This reflex is nothing but the ability of each eye to fix a definite object independently. Fixation reflex is dependent on the presence of adequate field of vision and adequately functioning fovea.

Re-fixation reflex: It concerns with the ability of eye to retain fixation on a moving object (passive re-fixation) or to change fixation from one object to another object (active re-fixation). This develops shortly after fixation reflex in young age.

Conjugate fixation reflex: This reflex is concerned with the application of fixation reflex of both the eyes simultaneously to retain the fixation during the conjugate movements. Usually present within 5–6 weeks of life and is well established by 6 months of age.

Disjunctive or vergence fixation reflex: This reflex is use of fixation reflex of both the eyes simultaneously to retain the fixation during the disjunctive movements. Even though these reflex appear later than conjugate reflex in life, but is also well established by the age of 6 months.

Corrective fusion reflex: This reflex is an expansion of both conjugate and disjunctive fixation reflexes. Process of fusion reflex enables the eyes to retain fixation and function binocularly even during stressful conditions. It is present since one year of age but is well established by 5 years of age.

Note: First two factors, the fixation and re-fixation reflexes, are uniocular, whereas the other three factors, conjugate, disjunctive and corrective fixation reflexes, are binocular in function.

Kinetic reflex: These reflexes are dependent on a controlled relationship between accommodative and convergence and are related with the maintenance of correct position of two eyes within the orbit. Process of accommodation is followed by an appropriate amount of convergence and vice-versa; so both of these reflexes are dependent on each other.

C. Central Mechanism

Factors which contribute in development of binocular vision by process of central mechanism are

- Fusion which is a sensory phenomenon and referred as proper overlapping of two images from each eye.
- Cortical control of ocular movement which is a motor phenomenon.

Development of normal binocular vision is dependent on these factors such as

- Transparent ocular media so that visual axes of both the eyes receive uninterrupted clear vision.
- Retinal and cortical elements of visual system should be capable of working together so that they can fuse the slightly dissimilar images as single image, means sensory fusion.
- Two eyes should be accurately coordinated in all directions of gazes so that retinal and cortical element of ocular system remain in a coordinated positions to handle the two images, means motor fusion.

Terminologies in Binocular Single Vision

Following terminologies are frequently used in relation to BSV, hence it is important to understand them in detail.

- Retinal correspondence
- Retinal rivalry
- Suppression

- Diplopia
- Horopter
- Panum's area

Retinal Correspondence

When visual axes of two eyes corresponding to their respective retinal components (fovea) share a common visual direction, then these two retinal points represent retinal correspondence. This retinal correspondence is of two types

- Normal retinal correspondence (NRC)
- Abnormal or anomalous retinal correspondence (ARC)

NRC: Retinal correspondence is termed normal retinal correspondence when these conditions are fulfilled

- Fovea of two eyes must share a common visual direction.
- The retinal component situated nasally to fovea of one eye should correspond with retinal component of other eye situated temporal to its fovea.

ARC: When fovea of one eye share common visual direction with an extra-foveal region of other eye, then retinal correspondence is referred as abnormal retinal correspondence. Usually ARC is present in low degree strabismus and condition where foveal and extra-foveal points lies very near thus two eyes try to regain binocular vision. Hence, in spite of manifest strabismus two eyes in ARC may have single binocular vision. During binocular vision in an ARC situation foveal point of one eye corresponds to extra-foveal point of other eye; however, when normal eye is closed, then extra-foveal point of other eye has no visual advantage over fovea of the same eye. So other eye will regain its original visual direction, means in monocular conditions the fixation is achieved by fovea.

Note: Cover test is based on this principle.

Retinal Rivalry

This is also called binocular rivalry because fusion is not possible when dissimilar shape forms are presented to corresponding retinal elements. These dissimilar objects will stimulate corresponding retinal area together, so in place of fusion there is confusion. To overcome this confusion visual cortex suppresses the image of one eye. Although by suppression retinal rivalry is seized but constant foveal suppression of one eye will cause a total sensory dominance of fellow eye. This dominance of one eye produces a significant obstruction in the development of binocular vision. In these cases restoration of binocular vision requires return of retinal rivalry.

Suppression

When dissimilar objects stimulate two corresponding retinal elements in the eye, then confusion will occur. Similarly, when similar objects stimulate two non-corresponding retinal elements, then diplopia will occur. As discussed above to remove either the confusion or diplopia, the image of one eye is suppressed by a central or peripheral inhibitory mechanism. It means to overcome the confusion suppression is foveal (central) and to overcome diplopia, suppression is extra-foveal (peripheral).

Suppression can be grouped as

- Facultative suppression
- Obligatory suppression

When suppression happens only in binocular situation with no residual monocular effects, it is called facultative suppression. Hence, monocular visual acuity remains good and no scotomas in visual field are seen in uniocular examination.

On contrary, when effects of suppression is seen even in monocular situation and there is residual monocular diminished vision. It is termed as obligatory suppression. This type of suppression will lead to amblyopia.

Diplopia

Diplopia or double vision occurs due to retinal disparity. It occurs when two non-corresponding retinal elements (fovea in one eye and nonfoveal point in other eye) are stimulated simultaneously by a point object. As a result image of object is localized in two different visual directions and the same point object appears as double when seen in two directions simultaneously.

Horopter

In the year 1613, Aguilonius coined a term Horopter, which means horizon of vision. Horopter is the plane of position of all object points which forms images on corresponding retinal points for a given fixation distance and create single vision. Different models proposed for horopter are

- Geometrical or theoretical horopter
- Longitudinal or empirical horopter

When corresponding points from retina has a regular horizontal distance, then the horopter formed would represent a circle passing through nodal points of the two eyes and fixation point (O) as shown in Fig. 6.1. This is also called Vieth Muller Horopter (VMH) and circle in this model becomes smaller when fixation points come closer.

A few decades later after invention of stereoscope by scientist Charles Wheatstone, several experimental studies concluded that many points in the space (not lying on VMH) also formed single images on retinal elements. So these researchers discovered another horopter called longitudinal horopter or empirical horopter curve which has more radius of curvature (means it is flatter) as compared to VMH (Fig. 6.1).

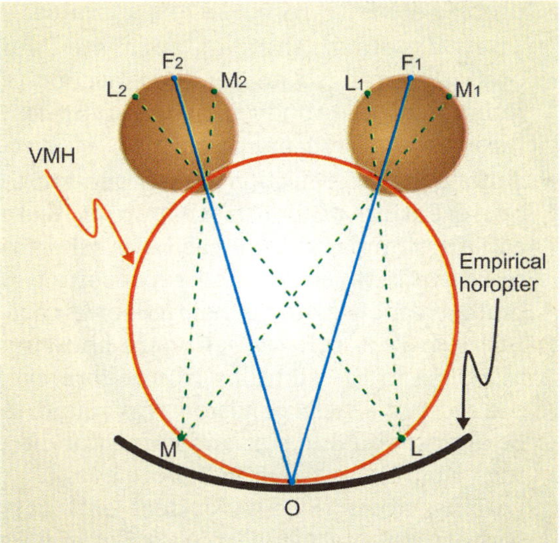

Panum's Area

As discussed above all the points which do not fall on horopter can produce physiological diplopia because these points will be imaged by non corresponding retinal areas, hence are seen as double. However, in normal ocular conditions we do not appreciate physiological diplopia, which can be explained by Panum's fusional area. Panum's area is the zone which surrounds the horopter and in this zone fusion of retinal images occur so that stimulus is perceived as single. This is a narrow band area situated around horopter and is narrowest at fixation point and broadest in peripheral region as shown in Fig. 6.2.

Fig. 6.1: Vieth Muller Horopter (VMH) and empirical horopter

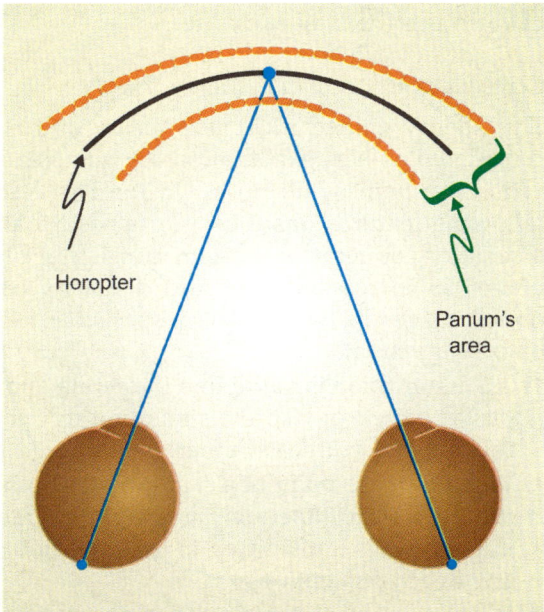

Fig. 6.2: Panum's fusional area

Increased width of Panum's fusional area in peripheral visual portion is advantageous as follows

- Peripheral diplopia generated during fixation of closely held flat targets is prevented by increased thickness of Panum's area.
- Increasing peripheral blurring is in correlation with increased size of Panum's area because visual acuity decreases with increase in size of receptive visual field.
- Increased peripheral extent of Panum's area potentiates cyclofusion, although cyclovergence of up to 2–3° is present between two eyes.

Panum's area may increase or decrease in accordance with the size, speed and sharpness of the stimulus. For example, extent of Panum's area for a slower, dimmer stimulus may be ten times wider than that of a faster and brighter stimulus.

Theories of Binocular Vision

Following theories of binocular vision has been proposed on the basis of development of various reflexes in early life.

Correspondence and Disparity Theory

This theory gained most popularity and is considered as best explanation for binocular vision mechanism till now. On the basis of following features this theory proposed that a sensory cooperation system consisting of binocular correspondence and disparity of object images in two eyes is responsible for binocular vision.

- An assumption is made that the retina and visual cortex of two eyes has one to one relationship with each other.
- When a single-point object stimulates both the eyes simultaneously, a single visual impression is transmitted to brain without any depth perception.
- When two-point objects differing slightly in character stimulate both the eyes

simultaneously, a binocular rivalry will occur in brain.
- When single-point object stimulate disparate retinal elements in two eyes, diplopia will occur.
- When horizontal disparity of image in two eyes is limited to Panum's area, usually a single visual impression is transmitted to brain with an associated depth perception or stereopsis.
- This depth and quality of perception is in correspondence with the amount of disparity, means the stereopsis increases, whereas perception quality decreases with an increase in disparity of image however after certain limit of disparity the stereopsis quality is very poor and diplopia will occur.

Neuro Physiological Theory

On the basis of physiology of neurons and distribution of cells in nervous system this theory tried to explain the mechanism of binocular vision and stereopsis. Salient features of this theory are

- Various experimental studies conducted by renowned scientists conclude that nearly 80% of total neurons from each eye situated in striate visual cortex get stimulated in the process of visual response to a stimulus.
- They assumed that an accurate and properly arranged neuronal connection of retina, geniculate body and cortex is present throughout the visual pathway.
- Among these connections nearly one-fourth representing binocular responses were equally stimulated from each eye, whereas remaining three-fourths represented a graded response from either right or left eye.
- In these 75% cells which were showing response to the stimulus from either eye, the receptive field of vision was found to be almost equal in size and corresponding the visual fields position in both eyes.
- During normal BSV cortical cell gets stimulated only when an optical stimulus is simultaneously presented to its two receptive visual fields.

- However, in some cells these two receptive visual fields may not necessarily be situated in the identical anatomical position in retinae of two eyes.
- So for a given location in retino-optic cortical map there are cells whose visual fields have perfectly corresponding points in two retinal elements and also cells whose visual fields have slightly different position in two retinal elements.
- This retinal field disparity caused by difference in direction or distance of field in retina of each eye is the basis of Panum's fusion area.
- Sensitive binocular neurons detect this fusion area of Panum and produces binocular vision and streopsis.

Depending on the position of images on retinal elements the BSV can be classified as

- Normal BSV: When the binocular single vision is bifoveal in nature and there is no associated manifested squint, it is termed normal BSV.
- Abnormal or anomalous BSV is seen due to alteration in the visual direction of retinal elements. In this type of BSV the image of fixating object in one eye is perceived from fovea while in other eye from extra-foveal area. This condition is always associated with a small degree of manifested squint.

Grades of Binocular Single Vision (BSV)

BSV occurs in following stages:

1. Simultaneous macular perception (SMP) or grade 1
2. Fusion or grade 2
3. Stereopsis or grade 3

Simultaneous Macular Perception (SMP)

Simultaneous perception of objects is most primitive type of binocular vision which is developed in a newborn. This ocular function requires a proper development of an efficient macula of both the eyes; so that two clear and almost equally distinct images can be formed by each eye. Once two images are perceived on the retina, then an efficient nervous system is required to receive and interpret these two clear images as one image. In simpler words, SMP is the first grade of BSV and is considered as present when the signals transmitted from two eyes are received as one by visual cortex of the brain at the same time. Simultaneous perception does not mean that there is overlapping of the images of the same object or pictures rather, it simply means that two dissimilar objects are seen simultaneously as one. For example, two eyes are given separate stimuli like picture of a lion and picture of a cage, if simultaneous macular perception is present then the lion will look inside the cage as shown in Fig. 6.3 while in absence of SMP only one image will be seen at one time.

Fusion

Fusion or second grade of BSV is an ability of two eyes to compose a single picture from two similar pictures, each one of them is lacking

Note: Macular dominance is a condition where one eye sees the images of both the objects most of the time. Similarly, if both the images are seen alternatively by each eye then equal macular function is present.

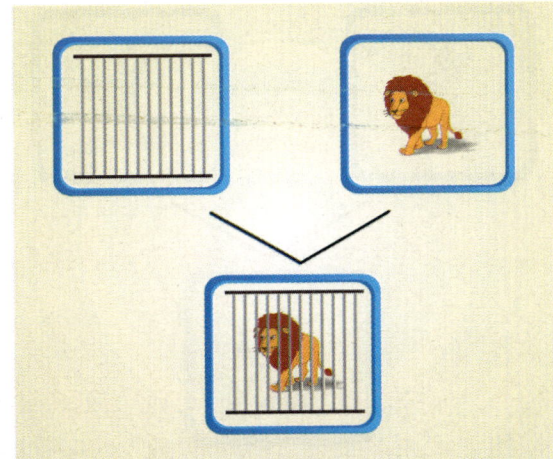

Fig. 6.3: Simultaneous macular perception

in a small detail. It simply means visual cortex combines two almost similar pictures as single complete picture. Facility of an ocular system to perceive two almost similar images from each eye as one single complete image is termed as sensory fusion and an ability of system to keep the eyes in alignment to maintain a sensory fusion is termed motor fusion.

Sensory fusion of images occurs only when two images are situated on their corresponding retinal area and are sufficiently similar in their size, brightness and sharpness. Sensory fusion is a foveal function and on contrary, motor fusion is an extra-foveal peripheral retinal function of ocular system.

Note: Both sensory and motor fusion occurs in visual cortex; so purely are central in origin.

For example, if eyes are presented with two pictures of rabbits, in which one rabbit is missing the tail and another is missing the bunch of flowers. If fusion is present, then only one rabbit will be seen having tail and holding a bunch of flowers (Fig. 6.4). Similarly, when two resembling letters like L and F are presented, then due to fusion only single letter E will be seen.

Similar to objects, the ocular system can also fuse two dissimilar colors when presented to both the eyes at the same time and the resultant color will be a different color (mixture of the two presented colors). This process is termed color fusion. For example, when red and yellow colors are presented together, then an orange color will be perceived by the visual system.

Stereopsis

This is the third grade of BSV and is an ability of two eyes to superimpose to a single picture from two pictures of the same object, each one of them are taken from slightly different angles. In horizontal plane eyes are slightly separated from each other and sensory fusion of two slightly separated unequal images in horizontal plane gives tridimensional perception. This is also called tridimensional vision because it gives an effect of depth perception. Objects lying on horopter are appreciated as flat because they causes zero horizontal disparity, however, objects situated in front or behind the horopter will give rise to non-zero disparities. When object is in front of the horopter, it produces crossed disparity because image of object from right eye is displaced towards left side and vice versa from left eye towards right side. Similarly, when object is behind the horopter, it produces an uncrossed disparity because when viewed monocularly the image of object viewed from right eye is displaced towards right and in left eye towards left.

For example, pictures of two buckets kept at slightly different angles are seen as a single bucket having three dimensions as shown in Fig. 6.5. Stereopsis is not synonymous with depth perception because depth perception is an assessment of distance of an object from observer or between two objects, whereas stereopsis means appreciation of three dimensions of an object during binocular vision.

Stereoscopic acuity: Ability of an ocular system to detect the smallest binocular disparity present in field of view is termed stereoscopic acuity (stereoacuity) and represents the minimum amount of disparity beyond which no stereopsis effect is seen. Usually a stereoscopic

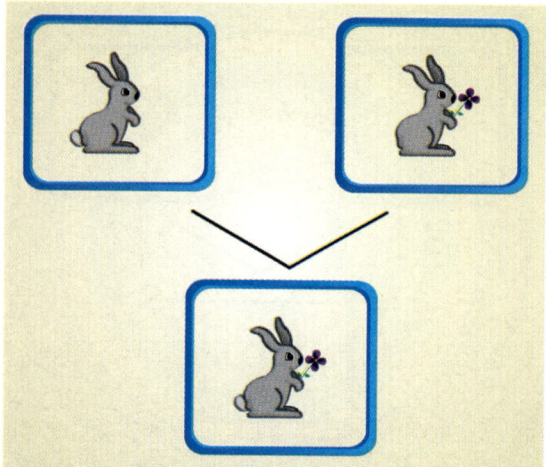

Fig. 6.4: Fusion

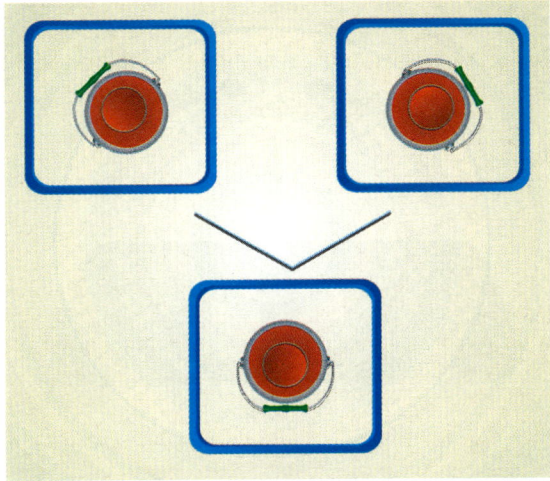

Fig. 6.5: Stereopsis

threshold of 20–30 arc seconds is considered as normal and a distance of about 150–200 meters is considered as critical distance beyond which streopsis effect is not appreciable. Stereoscopic acuity for stationary target is about 2–10 arc second, whereas for kinetic target it is in the range of 40–50 arc seconds.

As discussed above for perception of depth, stereopsis is must, however, several monocular clues which develop as a result of experience also give spatial orientations such as:

- *Geometric perspective:* At horizon the two parallel lines appear as if they are converging and ultimately vanishing. For example: Railway tracks.
- *Apparent size or linear perspective:* Large retinal images are interpreted as near objects while small retinal images are interpreted as distance objects. So, an object moving away from us appears as if progressively decreasing in size.
- *Relative velocity:* When a target is moving at far distance its image velocity appears lower as compared to image velocity of this moving target at near distance.
- *Aerial or Atmospheric perspective:* Distance objects appear indistinct due to scattering of light in atmosphere.
- *Motion parallax:* When focused at an intermediate distance the motion of

head leads to an opposite directional movement of near object image and same directional movement of distant object image, as that of head movement.
- *Overlapping contours or interposition:* Overlap in images determines the position of other object. For example, nearer objects have tendency to conceal distant objects and appear in front of distant objects.

Advantages of BSV

- Optical defects of one eye, if present, are masked by the image of opposite normal eye.
- Defective vision in a part of visual field of one eye is masked by other eye, because the same defect may not present in identical parts of two retinae. For example, blind spot caused due to optic nerve head is not seen in binocular visual field because image of the object which falls on blind spot of one eye is seen by retina of other eye and vice-versa.
- Binocular field of vision is larger than either field of one eye.
- Mobility of two eyes permits the person to converge the line of sight on a distant object and also helps to see a near object in its absolute distance.
- Stereopsis is most important and only advantage of BSV over monocular vision.
- Second eye is a safety factor against partial or complete loss of vision in one eye.

Evaluation of Binocular Vision

Following instruments are used to evaluate binocular vision and also sometimes to correct visual deficiency, if present.

- Synoptophore
- Stereoscope

Synoptophore

This instrument is used for the assessment of the degree of binocular function in terms of grades. Synoptophore is very useful for orthoptic exercises, which are required for development of the binocular function in cases of defective binocular vision (Fig. 6.6).

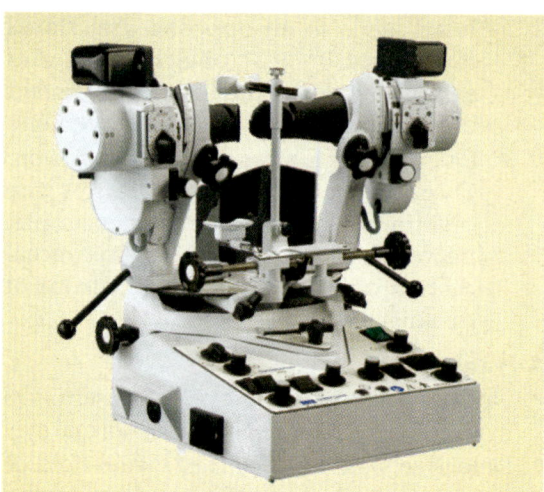

Fig. 6.6: Synoptophore

Synoptophore can also be used in cases of strabismus for

- Measurement of subjective and objective angles of strabismus.
- Diagnosis of latent or manifest strabismus.

Stereoscopes

In cases of binocular function deficiency, stereoscopes are very useful instruments for testing, training and home exercise purposes. Various types of stereoscopes are

- Fixed stereoscopes
- Kinetic stereoscopes
- Variable prism stereoscopes

Fixed stereoscopes: These instruments (e.g. Pigeon-cantonment stereoscope and Holme's and Whittington's stereoscope) are used to promote fusion and to treat uniocular suppression. Pigeon-cantonment instrument has two boards fitted with scales for measurement of angle of deviation. These boards are separated by a septum placed hinged book-wise and also has a mirror fixed in upper portion of septum. Patient has to place his/her nose against septum and tries to fuse the objects present on slides as shown in Fig. 6.7. Mirror present on septum can be covered if not required.

Kinetic stereoscopes: These instruments are used for fusion and stereopsis. In cases of

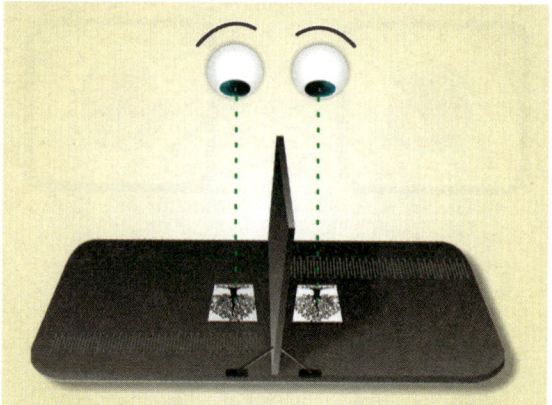

Fig. 6.7: Pigeon-cantonment stereoscope

small degree of incomitance deviation, it can be used for exercises at home because it facilitates swinging movement in all directions (fixed stereoscopes cannot be moved). Kinetic stereoscopes are only stereoscope which can be adjusted for both cyclophoria and hyperphoria.

Variable prism stereoscopes: These instruments (e.g. Cruise's stereoscope) are used for both testing and training purposes and utilize prisms which can be varied in strength as per requirement. Cruise's stereoscope (Fig. 6.8) is

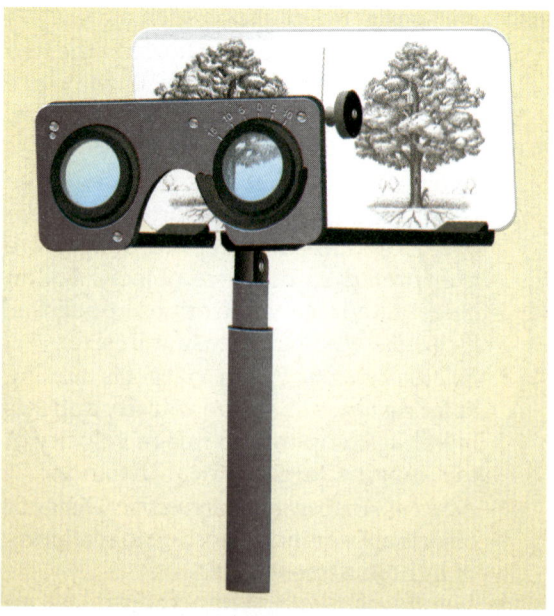

Fig. 6.8: Cruise's stereoscope

convenient for home teaching and training of amplitude of fusion in case of small degree strabismus. Prisms available in this instrument can be varied in strength up to 20 dioptres and can also be added for convergence if required. One of these prisms can be detached for providing vertical adjustment in cases of hyperphoria.

Various tests done for binocular vision are performed to assess
- SMP
- Fusion
- Stereopsis
- Retinal correspondence
- Suppression

Tests done to evaluate binocular single vision are summarized in Table 6.1.

Tests for SMP (Grade 1 BSV)

To test this primitive grade one binocularity, various slides having dissimilar pictures called SMP slides, are used in synoptophore. Commonly used SMP slides have pictures of lion and cage, parrot and cage, butterfly and net, etc.

These slides are projected in synoptophore and examine the superimposition of object images. Suppose superimposition is present for normal SMP slides, then by using SMP slides having targets of different sizes are presented to assess more accurate degree of simultaneous perception.

According to the size of target and angle subtended at nodal point of eye, these simultaneous perception slides are grouped as
- Foveal perception slides (1° angle)
- Parafoveal perception slides (1–3° angle)
- Paramacular perception slides (4–5° angle)
- Peripheral perception slides (more than 5° angle)

Tests for Fusion

Various tests done to evaluate the presence of fusion are
- Synoptophore test
- Worth four dot test
- Bagolini's striated glass test

Synoptophore test: Similar to SMP, fusion can be tested by synoptophore using fusion slides. These slides have two similar pictures differ in few details. For example, picture of rabbit in one slide missing tail and in another slide missing flowers in hand. When such slides are presented in synoptophore, then in presence of normal fusion the person will see a single rabbit having tail and flower in hand. Similarly, slides with letter L and with letter F will be fused as letter E when presented in synoptophore. Amplitude of fusion can be measured by help of synoptophore.

Table 6.1: Various tests done for binocular vision				
Tests for SMP	Tests for fusion	Tests for stereopsis	Tests for retinal correspondence	Tests for suppression
Synoptophore using SMP slides	• Synoptophore test • Worth four dot test • Bagolini's striated glass test	• Lang two pencil test • Titmus stereo tests • Random dot test • Lang test • Frisby test	• Worth's four dot test • Bagolini's striated glasses test • Synoptophore using SMP slides • Red filter test • After image test • Binocular visuoscopy test	• Bagolini's test • Red filter test • Worth's four dot test • Friend test • Synoptophore method • Four dioptre base out prism test

Table 6.2: Normal fusional amplitudes for different types of vergence

Vergence		Fusional amplitude (in prisms)
Horizontal	Convergence	35–40
	Divergence	5–8
Vertical	Supravergence	2–3
	Infravergence	2–3
Cyclovergence		4–5

Range of normal fusional amplitude in prisms is shown in Table 6.2.

For restoration of BSV fusion is must and assessment of fusion is required to manage and evaluate the prognosis of squint.

Tests For Stereopsis

Based on presentation of targets stereopsis tests are

- Three-dimensional targets are used in Lang's two pencil test. Gross stereopsis (either present or absent) of threshold 3000–4000 arc seconds can be tested by this method. Examiner and patient both hold the pointed tip pencils in their hand. Examiner holds the pencil vertically in front of the patient and instructs him/her to touch the tip of his pencil by the tip of his/her pencil; first with both eyes open and then with one eye closed.

    Interpretation: When patient touches the pencil tip with both eyes open, then gross stereopsis is present. However, with one eye closed patient will not be able to touch the pencil tip of examiner. In the absence of stereopsis even with both eyes open patient will not be able to touch the pencil tip of examiner.

- Two-dimensional targets are constructed in such a manner that they stimulate disparate retinal area and produce the effect of three dimensions. Following tests utilize this principle
    - Titmus stereo tests
    - Random dot tests
    - Lang test
    - Frisby test

Titmus stereo test and random dot tests require special types of glasses like Polaroid or red green, whereas Lang test and Frisby test can be performed with or without special glasses. These tests can also be grouped under vectographs tests and stereogram tests, respectively.

Vectographs tests: Principle of vectographs: The vectographs consist of plates made up of polarized materials on which target pictures are imprinted. These targets are polarized in such a manner that they are at 90° to each other and hence when viewed through special polaroid glasses they appear as two separate targets.

Titmus stereo test: Titmus stereo test is done by using a booklet made up of two plates consisting a three-dimensional polaroid vectographs. One plate on right side of this booklet is imprinted with a picture of house fly, whereas left sided plate is imprinted with pictures of animals and circles. Hence, Titmus stereo test consists of three components of examination. This booklet is viewed wearing polaroid glasses (Fig. 6.9).

- Titmus fly test is the first component of test which can evaluate gross stereopsis of 3000 arc seconds. Picture of a large housefly is imprinted on the plate, hence very useful in assessing stereopsis in young children. Booklet is kept at reading distance and polaroid spectacles are worn by patient. To test instruct the patient to hold the wings of housefly on the plate.

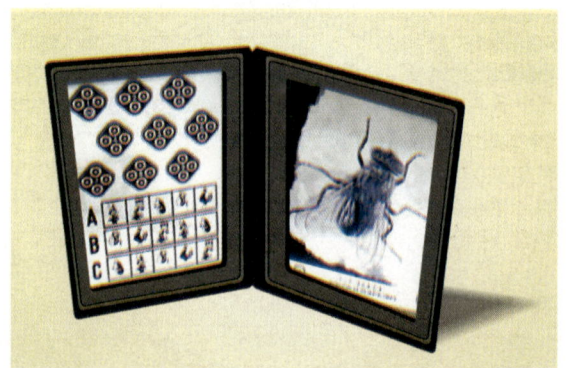

Fig. 6.9: Titmus stereo test

Interpretation: If stereopsis is present, the patient will reach above the plate and try to hold wings, however, in absence of stereopsis the picture appears as flat housefly. This test can assess only gross near stereopsis, distance stereopsis cannot be tested by this Titmus fly test.

- Titmus animal test is the second component of test and consists of three rows of animal pictures, representing threshold of 100, 200 and 400 arc seconds, respectively. Each row has pictures of five animals, among these five animals one animal is imaged disparately and one animal is outlined darker serving as misleading clue. Patient is asked to select that animal which stands out compared to other animals from each row.

Interpretation: If stereopsis is present, then patient will select the animal imaged disparately and if stereopsis is absent, then patient will select the darker outlined animal.

- Titmus circle test is the third component of test and contain set of nine squares, arranged three in each row. Each square has four circles arranged in the form of a rhomboid as shown in Fig. 6.9. At random, one circle out of four circles in each square is imaged disparately, producing a threshold in the range of 40 to 800 arc seconds.

If the patient has successfully cleared initial two components of Titmus stereo test, then ask him/her to push down the circle which is standing outwards as compared to other circles in each square. Remember to start testing from first square because threshold gradually decreases from first square to last.

Interpretation: Amount of stereopsis threshold is represented by the number of circle pushed down correctly by the patient. Lowest limit of fine stereoacuity is assumed as 100 arc seconds and is represented by circle of square number 5. Any stereoacuity below this limit (represented by circle of square number from 6 to 9) is considered as excellent.

Advantages
- Titmus stereo test is simpler and convenient.
- Useful to assess stereopsis even in young children
- Results can be easily interpreted in terms of stereoacuity threshold

Disadvantages
Require polaroid glasses, sometimes very young child may resist to wear glasses.

Stereogram tests: Principle of stereogram: These tests utilize a stereogram target. These stereogram tests give no monocular clues to the patient hence, the patient is unable to presume the type and location of stereogram picture in the test plate. So, these tests are considered as real assessment of stereoacuity as compared to Titmus stereo tests. This principle is used in these following tests.

Random dot tests: These tests utilize the random dot stereogram for testing of stereopsis. Following tests are included in random dot test
- Random dot E test
- TNO random dot test
- Lang test

Random dot E test: This test is performed by using three test cards having random dots patterns. The first card is a model E, second card is a stereo E and third card is a blank card. Model E card has letter E with random dot background and is shown to patient as reference card for him/her to understand what they should look in the coming cards. Second card is a stereo E card contains a letter E with random dot background, where letter E is visible only with Polaroid spectacles. Third card is a blank card having similar random dot background as that of stereo E card (Fig. 6.10).

To test stereopsis, ask the patient to wear polaroid spectacles, then show him/her model E card and explain the procedure. Now, from 20 inches distance show the stereo E card and blank card at random to the patient and ask

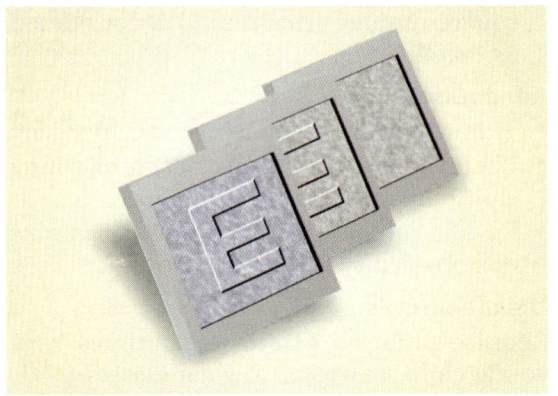

Fig. 6.10: Random dot E test (*see* text)

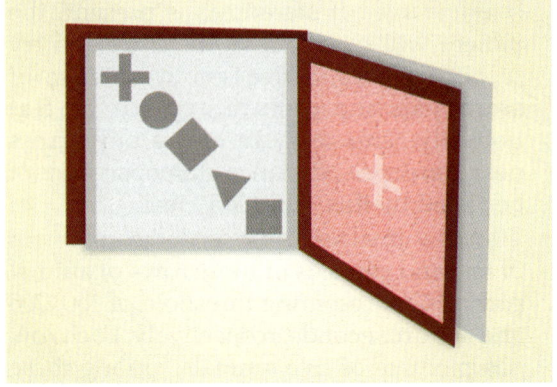

Fig. 6.11: TNO random dot test (*see* text)

the patient whether he/she can see the letter E or not.

Interpretation: If patient is able to tell correctly in which card letter E is present, then stereopsis is present. When stereopsis is present, to quantify the stereoacuity increase the testing distance of card from patient.

TNO random dot test: This test is based on the similar principle as that of random dot E test and it provides stereoacuity threshold in the range of 480 to 15 arc second. In this test stereoacuity can be quantified without altering the testing distance.

This test utilizes a booklet having seven stereogram plates, among them first set of three plates are for screening purposes and second set of remaining four plates are used to quantify the stereopsis. First set of plates can be tested with or without wearing the red green spectacle and used to assess only the gross stereopsis. For second set of stereogram plates red green glasses are required to visualize the stereogram figure. Each test plates has stereogram of various shapes like square, circle, triangles or crosses, made by the help of random dots in complementary colors (Fig. 6.11).

Patients are first shown the screening sterogram plates and if patient qualifies then the second set of stereogram plates are shown. Patient is asked to wear red green glasses and from a distance of 40 cm second set of stereogram plates are shown.

Interpretation: If patient see all the stereogram figures in first set of three plates then gross stereopsis is present. Quantification of stereoacuity is done by identification of correct stereogram pictures in second set of plates.

Lang test: This test comprises Lang I (Fig. 6.12A) and Lang II (Fig. 6.12B) tests. Both these tests are done by the utilization of random dot stereogram test cards having different sets

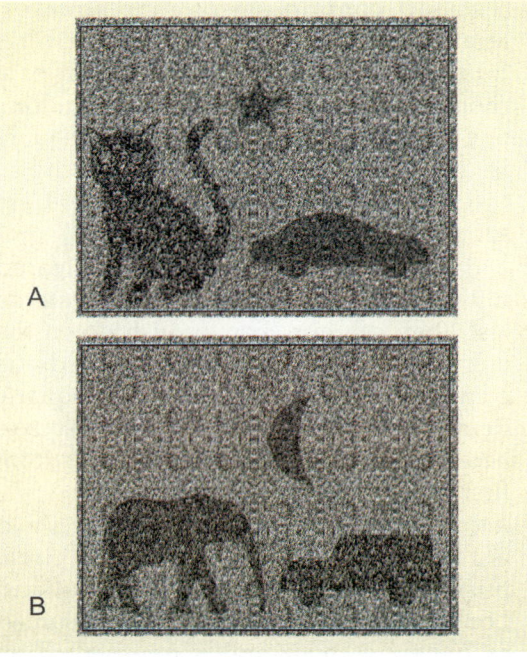

Fig. 6.12: Lang test (*see* text). A. Lang I test card; B. Lang II test card

of stereoscopic images. Lang I test card has stereoscopic images of cat (1200 arc seconds), car (600 arc sec) and star (550 arc second); whereas Lang II test cards has stereoscopic images of elephant (600 arc seconds), car (400 arc sec) and moon (200 arc sec). These images are embedded in random dots pattern on test card and are seen disparately by each eye through cylindrical lenses imprinted on laminated surface of test card; so no special glasses are needed to perform this test.

Patient is asked to hold the test card at 40 cm distance and identify the stereoscopic image and its relative position in card.

Interpretation: If patient correctly identifies the image and its location on test card means stereopsis is present. Stereoacuity threshold can be measured by the different size images identified by the patient.

Frisby test: In this test three plastic plates of various thickness (6 mm, 3 mm and 1.5 mm) are used as stereogram, and each plate consists of four squares in it. Arrow heads of various size and orientations are imprinted on both the sides of these plates in different positions. One of the square in each plate has a hidden circle which can be seen disparately (Fig. 6.13).

The disparity is produced by the displacement of random shape arrow heads due to thickness of plastic plates. There is no need of special glasses for this test and hence is very useful in young children who resist wearing of spectacles. Initially these plates are shown from a 40 cm distance starting from 6 mm thickness and if stereopsis present then it can be quantified by increasing the test distance to 80 cm.

Tests For Retinal Correspondence

Retinal correspondence can be tested by the following methods

- Evaluate the relationship between retinal elements of fixating eye and deviated eye which are stimulated simultaneously. Based on this principle following tests are done
  - Worth's four dot test
  - Bagolini's striated glasses test
  - Synoptophore method using SMP slides
  - Red filter test
- Evaluate the direction of visual axes in two corresponding fovea. Based on this principle following tests are done
  - After image test
  - Binocular visuoscopy test (foveo-foveal test of Cuppers)

Bagolini's striated glasses test: This test utilizes Bagolini's striated glasses and the examiner observes the ocular movements during test procedure. During this test, eyes are not dissociated hence it represents normal visual atmosphere. Bagolini's glasses are glass plates which are striated very finely in different orientation and are commonly referred as

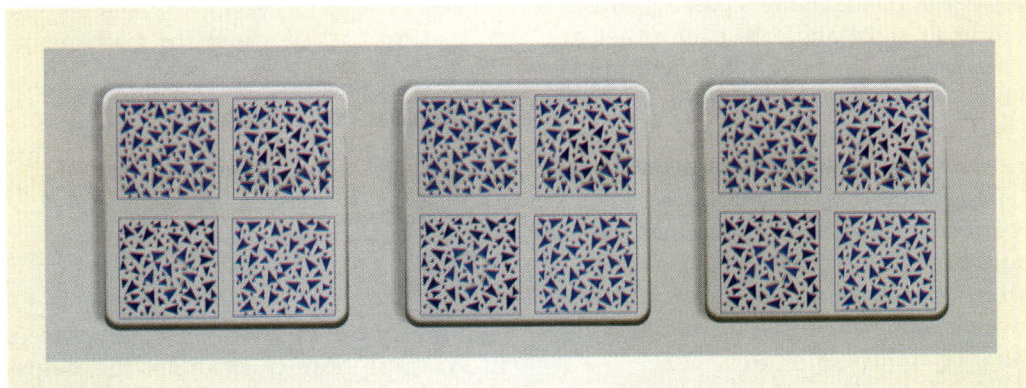

Fig. 6.13: Frisby test (*see* text)

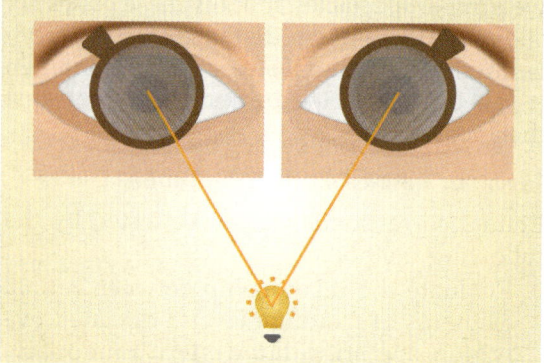

Fig. 6.14: Bagolini's test (*see text*)

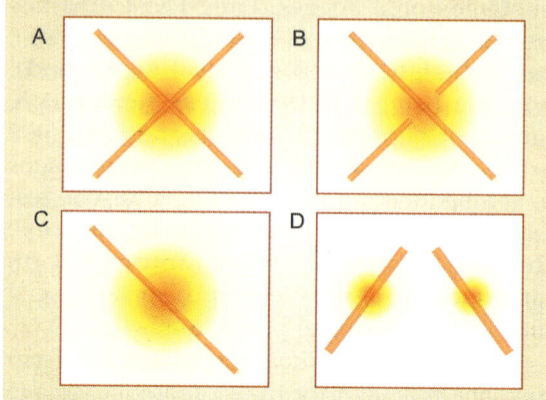

Fig. 6.15: Interpretation of Bagolini's test. A. NRC or harmonious ARC; B. Unharmonious ARC or NRC with suppression; C. Suppression; D. NRC without suppression

Bagolini's lenses (without refractive power). These glasses are mounted in a frame so that can be used in a trial frame for testing purposes. Light spot will appear as fine line perpendicular to the orientations of striations (similar to Maddox rods) and hence forms the basis for testing the retinal correspondence.

- Place two Bagolini's lenses in trial frame one in front of each eye, oriented at angles of 45° and 135° as shown in Fig. 6.14.
- Patient is asked to fixate at a small bright point light source shown by examiner from distance of 20 feet for distance and from 40 cm for near examination.
- Ask the patient about the orientation of lines seen through glasses.
- Now cover one eye with occluder and again ask the patient about orientation of lines.
- Results are interpret as follows
  a. A perfect cross of lines passing through light at right angle to each other and no deviation on cover test will be seen by a patient in case of NRC as shown in Fig. 6.15A.
  b. Patient with manifest squint will show any one of these results.
- A perfect cross with crossing lines passing through central light will also be seen by patient in case of harmonious ARC, however, on cover test a deviation will be seen (Fig. 6.15A).
- Cross of lines where one line is not passing through central light will be seen by patient

having unharmonious ARC or suppression with NRC (Fig. 6.15B).
- Single line will be seen by patient in case of complete suppression. This single line will be seen towards non-suppressed eye (Fig. 6.15C).
- Two lines having two light sources, not crossing each other will be seen by patient having diplopia without suppression in NRC situation (Fig. 6.15D).

Advantages
- Simple and easy test
- No requirement of expensive equipment
- Eyes are not dissociated, hence resembles with normal conditions during testing.
- Testing can be done for both near and distance vision.

Disadvantages
- Test results are only qualitative. Quantitative analysis (measurement of angle of deviation) is not done.
- Small degree of deviation is not assessed because it gets unnoticed.

Synoptophore method: SMP slides are used in synoptophore to evaluate the degree of deviation in visual axis by measuring the angle of anomaly. Subjective and objective angles of deviation are calculated by synopto-phore method and difference between these two angles represents the angle of anomaly.

- Patient is instructed to look inside the synoptophore tubes by placing chin over chin rest and fixing the forehead against head rest.
- Both the arms of synoptophore are adjusted at zero mark.
- Examiner places the SMP slides in their respective slots and flashes the light of instrument alternately. Simultaneously examiner rotates both the arms of synoptophore till there is no fixation movement done by eye of patient. This serves as alternate cover test.
- Record the reading of both the arms of synoptophore. Sum of these two reading is equal to the magnitude of objective angle of anomaly.
- Now slowly move one arm of synoptophore till the patient superimposes the targets (say lion and cage). Record the reading on arm of synoptophore; this is equal to magnitude of subjective angle of anomaly.
- Results are interpreted as
  - Difference between objective and subjective angles give the angle of anomaly
  - When subjective angle is equal to objective angle, then patient has NRC
  - When objective angle is more than subjective angle, then patient has ARC
  - When objective angle is equal to angle of anomaly (means subjective angle is zero), then patient has harmonious ARC
  - When objective angle is more than angle of anomaly, then patient has unharmonious ARC

Red filter test: This test utilizes a red filter to evaluate the status of visual field in cases of manifest strabismus and various responses are interpreted in terms of retinal correspondence.

- Place a trial frame on patient's eyes and instruct the patient to fixate on a white point light source situated at distance of 20 feet.
- Place a red filter in trial frame in front of deviating eye and ask the patient about the light perceptions. Results are interpreted as follows
  - If only one pink color (mixture of white and red color) light is seen by patient at the position of white light, then it indicates presence of harmonious ARC. Because in presence of manifest squint single light with mixed color indicates an ARC.
  - Two lights (one white and other red) will be seen by patient in case of NRC. Suppose if red filter is placed in front of the right eye and the patient see red light on the right side of white light, then it indicates presence of uncrossed (homonymous) diplopia as seen in case of esodeviation. In contrary, when red light is seen on the left side of the white light, then it indicates crossed (heteronymous) diplopia as in case of exodeviation.
  - In above situation when distance between two images is measured and found to be lesser than the magnitude of deviation of eyes, then it represents a case of unharmonious ARC.
  - Only one light (usually white) is seen by patient in case of suppression, however, occasionally single red light may be seen by patient depending upon density of red filter and amount of dominance of other eye.

After image test: Hering Bielschwsky discovered an orthoptic test by dissociating two after images of two eyes, which is popularly called Hering Bielschwsky after image test. He utilized two bright glowing filaments having central black spot (to protect fovea), among them one filament is oriented vertically and another horizontally. These vertical and horizontal filaments produced vertical and horizontal after images, respectively (Fig. 6.16).

- Patient is made to sit comfortably in examination room with dim illumination.
- Patient is instructed to cover his/her left eye with palm of hand and right eye is illuminated with a horizontal glowing

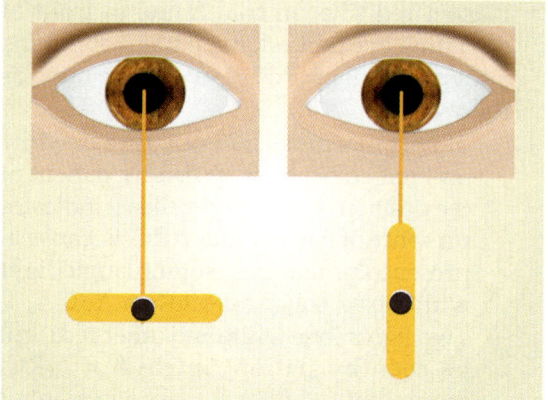

Fig. 6.16: After image test (*see* text)

filament (preferably camera flash light) for 20 seconds. Patient is instructed to fixate at central black spot of filament.

- Similarly, left eye of patient is illuminated with vertical light for 20 seconds, while patient is fixating the central black spot.
- Patient is asked either to close the eyes or look at blank screen at distance and draw the after images as he/she perceives.
- Results of patient's drawing of after images are interpreted as:
  - Symmetrical cross with blank central area (representing fovea) is drawn by patient having NRC. Even if there is a presence of either esodeviation or exodeviation with NRC, patient will still draw a symmetrical cross (Fig. 6.17A).

- Asymmetrical cross is drawn by patient having ARC, where central blank area is separated. The distance of separation of central blank area depends on the magnitude of angle of anomaly. For example, in case of patient having left esotropia with ARC will draw after images of vertical line towards right side of horizontal line as shown in Fig. 6.17B.
- Similarly, in case of patient having left exotropia with ARC will draw after images of vertical line towards left side of horizontal line as shown in Fig. 6.17C.
- Single horizontal line with a central blank area is drawn by patient having suppression in the left eye as shown in Fig. 6.17D.

Binocular visuscope test: This test is also known as foveo-foveal Cupper's test because invented by eminent scientist Cupper and this test determines the retinal correspondence by stimulating fovea of two eyes. In case of eccentric fixation the quantitative analysis of angle of anomaly can be done by assessing the visual directions of two fovea.

- Patient is made to sit comfortably at 15 feet distance from a Maddox tangent scale.
- Examiner instructs the patient to fixate at central light on scale with fixating eye while, examiner looks into the macula of deviated eye by a visuscope.

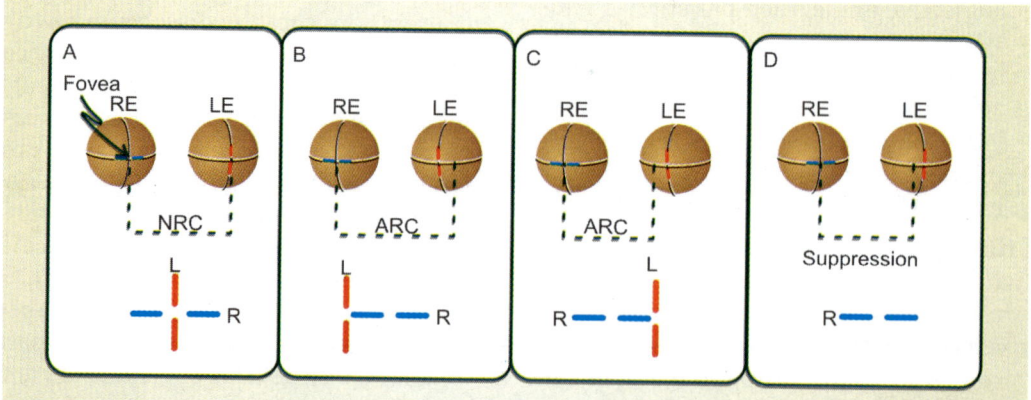

Fig. 6.17: Interpretation of after image test

- Practically, it is difficult for examiner to look into visuscope without blocking the view of patient. Hence, patient is asked to fixate via looking in a plane mirror or prism placed in front of his/her fixating eye.
- Now examiner projects an asterisk of visuscope on the retina of the deviated eye of patient.
- Once asterisk is focused on retina of the patient, the examiner asks the patient to visualize the position of asterisk on tangent scale in relation to fixating light (Fig. 6.18).
- Results are interpreted as
  - When asterisk of visuscope is seen coinciding with fixation light of tangent scale by the patient then it is a case of NRC as shown in (Fig. 6.19A).
  - When asterisk is seen either right or left of fixation light of scale by the patient then it is a case of ARC as shown in Fig. 6.19B. The number corresponding with the position of asterisk on tangent scale is equal to the magnitude of angle of anomaly.
- After confirmation of ARC the corresponding position of peripheral retinal element in the deviating eye having common visual direction with fixating eye can be examined by further modifying this test.
- Examiner moves the visuscope until the patient see the asterisk is coinciding with central light of tangent scale.

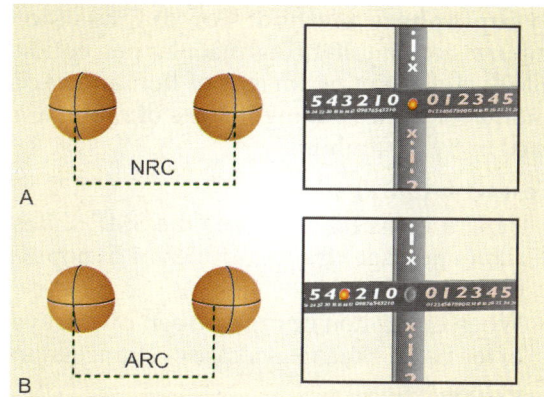

Fig. 6.19: Interpretation of binocular visuscope test

- At this point of examination position of asterisk on patient's retina is seen by examiner through the visuscope.
- The position of asterisk on the retina in the deviated eye of patient indicates the retinal element of this squinted eye corresponding with the common visual direction of fixating eye.

Disadvantages
- It is very complex test and cannot be performed on young children.
- This test requires sophisticated instruments and reasonable amount of practice to perform.

Tests For Suppression

As discussed to prevent confusion and diplopia due to unwanted stimuli, the image of one eye is suppressed by a central or peripheral inhibitory mechanism. Various tests done to evaluate the suppression in eyes are as follows
- Bagolini's test
- Red filter test
- Worth's four dot test
- Friend test
- Synoptophore method
- Four dioptre base out prism test

> **Note:** We have discussed Bagolini's test and red filter test, on page no 120–121, whereas Worth's four dot test and Friend test will be discussed later.

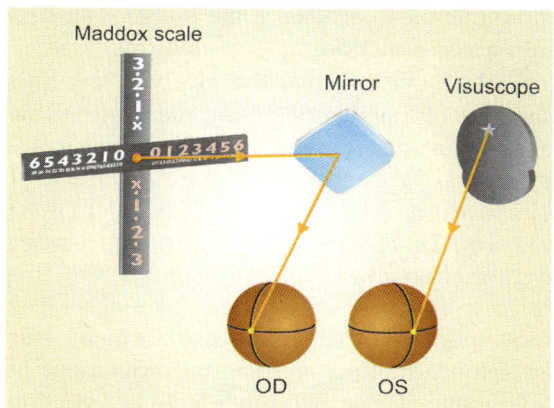

Fig. 6.18: Binocular visuscope test (*see text*)

Synoptophore method: For diagnosis of suppression simultaneous macular perception (SMP) slides having images of lion and cage and fusion slides having images of rabbit are used in Synoptophore.

Test with (SMP) slides

- Patient is instructed to see the SMP slides (lion and cage) through tubes of Synoptophore.
- When either lion or cage is seen by the eye of the patient then it is a case of suppression of that respective eye.
- Suppose suppression is present, then to quantify it we can modify this method as follows
  - Start with foveal slides and suppose foveal suppression is present then show the macular slides.
  - When patient has suppression in macular slides, then show the Paramacular slides.
  - When patient shows suppression even in Paramacular slides, then it is a case of total suppression of one eye.

Test with fusion slides

- Patient is instructed to see the fusion slides (rabbit with tail and rabbit with flower) placed in Synoptophore slots.
- When patient sees single image of rabbit with tail holding flowers means NRC is present.
- When patient sees rabbit is missing either in tail or flower, then suppression is present of respective eye.
- Grading of fusion slides can be done by decreasing the size of images similar to SMP slides.

By Synoptophore method suppression scotoma can be mapped in horizontal meridian as follows

- One arm of Synoptophore is moved and asks the patient at what point the target of that side disappears and reappears. Record the values at this point of disappear and reappear of target on Synoptophore. This point indicates the position of scotoma in visual field.

Four dioptre base out prism test: This test is based on the principle of image displacement and then evaluation of the resultant ocular movements whether binocular or monocular. This is an easy and fast screening test to evaluate the presence and absence of bifoveal fusion and suppression of one fovea.

- Patient is instructed to fixate a point light source at 20 feet distance.
- A 4Δ is placed in front of one eye (say right eye) keeping it in a base out position.
- Examiner observe the binocular movements (version) and monocular (left eye in our example) movement (fusional) after placing this base out prism in front of patient's eye.
- Results are interpreted as
  - In normal condition a biphasic movement of left eye (in our example) will be seen by examiner.
  - In case of central suppression scotoma no biphasic movement will be seen, rather only an outward (version) movement of left eye will be seen.
  - Repeat this procedure for other eye (left eye in our example) to check the biphasic movement of fellow eye.

Biphasic movement of the eye is elicited due to sudden displacement of a foveal image by the effect of base out prism. This sudden displacement of image leads to a refixating movement of eye when image is shifted into a normally functioning fovea, however, no movement will be seen if the image is shifted into a non-functioning (scotomatous) area.

Fellow eye follows the Hering' law and shows a biphasic movement; means first this eye moves simultaneously and symmetrically in outward direction with the movement of eye under examination. This is termed version of fellow eye. When eye under examination takes a refixating movement, this fellow eye will show an opposite slow movement to correct image displacement. This is termed duction or fusional movement of fellow eye. These two movements of version and duction in a phasic manner is termed biphasic movement of fellow eye. However, when a central scotoma is present, the second fusional movement is absent due to an impaired function of fovea and as a result eye remains slightly outward rotated.

ANISOMETROPIA

Introduction

The optical condition of the eyes where both the eyes have equal refractive power is called isometropia. Anisometropia or Asymmetropia means that the refractive power in two eyes is not equal so that focus formed are also different in two eyes. A small amount of anisometropia is very commonly seen in population but it has no visual concern. For example: The difference of 1 D refractive power in two eyes will produce unequal size and image on the retina of 2% only.

A person can well tolerate the anisometropic difference of up to 2.5 D at which retinal images of two eyes have a difference of about 5% in size of image. Whereas, anisometropia of 2.5 to 4 D can be tolerated by some but the difference of more than 4 D in both eyes is not tolerated and produce symptoms.

Classification

Anisometropia can be classified as shown in Table 6.3.

Etiological types

- *Congenital or developmental anisometropia:* It is hereditary in origin and develops due to disproportional growth between two eyeballs.

Table 6.3: Classification of anisometropia	
Etiological types	Clinical types
• Congenital or developmental anisometropia	• Simple anisometropia
	• Compound anisometropia
• Acquired or iatrogenic anisometropia	• Mixed anisometropia (antimetropia)

- *Acquired anisometropia* may develop as a result of various surgeries performed on eyeball or other reasons, ultimately causing change in the axial length of the eyeball.

It can be caused by:
  - Uniocular keratoplasty
  - Improper refractive surgery
  - Uniocular aphakia, i.e. lens is extracted from one eye due to various reasons like trauma or cataract.
  - Pseudophakia with placement of inaccurate intraocular lens power
  - Uniocular traumatic injury

Clinical Types

- *Simple anisometropia:* In this type only one eye is affected with refractive error while the other eye is normal (emmetropic). Depending on the type of refractive error present in affected eye it can be
  - Simple hypermetropic: One eye is normal and the other eye is hypermetropic.
  - Simple myopic: One eye is normal and the other eye is myopic.
  - Simple astigmatic: One eye is normal and the other eye is having simple hypermetropic or myopic astigmatism.

- *Compound anisometropia:* In this type of anisometropia both the eyes have same type of refractive error, i.e. myopia, hypermetropia or astigmatism, but there is significant difference in their refractive power. It may be
  - Compound myopic: Both eyes have myopia with different power
  - Compound hypermetropic: Both eyes have hypermetropia with different power
  - Compound astigmatic: Both eyes have astigmatism with different degree.

- *Mixed anisometropia (antimetropia):* In this type both the eyes have different types of refractive errors, means one eye is affected with myopia and the other with hypermetropia. Similarly, in mixed astigmatic anisometropia one eye is affected with hypermetropic astigmatism and the other with myopic astigmatism.

Effects of Anisometropia on Binocular Vision

Depending on the difference of refractive power and refractive error in both eyes binocular vision may be affected in the following ways:

- **Difference of small degree (<2 D) of aniso-metropia:** Binocular single vision take place.
- **Difference of high degree (>4–5 D) of anisometropia:** Binocular vision is lost and only uniocular vision is present. The eye which has refractive error of high degree is suppressed by other eye, and patient develops suppression amblyopia (termed anisometropic amblyopia) and strabismus, leading to poor vision in this eye.
- **Different types of refractive error in both eyes:** When one eye is either emmetrope or low degree hypermetrope while the other eye is myopic, then alternate vision is present. Person will see the distant object with emmetropic/hypermetrope eye and the near objects with myopic eye. Usually these patients remain asymptomatic and do not use any optical correction.

Examination Methods

- **Retinoscopy:** Patients complaining of defective vision either in one eye or both eyes need retinoscopic examination to confirm the diagnosis of anisometropia.

  Tests to check status of binocular vision
  - *FRIEND test:* In this test the word FRIEND is incorporated in Snellen's chart. Letters FIN are written in green color, whereas RED are written in red color. Now patient is advised to sit at 6 meters distance wearing a red green goggle (diplopia goggle). The red color lens of goggle is kept in front of the right eye and green in front of the left eye. Ask the patient to read the letters (Fig. 6.20).

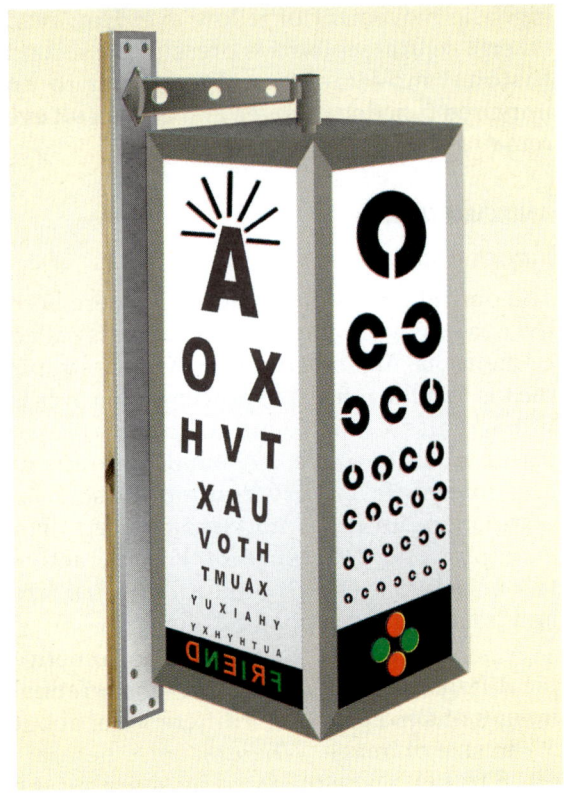

Fig. 6.20: FRIEND test (*see* text)

Result is interpreted as

- If patient read all letters as FRIEND at once, then binocular vision is present.
- If patient read either FIN or RED letters, then uniocular vision is present in the corresponding eye.
- If patient read FIN at one time and RED other time, then alternate vision is present
  - *Worth's four dot test:* This test comprises a view box having four lights, i.e. one red, two green and one white. This view box is placed at 6 meters distance. Patient is asked to wear diplopia goggle keeping red lens in front of the right eye and green lens in front of the left eye as shown in Fig. 6.21.

Patient is asked to see the four dot lights and possible outcomes are interpreted as

- If no manifest squint is present and patient sees all four lights as they are seen in Fig. 6.21A

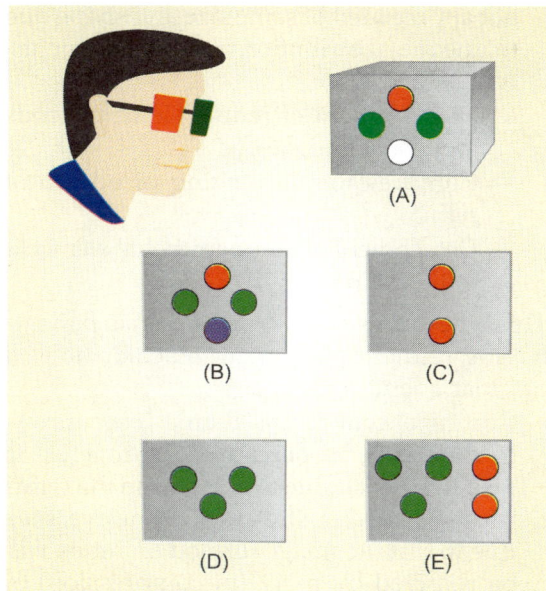

Fig. 6.21: Worth four dot test (*see* text)

means this individual has normal binocular single vision.

- When squint is manifested and patient sees all four lights where white light is seen as violet as shown in **Fig. 6.21B** means patient has abnormal retinal correspondence.
- Suppose the patient sees only two red color lights as shown in **Fig. 6.21C** means the left eye suppression is present.
- When the patient sees only three green color lights as shown in **Fig. 6.21D** it means that the right eye suppression is present.
- If patient alternately sees two red lights and three green lights as shown in **Fig. 6.21E** means an alternate suppression is present.
- Similarly when patient sees five lights, i.e. two red and three green as shown in **Fig. 6.21E** but continuously, it means that this patient has diplopia.

Treatment of Anisometropia

Optical Correction

Optical correction can be given in the form of spectacles or contact lens

- **Spectacles:** Corrective glasses can be prescribed in anisometropia up to a

difference of 4 D because difference of > 4 D will not be tolerated by patient and will produce diplopia. In case of difference > 4 D, alternate methods like contact lenses must be prescribed. In children, it is preferred to give full correction to prevent amblyopia. In anisometropic adults best correction of visual acuity can be achieved with some compromise and usually the eye having more refractive error is undercorrected. For example, a patient having best corrected visual acuity with powers of +4 D and +9 D and is not able to tolerate these lenses then a spectacle with power of +4 D and +7 D can be prescribed.

Anisometropic spectacles are special types of spectacles used to treat anisometropia. In these types of spectacles to minimize the peripheral prismatic effect (occurring due to strong lens) the margins of stronger lenses are kept weaker **(Fig. 6.22)**.

- **Contact lenses:** Use of contact lens is a better mode of treatment than spectacles as they are better tolerated and has less chances of diplopia. Contact lenses are useful in young children and patients having high degree of anisometropia.

Surgical Correction

Various surgical modalities are widely used and are very effective for correction of high degree of anisometropia. They include

- Intraocular lens implantation in cases of uniocular aphakia.

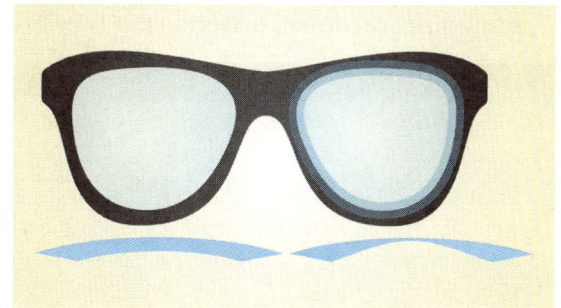

Fig. 6.22: Anisometropic spectacles

- Corneal refractive surgery for high degree uniocular myopia, hypermetropia or astigmatism.
- Clear lens extraction in cases of high degree unilateral myopia.

ANISEIKONIA

Introduction

Aniseikonia (An = not, iso = equal, ikon = images) is a binocular vision abnormality wherein the ocular images presented to the visual cortex from both the eyes are unequal in size and/or shape. It is not an uncommon condition and can cause distressing symptoms to patient.

Classification

Aniseikonia can be classified as shown in Table 6.4.

Etiological Types

The formation of unequal images may be due to:

- Optical or dioptric aniseikonia: It occurs due to difference in the dioptric size of images formed on the retina of two eyes. It may be inherent (congenital defect in the dioptric system of eye) or acquired (may arise due to difference in the power, shape or position of the corrective lens worn for refractive conditions, aphakia or uncorrected anisometropia).
- Anatomical or retinal aniseikonia: It occurs due to difference in the distribution of retinal elements (rods and cones) in the eye. Due to this even if the dioptric images of same size are formed on retina but they are not appreciated of same size and shape due to unequal distribution of retinal elements. It may be due to:
  - Displacement of retinal elements (rods and cones) in one eye
  - Compression, stretching or edema of retina
  - Detachment of neuroepithelial elements of the retina

This type of aniseikonia can be seen in patients having retinal detachment, macular hole or macular edema, etc.

- Cortical or central aniseikonia: It occurs due to difference in perception of images on visual cortex. If due to any reason the retina is compressed or stretched in one eye, then due to this the image formed on retina will be received by more (in compression) or lesser (in stretching) number of receptors or retinal elements (rods and cones) in that eye, leading to asymmetrical perception of images from both eyes through visual pathways. The image received by visual cortex would appear smaller (micropsia) if fewer elements were stimulated and vice versa if more retinal elements are stimulated.

Clinical Types

Aniseikonia can also be classified on the basis of types of images seen by the patient. Suppose if in a patient right eye is affected and he/she has normal vision in left eye (Fig. 6.23), then various images seen by him/her can be classified as:

Symmetrical aniseikonia (Fig. 6.23): It means the size of image in one eye differ from other eye in all meridians or in one meridian. It may be

- *Spherical or overall:* In this type the size of image is symmetrically increased or decreased in all directions or meridians.
- *Cylindrical or meridional:* In this type size of image is symmetrically increased or decreased in one meridian only (may be horizontal, vertical or oblique).
- *Compound:* In this type the image formed is a mixture of both as spherical and cylindrical.

Table 6.4: Classification of aniseikonia

Etiological types	Clinical types	
	Symmetrical	*Asymmetrical*
• Optical aniseikonia	• Spherical	• Prismatic
• Retinal aniseikonia	• Cylindrical	• Pin cushion
	• Compound	• Barrel
• Cortical aniseikonia		• Oblique

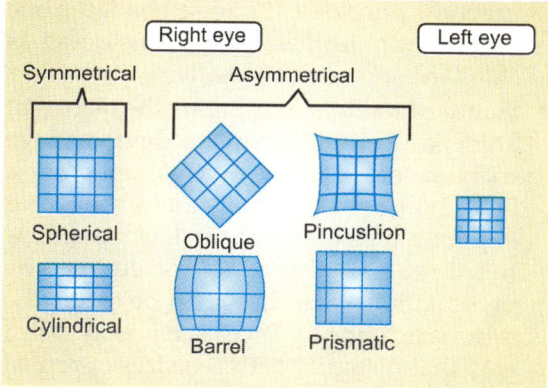

Fig. 6.23: Right-sided aniseikonia

Asymmetrical aniseikonia (Fig. 6.23)

- *Prismatic:* The image distortion increases progressively in one direction or meridian only.
- *Pincushion:* The image difference progressively increases in both the directions (as seen in aphakia after high plus correction).
- *Barrel distortion:* It is reverse of pincushion effect. The image distortion progressively decreases in both the directions. For example, giving high minus correction.
- *Oblique distortion:* Here size of images remains same but shape is obliquely distorted.

Clinical Presentation

Aniseikonia is well tolerated by many patients without causing any symptoms; on the contrary, a few patients may develop severe symptoms even with small amount of aniseikonia. When the difference in size of retinal images or the distortion of images reaches the tolerance limit of person these symptoms become a clinical entity and need treatment for aniseikonia. Usually, difference of more than 1% in image size and meridional distortion of >0.30 is associated with symptoms and require corrections.

Symptoms

Various symptoms of aniseikonia can be grouped as

- **Subjective symptoms:** Manifest in the form of asthenopic or eye strain symptoms due to difference in image size of more than 1% between two eyes. Person may complaint of blurred vision, photophobia, difficulty in reading, poor fixation and neurological manifestations such as headache, nausea, vertigo, nervousness, fatigue, etc. Visual fatigue is usually precipitated while patient is watching movies or reading books for longer duration. Severity of these symptoms are not related to the amount of aniseikonia rather depends on individual's tolerance to aniseikonia.

- **Symptoms due to binocular vision disturbances:** Most common binocular visual disturbances seen in aniseikonia are diplopia and confusion. If difference in image size is of small amount (0.25%), then it is ignored by the retina, however, as the difference of image size is more than 5%, then diplopia will occur. Younger patients try to avoid this diplopia by suppressing one eye, hence a uniocular vision will develop. But in adults once the binocular vision is well established and if there is sudden difference in the image size (e.g. unilateral surgical aphakia) then diplopia will occur.

- **Defect in spatial perceptions:** Stereoscopic visual effect perceived by our eyes in space is obtained due to formation of two slightly incongruent images on the retina. The formation of slight incongruent image on retina is due to location of two eyes on different lateral position on the head, resulting in physiological aniseikonia. The images which are projected in two eyes usually differ in their relative horizontal position (horizontal disparity) and this horizontal disparity of retinal images is the basis for the perception of depth. Aniseikonia due to any reason may disturb the normal incongruity of images on retina and results in anomaly of stereoscopic visual function (spatial disorientations). These spatial disorientations are more pronounced when horizontal meridian is involved. Most of time the disturbances in stereoscopic visual functions are not evident because a considerable amount of psychological adaptation for this visual incongruity develops especially if present since childhood. However, if the patient is tired or shifted to the environment where uniocular perception occurs (e.g. aviation and motoring), then spatial disorientations become very significant and lead to the misjudgement of the actual distances and may result in diplopia, ocular tiredness and ultimately accidents.

Common presentations of spatial disorientations can be explained by these examples:

– Right hand is larger than left hand

– Objects present in one-half of visual field will appear larger and further away as compared to other half of visual field; which has an object of same size situated at same distance.

– Face may appear asymmetrical with its left side protruding.

– Squares become rectangular; circles look elliptical and top of table as trapezoid.

– Plane ground appears tilted to the observer and gives a feeling as if he/she is climbing the hill; although in reality the patient is walking on plane surface.

– Flat surface of a table will appear as slant down on left side and up on the right side.

Measurement of Aniseikonia

Various methods adopted to measure the degree of aniseikonia are:

• Dartmouth studies introduced a method for measurement of degree of aniseikonia, which is well followed by majority of the practitioners. This method implies a 'rule of thumb' for the rough estimate of degree of aniseikonia. This rule states that if difference in the size of image due to anisometropia is refractive in nature, then the amount of aniseikonia produced due to this will be approximately 1.5% for every dioptre of anisometropia. However, for all practical purposes 1% aniseikonia for one dioptre of anisometropia is considered as standard and used clinically.

• Standard method to estimate the degree of aniseikonia is by using a device space Ekinometer designed by Ogle and Ames. However, being time consuming and expensive procedure, it has very less therapeutic value. In this device the presentation of the dissimilar objects of the same size to the two eyes is made in such a way that disparity between sizes of retinal images can be assessed accurately. This instrument can give information about following measurements

– Difference in size of image in horizontal meridian

– Difference in size of image in vertical meridian

– Amount of correction needed for inclination (indicates meridional aniseikonia)

Ekinometer consists of four vertical elements (lines A, B, C, and D shown in blue color in **Fig. 6.24**). Two lines (A and B) are in front and two lines are behind (C and D) a cross element (red color in **Fig. 6.24**). This cross has two cords F and G, lying right angles to each other. There is a fifth vertical line E (green color), which passes through the centre of the cross. This whole system is viewed through a test lens unit against a uniform black background.

If there is no incongruity of images, then all the elements in Ekinometer will appear in their normal relationship, and if incongruity of images is present then elements will appear displaced by an amount proportional to the degree of aniseikonia as well as in the direction related to type of incongruity. By neutralizing the displacement using iseikonic lenses, set in trial test unit, the elements can be made to appear normal. This will give the degree of aniseikonia by seeing the reading of test lenses settings. Various appearances of elements on the basis of displacement will be as follows:

• When all the elements are seen in their respective position or no displacement

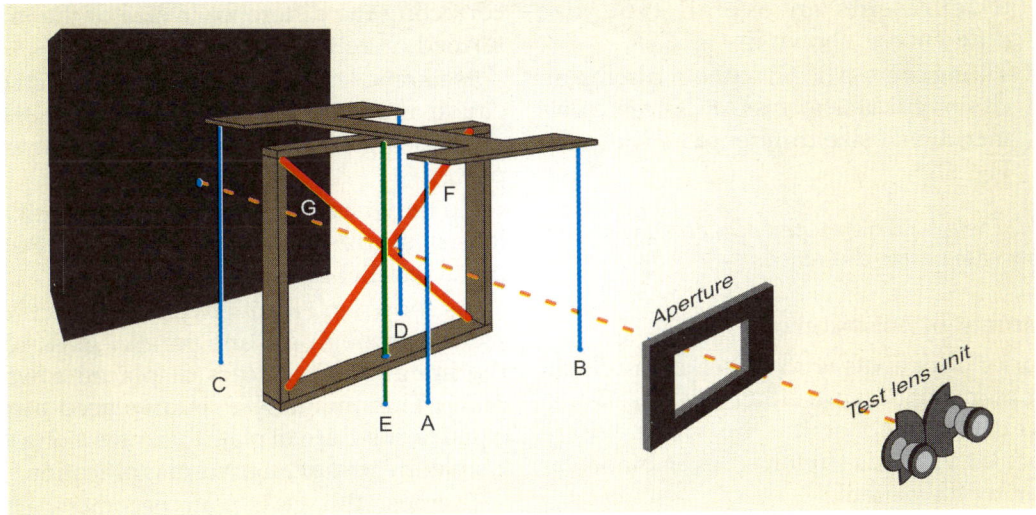

Fig. 6.24: Ekinometer

of elements is seen, it is considered as normal appearance as shown in Fig. 6.25.

- When front (A, B) and back (C, D) vertical elements appear displaced and cross (F, G) appears as if rotated in vertical axis in the same direction, it represents the horizontal size difference in images as shown in Fig. 6.26.
- Correct orientation of vertical elements (ABCD) with rotation of cross indicates the vertical size difference in images as shown in Fig. 6.27.
- As contrary to vertical size difference when there is rotation of vertical lines (ABCD) without rotation of cross (F, G)

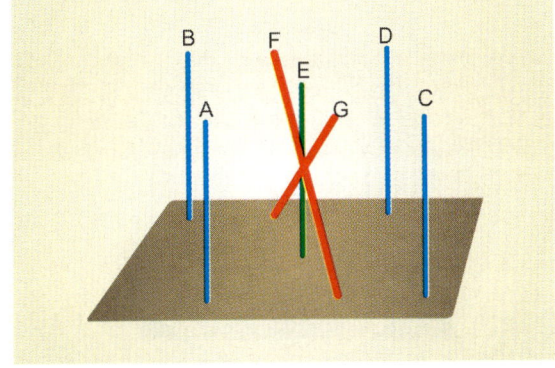

Fig. 6.26: Horizontal size difference appearance through Ekinometer

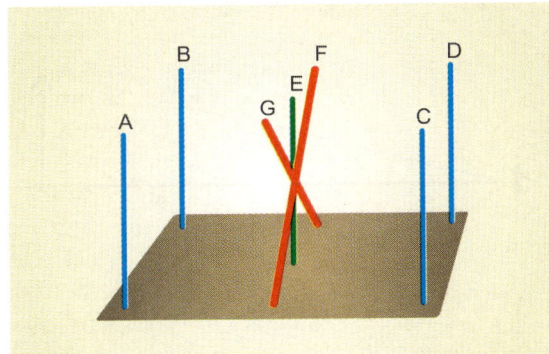

Fig. 6.25: Normal appearance through Ekinometer

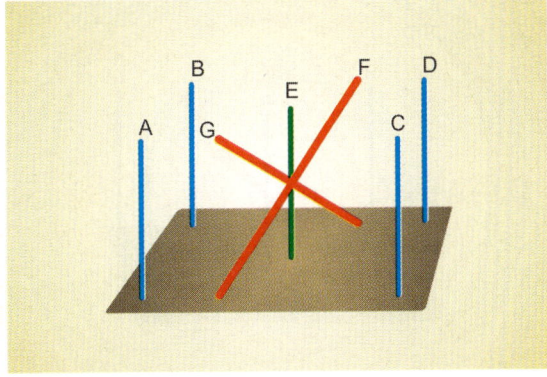

Fig. 6.27: Vertical size difference appearance through Ekinometer

it represents an overall type size difference as shown in Fig. 6.28.

- Tilting of cross (F, G) without discrepancies in vertical elements (ABCD) represents meridional size difference as shown in Fig. 6.29.

Note: There is no displacement of central cord (E) in any case of size difference.

Treatment of Aniseikonia

Majority of patients with aniseikonia remain asymptomatic because either the aniseikonia is well tolerated or has no value where uniocular vision is preferred over binocular vision by the patient.

Moderate degree aniseikonia requires correction by use of iseikonic lenses or contact lenses which treat the aniseikonia by

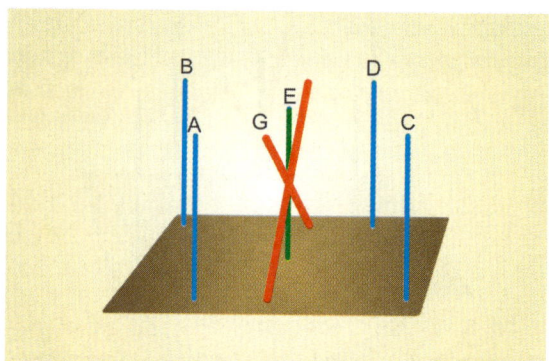

Fig. 6.28: Overall size difference appearance through Ekinometer

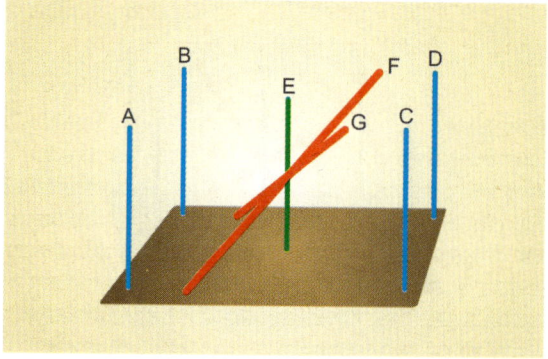

Fig. 6.29: Meridional size difference appearance through Ekinometer

correcting the difference in size of the image formed on retina.

Iseikonic lenses, when fitted in spectacles, cause magnification of images without introducing any obvious change in refractive power.

To understand the functioning of iseikonic lenses, study the illustration (Fig. 6.30) on plane parallel glass plate.

As shown in Fig. 6.30 when an object XY is viewed through a plane parallel glass plate, the image X'Y' appears displaced towards plate. This image X'Y' is displaced almost equal to one-third of plate thickness along with a small degree of angular magnification.

Suppose this glass plate becomes curved, then this angular magnification will get increased because magnification depends on the refractive power of the front surface and thickness of glass plate. However, to keep the image location same as that of the object, the refractive power of the front surface can be neutralize by a proportionate refractive power of back surface; means lens becomes of zero power. By using this principle image can be magnified in one or all meridians without changing the refractive power of lens. These types of lenses were used by several researchers with variable results for relief of visual disturbances seen in aniseikonic cases. Iseikonic lenses were prescribed in small number of patients and favorable symptomatic relief from distressing visual disturbances was seen in very limited patients.

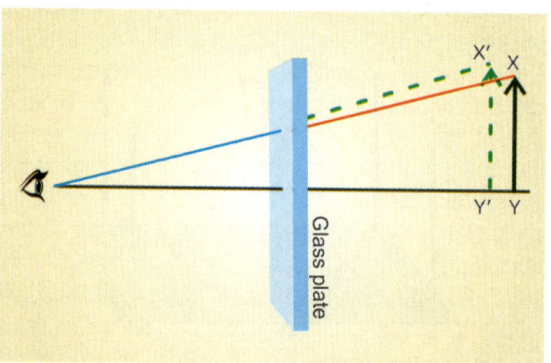

Fig. 6.30: Glass plate causing image magnification

Various treatment modalities can be used for different types of aniseikonia.

- **Optical aniseikonia:** Following modalities can be used to correct optical aniseikonia
    - Implanting of intraocular lenses in cases of unilateral aphakia.
    - Contact lenses can be successfully used to correct anisometropic aniseikonia and is more preferred than spectacles.
    - Corneal refractive surgery remains the best treatment choice for all types of optical aniseikonia.
    - Spectacles fitted with iseikonic lenses gives symptomatic relief in some selective cases of aniseikonia. However, these lenses are quite expensive and technically difficult to manufacture; hence are not used very commonly for correction of aniseikonia.
- **Retinal aniseikonia:** This is quite rare cause of aniseikonia and can be corrected by treating the underlying retinal disease.
- **Cortical aniseikonia:** It is very difficult to treat cortical aniseikonia, although symptomatic relief can be given by prescribing iseikonic lens spectacles.

Accommodation and its Anomalies

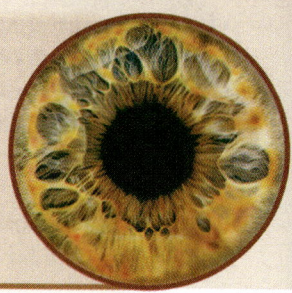

Chapter Outline

ASTHENOPIA

Introduction

Most common diagnosis made in ophthalmology practice, especially in patients having vague ocular symptoms is asthenopia. Commonly, it is also termed eye strain. The range of symptoms of asthenopia may vary from mild ocular discomfort to nonspecific headache of any severity, so it can be considered as syndrome. Generally patients suffering from asthenopia complaint of indistinguishable headaches associated with ocular symptoms like heaviness of eyelids, ocular fatigability or sleepiness feeling while watching TV or reading books and brow ache. Several gastrointestinal disturbances like nausea, stomach ache and neurological disturbances like giddiness, depression are also complained by many asthenopic patients.

Types of Asthenopia

As discussed asthenopia is presented with vague symptoms so various ocular and/or systemic conditions may cause this wide range of asthenopic syndrome. However, on the basis of etiology, asthenopia can be classified as shown in Table 7.1.

Accommodative asthenopia: It is most common cause of asthenopia and arises due to strain on ciliary muscles; usually seen in uncorrected refractive errors of the eyes.

Muscular asthenopia: Arise due to weakness of extraocular muscles as occur in heterophoria, intermittent heterotropia or convergence insufficiency.

Table 7.1: Etiological types of asthenopia	
Accommodative asthenopia	*Muscular asthenopia*
• Refractive errors	• Heterophoria
• Presbyopia	• Intermittent heterotropia
• Accommodative and /or convergence insufficiency	• Convergence insufficiency

Refractive Errors and Asthenopia

Asthenopic symptoms are usually observed more in persons having mild or moderate degree of refractive errors because patient tries to correct this small amount of error by using the increased efforts of ocular musculature. This excessive muscular effort will lead to fatigue of ocular muscles and subsequently asthenopic symptoms.

In persons with high refractive error the asthenopic symptoms are not so common because these persons either develop monocular vision or adjust their life according to diminished amount of visual acuity.

- **Myopia:** In myopes the far point is at a finite distance situated in front of the eye and far point distance is inversely proportional to the amount of refractive error. Hence, in an uncorrected myope blurring of letters will occur while they read a book kept at normal reading distance from their eyes. Because in myopic patients normal reading distance is farther away from their far point and also in a myope always a blur image is formed at any point situated beyond the far point of eye. So to read clearly, the myopic patients tries to keep the book nearer to their eyes (nearer than far point). This decreased distance of reading or the greater proximity of near object will increase the demand of convergence. Usually positive accommodative convergence reflex (means eye accommodate when convergence occurs) is absent in myopes so these myopic patients have to exert a positive fusional convergence to see the near object clearly and distinctly. This event of excessive exertion of fusional convergence will develop asthenopic symptoms in uncorrected myopes. Commonly uncompensated myopes develop an accommodative response which is lesser than response seen in an emmetropic person. It means in uncorrected myopes lower accommodation (as compared to emmetropes) is produced when eyes converge to see the near object. So, correction of myopic error in this type of patients will force them to use their accommodation (which otherwise was poorly used) to see the near objects clearly hence can produce asthenopic symptoms.

- **Hypermetropia:** On contrary to myope, in hypermetrope far point is beyond infinity, so in uncorrected hypermetropes only blurred images are received by retina when accommodation is at rest. To see the clear images hyperopes has to increase their refractive power by increasing the activity of ciliary muscle. More near will be the object, more ciliary muscle power will be required to see it clearly, so uncorrected hypermetropes produce significant amount of asthenopic symptoms due to excessive ciliary muscle efforts. Similarly, the presbyopic patients try to stimulate the accommodation by extra ciliary muscle efforts and when these attempts become physiologically difficult then the asthenopic symptoms precipitates.

- **Astigmatism:** Uncorrected astigmatism is more common cause for asthenopia than uncorrected spherical refractive errors especially, a small degree of hypermetropic astigmatism produces more severe asthenopic symptoms because in these cases accommodational efforts try to overcome the hypermetropia, which results in severe asthenopic symptoms. Patients having "with the rule" astigmatism are more symptomatic than the patients having "against the rule" astigmatism. Although the images formed in patients having "with the rule" astigmatism is clearer than "against the rule" astigmatism. Asthenopic symptoms are more severe in patients with low degree astigmatic error because the accommodation efforts exerted by these patients are of greater intensity.

- **Anisometropia:** In anisometropia an unequal amount of refractive error is present in both the eyes, so an unequal amount of blurring of images are seen by anisometropic patients. To clear these unequally blur images an imbalance in requirement of accommodation will arise. This difference in need of amount of accommodation will produce asthenopic symptoms in some patients having anisometropia.

- **Presbyopia:** Persons doing near work for long period like tailors, weavers, etc. may develop premature presbyopia and will complain of asthenopic symptoms due to uncorrected presbyopia.

Accommodation Insufficiency (AI) and Asthenopia

Accommodation insufficiency is a sensory motor abnormality of visual system in which the amplitude of accommodation is less than the expected for patient age. Normally, in the patients with accommodation insufficiency the uncorrected visual acuity is not so poor and refractive error is negligibly small but they show an inability to focus or sustain focus on near objects. So these patients usually complain of headache, blurring of objects, eyestrain or brow ache after reading continuously for a period of 30–40 minutes. In presence of accommodation insufficiency to compensate and to maintain the focus on near objects these patients either squint or frown while reading a near vision chart, however, usually they can even read up to N6 line. Following simple clinical tests can be performed to confirm the diagnosis of AI as well as to differentiate from presbyopia

- ± 2 dioptre flipper test
- Positive relative accommodation test
- Monocular estimated method (MEM) dynamic retinoscopy

Patients having AI show difficulty in clearing ± 2 dioptre flipper test, with minus lenses both in monocular and binocular examination. In patients of AI the value of positive relative accommodation is usually lower than −1.5 D and finding on MEM dynamic retinoscopy is higher than +1 D.

Convergence Insufficiency (CI) and Asthenopia

Convergence insufficiency, a sensory motor dysfunction of visual system, which is seen when patient is unable to converge properly or maintain the convergence to focus the near objects. In simpler words, convergence insufficiency is inability to converge properly while focusing on near objects. Criteria described on clinical evaluation for CI includes:

- Exophoria is more at near than distance
- Near point of convergence (NPC) is far away (more than 3 inches). Normal NPC is 8–10 cm.
- Reduced positive fusional vergence

Convergence insufficiency may occur due to refractive error (as seen in uncompensated myopes, first time corrected hypermetropes), presbyopia, or in patients having accommodation insufficiency. Systemic diseases or general debility due to chronic illness, metabolic disorders, and toxemia or endocrine disorders may also cause convergence insufficiency. Most common asthenopic symptoms associated with CI are frontal headache, loss of concentration, blurred vision and orbital pain. Sometimes CI patients may complain of poor stereopsis (depth perception) and also migraine headache. The episodes of migraine headache usually occur after doing excessive near work, however, these symptoms get relived after treatment of CI.

Heterophoria: Asthenopic symptoms in heterophoria do not appear until there is no interference with amplitude of motor fusion and deviation. Development of asthenopic symptoms in these persons will depend on the general health condition of person, state of sensory motor system and the type of work done by person. In heterophoria, frequency of asthenopic symptoms usually increased following a debilitating disease, even if the amplitude is normal. Symptoms are more in near vision than distant vision because there will be more strain on sensory motor system. Furthermore, chances of symptoms are more with vertical deviation because of limited amplitude for vertical fusion.

Clinical Features of Asthenopia

Asthenopic symptoms are variable in nature and are dependent on the amount of use of ocular system because the asthenopic symptoms are secondary to the muscular fatigue that may occur due to increased efforts of ocular muscles.

- **Pain around orbit and head:** Headache is most common symptom of asthenopia. The exact cause of it is not known but it can be considered as a referred pain. Pain in asthenopia arise due to increased effort of ciliary muscle which is then referred into those areas which are associated with cervical segments like superior cervical ganglion, bulbo-spinal root of trigeminal nerve, and upper cervical nerves. Pain is more noticed in frontal and occipital regions because ophthalmic division of trigeminal nerve is represented most caudally. Pain may vary in terms of location and severity.
  - An ache may be present locally around eyes or orbit, or may be localized in frontal, temporal, or occipital region or may be diffuse in nature. Sometimes these aches may radiate up to neck or into arms.
  - Ache may be limited to any part and may be associated with tenderness over that area, e.g. commonly on vertex or temple of head or in the orbital area near eyes (brow ache).
  - Nature of headache may be variable from superficial to deep seated.
  - Similarly, headache may be in form of dull heavy ache or sharp, shooting and piercing in nature (resembling neuralgic pain).
  - Headache may be intermittent or permanent type and may be at regular or irregular intervals.

- **Vague ocular symptoms:** General ocular symptoms such as eye strain, ocular fatigue, ocular aches, and tired eyes may occur, usually seen after doing continuous near work or reading book for more than 30–40 minutes. Continuing near work in spite of ocular strain can result into actual pain or severe headaches. Normally, these ocular symptoms get relived by taking rest or rubbing eyes or relaxing the eyes by looking at distant objects. However, asthenopic eyes generally have a typical look (watery, suffused and dull) due to continuous status of irritability and congestion. Rubbing of eyes, especially in children may lead to development of recurrent blepharitis, styes or conjunctivitis and an accurate cycloplegic refraction must be done to know the refractive status. Once refractive error is corrected, then these vague ocular symptoms subside automatically.

- **Diminution of vision:** Visual symptoms may vary depending on the refractive error of patient. Most of the time small degree of refractive errors are fully compensated by the efforts of ocular system of an individual and thus visual acuity remains unaffected and patients do not complain of visual symptoms. However, in the presence of stressful conditions (e.g. poor general health, eyes are being used too much like for reading book, jobs demanding high degree of visual acuity for long period, fine tailoring work, etc.), or when refractive errors cannot be compensated by ocular system, then the visual acuity remains poor and visual symptoms (blurring or diminution of vision) will appear. During unusual strain on eye both the ciliary muscles and ocular muscles of eye initially try to compensate it by excessive efforts of contraction but finally the muscles get tired and undergo in the state of relaxation, leading to blurring of vision and diplopia, respectively.

- **Associated symptoms:** Sometimes patients along with visual symptoms may also complaint of various vague general symptoms in the form of digestive upset (nausea, dyspepsia), neurotic (dizziness, insomnia, depression, etc.) and abnormal sensitivity to light, etc.

Management

Management of asthenopia includes identification and treatment of multiple causative factors by means of

- Refraction
- Correction of accommodation insufficiency
- Visual training
- Prism therapy
- Improvement in general health status

Refraction: Refractive status of every patient having asthenopic symptoms should be checked by performing cycloplegic refraction and if error is present it should be fully corrected. Correction of the refractive errors will decrease the muscular efforts of eye and thus help to relieve the asthenopic symptoms.

Accommodation insufficiency: Patients diagnosed with accommodative insufficiency can be prescribed with plus lenses (+1 or + 1.25 Dsph power) to decrease motor demand on accommodation system. These glasses are prescribed as half eye glasses so that near vision is improved without disturbing distance vision.

Eye exercises: Patients having muscular type of asthenopia are advised for visual training, which is given in the form of orthoptic exercises like adduction exercise gives best results in cases of convergence insufficiency. These exercises help in development of range of fusion and accommodative efforts. Improvement in these factors will be added for the convergence facilitation and hence improves convergence abilities of patient. However, the results of these orthoptic exercises are not visible immediately rather these exercises take some time to show the desired results perhaps patient perform them regularly and judicially.

Prism therapy: If orthoptic exercises do not work to relieve asthenopic symptoms due to convergence insufficiency, then prism therapy in form of base-in (BI) prisms fixed in spectacles for near work can be prescribed.

General measures to improve health: For a successful treatment of asthenopia an improvement in general health, management of systemic diseases and debility due to illness is equally important to relieve the symptoms. For severe headaches pain relieving tablets can be prescribed for immediate symptomatic relief however, extensive search should be done to find the root cause of headache.

ACCOMMODATION

Introduction

Human eye has developed such a mechanism by which parallel rays of light from infinity get focused at macula of the retina. This phenomenon is accomplished by refractive system of an emmetropic eye without exerting any effort and as a consequence, the objects which are present at a considerable distance are seen clearly and distinctly. So, it is obvious that if eye has to function properly it should be able to vary its focus from distance to near objects in very short interval of time. Hence eye needs to adopt its refractive mechanism in such a manner that it allows even near objects to be seen clearly and distinctly.

In emmetrope eyes the parallel rays of light coming from infinity are focused on the retina while accommodation is at rest. Human eyes have a unique mechanism by which it can even focus the diverging rays coming from a near object on the retina so that object is seen clearly. This mechanism is known as accommodation.

As shown in Fig. 7.1 that parallel rays coming from infinity are getting focused on

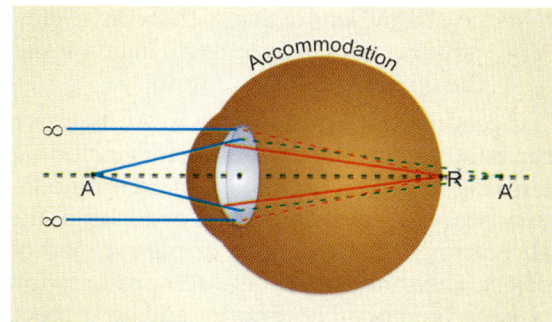

Fig. 7.1: Accommodation causes focusing of near object on retina

the retina (R). Suppose the object under examination is now brought at point A, when eye is in nonaccommodative state then the conjugate image will be formed at point A' which is situated behind the retina and hence a large blur circle of diffusion is seen on the retina. Now if by any means we can increase the converging power of the eye so that the focus A' is formed at R, then the object will be seen clearly while still keeping the distinct image clear. This mechanism which causes change in the power of focusing is called accommodation.

Various possible mechanisms by which accommodation can be achieved are:

- *Change in axial length of eye:* If eye could be made elongated (i.e. its axial length increased) so that retina (R) moves out to point A' (Fig. 7.1), i.e. image falls on retina.

- *Curvature of cornea:* Another possible mechanism is that an increase in converging power can be attained by changing (more steep) the curvature of cornea.

- *Position of lens:* Accommodation could be attained by altering the position of lens and making it to move forwards (i.e. towards cornea).

  However, all these possibilities in human eye are not possible in real life.

  The most possible mechanism to achieve accommodation is

- *Change in refractive power of lens:* There is increase in the refractive power of crystalline lens of eye so that converging power of ocular system will increase and the image will form at retina.

Accommodation response in human eye can be stimulated by various factors including blurring of image, oscillation of accommodation, scanning movements of eye, chromatic aberrations, distance and apparent size of object. The time period between presentation of an accommodative stimulus and occurrence of an accommodation response is known as reaction time of accommodation. Average reaction time for 'far to near' and for 'near to far' accommodation is 0.64 and 0.56 second, respectively.

Mechanism of Accommodation

Though there is a considerable amount of controversy about the precise nature of mechanism during accommodation, however, majority of researchers agreed that it is essentially the increase in the curvature of crystalline lens (mainly of the anterior surface of lens) which causes accommodation in human eye. Mechanism of accommodation also varies species to species like snakes and frogs have mechanism by which they can move their lens forward to see near objects clearly or Mollusc pecten species can elongate their eye to focus on the near objects.

There was a long debate since 19th century that how humans are able to shift the focus from far to near and near to far objects, without moving their body. Many researchers have presented various theories for the mechanism of accommodation in past years. Some popular theories are:

- Cramer's vitreous theory
- Helmholtz theory of relaxation
- Tscherning's theory of increased tension
- Coleman theory of accommodation
- Schachar's theory of contraction

Cramer's Vitreous Theory

In year 1853, Cramer studied the size of Purkinje's image during accommodation process. He concluded that size of image became smaller during accommodation as compared to resting state of eye as shown in Fig. 7.2.

He also observed change in the anterior surface of the crystalline lens during accommodation which became more convex, whereas there was minimal change in the posterior surface of crystalline lens (which he concluded because image of candle from anterior surface of lens became significantly smaller as compared to the image of candle from posterior surface of lens as shown in Fig. 7.2. Based on his observations Cramer proposed a theory called vitreous theory. Cramer's vitreous theory for accommodation states that during process of accommodation there is contraction of ciliary muscle which

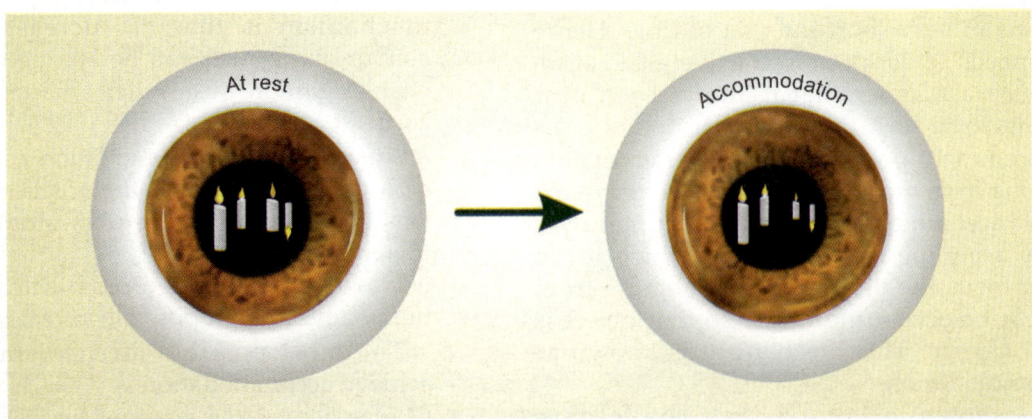

Fig. 7.2: Purkinje images (becoming smaller) as seen during accommodation process

acts upon choroid. The choroid in turn causes compression of vitreous gel body against posterior portion of crystalline lens. As a result pressure on posterior crystalline lens is increased; in response to this the iris tries to resist this increased pressure, leading to increase in the curvature of anterior surface of lens in pupillary area.

Points not in favor of vitreous theory

- Later on a few studies concluded that accommodation also present in those patients who are not having iris (aniridia), hence counter pressure by iris is not the probable cause for increase in the curvature of crystalline lens.
- Moreover, accommodation is also possible in those cases where complete vitrectomy has been done.

Points in favor of vitreous theory: Subsequent studies supported the statement of Cramer's that lens is involved for process of accommodation.

Helmholtz Theory of Relaxation

This theory was initially proposed by Thomas Young which was further explained in details by Helmholtz (1885). This theory is also known as Young-Helmholtz theory of accommodation or capsular theory. This theory of accommodation was the most widely accepted and later on modified by various other researchers like Fincham in the year 1937.

Relaxation theory comprises these points:

- During rest phase (unaccommodated state of eye, i.e. during distant vision), the soft substances of crystalline lens remains compressed inside the lens capsule due to increased tension of zonular fibres. Due to this increased tension of zonules, the lens is pulled backwards towards equator. As a result, the anterior surface of lens is less curved means maintain a flat shape to increase the focal length (as shown in Fig. 7.3). Helmholtz proposed that zonules remain under tension due to pull exerted on them by elastic choroid, however, later on several studies conclude that zonules fibers remain in state of tension due to the relaxation of ciliary muscle fibers.
- During accommodation phase there is contraction of ciliary muscle and the choroid is pulled forwards which result in uniform reduction of tension (relaxation) on all anterior, posterior and equatorial zonular fibers. Due to relaxation of zonular fibers the lens being elastic, mould itself and undergo following changes:
  - Increase in the curvature of lens (mainly of anterior surface)

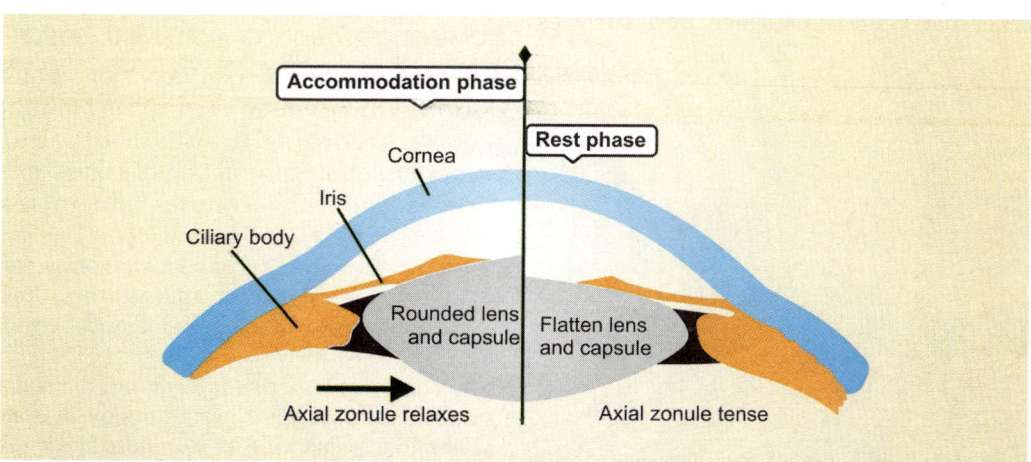

Fig. 7.3: Showing accommodation and rest phase

– Increase in the anterio-posterior diameter of lens
– Increase in axial thickness of lens
– Decrease in equatorial diameter of the lens
– Forward movement (bulging) of the anterior pole of the crystalline lens
– Equatorial edge of lens moved away from sclera

Due to all these changes the lens becomes more spherical or round in shape and dioptric power of the eye is increased which enable the eye to see the near objects clearly (Fig. 7.3).

Helmholtz considered that lens capsule and lens matrix act as an elastic body. In normal state the lens is kept stretched and remains more flat due to tension of zonular fibers (suspensory ligaments). Thus, in state of rest the radius of curvature of anterior surface of lens is about 10 mm, whereas during state of accommodation it decreases to 6 mm. This change in curvature of lens increases the converging power of the eye and focus can be altered as per requirement (Fig. 7.4).

Helmholtz's theory was widely accepted. However, this theory could not explain reason for change in shape of lens during accommodation. Later on, Fincham suggested that peculiar form attained by lens during process of accommodation is due to structure of lens capsule. He suggested that thickness of lens vary at different places. The anterior surface is thicker than posterior surface. Both surfaces are thicker in periphery (site of attachment of zonules) than centre or pole of lens. Due to this variable thickness of lens, on application of increased tension of zonules the peripheral portion of lens will preferentially become flatter than central part, so there is bulging of central part of capsule. On the basis of these observations, Fincham concluded that variation in thickness is responsible for change in shape of lens during accommodation. Helmholtz theory was modified by other researchers also. Gullstrand proposed that along with the change in elasticity of lens, change in the intracapsular forces also play role in accommodative process.

Points against relaxation theory

- As per Helmholtz hypothesis, with aging the zonules should relax because equatorial diameter increases (as crystalline lens and equator comes closer to ciliary muscle) with process of ageing. So, the power of crystalline lens should increase as age advances for seeing the distant objects during accommodation and person should become more myopic with an unstable lens position. But in reality with advancing age the person becomes hypermetropic and lens position remains stable.
- Helmholtz theory could not explain the decrease in spherical aberrations, which occurs during the process of accommodation.

Tscherning's Theory of Increased Tension

Tscherning's proposed a theory of accommodation which was opposite of Helmholtz theory. According to this theory, during accommodation contraction of ciliary muscle directly pulls the zonules and increases

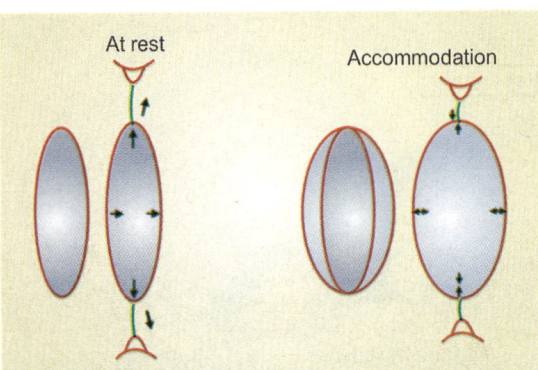

Fig. 7.4: Helmholtz's theory showing mechanism of accommodation

Note: Since majority of anatomical and physiological evidences were found against this theory; Tscherning's view of increased zonular tension is not accepted widely.

According to Tscherning's theory, accommodation results due to increase in the tension in zonules rather than relaxation of zonules (Helmholtz's theory).

tension on zonules which in turn will increase tension on the capsule of lens. Hence, the lens will become more flat at periphery due to compression of lens capsule at equator and simultaneously it will buldge out from central pupillary zone (at pole).

Coleman's Theory of Accommodation

In 1970 Coleman proposed a theory for accommodation known as the 'Coleman's hydraulic suspension theory of accommodation'. Although by the time Coleman's proposed his theory, already two popular theories were existing, i.e. Helmholtz's relaxation theory and Tscherning's zonular contraction theory. However, these theories were not able to explain some queries like

- How convergence potentiate the accommodation process?
- What is the exact cause of reduction of accommodation during presbyopia?
- What is the relationship of accommodation process with progression of myopia and glaucoma?
- How the optical surfaces of crystalline lens rapidly gains functionality, even in associated accommodation hysteresis, where time is limited?
- What is the reason for forward movement of lens during accommodation?
- How the zonular ciliary body attachments can flatten the lens without involvement of vitreous?

Coleman proposed that lens and zonular fibers in the eye acts as a diaphragm between anterior and vitreous chamber of the eye and remain in a catenary shape (hydraulic suspension bridge), because of pressure difference of aqueous and vitreous bodies of the eye. The movement of posterior pole of crystalline lens is prevented by vitreous gel body. During accommodation when ciliary muscle contracts, the pressure in vitreous chamber is increased while the pressure in

Note: There is no change in curvature of posterior surface because of vitreous.

anterior chamber is decreased. This pressure difference creates a hydraulic shift of crystalline lens. As a result, the vitreous applies a force on the posterior surface of lens and causes change in the shape of catenary which in turn changes the curvature of anterior lens (makes anterior central curvature of lens more steep).

Points not in favor of Coleman's theory:

- Later on some studies found that no significant difference in the amplitude of accommodation is seen in cases having vitreous body or in cases without vitreous (after vitrectomy), and suggested that vitreous plays no essential role in accommodation process or forward displacement of crystalline lens.
- Some studies compared Coleman's hydraulic suspension theory and Helmholtz's capsular theory to determine changes in refractive power during mechanism of accommodation. They found that change in refractive power during accommodation process was consistent with Helmholtz's capsular theory, not with Coleman's hydraulic suspension theory.

Schachar's Theory of Contraction

Schachar (1992–1995) gave another theory for the process of accommodation which resembles with Tscherning's theory of increased tension. Theory of Schachar's also became basis for surgical treatment of presbyopia done to restore accommodation. Schachar suggested that during accommodation process the active role is played by equatorial zonular fibres, while the anterior and posterior zonular fibres only provide passive structural support to lens just like supportive ligaments of skeletal joints. Thus, the equatorial zonular fibres are main component to decide the optical power of lens in the eye. Anterior and posterior zonular fibres get tense during distant vision, whereas they are relaxed during accommodation. According to this theory, during accommodation there is contraction of ciliary muscle which leads to increase in the tension of

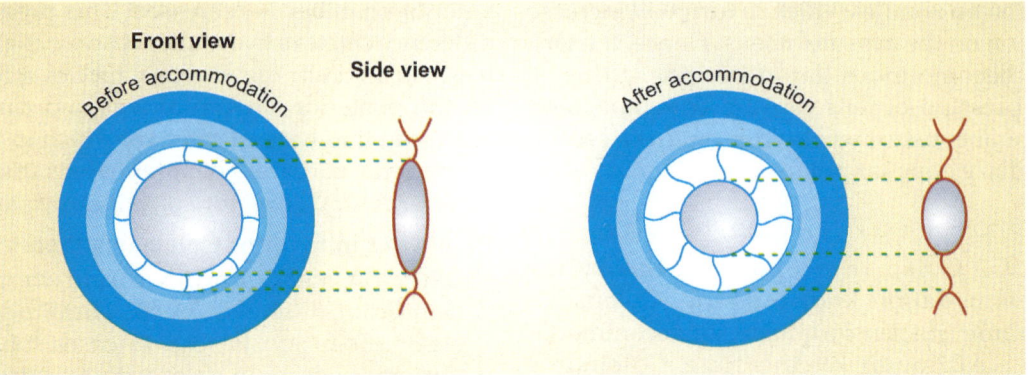

Fig. 7.5: Schachar's theory—ciliary muscle contraction causing relaxation of equatorial zonules

Note: Schachar's theory challenged the classical and most widely accepted theory of Helmholtz where contraction of ciliary muscle caused decrease in the tension (relaxation) of the zonules and allowed centripetal elasticity of lens capsule to change the shape of crystalline lens. As per Helmholtz's theory the equatorial or coronal diameter of lens is reduced and equatorial edge of crystalline lens moves away from sclera and entire lens becomes spherical shape which is just opposite to theory proposed by Schachar.

Note: As discussed there are lots of controversies about various theories of accommodation, but Von Helmholtz's capsular theory is probably the most widely accepted, because various experimental physiological studies done in last century provided enough evidences to prove the fundamental elements of mechanism of accommodation still holds good.

equatorial zonular fibres (as also suggested in Tscherning's theory) while of tension on anterior and posterior zonules is decreased (Fig. 7.5). As a result there is equatorial displacement of lens. Biomechanical property of crystalline lens is such that, central portion of lens rounds up when equatorial region stretches and hence central portion moves anteriorly, i.e. the central surface of lens becomes more convex and peripheral surfaces become more flat due to more increase in central volume of lens than peripheral volume (Fig. 7.5). Due to all these changes the equator of lens is pulled towards the sclera leading to increase in the refractive power of the lens.

- Schachar's theory also states that growth in equatorial diameter of crystalline lens with age results in presbyopia. He proposed that presbyopia happens due to reduction in the distance between lens equator and ciliary muscles. He thought that with aging, the area surrounding the crystalline lens

(perilenticular space) is reduced and contraction of ciliary muscle is not so effective so that lens become unable to expand coronally. Based on this principle, Schachar (1992) introduced a new surgical method for correction of presbyopia, known as sclera expansion procedure. The scleral expansion will increase the zonular tension and hence should re-establish the accommodation in presbyopia. He used bands for sclera expansion with an aim of increasing the distance between lens equator and ciliary muscle. As per his theoretical calculations this increase in distance will provide more space for the ciliary muscle to work on zonular tension.

- However, various reports had shown conflicting results about sclera expansion bands procedure and challenged the authenticity of Schachar's theory of zonular tension during accommodation.

Comparison of accommodation theories: Salient features of various accommodation theories are summarized in Table 7.2.

Table 7.2: Comparison of salient features among various accommodation theories

Cramer's vitreous theory	Helmholtz theory of relaxation	Tscherning's theory	Coleman theory	Schachar theory
Contraction of ciliary muscle ↓	Contraction of ciliary muscle ↓	Contraction of ciliary muscle ↓	Contraction of ciliary muscle ↓	Contraction of ciliary muscle ↓
Acts upon choroid ↓	Choroid is pulled forwards ↓	Directly pulls the zonules ↓	Pressure in vitreous chamber is increased and in anterior is decreased (pressure difference) ↓	Increase in the tension of equatorial zonular fibres ↓
Choroid causes compression of vitreous on posterior portion of lens ↓	Uniform reduction in tension on all zonular fibres ↓	Increases tension on zonules ↓		Equatorial displacement of lens ↓
Pressure on posterior lens increased ↓	Lens undergo changes: • Increase in the curvature of lens • Increase in the anterioposterior diameter • Increase in axial thickness • Decrease in equatorial diameter • Forward movement of anterior pole • Equatorial edge of lens moved away from sclera	Increase tension on the capsule of lens ↓	Creates a hydraulic shift of crystalline lens ↓	Central surface of lens becomes more convex and pulling of the equatorial lens toward the sclera
Iris tries to resist this increased pressure ↓		Lens is more flat at periphery and bulge out from central pupillary zone	Vitreous applies force on posterior surface of lens ↓	
Increase in the curvature of anterior surface of lens			Changes the curvature of anterior lens	

Physical and Physiological Accommodation

Efficiency of process of accommodation is dependent on two factors:

• Ability of lens to change its shape
• Contractile power of ciliary muscle

With advancing age the elasticity of lens is decreased and it no longer can change its shape as efficiently as in younger age. In this situation accommodation will not be effective even if ciliary muscle contracts powerfully. Similarly, a weak or paralyzed ciliary muscle will not cause change in the shape of lens, even if lens substance elasticity is normal. On the basis of these two facts mechanism of accommodation has two components:

Physical accommodation: The physical accommodation indicates actual deformation in the shape of lens and is measured in dioptres (D). It means to increase the converging power of eye by 1 D, an expenditure of 1 D accommodation is needed.

Physiological accommodation: The physiological accommodation indicates the contractile power of ciliary muscle and is expressed in myodioptre. One myodioptre unit is the amount of contractile power of ciliary muscle which is required to bring a change in the refractive power of lens by 1 D.

Though these two elements normally correspond to each other during first half of life (nearly 40–45 years) but they are fundamentally distinct elements. These factors may dissociate due to various precipitating factors and if this happens they produce pathological effects in life.

For example, when lens becomes hard in later years of life (nearly 40 years) as in presbyopia, the physical accommodation gets fail. It is known that alteration in the physical properties of lens alone lead to this condition and accommodation become difficult in presbyopia, however, the ciliary muscle power is unaffected during this phase of early presbyopia.

In contrary, if contractile power of ciliary muscle decreased due to any debility in life (at any age) also lead to reduced or abolishing accommodation, although lens is being able to change its shape with normal elasticity. Person may try to overcome this muscle deficiency by exerting excessive ciliary efforts which may manifest in form of asthenopia or eye strain symptoms.

Range and Amplitude of Accommodation

Far point of accommodation (punctum remotum) is referred as the maximum distance at which an object can be seen clearly when accommodation is relaxed and refractivity of the eye is at minimum. Near point of accommodation (punctum proximum) is referred as the nearest distance at which eye can see the object clearly with maximum effort of accommodation and refractivity of the eye is at maximum. The distance between far point of accommodation and near point of accommodation is termed the range of accommodation, i.e. this is the distance over which the accommodation of a person is in active form. The difference between the refractivity (dioptric power) of eye in these two conditions, i.e. when eye is at rest with

minimal refraction (eye is focused for far point i.e. static refraction) and when eye is in fully accommodative state with maximum refraction (eye is focused for near point, i.e. dynamic refraction) is called the amplitude of accommodation.

The range and amplitude of accommodation can be calculated by following formula as follows:

$$a = r - p$$
$$A = P - R$$

Where,

r = distance of far point (punctum remotum) in meters

R = refractive power of eye or static refraction (dioptres) when accommodated for r.

p = distance of near point (punctum proximum)

P = refractive power of eye or dynamic refraction (dioptres) when accommodated for p.

a = range of accommodation (meters)

A = amplitude of accommodation (dioptres).

Amplitude of Accommodation

As discussed above difference in the refractivity of eye during accommodative and resting state is considered as amplitude of accommodation. Normally, we have certain amount of accommodation since birth, which gradually decreases with advancement of age. An average value of amplitude of accommodation according to age has been standardized by conclusions drawn from several studies as shown in **Table 7.3**.

Amplitude of accommodation can be assessed by measuring the near point of accommodation (NPA) which is defined as the nearest distance till which an eye can see small objects clearly. The tests should be done with both eyes together (binocular) as well as with each eye (monocular) separately. Before testing full optical correction of refractive error

Table 7.3: Average amplitude of accommodation at different ages	
Age in years	*Amplitude in dioptres*
6–10	13.5–14.5
11–15	12–13.5
16–20	10–12
21–30	8–10
31–40	6–8
41–50	4–6
51–60	2–4
Above 61 years	0.5–1.5

must be done in ametropic or presbyopic eyes. NPA can be measured by three methods.

1. The simplest way to measure the NPA is by using a linear target (e.g. a line drawn on piece of paper). This target is brought forwards towards the eye of the patient and the distance at which the target appears blur to the patient, that point is called NPA. The reciprocal of this distance gives measurement of amplitude of accommodation. Near point of convergence (NPC) is the point at which the target appears double to the patient.

2. Measurement by using instruments like prince rule or Royal Air Force (RAF) rule or Livingstone gauge or near point ruler: The instrument consists of a binocular gauge which can be used for measurement of both subjective and objective NPC and NPA.

As shown in Fig. 7.6 RAF rule has a long ruler (50 cm) with a slider which holds a rotating four-sided cube. A cheek rest is provided on one end of ruler which ensures a consistency and proper height of target to the patient's eyes. Other end has a handle to hold the ruler straight while examining the patient. The instrument bar is marked on three sides as follows:

- one side is graded in centimeters for measurement of range of accommodation
- second side is divided in dioptres for measurement of amplitude of accommodation
- Third side is marked with number of years which indicate the standardized corresponding age of the patient.

Similarly, each side of cube has different targets

- First side of cube contains a vertical line with a central dot for convergence fixation.
- Other three sides provide a limited number of lines of near reading examples.

Test procedure

- Full optical correction of refractive error is provided by spectacles. The cheek rest of the RAF rule is placed on cheeks of the patient and a sliding target with 6/9 size letters, numbers

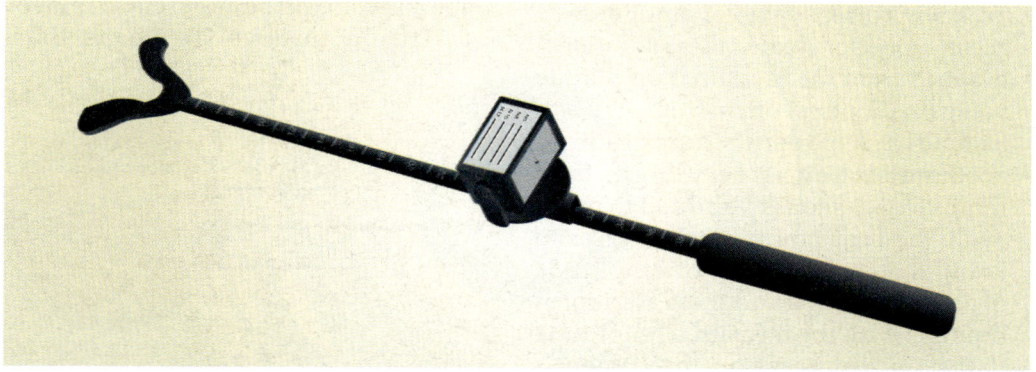

Fig. 7.6: RAF rule

or fine lines are presented towards eye.

- Slowly the target is moved towards the eyes of patient till he/she is able to read it clearly. Once the patient feels difficulty in reading the 6/9 size letters clearly, at this point stop the movement of sliding. Repeat the testing procedure first by only one eye (monocularly) and then for both the eyes together (binocularly). Record the distance of target in centimeters.

- The NPA is value (in centimeters) measured at the mark on instrument bar where target is present. Instrument bar also has measurements on other side, for amplitude of accommodation in dioptres and a third side which corresponds to the age in years. For example, if the patient sees the blurring of target objects at a distance of 25 cm, then the corresponding dioptre marking will show +4 D and age marking will be at 40 years.

On the basis of amplitude of accommodation two situations may arise. If the patient's amplitude of accommodation is very low (so much so that his/her near point lie beyond the total length of instrument), then plus lenses should be added with his/her full refractive correction until the near point comes within the range of length of instrument. To know correct value of amplitude of accommodation deduct these additional dioptres from the measured amplitude value (in dioptres) on instrument's bar. Secondly, if patient's amplitude of accommodation is very high, then minus lenses should be added to move away the near point. In these cases to know the correct value of amplitude of accommodation add these additional dioptres with the measured amplitude value (in dioptres) on instrument's bar.

3. *Measurement by using minus lenses:* Patient is asked to wear his/her full refractive correction, then test is performed first for each eye and then for both eyes. Make the patient to sit comfortably at 6 meters distance from the Snellen's chart. Place the trial frame, occlude one eye and now instruct the patient to fixate at 6/60 target on Snellen's chart. Once patient visualizes the 6/60 target clearly, gradually add minus power lenses with increasing powers till this 6/60 target becomes blur. Power of these added minus lenses is equivalent to the amplitude of accommodation.

Refractive Status of Eye versus Far or Near Point

Knowledge of relationship between refractive status of eye and far or near point of eye is important for calculating range and/or amplitude of accommodation. The position of far point or near point of eye is dependent on refractive status of eye as follows

- In emmetropic eye far point (r) is at infinity and near point (p) varies with the age of person (Fig. 7.7). As discussed in Table 7.3 at an age of 10 years, the average amplitude of accommodation is 14 D, so near point will be situated at 1 meter (100 cm)/14 D cm distance (i.e. about 7 cm) in front of the eye. Similarly, at an age of 40 years it will be at 100 cm/4 D (about 25 cm) and at an age 45 years will be at 100 cm/3 D (about 33 cm) from the eye. It means that the

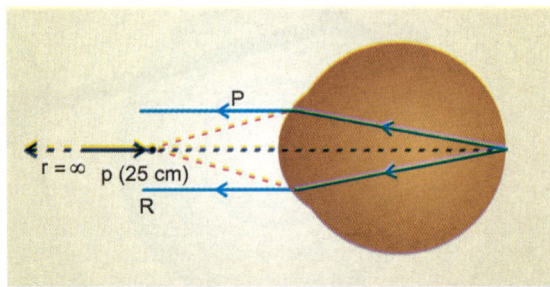

Fig. 7.7: Emmetropic eye (far point is at infinity)

refractive power can be compensated with accommodation of eye; greatest during childhood and least after middle age.

For example, for a 40 years emmetrope r = infinity and p = 25 cm

As we know that

Range of accommodation $(a) = r - p$

Amplitude of accommodation $(A) = P - R$

So, the range of accommodation (a) = infinity – 25 = infinity

Similarly, $R = 0$ and $P = 100/25$, i.e. + 4 D

So, the amplitude of accommodation (A) = 4 – 0 = + 4 D

- In hypermetropic eye the far point (r) is a hypothetical point beyond infinity or behind the retina (Fig. 7.8). Hence, to see the objects clearly at far point, hypermetropic eye has to exert accommodative efforts equal to degree of hypermetropia.

For example, in +4 D hypermetrope, hypothetical point (r) lies beyond infinity or 25 cm behind the retina, whereas the static refraction (R) is of +4 D power. Suppose, for an adult if near point (p) in front of the eye is 20 cm then P will be +5 D $(P = 100/20 = +5$ D).

So, range of accommodation (a) = infinity –25 = infinity and

Range of amplitude $(A) = 5$ D – (–4 D) = 5 D + 4 D = +9 D

Note: Distances behind the retina are calculated as negative.

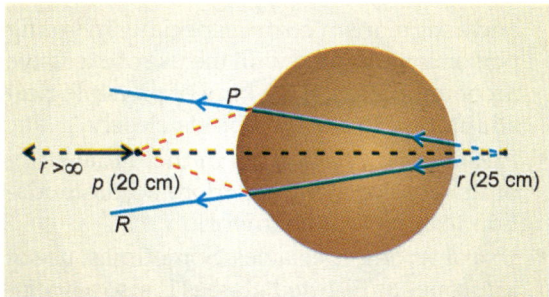

Fig. 7.8: Hypermetropic eye (far point is beyond infinity or behind eye)

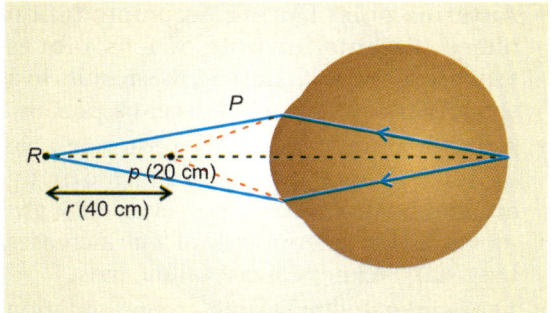

Fig. 7.9: Myopic eye (far point lies in front of eye)

- In myopic eye the far point (r) lies in front of the eye and is real. Hence, the distance of far point (r) from the eye is fixed, for example, 40 cm (for – 2.5 D myopia) (Fig. 7.9). Suppose, the near point (p) is at 20 cm for an adult, then R is 2.5 D and P is 5 D. Now, as per formula

Range of accommodation $(a) = 40 - 20 = 20$ cm; and

Amplitude of accommodation $(A) = 5$ D – 2.5 D = 2.5 D.

Ocular Changes During Accommodation

Ocular changes especially in crystalline lens happening during the process of accommodation can be summarized as follows:

- **Zonular loosening:** Normally zonules remain in tension and keep the lens flat. During accommodation there is contraction of ciliary muscle which causes relaxation of these zonules.

- **Curvatural change in lens surface:** During rest phase, the curvature of anterior surface of lens is 11 mm and of posterior surface is 6 mm. During accommodative phase the curvature of posterior surface remains almost same, i.e. 5.7 mm but that of anterior surface changes significantly. In strong accommodative phase the anterior surface curvature becomes 6 mm in periphery and nearly 3 mm in central portion of the lens. Central portion of lens bulges more probably due to the less thickness of capsule in central portion as compared to peripheral portion of capsule.

- **Anterior pole:** During accommodation phase the anterior pole of lens moves forward along with the iris, this results in a shallow anterior chamber in centre portion.
- **Axial thickness:** Normally posterior pole of lens shows no movement during accommodation phase, however, forward movement of anterior pole of lens increases the axial thickness of crystalline lens.
- **Lens sinks down:** During accommodation as the lens is less firmly held by its zonular attachments so due to gravitational pull the lens sinks downwards within the globe.
- **Lens substance changes:** Along with change in curvatures of lens, the change in the substance of crystalline lens also produces a change in refractivity of lens. Changes in curvature of various portions of lens happen due to internal changes in substances having different refractive indices.
- **Pupillary constriction and eye convergence:** During accommodation constriction of pupil and convergence of eyes takes place almost simultaneously with the above mentioned changes in crystalline lens and zonules. These all changes occur together in a bid to see near objects clearly. Pupillary constriction is just a synkinesis reflex (not a true reflex) because it is neither dependent on alone accommodation or alone convergence of the eye.
- **Choroid:** Ciliary muscle contraction cause forward stretching of the choroid.
- **Ora serrata:** Each dioptric power of accommodation moves ora serrata forwards to about 0.05 mm.

ACCOMMODATION ANOMALIES

Introduction and Classification

As per our previous discussions the amplitude of accommodation varies with age and has wide range, which may be considered as variant of normal range. Any variation above or below of this normal range is not common and is considered as an accommodation anomaly, which can be classified as shown in Table 7.4.

Table 7.4: Classification of accommodation anomalies

Increased accommodation (Hyperaccommodation)	Decreased accommodation

• Excessive accommodation
• Accommodative spasm
	• Physiological: Presbyopia
	• Pathological
	  – Insufficiency of accommodation
	  – Inertia of accommodation
	  – Ill-sustained accommodation
	  – Paralysis of accommodation
	• Pharmacological: Cycloplegia by drugs
	• Fatigue of accommodation

Increased Accommodation

Excessive Accommodation

As the name explains this is a situation where an individual apply more than normal accommodation to see the near object clearly, this situation is termed an excessive accommodation. This is under the voluntary control of a person and is discontinuous phenomenon, whereas spasm of accommodation is nonvoluntary and is a continuous process.

Etiology: Under following conditions person may use excess accommodation:
- Refractive errors: Hypermetropia, myopia and astigmatism errors especially in young person is associated with the use of excessive accommodation. It is a kind of physiological adaptation to see the objects clearly.
- Presbyopia: Presbyopes in the initial stage of its development use more accommodation to carry out near work.
- Use of wrong spectacles: Sometimes, use of improper or ill-fitted glasses is also associated with an excessive use of accommodation.

- Prolonged near work: Near work carried out in presence of poor/excessive illumination for long duration may cause an excessive use of accommodation. In addition, most of the time the general health conditions (physical and mental) of these patients are also poor.

Symptoms

- Diminution of vision: Due to increased tone of ciliary muscles a condition like pseudo myopia develops so that emmetrope becomes myopic, a myope becomes more severe myopic and a hypermetrope may appears myope, less hypermetrope or emmetrope. There is blurring of vision of variable degrees mainly for distant vision.
- Both the far and near point becomes nearer to eyes and distant vision becomes blur, so concave lenses are prescribed for improvement in vision. However, improving the pseudo myopia by use of concave lenses will worsen the situation.
- Near vision usually not affected but in advanced cases the near vision is also affected and after reading a few pages the print becomes blurred and letters get confused. This condition will improve after taking the rest or closing the eyes for some time.
- Ocular asthenopic symptoms like headache, fatigue, discomforts in eyes and tiredness are usually present especially when doing near work.

Treatment

It can be treated effectively with a good prognostic outcome.

- **Correction of refractive errors:** Refraction should be done under full cycloplegia and correction of refractive error done by prescribing glasses of power having 1 D less than the total correction. In recalcitrant cases to ensure absolute visual rest, eyes are kept mildly under the influence of atropine for a period of one to two weeks. This will allow the overexcited ciliary muscle to recover from its irritable condition.

- **General treatment:** Treatment of general condition is equally important for an effective outcome which includes
  - Near work is stopped completely for some period of time. Once the near work is restarted, the amount, duration and conditions in which near work is done should be supervised.
  - General health conditions of these patients are taken care because most of them are in poor health or overworked or neurotic. Hence a plan of holiday or trip with change of weather has a great beneficial effect than any medical treatment.

Accommodative Spasm

Accommodation spasm is a condition where an individual exerts an abnormally excessive accommodation non-voluntarily.

Etiology: Accommodative spasm may occur due to various functional or organic reasons.

- Spontaneous spasm of accommodation is rarely seen in young children with decreased visual acuity who try to compensate for their refractive error (usually hypermetropia, may be astigmatism or myopia also) especially when doing prolonged near work in conditions such as poor illumination.
- Use of miotic drugs: Certain strong miotic drugs like echothiophate and Di-isopropyl fluoro phosphate (DFP) on instillation may cause spasm of accommodation. Young glaucoma patients using pilocarpine having associated myopic error may also develop accommodative spasm.
- Brain stem lesions such as meningitis, tabetic crisis and epidemic encephalitis, in their irritative phase may be associated with spasm of ciliary muscle.
- Toxic adverse effects due to some drugs like sulphonamides, arsenic or even excessive smoking may sometimes induce accommodation spasm.
- Spasm of near reflex is characterized by miosis, excessive accommodation and

intermittent convergence strabismus, usually functional in origin (seen in hysteria or tense individuals).

- Inflammatory condition of eye: Iridocyclitis or other inflammatory condition of eye may cause spasm of accommodation.
- Other conditions: Trigeminal neuralgia, dental wound, sympathetic and parasympathetic imbalance are other precipitating factors of accommodative spasm.

Symptoms

- Blurred vision for distant objects because of pseudo myopia. Near point is shifted abnormally close to eye.
- Asthenopic symptoms: May be more than visual symptoms in the form of headache and brow ache.
- Macropsia, a condition where objects appear larger than they really are, may appear due to optical delusion.
- Sometimes patient may complain of gastric problems due to reflex mechanism.

Treatment

- Medical treatment is done by inducing relaxation or paralysis of ciliary muscle. Complete paralysis of ciliary muscle is done for a long period (≥ 4 weeks) by using cycloplegic drug like atropine. Sometimes, spam may reappear, once the effect of cycloplegic is over. In this situation, it is advised to start atropine again for further period of time.
- Post cycloplegic optical correction: Glasses of appropriate power should be prescribed immediately after the effect of atropinization is over.
- General measures should be taken to prevent spasm as described in excessive accommodation section.

Decreased Accommodation

Physiological: Presbyopia

Presbyopia or eyesight of old age is not considered as refractive error; rather it is an age related decline in visual acuity, occurs due to physiological deficiency of accommodation, which leads to a gradual diminution of near vision.

Changing pattern of amplitude of accommodation with age: Age related change in the power of accommodation can be understood easily by the graph (Fig. 7.10) composed by Fisher.

This graph is representing average amplitude of accommodation (the ordinate) in relation to advancing age (the abscissa). We know that far point in emmetropes is at infinity, while near point varies with the age of person. During early childhood (10–12 years) the amplitude of accommodation is about 14 D, and near point (punctum proximum) is at a distance of about 7 cm. Thereafter, with advancing age there is gradual reduction of the amplitude of accommodation in linear fashion and by the age of 30–36 years amplitude becomes nearly 50% of original, i.e. about 7 D while near point moves away at distance of about 14 cm. By the age of 45 years amplitude remains only 4 D and near point reaches about 25 cm. At age of 60 years the amplitude remains only 1 D. Normally, we do near work at an average distance of 28–30 cm and in emmetropes this final limit to see the near objects clearly is achieved at about 40–45 years of age when the power of accommodation remained only of 4 D. Hence to work continuously at the near point of

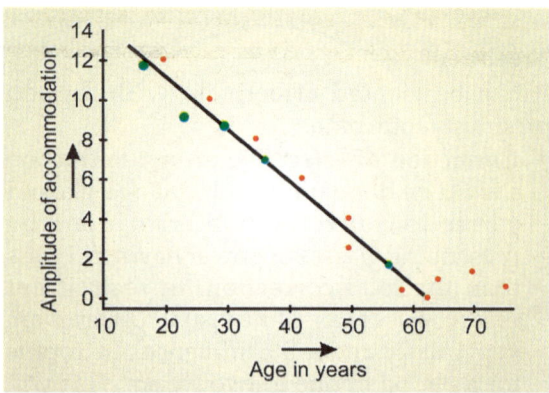

Fig. 7.10: Graph showing variations of accommodation with age

25–30 cm at this age, the person has to use whole of the available accommodative power which puts a substantial strain on the eye and produce asthenopic symptoms. To avoid these symptoms due to eye strain it is necessary that about one-third of total accommodation must be in reserve. It is clear that as the near point reaches to 25–30 cm, it means presbyopia has started and the person needs visual aid for near work at this point. Presbyopia in emmetropes usually starts at the age of 40–45 years. However, depending on the refractive status of person also, the age of onset of presbyopia may vary. For example, in uncorrected hypermetrope the symptoms of presbyopia appear at earlier age because in hypermetrope near point is significantly away from the beginning of life thus hypermetrope person exerts own voluntary effort in the form of increased accommodation to correct the error. In contrary, the myopes rarely or never develop presbyopia because near point distance of myopes lies within working distance.

Age of onset of presbyopia also depends on reading habits and profession of an individual. For example, if a person has a habit of reading books more closely, has greater chance to develop presbyopia at early age than who maintain some distance while reading. Similarly, the professionals who are musicians, carpenter, etc. (who do work at 30–35 cm distance) will need visual aid for presbyopia at later age as compared to professionals goldsmiths, compositors , engravers, etc. (work at small distance of about 20–25 cm).

Etiology of Presbyopia

Presbyopia occurs due to loss of accommodation with advancement of age. This decline in accommodative power may occur due to

- **Age related changes in crystalline lens and its capsule:** With advancing age sclerosis (hardening) of the lens tissue is increased and there is change in the ratio of elasticity of lens capsule and lens matrix, as a result the capsule is not able to mold the hardened lens. There is also change in size and volume of the lens.
- **Age related decrease in ciliary muscle activity:** With increasing age the contractile power of ciliary muscle is decreased and angle of insertion of zonules on lens changed.

Usual age of onset of presbyopia is 40–45 years. However, in some situations premature onset of presbyopia may occur, like in

- Uncorrected hypermetropia
- Chronic simple glaucoma
- General debility and chronic illness: Poor nutrition and more exposure of sunlight predispose early changes in lens.
- Premature nuclear sclerosis of lens

Symptoms

- Difficulty to focus on near objects: As the amplitude of accommodation declines, it becomes difficult for person to do near work at usual distance. In initial stage, presbyopes feel difficulty in reading of small fonts or to see finer objects, especially in dim light (e.g. evening). To get clear vision they usually try to hold their head backwards, keeping the book at more distance and prefer to read in bright light. However, with decrease in accommodation the vision is reduced even in bright light and finally it becomes impossible to do near work.

Note: There is less difficulty in bright light because constriction of pupil (miosis) occurs in bright light which will further increase the depth of focus.

- In more old age, when there is no accommodative power in the eye but the person can see the near objects clearly up to some extent. This is because of decrease in the size of pupil (senile miosis) at this age.

Note: Presbyopic symptoms are exaggerated by associated systemic illness, fatigue, or debilitating diseases.

- Asthenopic (eye strain) symptoms may appear due to decrease of ciliary muscle power and its fatigue. Headache and tiredness of eyes are common after reading for a longer duration or doing near work continuously.
- Sometimes, person may experience diplopia due to dissociation between accommodation and convergence.

Treatment of presbyopia

Presbyopia can be treated by:
- Optical correction
- Surgical correction

Optical correction: Glasses should be prescribed after evaluation of static refraction in both eyes (binocular) and in individual eye (monocular). Convex lenses of suitable power should be added for clear and comfortable near vision. The purpose of prescribing addition is to reinforce accommodation so that the near point lies into a useful working distance after addition. Thus, an addition or add is the difference between distance correction and near correction, in terms of power of lenses.

Some basic rules which should be followed for optical correction in presbyopes are

- First do the refraction under cycloplegia and mydriasis and correct the refractive error for distance, if present.
- After correction of distant vision, estimate the amount of correction required for presbyopic error in each eye separately, i.e. find out the working distance and amplitude of accommodation. Add this correction with the distance correction.
- Presbyopic correction should be given in such a way that at least one-third of accommodation remains in reserve for symptom free reading and near point of presbyope comes into useful working distance.
- However, the limit of accommodation and working distance vary in individuals according to profession and age. Hence, near point is decided on the basis of individual requirement (e.g. working distance for an executive will be more, so lesser add is required) and correction should be done on individual basis.

A rough estimate of addition power requires at various age groups especially in emmetropes is shown in Table 7.5.

- Power of presbyopic addition is prescribed as per the need of working distance required by a particular person. According to working distance the power of addition will change among the patients having similar type of refractive status.

An emmetropic person in his/her late 40s has been left with only 4–6 D total amplitude of accommodation. For various working distances addition given to this person is shown in Table 7.6, sparing him/her with a comfortable 50% of accommodation.

- In all cases, it is advised that convex lens of weakest power (under correction) with which a person can see the near object clearly and comfortably should be given. As overcorrection or prescribing of strong lenses will disturb the association of accommodation and convergence and lead to asthenopic symptoms, i.e. headache.

Table 7.5: Presbyopic addition at various age groups

Age in years	Addition in dioptre
40–45	+0.75 to + 1.25
46–50	+1.5 to +1.75
51–55	+2.0 to +2.5
56–60	+2.5 to +3.0
> 60	Variable

Table 7.6: Estimated addition in relation to working distance

Working distance	Add power (dioptres)
1/4 meter or 25 cm	+ 2.5
1/3 meter or 33 cm	+ 1.75
0.4 meter or 40 cm	+ 1.0
Half meter or 50 cm	+ 0.5

Note: For an intermediate distance vision an additional correction may be required if patient wants to see the objects at an intermediate distance.

Addition for intermediate vision: When amplitude of accommodation decreases the addition power will increase, so that the range to see near objects also decreases and it may produce dissatisfaction in an aging person. In simpler words, the range of near vision decreases with increase of addition power.

For example, if we consider a 42 years old emmetrope who works normally at distance of 38 cm, will have total amplitude of accommodation of about 4 D. Suppose if this person has been prescribed with reading glasses of power +1 D bilaterally, then his range to see the near objects clearly through these reading glasses will begin from point A at a distance of 1.00 meter (or 1/1 D) from eye and will extend up to point B at a distance of 0.2 meter (1/(4 + 1) D = 1/5 D) as shown in Fig. 7.11.

The same individual after 20 years (about 62 years) will be left with only 1.25 D of total amplitude of accommodation. Suppose , if the working distance of this individual is still 38 cm, and an addition power of +2.5 D has been prescribed for near vision, then his range to see the near objects clearly through these glasses begins from point A at a distance 1/ 2.5 D or 0.4 meter from eye and extends up to point B at a distance 1/(2.5+1.25) = 1/3.75 or 0.26 meter as shown in Fig. 7.12.

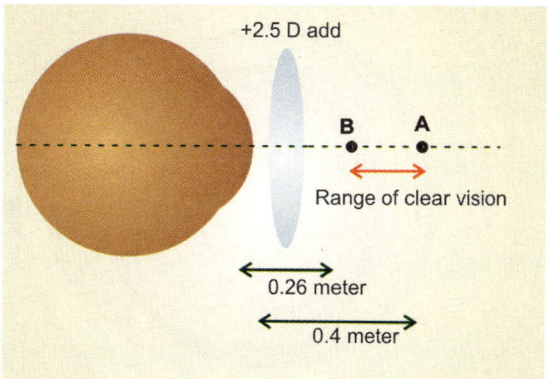

Fig. 7.12: Range of clear near vision with +2.5 D lenses

Being an emmetrope even at an age of 62 years this person will see the distant objects clearly without wearing glasses, however he/she can see near objects clearly in very small range (as shown in Fig. 7.12) after wearing reading glasses.

If this person desires to see the objects situated at an intermediate distance (say at 50–60 cm) after wearing the reading glasses, then the objects will appear blur because they are situated out of the range of clear vision. To increase the range of clear vision in this patient we need to prescribe an intermediate additional power, along with near add. These intermediate additions are usually one-half the power of near correction. Hence, in this emmetropic patient the range for intermediate objects can be widened by giving an intermediate addition of +1.25 D along with +2.5 D near add. With this prescription person can see clearly an additional range which starts from point A at a distance 1/1.25 D or 0.8 meter up to point B at 1/(1.25 + 1.25) = 1/2.5 D = 0.4 meter also. However, the near add of +2.5 D give total near vision range up to point C at 0.26 meter as shown in Fig. 7.13. In a nutshell, near vision range with only +2.5 D was 0.26 to 0.4 meter, which widened to 0.26 to 0.8 meter after adding intermediate power of +1.25 D in glasses.

Modes of prescribing presbyopic correction

Various types of following optical glasses

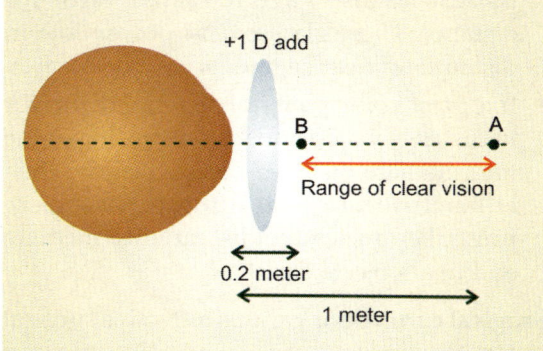

Fig. 7.11: Range of clear near vision with +1 D lenses

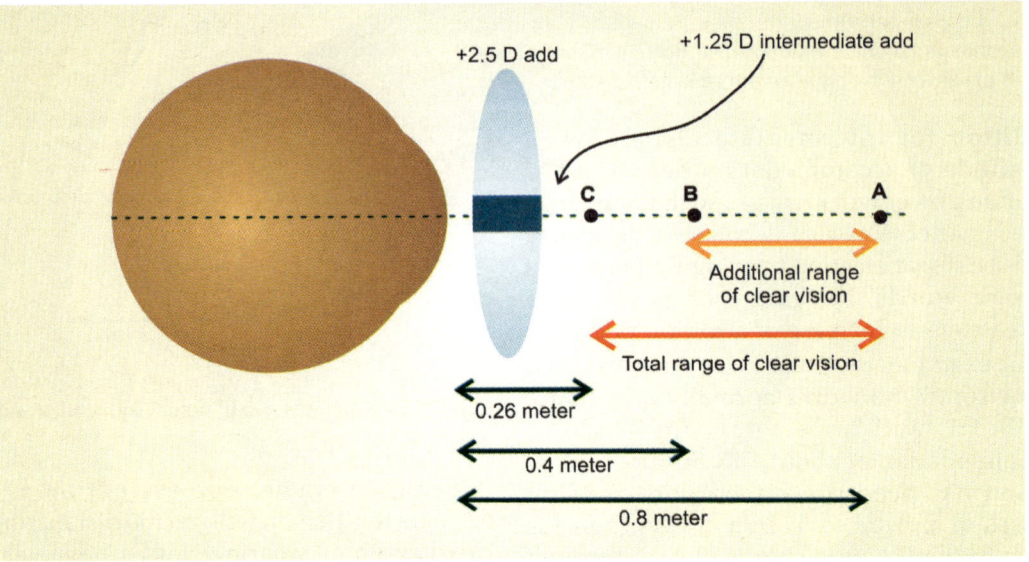

Fig. 7.13: Increased range of clear near vision by adding intermediate power +1.25 D with existing near addition +2.5 D power lenses

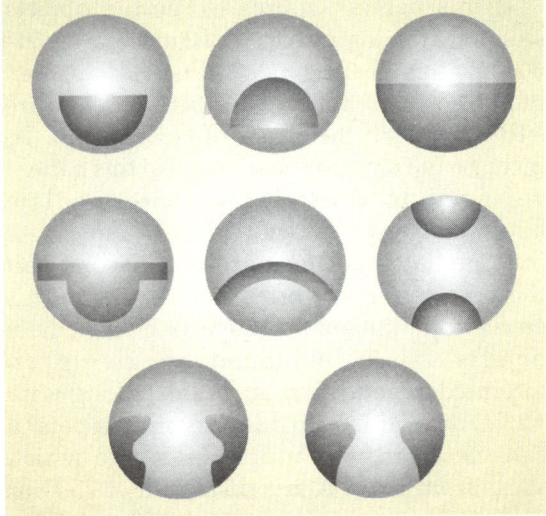

Fig. 7.14: Various optical glasses for presbyopia correction

(Fig. 7.14) can be prescribed in presbyopes as per the requirements of patient
- Monofocal reading glasses
- Plano focal glasses
- Bifocal glasses
- Trifocal glasses
- Multifocal glasses

- If the patient is emmetrope or having a non-significant distance error, then single vision reading glasses are the best choice for near vision. Because the distance vision becomes blur through these reading glasses, so to see the distant objects clearly patient can remove these glasses or can look from above these reading glasses. Alternatively, plano focal or bifocal glasses can be prescribed. Plano focal glasses have no power for distance in upper segment and have suitable near addition power in lower segment. Bifocal glasses are prescribed to those who also have refractive error for distance. These glasses have power both in distant and near segments.

- If a presbyopic patient has refractive error in distance vision and also wants to see the intermediate distance objects clearly, then either trifocal or multifocal glasses are prescribed to see the distant, intermediate and near objects clearly.

Surgical correction: Various refractive surgical correction procedures of presbyopia are described in Chapter 15.

Pathological

Insufficiency of Accommodation

When accommodative power of eye is significantly less than that of normal physiological limits adjusted for his/her age, is called insufficiency of accommodation.

Note: In presbyopia physiological limits of accommodation are normal according to the age of person.

Aetiology

- Ciliary muscle weakness or fatigue: May occur due to
  Systemic illness causing muscular fatigue: As seen in anemia, malnutrition, diabetes mellitus, stress, debilitating diseases, toxemia due to infections or chronic alcoholism, etc. Excessive near work done in unfavorable conditions in presence of ciliary muscle fatigue may lead to failure of accommodation followed by asthenopic symptoms.
  Ocular diseases: Ciliary muscle weakness may also occur due to ocular causes such as primary open angle glaucoma, sympathetic ophthalmia causing mild cyclitis.
- Lenticular changes such as nuclear sclerosis of lens which indicate onset of premature presbyopia and only physical accommodation is affected. Hence this is a stable condition and gives rise to no symptoms except those of presbyopia, which sets in unusually at early age.

Symptoms

Symptoms of this condition are similar to presbyopia except that asthenopic symptoms are more pronounced than visual symptoms. Patients usually present with following symptoms

- **Asthenopic symptoms while doing near work:** Patient may complaints of headache, irritability, tiredness, early fatigability of eyes while making an effort to do near work. Normally, the patients remain asymptomatic if they do not perform any near work.

Note: Symptoms of accommodation insufficiency developing due to lenticular changes usually remain stable, however, if they occur due to ciliary muscle weakness they may show improvement when general and ocular condition of patient is improved and excessive near work or strain due to near work is reduced.

- **Blurring of vision:** Occur during near work and sometimes it becomes impossible to perform the near work.
- **Intermittent diplopia due to disturbance in convergence:** Usually the accommodation insufficiency is associated with convergence failure, but occasionally, if a patient tries to overcome accommodation insufficiency then excessive amount of convergence may occur.

Treatment

Treatment of insufficiency of accommodation is done on following guidelines:

- **Proper treatment of the systemic and ocular causes:** All the systemic or local causes responsible for accommodative failure should be detected and treated accordingly to give improvement in accommodation. Work conditions (avoid overwork or worry) should also be regulated with improvement in general health for good results. If the same conditions prevail again, then there are chances of recurrence of symptoms.
- **Optical correction for near vision:** In every case any refractive error for far should be corrected first. If still vision for near work is blurred, then spectacle with weakest convex lenses is prescribed which give the adequate amount of vision, till there is an improvement in power of accommodation.
  - If an associated convergence insufficiency is present, then base in prism of adequate

Note: In a nutshell any type of refractive error should be fully corrected and when a recovery in accommodation is seen, then the additional power for near is made weaker gradually at regular intervals of time.

power are added to improve the comfort of patient.

– If an associated convergence excess is present, then full spherical correction is done.

• **Exercises for improvement of accommodation:** Accommodation exercises are helpful in those cases

  – where accommodation insufficiency is due to decreased activity of ciliary muscles.

  – who are not having lenticular sclerosis (early cataract) and state of general debility or has recovered from it

Methods to perform accommodation exercises are

• Distance correction glasses should be worn during accommodation exercises.

• Exercises can be done with the help of a simple accommodation test-card. The test card simply has a black vertical line drawn on a white background card. These exercises should be done at short periods throughout the day.

• The patient is asked to hold this card at a considerable distance and then bring this card closer to the eyes until the black vertical line of card becomes blur and indistinct. Encourage the patient to repeat this procedure in an attempt to bring his/her near point as close as possible to eyes. Along with this ask the patient to maintain his/her accommodation efforts as long as possible with comfort, while keeping the vertical line clear.

• Exercise should be done with both eyes simultaneously if there is convergence deficiency. However, in case of convergence excess only one eye should be used for exercise at a time, other eye should be covered.

Inertia of Accommodation

This is relatively a rare condition, where patient feels some difficulty in altering the accommodation as per the distance or range of the desired object. Normally the accommodative response occurs within one second to change focus. In inertia of accommodation patient takes some time along with some extra efforts to focus a near object, after looking a distant object for some period.

Symptoms: Typically patients complain that they need some time and some extra efforts to focus near object after looking a distant object for long duration. Some frustration and trouble may be created by this condition although it rarely poses any serious problem.

Treatment

• For symptomatic relief optical correction of associated refractive error should be done.

• Accommodation exercises are advised for relief for long duration.

III Sustained Accommodation

This is also termed condition of accommodation fatigue and mainly refers to a situation where range and amplitude of accommodation is normal but patient is not able to maintain the accommodative efforts for a long time period. Hence, in an effort to use eyes for a near work over a prolonged period weakens the accommodative power so that the near point progressively recedes and blurring of near vision occurs.

Causes

Ill sustained accommodation is considered the initial stage of true accommodation insufficiency hence causative factors is same as in true insufficiency. However, accommodation fatigue characteristically seen in following situations

• Person is recovering (convalescence stage) from debilitating illnesses.

• Person is in a state of general tiredness

• Person is reading in physically relaxed situations or in the evening time.

Symptoms

Patients mainly complain that while performing near work they feels tired very soon. Their near point of accommodation gradually recedes, which leads to blurred near vision.

Treatment

- Patients are directed mainly to reduce the near work within their capabilities and limits of duration especially during convalescence and tiredness.
- Improvement in visual hygiene especially improvement in illumination conditions and posture while reading.

Paralysis of Accommodation

Paralysis of accommodation means the accommodative system of eye does not respond to any stimuli, i.e. complete absence of accommodation. It can be unilateral or bilateral, sudden or insidious in onset and may or may not be associated with palsy of extraocular muscle and fixed dilated pupil (paralytic mydriasis).

Aetiology

Paralysis of accommodation may be due to
- **Ocular causes**
  - Exposure of eyes to parasympatholytic drugs like atropine, homatropine, etc.
  - Traumatic injury, glaucoma and cyclitis in eye.
- **Systemic causes**
  Systemic causes may cause paralysis of accommodation by affecting oculomotor nerve, ciliary muscle, sphincter pupillae and midbrain region. Causes may be
  - Infectious diseases may act either centrally or via peripheral neurotoxin mechanism includes mumps, herpes zoster, tonsillitis, infectious mononucleosis, pneumonia, diphtheria and typhoid.
  - Central neurological disease and infections: Vascular disorders, cerebral syphilis, epidemic encephalitis.
  - Non-infectious toxic conditions like chronic alcoholism, diabetes mellitus, botulism, lead poisoning or belladonna intoxication may also be responsible.
  - Intracranial or orbital lesions such as traumatic, inflammatory or neoplastic conditions causing third nerve paralysis are also responsible for paralysis of accommodation.

Symptoms

- **Near vision blurring:** As the near point in paralysis of accommodation get recedes gradually, the emmetropic or hypermetropic person complaint of blurring in near vision although it is less marked in myopes.
- **Photophobia or glare:** This happens due to the dilatation of pupil or mydriasis, which is generally associated with paralysis of accommodation.
- In cases of paralysis of accommodation, ocular examination shows an abnormal receding of near point (which approximates the far point) and a decreased range of accommodation.
- Phenomenon of micropsia may also occur because a delusion of distance may be induced by accommodative anomaly and objects will appear smaller than their actual size.

Treatment

- Primarily this condition is resolved once the treatment of its cause is done. For example, in drug induced paralysis once the effect of drug is over, self recovery occur. Similarly treatment of toxemic conditions like diphtheria, diabetes or poisoning, etc. will give favorable results.
- However, in some cases of traumatic injuries, the recovery may be incomplete or totally absent. Presbyopic spectacles (convex lenses) may be prescribed in these cases for near work or for reading purpose.
- Photophobia or glare can be reduced by use of dark glasses.

Pharmacological Deficient Accommodation

Cycloplegia

Cycloplegia (cyclo = ciliary and plegia = palsy) means paralysis of the ciliary muscle or paralysis of accommodation of the eye. Cycloplegia can be produced by administration of anticholinergic (parasympatholytic) drugs like atropine, homatropine, scopolamine, etc. (termed cycloplegics) into the conjunctival sac. These anticholinergic drugs also cause mydriasis, i.e. dilatation of pupil by relaxation of the sphincter pupillae (constrictor pupillae) muscle of iris. Hence, these drugs along with dilatation of pupil also cause some degree of paralysis of accommodation. In contrast, the drugs (cholinergic drugs like physostigmine or pilocarpine) which cause the constriction of pupil, i.e. miosis will induce some degree of spasm of accommodation by causing spasm of ciliary muscle. Ideally a cycloplegic agent should have fast onset of action, short duration of action, must produce full cycloplegia and should produce less or no ocular and systemic adverse effects.

Uses of cycloplegics
- Both cycloplegia and mydriasis are required for accurate estimation of refractive errors. Due to cycloplegic action the accommodation efforts to see near objects is abolished and the refractive error which was latent before gets obvious (latent to manifest hypermetropia). It is especially required in children because they have high amplitude of accommodation.
- Due to dilatation of pupil (mydriasis) caused by these drugs, the estimation of the amount of refractive error by retinoscopy become easier especially in persons having small pupil.
- Mydriasis is also necessary for detailed examination of interiors, i.e. fundus of eye.
- Symptoms of asthenopia or eye strain occurring due to spasm of accommodation can be improved by using long-acting drugs, e.g. atropine or homatropine which imparts a state of rest on the eye and thus helps it in recovery from the fatigue.

Cycloplegic drugs
Various cycloplegic drugs of ophthalmic interest are:
- Atropine
- Homatropine
- Scopolamine (Hyoscine)
- Cyclopentolate
- Tropicamide

Atropine
Mechanism of action: Atropine is the most potent cycloplegic agents as compared to others. After administration into conjunctival sac, it gets absorbed into the anterior chamber of eye. Being parasympatholytic drug it blocks action of acetylcholine on ciliary muscle and sphincter pupillae muscle of iris. Thus, all the muscle fibers in eye which are supplied by parasympathetic nervous system get paralyzed resulting in cycloplegia along with mydriasis.

Duration of action: It causes dilatation of pupil within about 15 minutes but cycloplegic action is slow in onset. Hence, it is advised to prescribe atropine 3–4 days prior to examination especially in young children so that full paralysis of accommodation is achieved. For young people having strong accommodation, atropine should be given thrice daily for three consecutive days to achieve desired results. Atropine has long duration of action and complete recovery of accommodation occurs in about 7–10 days and mydriasis in 9–12 days. Effect of atropine is usually not counteracted by miotic drug like pilocarpine, hence it is advised that post mydriatic test should be carried out after 10 days in atropine treated patient.

Dosage: It is available as 0.5% or 1% either in the form of drops or ointment. Usually, drops are watery solution of atropine sulphate, whereas ointment contains a 1% solution of alkaloid form with soft yellow paraffin base. Drops can be used three times daily for 3 days and ointment is used specially in children once daily (usually at night) for 3–4 days before examination.

Clinical effects: Ointment is more preferred in young children because ointments can be rubbed easily into the eyes as children resist strenuously for instillation of drops and frequency of administration of ointment is also less. Moreover, it is slowly and continuously absorbed as compared to drops. Sometimes, symptoms of atropine intoxication may occur because of passage of drugs through lacrimal duct.

Precautions: Application of ointment should be avoided a few hours before examination of eye because being greasy in nature ointment may remain over the cornea and interfere with its transparency which in further will affect the estimation of refractive error.

Atropine should not be used in patients with closed-angle glaucoma and in hypersensitive patient.

Homatropine

Mechanism of action of homatropine is similar to atropine, however, onset of action is rapid and less potent as compared to atropine.

Duration of action and dosage: As compared to atropine its action starts within 5 minutes and reaches its maximum within 45–50 minutes and also the duration of action is short, its effects usually last up to 24 hours, however, some residual impairment in accommodation may persist for 2–3 days. Homatropine eye drops are available as watery solution of homatropine hydro bromide in strength of 1% or 2%. Drops are installed 3–4 times at an interval of 15 minutes to produce desired effect on accommodation for examination purpose or are given as twice daily dosage for therapeutic purpose.

Cyclopentolate and tropicamide

Cyclopentolate and tropicamide (bistropamide) have rapid onset of action, with a satisfactory cycloplegic effect. One drop of drug (0.5% and 1% solutions) instilled in each eye and is repeated every 10 minutes for 3–4 times will produce intense mydriasis and cycloplegia in about 30–45 min. Effect of cyclopentolate remains for a period of 24 hours but some amount of accommodation insufficiency can persist till 3–4 days. Action of tropicamide lasts for about 4–7 hours.

Note: In very young children cyclopentolate due to its irritant action can produce spasm of accommodation for a temporary period. In these cases it is better to use atropine for cycloplegia.

Scopolamine (Hyoscine)

Hyoscine or scopolamine bromide in 0.5% solution has a similar action as that of atropine. It has an advantage over atropine because of transitory action which lasts only for a period of about 4–5 days. It is a suitable cycloplegic for children.

Note:
- It is important to know that quantity and type of cycloplegia is not always same for each individual. The dosage of cycloplegics requires to produce the adequate degree of paralysis of accommodation may vary significantly in individuals. Sometimes, even the two eyes of same individual may show different degree of cycloplegia in response to same dose of a cycloplegic drug, a condition called anisocycloplegia (0.5 D difference in depth of cycloplegia is commonly seen, in exceptional cases it may reach up to 10 D)
- It has been recommended that before doing refraction, the depth of cycloplegia should be tested in each individual. This can be done easily by using accommodation cards which is used to test the remaining amplitude of accommodation. Normally, after cycloplegia it should not exceed 1 D. It means that line on test card should appear blur at a distance of 1 meter, if line is still clear at 1 meter then further instillation of cycloplegic drug is needed.
- Drugs like phenylephrine (directly acting sympathomimetic) and cocaine (indirectly acting sympathomimetic) also cause dilatation of pupil (mydriasis) but no cycloplegia. It has been suggested that combination of sympathomimetic drugs with atropine or homatropine may cause synergistic action and helps to produce quicker cycloplegia.
- Instillation of cycloplegics and mydriatic drugs may precipitate glaucoma in patients especially with shallow anterior chamber. Hence it is advised to measure intraocular tension before administration of these drugs especially in patient with more than 40 years of age.

Fatigue of Accommodation

Usually, in a normal eye fatigue of accommodation is rare; rather an excessive use of accommodation may cause increase in the amplitude of accommodation in many cases. However, when the visual tasks are repeated for a long time in the range which lies near punctum proximum, an accommodation fatigue can develop even in normal emmetropic eyes. The most common symptom is asthenopia. Most commonly adopted technique to measure the fatigability of accommodation was developed by Lucien Howe, which was further modified by scientist Berens. Test is done by repeatedly presenting a target carrying a dot or small object to the patient eye till that target appears blurred. The details of target movement pathways are recorded on a drum automatically. The target movement pathways should not be diminished for a minimum period of 15 minutes, because usually after 15 minutes duration a general fatigue will be noted.

Note: Fatigue responses of two eyes are different and either of the uniocular response again may differ from binocular response.

Convergence and its Anomalies

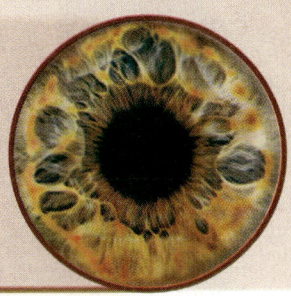

CONVERGENCE

Introduction

When an emmetrope person looks at a distant object, the position of visual axes is parallel to each other and there is no associated accommodative effort. However, as the fixation point change from distant point to a nearer point, then to see the near object clearly there is an effort of accommodation (increase in refractive power of eye) and also the visual axes rotate inwards to maintain a defined image formation on the retina or fovea. In other words, we can say that the angle formed between visual axes of two eyes will increase to maintain image of object at two foveae. This change in the relative position or movement of visual axes is known as convergence. Hence

Convergence means the simultaneous and synchronous inward rotation of both the eyes to maintain single binocular vision as the fixation point alters from more distant to a nearer point.

Amplitude of convergence is not influenced by the process of ageing as seen in case of accommodation (decline in accommodation occurs with increasing age). Usually, convergence does not change with progression of age. However, associated abnormal systemic and ocular conditions may decrease the power of convergence while various ocular exercises show positive influences on the power of convergence.

Types of Convergence

Convergence per se is a complex process and can be grouped as shown in Table 8.1.

Voluntary Convergence

Convergence is the only vergence movement of the eye that can be exerted at will also. Normal type of convergence which occurs during normal visual and ocular activities is essentially a reflex mechanism. However, it can be produced by voluntary rotation of both the eyeballs also, so that the visual axes of both the eyes intersect to focus on the object. With practice some person can maintain this

Table 8.1: Types of convergence	
Voluntary convergence	Involuntary or reflex convergence
	• Tonic convergence
	• Accommodative convergence
	• Fusional convergence
	• Proximal convergence

convergent position of eyes even in absence of fixation object. It is more commonly seen in children where it is done in an attempt to gain attention of their parents. Voluntary convergence is centered in frontal lobe of cerebrum. Every person is not skilled enough of converging at will, but if voluntary convergence is well developed, then reflex type of convergence usually becomes more automatic and efficient.

Reflex (Involuntary) Convergence

As the term implies the phenomenon of convergence is not under voluntary control. Rather it is a psycho-optical reflex controlled by peristriate area of occipital cortex and by centre for fixation reflex. It has four elements

- Tonic convergence
- Accommodative convergence
- Fusional convergence
- Proximal convergence

Tonic convergence: When a person is awake and alert, it is the tonic convergence which decides the relative position of visual axes and helps to maintain the parallelism of the eyes at infinity. This tonic convergence is considered due to presence of intrinsic innervational tone in extra ocular muscles of eye which arises because of various excitatory and inhibitory inputs arising to extraocular muscles from cortex, subcortex or vestibular center. Normally due to effect of this tone eyes become more convergent as compared to previous condition, however, anatomically still the eyes remain divergent in relation to each other. Tonic convergence does not depend on fusion or location of the object. However, amplitude of tonic convergence deceases with advancement of the age and is totally abolished under deep general anesthesia. Emotional status of a person can also affect tonic convergence.

Accommodative convergence: As the name implies an accommodative convergence is that component of convergence which occurs along with accommodation of eye. As discussed above disparity of retinal images is responsible for stimulation of fusional convergence. However, stimulus for accommodative convergence is blurring of retinal images, not retinal disparity. As a response to blur image, the impulse are discharged to eyes from central system for accommodation and then the visual system tries to clear the blur images by mechanism of accommodation. Hence we can say that both accommodation and convergence are related to each other and are in synkinetic relationship along with contraction of pupil (miosis). Thus, the central mechanism to focus the near object is governed by a synkinetic near reflex, which consists of three elements

- Accommodative convergence
- Accommodation
- Miosis

The quantitative relationship between accommodative convergence (AC) and accommodation (A) is denoted as AC / A ratio, i.e. it is the change in the amount of convergence due to change in specific amount of accommodation. The amount of accommodative convergence is measured in prism dioptre and that of accommodation is measured in lens dioptres, hence the ratio can be denoted as number of prism dioptre induced by per one diopter of accommodation.

An accommodative convergence of 3–4 prism dioptre for 1 D of accommodation is considered as a normal AC / A ratio. High ratio indicates that eyes are over converging for a specific amount of accommodation and responsible for more esotropia (convergent squint) and less exotropia on near vision,

whereas low ratio indicates that eyes are under converging for given amount of accommodation and may cause more exotropia (divergent squint) and less esotropia on near vision. The AC / A ratio states a linear relationship which usually does not change throughout life.

AC / A ratio is of two types:
1. Stimulus AC / A ratio: When eyes are stimulated with lens of different power or object at different distance (i.e. stimulus), then there is change in convergence capacity of eyes resulting in change in accommodation. Usually, the stimulus is presented at distance of 40 cm which require accommodation of about 2.50 D
2. Response AC / A ratio: It indicates the response of accommodation which occurs due to change in convergence capacity of eyes. As discussed above the stimulus for accommodation is of 2.5 D (40 cm) but the accommodative response is generally 10% less than this stimulus (2.5 D) and there is accommodation lag of about + 0.25 D to + 0.50 D.

Measurement of AC/A Ratio

Measurement of AC / A ratio can be done by following methods
- Heterophoria method
- Gradient method
- Fixation disparity method
- Haploscopic method

Heterophoria method: This test is based on the fact that changes in the accommodation cause change in amount of convergence and accommodation can be altered by changing the fixation distance of eyes. In this method the distance and near deviation of eyes are measured which are then compared to find out AC / A ratio. Deviation of eyes in distance vision (Δd in prism dioptre) is measured at 20 feet after giving full optical correction and assuming that accommodation is at rest. Deviation of eyes in near vision (Δn in prism diopter) is measured at 33 cm (or 3 D) assuming that the convergence applied is caused by accommodative convergence solely. Interpupillary distance (IPD) is measured in centimeters by using ruler.

Now AC / A ratio can be calculated by applying this formula using all these value as

$$AC / A = IPD + \frac{\Delta n - \Delta d}{D}$$

Here,

IPD = Interpupillary distance (cm)

Δn = Deviation of eyes in near vision (prism dioptres)

Δd = Deviation of eyes in distance vision (prism dioptres)

D = Accommodation for near fixation (dioptres)

Conventionally, for calculation purposes esodeviation are prefixed with a plus (+) sign and exodeviation are prefixed with minus (–) sign.

For example, if a patient has 12Δ exophoria for near and 6Δ exophoria for distant vision with an IPD of 6 cm, then by formula

$$AC / A = 6 + \frac{[-12 - (-6)]}{3\,D}$$

$$= 6 + \frac{(-12 + 6)}{3}$$

$$= 6 + \frac{(-6)}{3} = 6 - 2$$

AC / A = 4Δ

Means, 4Δ accommodative convergence is applied for each dioptre of accommodation.

Normal AC / A ratio for heterophoria method is considered as 4:1.

Gradient method: In gradient method the stimulus for accommodation is generated by use of ophthalmic lenses (plus or minus spherical lens) in place of distance variation. Hence, the calculation of AC / A ratio is based on theorem that plus lenses placed before the eyes will relax (decrease the requirement) the accommodation and due to less accommodation there will be less convergence and vice

versa a minus lens will increase the requirement of accommodation thus associated with increased convergence (eso-shift). This method measures the change in deviation of eye due to change in lens induced accommodation.

Moreover, a +1 D power lens will relax accommodation equivalent to 1 D while –1 D power lens will increase accommodation equivalent to 1 D, thus the accommodative response produced due to lenses and accommodative convergence will be in linear relationship in a certain range.

First, with full optical correction original deviation for near vision of patient is measured using prisms. Then measure patient's deviation for near vision after adding lenses (say +3 D power) in both sides of trial frame. AC / A ratio is calculated by using following formula

$$AC / A = \frac{\Delta_1 - \Delta_0}{D}$$

Here

Δ_0 = original deviation without additional power

Δ_1 = deviation with additional power of +3 D

D = dioptric power of additional lens (here +3 D)

For example, if a patient has original deviation of 4Δ exophoria for a given distance and deviation of 8Δ esophoria is induced after adding +3 D lenses, then AC / A ratio will be

$$AC / A = \frac{8 - (-4)}{3}$$

$$= \frac{8 + 4}{3}$$

$$= 4\Delta$$

Second way to calculate AC / A ratio is to measure original deviation (Δ_0) for a fixation distance of 33 cm with full optical correction. Then add –3 D power lens in front of both the eyes and again measure the deviation (Δ_1). Calculate the AC / A ratio as discussed above.

Note: AC / A ratio calculated by Heterophoria method is usually more than AC / A ratio calculated by gradient method, mainly due to the effect of proximal convergence. So, it is considered that only gradient method gives a true estimate of AC / A ratio because of presence of consistent tonic, proximal and fusional convergence.

IPD measurement is taken in calculation by heterophoria method but not in gradient method.

Fixation disparity method: This method was introduced by Ogle and coworkers however, being a complex method, it is not commonly used in clinical practice. The AC / A ratio is calculated indirectly on the basis of disparity of fixation object. This disparity is induced by changing the accommodative stimulus with help of ophthalmic lenses in one group while in second group forced convergence is induced with help of prism. The data collected from these two groups are then analyzed to find out those accommodation and convergence stimuli which produced same amount of fixation disparity.

Haploscopic method: Original haploscope instrument was designed by Herring's with the purpose to study the relationship between accommodation and convergence. In haploscope each eye is presented with a separate target to differentiate the visual fields of two eyes. Like fixation disparity method it is also not routinely used in clinical practice. However, instruments based on this design like Synoptophore are used clinically to study various conditions of the eyes.

Clinical significance of AC / A ratio

- In presbyopes, the AC / A ratio usually remains stable, indicates that it is dependent on stimulus for accommodation, not on amount of accommodation.
- AC / A ratio is normally higher in majority of myopes and lower in majority of hyper-metropes as compared to emmetrope. Although, magnitude of AC / A ratio has no association with degree of hypermetropia or myopia.

- Interpupillary distance (IPD) affects the AC / A ratio, because persons having wide IPD needs more convergence power as compared to persons having narrow IPD, to look at same fixation distance.
- AC / A ratio anomalies play an important role in etiology of strabismus. A high AC / A ratio will cause excessive convergence, which leads to a convergent squint or esotropia, whereas a low AC / A ratio will lead to a divergent squint or exotropia, when patient is focusing a near object.

Fusional (Positive) Convergence

Fusional convergence (positive convergence) is a type of optomotor reflex (involuntary) and it is stimulated by retinal image disparity. As we know fusion of two similar object images is important to achieve binocular single vision. Whenever there is retinal image disparity, the fusional convergence is stimulated to adjust the visual axes in such a form that similar retinal images are formed on two fovea of both the eyes to ensure bifoveal single vision. It is because of fusional convergence person does not feel diplopia. For example, if a person is having 4 prism diopter of esophoria then 4 D fusional convergence is required to avoid diplopia. During fusional convergence there is no change in the refractive status of eye. Studies show that fusional convergence is disrupted if one eye is occluded or there is extreme blurring of image on one eye. Normal range of amplitude of fusional convergence is 14–20 D for distance and 35–40 D for near. In normal circumstances the fusional convergence keeps the eyes in orthophoric position by controlling the lateral divergence of eyes; however systemic illness or ocular fatigue can lead to heterophoria and heterotropia. In simpler words, latent divergent squint (exophoria) can convert into manifest squint due to decreased fusional convergence. Hence, fusional convergence has important role in motor anomalies. Orthoptic exercises help in improving the amplitude of fusional convergence, hence are useful in management of heterotropia.

Proximal (Psychic) Convergence

Usually, during clinical examination the esodeviation measured by synoptophore is found more as compared to the esodeviation measured by prism bar and cover test. Similarly, if we measure near deviation in a patient (after full optical correction) by placing equivalent lenses for near distance, then theoretically, the near deviation should be equal to distance deviation because equivalent lenses had been used, however, actually the deviation is found larger for near than distance. Possible explaination for these two instances is that either accurate full optical correction was not given or the difference in deviation is caused by proximal convergence.

Proximal convergence is the convergence resulting due to proximity of an object or due to awareness that an object is placed nearby. In the above discussed instances the proximal convergence was stimulated because during measurement of near deviation there was proximity (nearness) of an object. While in synoptophore the awareness of nearness was present because in reality object was situated near but made to appear optically placed at infinity. Psychological status plays an important role in initiation of proximal convergence because even the thought of looking at near object will induce convergence of eyes; although in reality the object is not present or is placed at infinity. Like accommodative convergence an inverse relationship exists between proximal convergence and observation distance (indicate change in vergence, i.e. in dioptres). Hence change of vergence of 1 D means a change in fixation from infinity to 1 meter distance. Normally, an approximate 1.5 prism dioptre change occurs in proximal convergence with each dioptre change in distance.

Measurement of Convergence

Convergence angle: As it has been discussed above that when eyes are at rest the visual axes are parallel to each other but as the eyes focus on a object at a distance then an angle is formed.

Convergence angle is an angle formed between two primary lines of vision during convergence as shown in Fig. 8.1A. Value of convergence angle depends on two factors: Distance of fixation object from eyes and distance between two pupils, i.e. IPD. Size of angle is decreased with an increase in the distance of fixation object (Fig. 8.1B) and increased with increase in IPD (Fig. 8.1C). IPD shows no appreciable effect on convergence angle, so practically during measurement of convergence angle we can exclude IPD.

Convergence angle of eyes can be measured either as meter angle or prism dioptres.

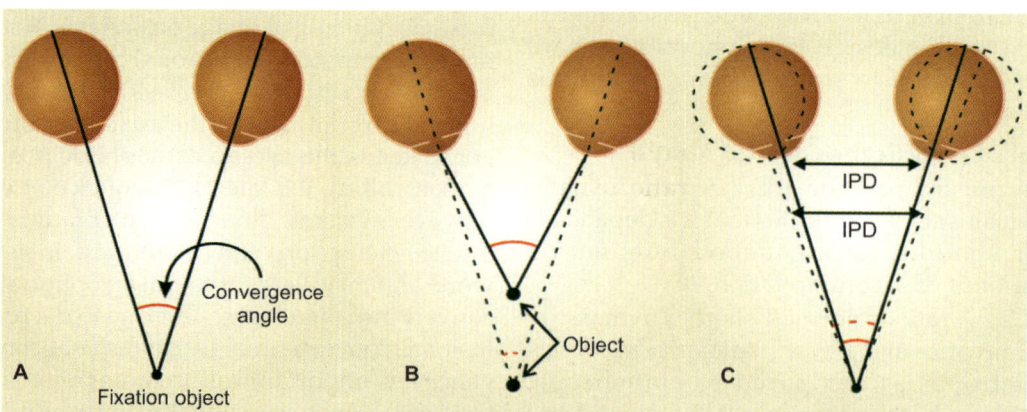

Fig. 8.1: A. Convergence angle; B. Convergence angle becomes smaller with increasing object fixation distance; C. Convergence angle becomes larger with increasing IPD

Meter Angle

Nagel introduced unit of measurement for convergence angle as meter angle. When eyes are directed to an object situated at distance of 1 meter (distance measured from a midpoint of meridian line drawn between two eyes), then the angle formed by visual axes of both eyes with the meridian line will be equal to one metre angle.

The convergence exerted by each eye in meter angle (ma) depends on the distance (meters) of object situated in front of eyes and on IPD. It varies inversely with the distance of object. For example, convergence will be of 2 ma for a distance of ½ meter and only ½ ma for a distance of 2 m, as shown in Fig. 8.2. It is based on the similar comparison for the dioptre. In an emmetropic eye to see an object clearly the amount of accommodation in dioptres is equivalent to value of meter angles exerted by each eye to converge and see the same object clearly. It means that 1 D of accommodation is associated with 1ma of convergence exerted by each eye.

Prism Dioptres

Convergence can be expressed in terms of prism dioptres (Δ) also, which is a tangent measurement. Consider if an adducting or converging prism (base out) is positioned in front of an eye then it will produce diplopia. Diplopia is produced due to deviation of rays of light in outward direction (depending on the strength of base out prism) by the prism before they enter the eye. In normal situations to avoid this diplopia, the eye will turn in inward direction and tries to maintain binocular single vision. The convergence (degree of inward deviation) of eye will be equal to the degree of outward deviation of light rays.

The amount of convergence exerted by the eyes to see an object (placed at 1 meter distance from eyes) as single, when base out prism of 1 prism dioptre power is placed in front of one eye, is termed 1 prism dioptre (Δ) convergence (Fig. 8.3). On convergence scale, 1 metre angle

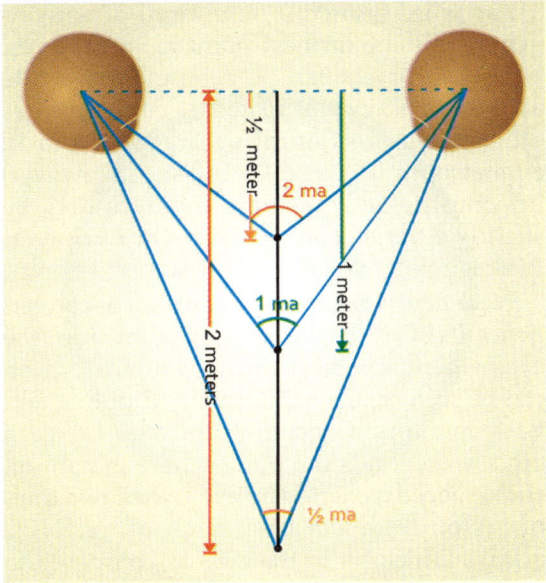

Fig. 8.2: Meter angle

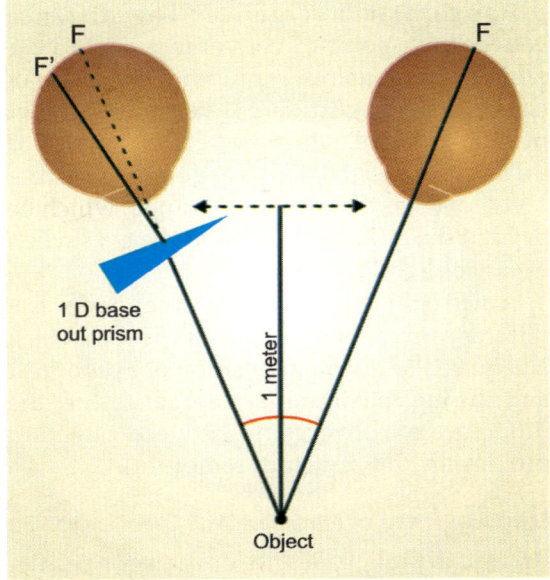

Fig. 8.3: Prism dioptric convergence

convergence is approximately equal to 3 prism dioptre convergence (1 ma = 3Δ).

Range and Amplitude of Convergence

To understand range and amplitude of convergence it is essential to know the far point and near points of convergence.

Far point (punctum remotum) of convergence: It is the farthest point from the eyes, where an object can be seen clearly while accommodation is at rest. It is considered as the relative position of eyes at rest and in emmetropes it is usually infinity. However, in complete rest position, the eyes may be slightly divergent so the far point of convergence is in negative value, i.e. it lies beyond infinity.

Near point (punctum proximum) of convergence (NPC): It is the nearest point from the eyes where an object during bifoveal vision can be seen clearly without any dipolpia and with maximum accommodative effort. In other words, it is the point where maximum convergence is exerted by eyes when two lines of vision intersect with each other. NPC always lies closer to the eyes as compared to near point of accommodation (NPA) and normally, it is less than 8 cm.

Range of convergence: The distance between far point of convergence and near point of convergence represents the range of convergence. Positive convergence is that portion of range, which lie between eyes and infinity. Negative convergence (relative divergence) is that portion of range, which lie beyond the infinity (i.e. behind the eyes when eyes are slightly divergent).

Amplitude of convergence: It is the difference in converging powers of eyes which is required to maintain position of eyes at rest and during maximum convergence (i.e. the difference of convergence between punctum proximum and punctum remotum).

Measurement of Near Point of Convergence

Practically all types of convergence, i.e. fusional, accommodative, proximal and even voluntary convergence (in later stages when patient exert voluntary converging efforts) are stimulated when a person tries to focus on an object which is actually approaching the eyes during testing.

A large number of instruments can be used to measure the near point of convergence. These instruments can be simple graded plastic ruler or metallic ruler where fixation target for test is common objects like tip of pencil or could be specially designed rulers, for example, Livingstone binocular gauge, Beren's rule, Prince's rule, Krimsky Prince near point rule and RAF (Royal Air Force) rule.

Beren's rule (Fig. 8.4) basically consists of a bar made up of plastic on which a rider is fixed with a test chart (fixation target). This target can be moved back and forth along the scale while testing. Sliding target has various targets for measurement of NPC. The bar is graded for measurements on two sides in centimeters and dioptres.

Prince rule (Fig. 8.5) consists of bar of 2 feet with 0.5 inch square in size. This square bar has different markings on four sides as follows
- One side is graded in centimeters for measuring NPA and NPC.
- Second side is divided into inches
- Third side is graded in dioptres to measure NPA in dioptres
- Fourth side of square indicates the corresponding age of patient in years.

Krimsky Prince near point rule (Fig. 8.6) is a modification where a sliding fixation target is mounted on a board. One end of board has a wing like support which rest against lower orbital margins and the other end is closed. One side of board is graded in dioptres for measurement of NPA and NPC and on the

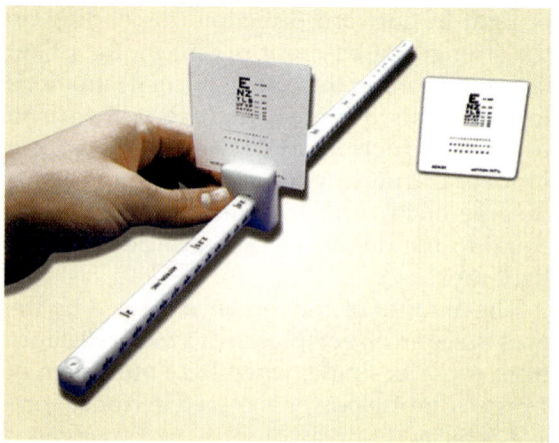

Fig. 8.4: Beren's rule (*courtesy:* Bernell Corporation)

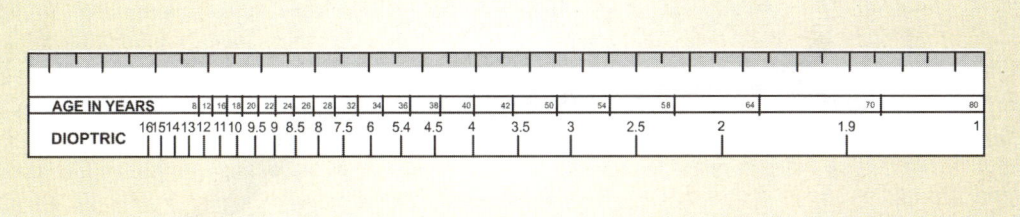

Fig. 8.5: Prince rule bar

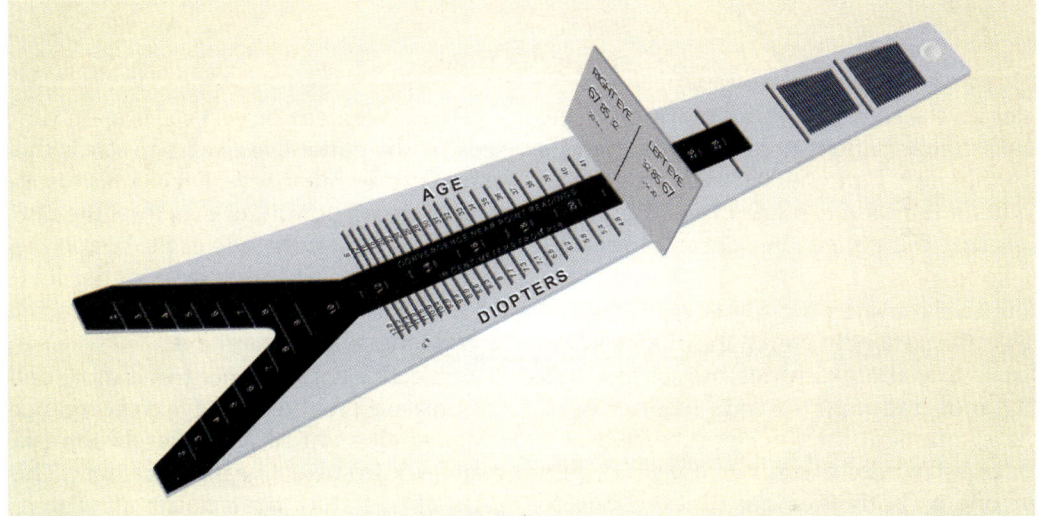

Fig. 8.6: Krimsky Prince near point rule

other side the age (years) is represented. Central back portion is graded for distance measurement in centimeters. Sliding target has optotypes for right eye and left eye.

RAF (Royal Air Force) rule consists of a binocular gauge which helps in measurement of objective and/or subjective convergence and accommodation in 1 mm increments. RAF rule (Fig. 8.7) is made of a metallic bar of 50 cm length which consists of a slider holding a rotating four-sided cube. Every side of this sliding target shows a different target.

- One side of ruler shows a vertical line having a central dot for convergence fixation.
- Other three sides have some limited number of lines indicating examples of near reading.

A cheek rest is present on one end of the ruler which ensures a consistency and proper height of target to the eyes. Other end has a handle to hold the ruler straight while examining the patient.

A few studies suggest that measurement of NPC with RAF rule provides more consistent result, compared to the measurements done by means of a pencil or finger.

RAF rule can be used to determine both objective and subjective convergence points, to observe the accommodation and to determine the master eye. It is also useful as a diagnostic and therapeutic device for detection of convergence or accommodation anomalies.

Objective Convergence

To measure objective convergence, the RAF rule box attachment should be positioned at distance of 36 cm. Examiner puts face-piece

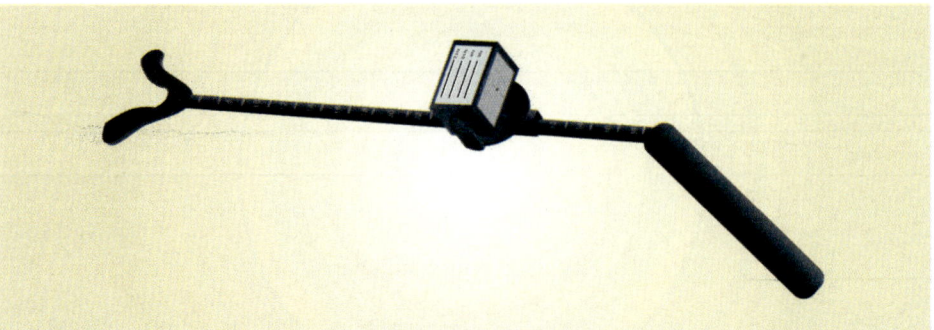

Fig. 8.7: RAF rule

of ruler on the inferior orbital margins of the patient, so that patient hold the ruler handle in his/her left hand while two fingers of examiner's hands are placed over the small dot, so that the patient is unable to see this dot.

Examiner removes the finger from the dot and asks the patient to watch the black section of dot, while the examiner moves the box slowly and gradually towards his/her eyes. The measurement on ruler is recorded at a break point where examiner observes that either one or both eyes get diverge due to failure of binocular fixation. The distance of break point recorded in centimeters or millimeters is termed as NPC. As in this test observations are made by examiner, hence it is known as an objective convergence. Normal reading of NPC ranges from 6 to 10 cm in an emmetrope young adult.

Subjective Convergence

For measurement of subjective convergence the ruler box is kept behind 36 cm mark on the ruler end. The position of this ruler box is adjusted in such a way that the patient will be seeing the black vertical line. Now patient is instructed to watch the line constantly, as the examiner moves the ruler box slowly and steadily towards his/her eyes. Patient is asked to report immediately as the line on box moves even slightly, either to the left or right, or it becomes double. This distance is recorded where movement or doubling of line occurs, it denotes the subjective convergence.

The movement of vertical line on the box, seen by the patient, is always towards the side of his/her dominant eye. For example, suppose if right eye is dominant eye, then the line will move towards right side of the box. If the line does not move on either side, rather it is seen as double then it indicates that no specific eye is working as dominant eye.

Subjective convergence test is more delicate as compared to the objective convergence test because element of accommodation plays a major role in subjective measurement. This test tells about that first point at which full binocular vision is not maintained and this point cannot be observed by the examiner. The reading of subjective convergence is normally less than 20 cm, but usually it is always more than that of reading in objective convergence.

Accommodation Test

The positive range of accommodation should be tested both uniocularly and binocularly. For accommodation test the ruler box is rotated, so that the text can be shown to the patient.

Keep this ruler box at 36 cm mark while examiner moves the ruler box slowly and steadily toward the eyes of patient. The patient is instructed to report, when he/she first

Note: A number of near point rulers have been designed having zero as starting point on their scales at the assumed spectacle point which is 27 mm away from the canthus. In these kinds of rulers a value of 27 mm is added in the recorded break point distance while measuring the distance of NPC.

notices that letters are becoming blurred. In an emmetrope young adult, normal reading distance is about 10 cm or lesser.

Measurement of Amplitude of Convergence

Amplitude of convergence can be measured by
- Prism bar method
- Synoptophore method

Prism Bar Method

In this method the prism bar is used to produce blurring or diplopia, either for near or distance targets. For convergence test, base out (BO) prism bar, and for divergence test, a base in (BI) prism bar is used. Three cardinal points such as break point, recovery point and blur point are recorded to measure amplitude of convergence.

For near test, patient is instructed to fixate a 6/9 symbol in a chart placed at distance of 33 cm. BO prism bar is placed in front of the eye of patient and by sliding the prism bar the power of prism is increased gradually until the eyes are converged to a maximum limit to maintain binocular single vision or the patient just start to realize diplopia. This point is known as break point and reading of this point (power of prism) is recorded.

Now, the power of prism is decreased gradually until the patient sees the 6/9 target clearly or diplopia get disappear. This point is known as recovery point and this point reading is also recorded.

During test before appearance of break point, a blur point should also appear because initially the patient consumes fusional convergence to avoid diplopia; however once this fusional convergence is completely used then the patient will start using the accommodative convergence to avoid diplopia. The point where fusional convergence is fully used and accommodative convergence started indicates blurring of image. This point is called as blur point, and it is important to record the distance of blur point to know about the fusional convergence.

For distance test patient is instructed to fixate a 6/9 target in a chart placed at distance of 20 feet and prism bar is placed in front of the eye to record the break point, recovery point and blur point in similar manner as described above.

Synoptophore Method

As discussed in Chapter 6 page 120–121 an objective angle of deviation can be estimated by using grade 1 simultaneous macular perception slides (SMP slides) in Synoptophore. Then grade II fusion slides, i.e. the fusion slides having similar kind of targets but an additional two control marks for each eye, are placed in Synoptophore. Suppose patient is able to fuse these targets and see them as single image simultaneously with both the control marks, means the objective angle is achieved. Now lock the arms of Synoptophore and measure the amplitude of convergence or divergence as follows

Measure the amplitude of convergence: As discussed above we need to record the breaking point and recovery point for measurement of amplitude of convergence. To record the break point, unlock the arms of Synoptophore and gradually converge them until the patient report about the disappearance of either one or both of the control marks or appearance of diplopia. This point where fusion is broken and patient report of disappearance of control mark is called break point and its value is recorded. Now the arms of Synoptophore gradually moved in backward direction in a less convergent position or divergent position, till the patient again fuses the target as single with both the control marks visible. This is called recovery point and value is recorded.

Measure the amplitude of divergence: On contrary to convergence, to measure divergence, diverge the arms of Synoptophore gradually till the fusion breaks and record the break point. Now, move back the arms of Synoptophore slowly in a less divergent or convergent position until the patient again fuses the target as single. Record this recovery point.

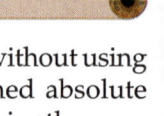

Table 8.2: Normal values of various vergence		
Vergence types	*Distance vergence (Δ) (20 feet)*	*Near Vergence (Δ) (33 cm)*
Convergence	14–20	35–40
Divergence	5–8	15–20
Vertical vergence	2–4	2–4
Incyclovergence	10–12	10–12
Excyclovergence	10–12	10–12

Measure the amplitude of vergence for near: Place –3 DS lenses in front of each eye (to overcome power of these lenses, the person has to apply his/her accommodation in order to see the object clearly, as if fixing an object at 33 cm). Orthoposition for near fixation is simulated by setting the tubes of Synoptophore according to a convergent requirement [in prism dioptres which is about 3 times of patient's IPD (cm)] for a target at 33 cm distance.

Now the procedure for testing, near convergence or divergence is similar as that for distance, which has been described above.

Normal values for distance and near vergence in various types of vergence conditions are shown in Table 8.2.

CONVERGENCE ANOMALIES

Convergence anomalies commonly seen are:
- Insufficiency of convergence
- Convergence insufficiency secondary to accommodative insufficiency
- Convergence excess
- Convergence paralysis

Insufficiency of Convergence

As convergence is valuable in maintenance of binocular single vision for all distances (which are optically nearer than infinity), so its failure can lead to clinically significant problems. Convergence insufficiency is known for many years and it is one of the common conditions responsible for muscular asthenopia.

Convergence insufficiency (CI) is defined as inability of ocular system to sustain or acquire an adequate amount of binocular convergence, for any time period without using the additional efforts. CI is termed absolute CI when in absence of presbyopia, the near point of convergence becomes greater than 11 cm from intraocular base line or when the person has difficulty in acquiring the convergence of 30° or more.

Broadly, we can group CI in two categories
- Primary or functional convergence insufficiency
- Secondary convergence insufficiency

Primary Convergence Insufficiency

Causes of Convergence Insufficiency

- *Idiopathic:* When the exact cause of convergence insufficiency is not identified. However, anatomical factors like more inter pupillary distance (IPD) and late development of acquired function may affect the convergence. Several precipitating factors for this type of CI are stress, overwork, systemic debilities and psychological disturbances.
- *Presence of accommodative difficulties or refractive errors:* Uncorrected high hypermetropia or myopia may also produce convergence insufficiency. As we know that accommodation and convergence acts synergistically and if accommodation of a person suffers due to any reason, then there is also disuse of accommodative convergence mechanism. Uncorrected refractive errors of high degree may decrease the accommodative convergence mechanism of person which ultimately lead to convergence insufficiency. Mechanism involved in these conditions are
  - High degree (>+5 D) hypermetropes use negligible amount of accommodative efforts, so they develop an associated accommodative convergence deficiency.
  - Myopes do not require accommodation to visualize the near objects clearly so they do not use even the minimum amount of accommodation and due to disuse of accommodation they develop poor accommodative convergence.

- Presbyopia: As discussed before, when a person approaches the presbyopic age, the near point of eye recedes, so there is decreased utilization of convergence. Hence, negligence in presbyopic correction can cause permanent convergence insufficiency. On contrary, the patients who use the presbyopic correction first time in their life can also develop convergence insufficiency. Proposed mechanism is that presbyopic correction gives a relaxation to these patients from a sustained accommodative effort; hence a decrease in accommodative convergence can lead to convergence insufficiency.

Note: In case of overcorrected hypermetropia the patient may utilize less accommodation and can develop convergence insufficiency.

- *Prolonged extraocular muscles imbalance:* convergence insufficiency may be associated with conditions like exophoria, intermittent exotropia and imbalances of vertical muscle if remained uncorrected for long duration.
- *Consecutive insufficiency of convergence:* As a consequence of squint surgery, i.e. either resection of lateral rectus or recession of media rectus muscle can lead to convergence insufficiency.

Symptoms of Convergence Insufficiency

The occurrence of symptoms due to convergence insufficiency (CI) mainly depends on the visual requirement of the person. CI is commonly seen in those persons who are involved in too much reading, or writing work and doing precise near work for longer durations especially, in young school going children excessive school work, long duration reading and writing homework can cause the problem of convergence insufficiency. On the other hand, it is uncommon in persons involved in manual work or field work or in profession not requiring a lot of precise near work.

Convergence insufficiency symptoms can be grouped as a symptom complex of asthenopia. Majority of the patients wearing glasses and having convergence insufficiency present with complain of asthenopia due to incompatibility of glasses they are using.

Asthenopic symptoms complex of convergence insufficiency can be grouped as

- **Symptom due to muscle fatigue:** Constant use of eye muscles especially to perform near work for long duration will result in muscular fatigue and asthenopic symptoms
  - Frontal headache and brow ache after continuous near work is felt by many patients, which may get relieved after closing the eyes or taking rest for some time. Headache of migrainous type or precipitation of migraine attack is experienced by some patients having convergence insufficiency which is usually not relieved by analgesics.
  - Eye strain and feeling of heaviness in and around the eyeball is commonly complained by many patients.
  - After prolonged near work tenderness of eyes, burning/itching or hyperaemia with conjunctival congestion may occur in some patients.
  - Sudden changing of focus from near to distance after continuous near work cause difficulty in a few patients having CI.
- **Symptoms due to breakdown of continuation in BSV**
  - A periodic closure or covering of one eye after prolonged book reading is characteristically seen in cases of CI which is usually done to attain some relaxation from visual fatigue.
  - Some patient may complain of sudden occasional blurring or crowding of words while reading books for long duration.

– Intermittent crossed diplopia due to ocular fatigue is quite commonly reported by many patients involved in professions requiring extensive near work.

Diagnosis of Convergence Insufficiency

Convergence insufficiency can be diagnosed by these factors

- *Fusional convergence:* An absolute convergence insufficiency is considered if the patient has a difficulty to achieve a 30° convergence, when fusional convergence for near is measured by using Synoptophore. Fusional convergence is decreased for near fixation.
- *Near point of convergence (NPC):* When NPC is more than 11 cm from the intraocular base line or 9.5 cm from the apex of cornea, in the absence of presbyopia.
- *Prism convergence:* When vergences are measured by ophthalmic prism, the prism convergence is low, whereas the prism divergence remains normal.
- *Near point of accommodation (NPC):* NPC is usually normal and also corresponds with the age of patient. However, clinically it is essential to measure the NPA in every case of convergence insufficiency for diagnostic and treatment purposes. As there may be combined convergence and accommodation insufficney and these patients may require different forms of therapy.

In nutshell salient features of convergence insufficiency for diagnosis are

- Majority of patients show varying degree of exophoria for near than distance
- Orthophoria for distance is also not uncommon
- Proximal fusional convergence amplitude for near objects remain poor
- Decreased adduction of approximately 5°–6° (8–10Δ) is seen; but rarely abduction goes below 10° (18Δ).
- Prism convergence usually decreased to 8°–12° (means lesser than 15–20 prism dioptres)
- Near point of convergence recedes to 3 inches or 7.5 cm.
- Periodic increase of relative divergence is seen when near point is approximately reached

Differential Diagnosis of Convergence Insufficiency

As discussed earlier, asthenopic symptoms in patients can be produced by many other conditions along with convergence insufficiency, so it becomes essential to exclude all other conditions like: accomodative effort syndrome and convergence paralysis.

Convergence insufficiency can be differentiated from accommodative effort syndrome on the basis of following factors as summarized in Table 8.3.

Convergence insufficiency can be differentiated from convergence paralysis on the basis of following factors as summarized in Table 8.4.

Table 8.3: Differences between convergence insufficiency and accommodative effort syndrome

Accommodative effort syndrome	Convergence insufficiency
• Patient usually present with esophoria at near vision	• Presents with exophoria in near vision
• Symptoms get improve on adding plus lenses (lenses cause relaxation of the accommodative convergence and hence decreases the efforts during accommodation)	• Symptoms get worse on adding plus lenses (relaxation of accommodative convergence leads to excessive convergence efforts.)
• Minus lens test (–3D): patient may develop diplopia due to sudden induction of deviation of eyes due to lens.	• Patients feel better because these lenses compensate for poor fusional convergence found in CI

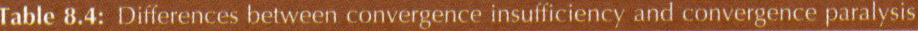

Table 8.4: Differences between convergence insufficiency and convergence paralysis

Convergence paralysis	Convergence insufficiency
• Eyes are totally incapable to converge, so in these cases patient is unable to counter the effect of base out prism of any dioptric strength	• Patient can show convergence ability for several dioptres of prism
• On receiving a convergence stimulus, there is pupillary constriction (miosis) but person is not capable to converge	• There is pupillary constriction along with convergence. However, patient is unable to sustain this convergence, so after some time dilatation of pupil (mydriasis) will occur.

Management of Convergence Insufficiency

In adults many a times convergence insufficiency (CI) remain subclinical or asymptomatic, so in adults treatment of CI is required mainly in those situations where annoying asthenopic symptoms are present and patient is uncomfortable. Children, on the other hand, having convergence insufficiency may develop poor fusional vergence due to constant under use of convergence. These children may have symptoms of exodeviation and require proper treatment of CI to improve the fusional vergence. Prognosis after treatment is exceptionally good in most of the cases of CI.

Various treatment modalities for convergence insufficiency are:

- Optical treatment
- Orthoptic/vision therapy
- Prism therapy
- Surgical treatment

Optical treatment: The cycloplegic refraction should be performed in all cases to find out any associated refractive errors. If any refractive error is present, then in cases of convergence insufficiency corrective glasses should be prescribed as follows:

- Hypermetropes are usually kept under corrected so that their accommodative efforts remain stimulated, which in turn keep the convergence stimulated. Overcorrection with plus lenses will worsen the CI in hypermetropic cases.
- On contrary, myopes should be given full correction with glasses to keep their accommodation in stimulation and hence convergence also stimulated. Under correction with minus lenses will worsen the CI in cases of myopia.
- Full amount of presbyopic correction as per patients working distance should be done to avoid any exertion on already reduced accommodation. Under correction or an inadequate correction will worsen the CI symptoms in presbyopes.

Orthoptic treatment

The main purpose of orthoptic trainings are

- Improvement in binocular convergence
- Increase the amplitude of fusional convergence

Various modalities of orthoptic treatment are summarized in Table 8.5.

Near point of convergence can be improved by

- *Advancement exercises:* These are simple and home based exercise to improve the convergence efficiency in near vision. Basic principle used is to advance the near target and increase the strength of convergence, hence the name advancement exercises. Patient is instructed to use a near target like pictures with some details or fine lines printed on a card. Then patient hold this card at an arm length so that the details of target are clear. Now slowly patient will advance this picture card towards his/her nose, so this exercise is also called picture-to-nose exercise. Once the details of target become blur the patient will hold the card at that point and try to converge to see those

Table 8.5: Orthoptic treatment for convergence insufficiency	
Mode of treatment	*Type of exercise*
To improve near point of convergence	• Advancement convergence exercises • Jump convergence exercises
To improve amplitude of fusional convergence	• Convergence card assisted convergence exercises • Stereogram card assisted exercises for uncrossed physiological diplopia • Prism assisted convergence exercises • Diploscope assisted convergence exercises • Synoptophore assisted convergence exercises
To improve control over physiological diplopia	• Voluntary convergence training
Relaxation exercises	• Stereogram card assisted exercises for crossed physiological diplopia • Prism assisted divergence exercises • Synoptophore assisted divergence exercises

details clear. If succeed, then patient can advance the card nearer to his/her nose. In case patient is unable to see the target details clearly, then he/she will move back the card away from nose till details become clear. This picture-to-nose exercise is repeated 10–15 times twice daily for improvement in near point of convergence.

• *Jump convergence exercises:* Once some amount of convergence get improve by picture-to-nose exercise, then these advanced versions of advancement exercises should be performed. Usually a month training of basic convergence exercises by advancement method is required to attain reasonable degree of convergence to perform jump exercises. In these exercises patient is made to learn to achieve a single binocular vision when there is a sudden change in the requirement of convergence.

Amplitude of fusional convergence can be improved by use of convergence card, stereogram card, prisms or diploscope.

• *Convergence card:* This is also called physiological card because it is based on the principle of improving the state of physiological diplopia and patient learn to appreciate the homonymous physiological

and heteronymous physiological diplopia. Convergence card has three dots which gradually reduces in size and are identically placed on either side of the card. On one side of card (side A) the dots are blue colored while on other side of card (side B) the dots are red in color. These dots are seen as large, medium and small size dots by patient as shown in Fig. 8.8.

Exercise procedure

– Examiner rests the convergence card on patient's nose like a septum so that patient will see red dots with one eye and blue dots with another eyes; keeping the large size dot farthest away from nose.

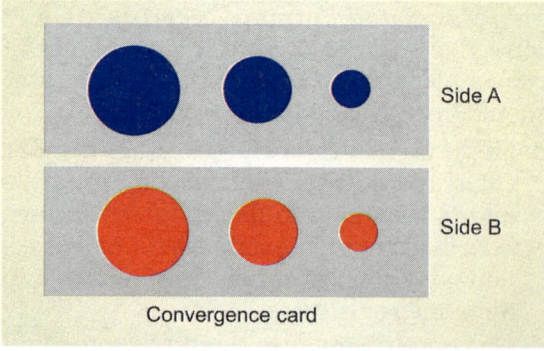

Fig. 8.8: Convergence or physiological card

- Patient is now asked to focus on large size dots of red and blue color and then try to fuse them in each other.
- Once patient is able to do so then ask him/her to repeat the same procedure for medium size dots and finally for small size dots.
- However, these convergence card evoke a large degree of retinal rivalry between two eyes, hence many a times patient is unable to fuse these dots. To increase the convenience of patient these three dots are joined by a black line on both sides of the card as shown in Fig. 8.9.
- Suppose with this modification patient is able to fuse large size dots on either sides, then the straight black line will appear as an inverted V(Λ) to the patient as shown in Fig. 8.10A.
- Once patient is able to fuse the large size dots and tries to fuse the medium size dots he/she will see the black line as X (Fig. 8.10B) and finally when patient is able to fuse medium size dots and tries to fuse the small size dots, then the black line will appear as V (Fig. 8.10C).
- **Stereogram card:** These cards have two identical pictures with a small variation in details (similar to fusion slides of synoptophore) as shown in Fig. 8.11.

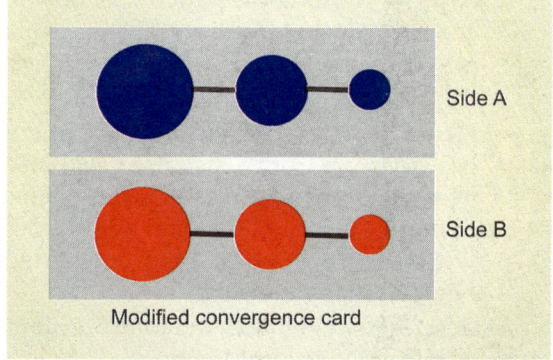

Fig. 8.9: Modified convergence or physiological card with black joining line

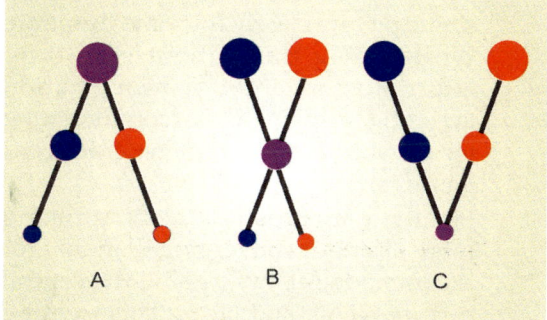

Fig. 8.10: Test results of a convergent card. A. Fusing large size dots; B. Fusing medium size dots; C. Fusing small size dots

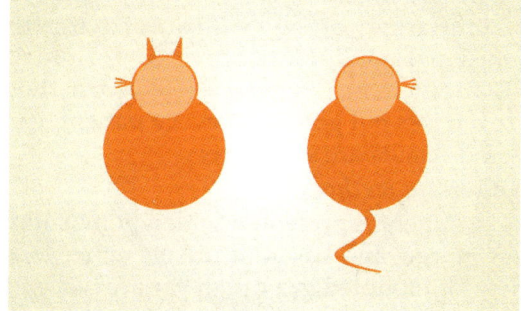

Fig. 8.11: Stereogram card

Exercise procedure

- Stereogram card is held at about one meter distance from the patient eyes at the level of glabella.
- Patient is instructed to look at the pictures on the card and then place a pen tip in between the stereogram card and patient's eyes.
- Patient is asked to shift the focus on tip of pen while simultaneously keep looking at the stereogram card. This will produce an uncrossed physiological diplopia and patient will see four pictures instead of two pictures on the card.
- Now patient is instructed to adjust the distance of pen tip such that he/she is able to fuse the two central pictures into one single and see only three pictures on the card.
- Gradually patient is trained in such a way that he/she is able to see the central

single picture clearly for some duration. While doing this patient is putting efforts to converge for near fixation target (i.e. pen tip) and accommodating for distance target (i.e. stereogram card pictures).

– Finally, patient is relatively applying more effort for converging than that for accommodating by keeping the central picture single and clear. This exercise can be performed at home about 3–4 times a day for 5–6 minutes.

• *Prism assisted convergence exercises:* convergence exercises using prisms are simple and effective in improving the fusional amplitude of convergence. Initially patient may not be able to learn these exercises but gradually every patient learn and results are satisfactory.

Exercise method
– Patient is presented with a point source target and base-out prisms either loose or mounted in a prism bar are placed in front of the patient's eyes
– Patient is instructed to converge and try to focus on the target. Check the convergence of patient while he/she is focusing on the target.
– Once patient is able to converge with small power prism, slowly and gradually the power of prisms are increased and convergence is checked.
– Repeat the exercise on weekly basis for a few minutes and measure the convergence status on follow-up visits.

• *Diploscope:* It is a simple instrument having a metallic bar with head rest at one end and a handle in the middle. Other end of bar has a card printed with letters D, O and G in the centre and on top and bottom of the card there are two squares, one red and other green in color. In front of card a metallic septum is attached which contains

Note: During exercise the examiner should observe the eyes of patient and make sure that patient is not either diverging or suppressing the eyes.

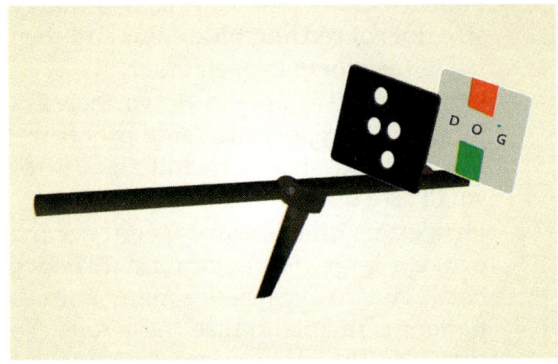

Fig. 8.12: Diploscope

four holes as shown in Fig. 8.12. In presence of binocular single vision the relative convergence can be improved by doing the exercises with the help of diploscope.

Exercise procedure
– Patient is instructed to hold the handle of diploscope and keep the head rest on his/her glabella or forehead.
– Now the convergence exercise is performed by moving the eyes relative to card and septum in four different positions.
– As patient moves his/her eyes in relative positions of card and septum, he/she appreciates a change in the relative position of letters and color of squares on card from each eye.
– This movement of letters and color squares in a definite pattern becomes basis for training the patient, i.e. how to control and appreciate the various positions of eyes and direction of their movements.
– Hence it helps in training the patient how to fixate from a distance vision to a near vision or vice versa, which helps in improvement of fusional amplitudes which is very vital for a contented binocular single vision.

As described in Fig. 8.13 the four positions during training with diploscope are

• *Position 1:* Patient is instructed to hold the diploscope as described above and

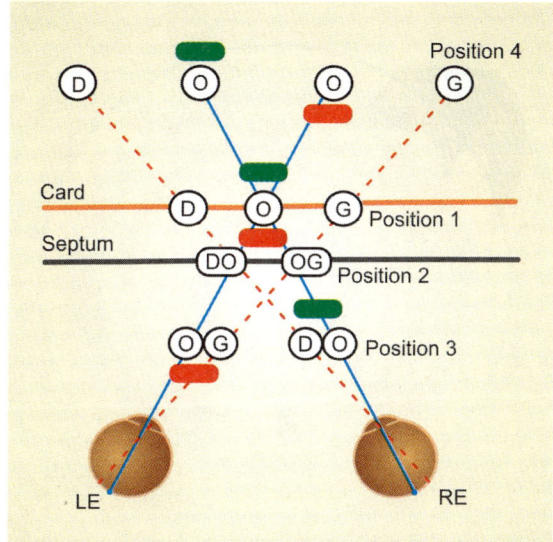

Fig. 8.13: Various positions during diploscope method

fixate on central letter 'O' written on the card. Once the patient focuses on letter 'O', then the letter 'D' will fall temporal to fovea of right eye (so projected left to letter 'O' on card). Whereas, letter 'G' will fall temporal to fovea of left eye (so projected right to letter 'O' on the card). As a result, letters DO are seen by right eye and OG by left eye. When binocular single vision (BSV) is present patient will see three holes in septum having the letters DOG, inside them (as shown in Fig. 8.13). The color square will be at their relative positions, i.e. green above and red below letter 'O'.

- *Position 2:* Now patient is instructed to fixate at the midpoint of the two horizontal holes in the septum. Once patient converges to this point of fixation the image of letter 'O' will fall on retinal component nasally to fovea of each eye (instead of fovea of both the eyes). So the letter 'O' will be seen in a homonymous uncrossed diplopia by the patient as DO and OG in two holes (as shown in Fig. 8.13). By exercising a huge amount of convergence power patient

may overlap the letters 'D' and 'O' and letters 'O' and 'G' with resultant letter 'D' and 'G' in each of two horizontal holes.

- *Position 3:* Instruct the patient to focus midway between the septum and his/her eyes on an object like on tip of a pen. As patients converge to focus the tip of pen, the images of letter 'D' and 'O' of right eye and letters 'O' and 'G' of left eye will fall on a retinal component nasally to fovea of respective eye; so these letters are projected temporal to fovea. Patient sees the letters 'O G D O' (as shown in Fig. 8.13). Green square will shift to right over 'DO' letters and red square to left under 'OG' letters.

- *Position 4:* Examiner asks the patient to fixate on an object like a wall mounting hanged far away from the card on a wall. As patients diverge to focus the distant object, the images of letters 'D' and 'O' of right eye and letters 'O' and 'G' of left eye will fall on a retinal component temporally to fovea of respective eye; so these letters are projected nasally to fovea. Patient sees the letters 'D O O G' (as shown in Fig. 8.13). Green square will shift to left over letter 'O' and red square to right under letter 'O'.

An unforced convergence and/or divergence can be established once patient is well trained to accomplish and sustain these four relative positions of diploscopic exercise with effortlessness. These exercises are done for 3–4 minutes about 3–4 times in a day to achieve good results.

- **Synoptophore assisted convergence exercises:** Synoptophore assisted convergence exercises are very effective and result oriented even in young children having mild to moderate amount of convergence insufficiency.

Note: For improvement of fusional divergence or negative convergence position 4 of diploscopic exercise is very helpful.

These exercises are carried out by the use of fusional slides in synoptophore. During these exercises the arms of synoptophore are gradually converged starting at an angle where patient is able to fuse the pictures on slides. These exercises are done twice or thrice per week for a period of 5–6 minutes. Minimum 15–20 settings are required to achieve the desired amount of convergence in mild to moderate cases of CI.

Voluntary convergence training: Voluntary convergence training gives very encouraging results in motivated and determined patients to improve voluntary control over relative positions of both the eyes. By this training the patient is made to learn, appreciate, maintain and then control over the physiological diplopia developed during the exercise method.

Exercise method:
- Patient is instructed to focus on a bright light source situated at a distance.
- Once eyes are focused on light, ask the patient to bring his/her finger in the field of vision in between the light and eyes (Fig. 8.14). A sudden breaking of fusion for distance will produce physiological diplopia.
- Patient will see two fingers when he/she is still focusing on the distant light. Patient is advised to learn this physiological diplopia.
- Now ask the patient to focus at finger tip and still looking at distance light. Then patient will appreciate two distance lights.
- Instruct the patient to move the finger to and fro and ask him/her to observe the increasing and decreasing distance between two distant lights as shown in Fig. 8.14.
- Patient is advised to maintain the two distance lights apart and moving with finger movement as long as possible. Patient is asked to remove the finger from field and continue to watch the distance lights.
- Once the distance light becomes single after removal of the finger from visual field, then patient is instructed again to focus on the

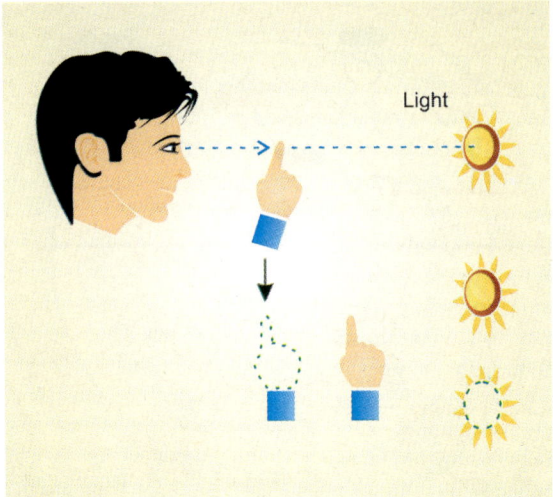

Fig. 8.14: Voluntary convergence exercise method (*see text*)

distance light for some time and reintroduce the finger to appreciate the physiological diplopia.
- Patient is asked to practice this exercise till he/she is able to appreciate two lights and can increase or decrease the distance between two lights without the addition of finger in visual field.

Relaxation exercises: These exercises are performed to relax the eyes hence are termed as negative convergence exercises. Various methods are adopted to relax the eyes apart from simple resting.
- **Stereogram assisted relaxation exercise:** As discussed before patient is made to learn, appreciate and control the crossed physiological diplopia prior to start the relaxation exercises for the convergence. Crossed physiological diplopia can be elicited with the help of a flash light or a pen tip, which patient should be able to learn and appreciate. Stereogram assisted relaxation exercise can be performed once patient is well trained to handle the crossed physiological diplopia.

Exercise method:
- Patient is instructed to fixate on a distant object, now place the stereogram card

at about one feet distance from his/her eyes.

- As patient focuses on stereogram card he/she will see four pictures (instead of two pictures) on card due to elicitation of crossed physiological diplopia.
- Patient is instructed to move the card to and fro to adjust the relative position of stereogram card, until the two central pictures fuses and become single. Now patient sees only three pictures on stereogram card in total.
- Tell the patient to maintain clarity of the joined central single picture for as long as possible. While patient is trying to keep the central picture clear and single he/she is accommodating for a near target (stereogram card) and simultaneously he/she is converging for a distant target (flash light). Thus, the accommodation is at work while convergence is relaxing during this exercise.
- After completion of learning and training patient can practice this relaxation exercise at home.

- **Synoptophore assisted divergence exercise**
  - To elicit fusion, stereopsis slides are used in place of fusion slides in synoptophore; because strongest stimulus for fusion is produced by stereopsis not by fusion of images.
  - Patient is asked to fuse both the slides and once the fusion of two pictures on slides is achieved, the patient is instructed to maintain the fusion while slowly tubes of synoptophore are diverged.
  - To maintain the fusion with diverging tubes of synoptophore patient needs to relax the convergence.
  - These diverging exercises are done for 4–5 minutes in a clinic per week for improvement in relaxation power of convergence.

- **Prism-assisted divergence exercise**
  - Patient is instructed to fixate on an object. If possible object must be situated

Note: Risley's rotatory prisms or even loose prisms can be used in place of prism bar to perform these exercises, though prism bar is most favored because of ease of use.

at such a distance where focusing will elicit largest degree of esophoria in patient.
- Examiner places a prism bar with base-in position in front of one eye of the patient and gradually increases the power of prism till two images are seen by the patient. Thus, the fusion gets dissociated and patient appreciates an additional blur image of object (Fig. 8.15).
- Now patient is advised to maintain a single clear image of distant object for as long as possible. This relaxes the convergence and helps in improvement of symptoms of convergence insufficiency. These relaxation exercises are done for about 4–5 minutes per week.

Prism therapy: If the asthenopic symptoms due to convergence insufficiency did not show any improvement by any of the above discussed orthoptic exercises, then prism therapy should be started to improve symptoms. Base-in prisms can be incorporated in the near vision glasses or bifocal glasses (here prisms are fitted in lower segments) to improve the symptoms of CI. These are also termed relieving prisms because they relieve the asthenopic symptoms.

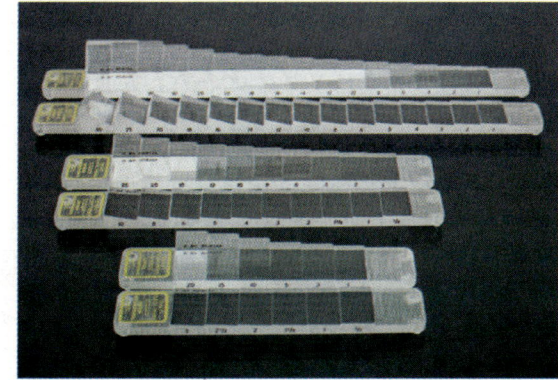

Fig. 8.15: Prism bar (*courtesy:* Bernell Corporation)

Note: The relieving prisms or bifocals with prisms are avoided in young patients as they can worsen the situation because of the associated accommodative changes.

Surgical management: CI insufficiency is usually a reversible condition, hence decision to perform any surgery should be taken only when all other therapeutic possibilities have failed. Depending upon the amount of exophoria resection of medial rectus in one or both eyes is considered most effective surgical treatment for convergence insufficiency. Patients must be informed that after surgery he/she may experience double vision for several weeks or months which is more at distance fixation (consecutive esotropia). However, this esotropia get resolved spontaneously with time.

Note: In some cases even after surgery recurrence of exophoria for near vision can occur which is usually asymptomatic.

Secondary Convergence Insufficiency

Patients can have convergence insufficiency due to an associated condition such as insufficiency of accommodation. As discussed before, accommodation and convergence mechanisms are very closely related to each other; hence it is always advisable to rule out any associated accommodation defects before treating the patient for a convergence problem.

A secondary convergence insufficiency having a primary accommodative insufficiency is seen in the following conditions such as

- Early Adie's syndrome
- Infectious mononucleosis
- Viral encephalopathy
- Diphtheria
- Following head injury
- Thyroid eye disease and Parkinson's disease are also associated sometimes with CI.

Clinical presentation

- Asthenopic symptoms are similar to those seen in primary convergence insufficiency
- Near point of convergence and near point of accommodation are reduced
- AC/A ratio is usually negligible or very low.

Management

- Orthoptic exercises
- Optical treatment
- Prism therapy
- Surgical treatment

Orthoptic exercises: Orthoptic exercises are done similar to those done in functional convergence insufficiency as discussed above. However, the result of orthoptic exercises alone is not very encouraging as compared to the results in primary convergence insufficiency. These exercises are advised with an additional optical correction using bifocal glasses for a satisfactory outcome.

Optical treatment: Reading glasses are prescribed after evaluating the requirements of the patient. Minimal plus power lenses which give comfortable near vision are prescribed. Although prescription of glasses for reading purposes alone is less effective, they need to be combined with prism therapy.

Prism therapy: Fresnel membrane prisms (Fig. 8.16A) are used with bifocal lenses which can be glued in the lower segment of spectacle bifocal lenses because adjustment may be required before determination of final power of glasses. Executive bifocals having a decentered plus lens serving as prism in lower half, is an alternative to Fresnel's prisms. Similarly press on bifocal prisms (Fig. 8.16B) are also available, which can simply be glued to spectacle lens, produces bifocal adjustment of images.

Surgery: Surgical treatment is rarely recommended to correct secondary convergence insufficiency however, strengthening of medial rectus muscle by resection procedure with subsequent prescription of bifocal glasses has shown some symptomatic relief in recalcitrant cases.

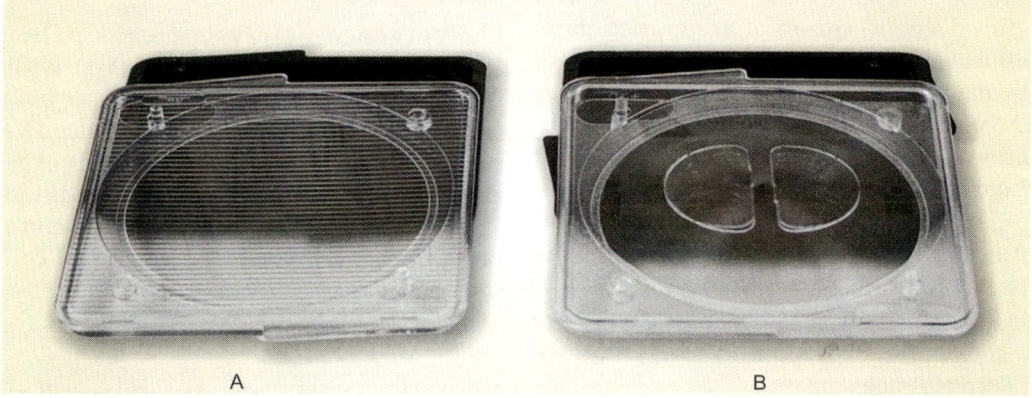

Fig. 8.16: Press on prisms (*courtesy:* Bernell Corporation). A. Fresnel's prism; B. Bifocal prism

Convergence Excess

An excessive convergence or spasm of convergence is not very uncommon.

Etiologically this condition may occur when

- Increased convergence is associated with increased accommodation: as both are synergic in action, hence change in one tends to cause change in other also. For example, commonly seen in uncorrected hypermetropes who use excessive accommodation, sometimes also in recently corrected myopes or early presbyopes.
- Diseases of central nervous system (e.g. meningitis or increased labyrinthine pressure): Leads to convergence excess because of irritation.

Convergence Spasm

It is a condition where intermittent episode of an excessive amount of convergence occur along with an accommodative spasm (ciliary spasm). It is in the form of triad of intermittent sustained convergence, spasm of accommodation and constriction of pupil (miosis) because there is synkinesis between convergence, accommodation and miosis.

Causes of Convergence Spasm

- *Functional:* Isolated episode of convergence spasm are usually functional in origin. Most commonly seen in hysteric or neurotic persons.
- *Organic:* Rarely an underlying organic condition may cause convergence spasm. Generally, the convergence spasm due to organic origin is associated with other abnormalities and neurologic impairment. It may appear secondary to conditions such as post head injury, pituitary adenoma, tumors of posterior fossa, viral encephalitis, tabes dorsalis, and Arnold-Chiari malformation.

Clinical Features

Convergence spasm is an intermittent condition and patient remains asymptomatic in between the attacks of spasm. During attack following symptoms may occur

- *Excessive convergence:* This condition resembles to bilateral abducent nerve palsy since both the eyes remain fixed and inwardly rotated (esotropia) in a state of extreme convergence spasm.
- *Blurred vision:* Convergence spasms are usually associated with spasm of accommodation, hence patient may complaint of blurring or loss of vision for near work and diplopia.
- *Induced myopic state (pseudomyopia):* Patient may also complaint of decrease vision for

Note: In abducent nerve palsy size of pupils and visual acuity remain normal.

distance because a state of myopia is also induced due to spasm of accommodation. Retinoscopic findings during an attack of spasm have revealed myopia of as high as 6D contributed due to associated accommodation spasm. It can be differentiated from true myopia by cycloplegic refraction.

- *Constriction of pupils (Miosis):* Being an inherent component of near reflex, the pupils undergo constriction.
- *Homonymous diplopia:* Patient may experience an intermittent diplopia during an attack of convergence spasm.

Investigations

Psychiatric evaluation: It is necessary as functional spasm is common in hysteria and neurosis which can be diagnosed on evaluation.

Neurological evaluation: Rarely, convergence spasm may be associated with an underlying organic lesion; hence all patients should also be evaluated for presence of any neurological condition.

Treatment

To relieve convergence spasm following measures are used:

- Treatment of associated cause, if any present.
- Perform cycloplegic refraction and presence of any refractive errors should be treated.
- Atropine 1% can be instilled for long term along with bifocal glasses having plus lenses in the lower segment (used for near work). This therapy may break the spasm cycle.
- Monocular occlusion of alternate eyes may be tried as an alternative treatment to abolish diplopia.
- Injection of botulinum toxin into medial rectus muscle for alignment of visual axes also tried.
- For long-term relief in selected cases psychiatric evaluation and counseling and treatment of any precipitating disease is useful.

Convergence Paralysis

Convergence paralysis means patient is unable to converge the eyes even with the strongest stimulus. In other words, an inability to overcome the effect of smallest power of base-out prism is termed convergence paralysis. Although, it is a rare condition but it may be confused with a very common condition like primary or functional convergence insufficiency.

Aetiology

Convergence paralysis is rarely primary in origin and not associated with any significant past history. It usually occurs secondary to organic brain lesions situated at corpora quadrigemina or at third cranial nerve nucleus region. Some organic brain lesions associated with convergence paralysis are

- Head trauma
- Disseminated sclerosis
- Tabes dorsalis
- Encephalitis
- Tumors
- Narcolepsy

Features

Convergence paralysis is characterized by features such as

- An acute onset convergence failure with total absenteeism of convergence.
- Exotropia with crossed diplopia will precipitate when patient tries to fixate a near object (due to absence of fusional convergence).
- Fusional divergence is not affected. Adduction remains normal.
- Mostly the accommodation remains normal however, in selective conditions accommodation may decrease or even absent. If accommodation is also affected, then symptoms are in more severe form because of deficiency of associated accommodative vergence.
- Eye movements may also affect when palsy is due to underlying neurological disease.

Diagnosis

Bielschowsky's described following criteria for diagnosis of convergence paralysis:

- Positive history of an acute onset crossed horizontal diplopia for fixation of near objects.
- Pupillary reflex and accommodation reflex remain present during convergence.
- Investigations favoring intracranial lesion.
- Consistency of these positive findings even on subsequent examination of case.

Treatment

- The underlying secondary cause should be identified, if present should be treated accordingly.
- To overcome diplopia for near vision in presence of normal accommodation function, base-in prisms can be prescribed.
- If patients having weakness of accommodation with convergence paralysis, then base-in prisms with plus lenses (minimum hypermetropic correction) can be prescribed.

Note: Conservative treatment is preferred for convergence paralysis. Surgery on the muscle has no role in convergence paralysis cases.

In some cases, for temporarily relief botulinum toxin is used, however, it has no role in long-term management.

- Monocular occlusion during near work is advised in patients who are unable to regain binocular single vision.

Associated Syndromes

- Parinaud's syndrome: Characterized by convergence paralysis with a vertical gaze paralysis.
- Pretectum-posterior commissure syndrome also called dorsal midbrain syndrome. This syndrome results due to a tumor present in pineal region of brain and is characterized by:
  - Parinaud's syndrome
  - Bilateral fourth cranial nerve paralysis
  - Pupillary reflex is absent with light near dissociation
  - Lid retraction in a few patients

Binocular Muscle Co-ordination Anomalies

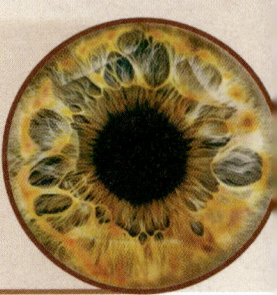

ORTHOPHORIA

In Greek *'orthos'* means straight or correct and *'tropos'* means turn or direction. Thus, orthophoria represents straight direction of two eyes and can also be called 'orthoposition' which means correct position of two eyes, where under the effect of fusion two visual axes intersect at the fixation point.

When eyes are at rest and a distant object is looked straight ahead, then the visual axes of both eyes remain parallel to each other. This is known as primary position of the eyes. Thus, during primary position of eyes the light rays enter in both eyes and fall on corresponding points on the retina (fovea centralis) of each eye, subsequently the two images get fuse together psychologically as single image and as a result binocular single vision is achieved.

Normally we can say that both eyes work simultaneously and are considered by brain as one, though retinal images formed in both eyes are not same because each eye observes different aspect of an object. For example, the right eye observes right portion of an object more, whereas left eye observes left portion more. Consequently these two images with slight disparity are fused together psychologically. Along with other factors which are derived from experience of person this psychological fusion allows a person to appreciate the solidity and depth of object and also helps in assessment of the distance of object from the eyes.

If the position of the object is altered, then the direction of vision will also change, and as a result, both eyes will occupy different position, which is called secondary position. To maintain binocular single vision in secondary position also there must be psychological fusion of two images as single and to achieve this fusion both the eyes must move in a perfectly coordinated manner. During these coordinated movement of eyes both conjugate and disjunctive movements (convergence and divergence) should remain accurately balanced so that if two eyes move or fix any object present at any distance, the primary lines of sight remain directed upon the fixation point, i.e. macula of each eye remains in the line of vision.

It is the perfectly coordinated oculomotor system of eye which allows free mobility of eyes in primary and secondary position through six pairs of extraocular muscles so that the visual axes of two eyes remain focused upon the fixation point.

This coordinated state of the eye where the actions of extraocular muscles are normally balanced in such a way that visual axes of two eyes remain in alignment and fusion of images occurs without any efforts is called orthophoria.

The condition where eye gets deviate from orthoposition due to ocular muscle imbalance so that visual axes of two eyes are not in alignment and do not meet at a fixation point is called strabismus or squint. It may be

Heterophoria or latent squint/strabismus: It is the condition where the tendency of eyes to deviate (due to imbalance) can be overcome by fusion, so that proper alignment of eyes remains maintained under stress. It means the squint remains latent during binocular vision due to fusion reflex.

Heterotropia or manifest squint/strabismus: It is the condition where the ocular muscle imbalance or deviation of eyes cannot be overcome by fusion reflex and the latent squint turns into manifest squint.

Although heterophoria and heterotropia are not directly related to optics but these are essential for knowledge because presence of various refractive errors play an important role in the etiology of squint especially in concomitant type squint and thus optical correction is required in their treatment.

HETEROPHORIA (LATENT SQUINT/STRABISMUS)

Introduction

Latent means under cover or hidden, hence in heterophoria the deviation of eyes during binocular vision remains hidden or covered due to presence of fusion mechanism. This states where the imbalance of extraocular muscle is overcome by effect of fusion, so that proper alignment of eyes is maintained under stress is termed heterophoria.

Mechanism: Usually the relative functional insufficiency of one or more extraocular muscle is the main cause of heterophoria. In order to maintain the parallelism of visual axes in both eyes during binocular single vision, the weak extraocular muscle remains in the state of continuous contraction to maintain its normal tone. Hence, a squint is potentially present but it is covered/hidden due to continuous activity of the muscle. This constant activity of muscle may produce eye strain and fatigue to the eye which may vary person to person. However, if the person develops state of debility, i.e. stimulus for fusion becomes poor or there is a great difference in visual acuity of two eyes or neurological pathway involved remain underdeveloped then latent heterophoria becomes manifest heterophoria. Muscular imbalance may also differ with age of person. For example, in children and young person, there is tendency of the eyes to deviate inwards because of increased convergence, whereas after presbyopic age an outward deviation of the eyes is more common.

Causes of Muscular Imbalance

Several conditions may disturb the normal muscular equilibrium of eye muscles such as:

- Deficiency in the function or tone of muscle may be due to any congenital cause or it may occur due to illnesses like generalized weakness, anemia, nervous disease, etc. Symptoms of phoria are periodic and usually appear when body is fatigued like in the evening, after doing excessive work or in the state of anxiety, etc. Symptoms tend to disappear after taking rest or vacation from work for sometime.
- Sometimes, spasm of antagonist muscle or an amplification of its tone may lead to the loss of muscle equilibrium.
- Various refractive errors and resultant accommodation convergence disturbances may cause muscular imbalance.
- Altered configuration of the orbits and anatomical variation in the origin and insertion of muscles may contribute for muscular imbalance.
- Disturbances in the nerve supply of muscle which affect the tone of muscles may lead to imbalance of extraocular muscles.

Classification of Heterophoria

Depending on the involvement of type of extra-ocular muscle and the direction of deviation of eyes heterophoria can be classified as shown in Table 9.1.

Esophoria

Esophoria is a common condition and is a type of heterophoria where visual axis of one eye has tendency to deviate inwards (nasally) relative to other eye when fusion is broken (Fig. 9.1). Esophoria may be caused by

- *Excessive convergence:* As convergence is more active during near fixation while divergence is more active in distance fixation, hence esophoria due to convergence excess is more pronounced for near vision than distant vision. This is the most common cause of esophoria but still gives rise to very few symptoms. As discussed previously that convergence excess is also associated with accommodation excess, hence this type of esophoria usually coexists with under corrected hypermetropic refractive state where the excess accommodative effort tend to stimulate adduction of the eyes. Cases

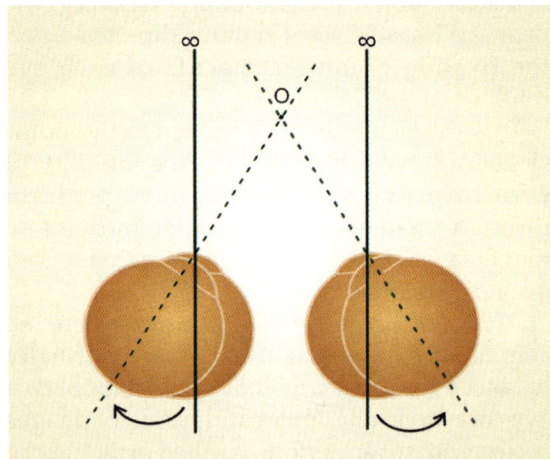

Fig. 9.1: Esophoria

Types of phoria	Type of heterophoria		Insufficiency of muscle	Latent deviation of eyes
Horizontal phoria		Esophoria	Lateral rectus muscle	Inwards
		Exophoria	Medial rectus muscle	Outwards
Vertical phoria	Hyperphoria	Hyperesophoria	Combination of	Upward and inwards
		Hyperexophoria	extraocular muscles	Upward and outwards
Rotational phoria	Cyclophoria	Incyclophoria	Combination of	Intorsion
		Excyclophoria	extraocular muscles	Extorsion

Table 9.1: Classification of Heterophoria

of bilateral congenital myopia with increased convergence may also present with esophoria.

- *Deficient divergence:* Esophoria due to divergence insufficiency is more noticeable for distant vision as compared to near vision. Divergence insufficiency is not so common cause for esophoria rather in normal situations two eyes generally remain in slight divergent position.

- *Innervational:* Disturbances in central distribution of innervations of extraocular muscles may cause esophoria.

Exophoria

Exophoria is referred to a situation where visual axis of one eye tend to deviate outwards relative to other when fusion is broken (Fig. 9.2). Exophoria is the most common type of muscular imbalance than any other types of heterophoria. As discussed before that at rest eyes exist in the position of slight divergence, hence when eyes converge for a near fixation, then there is tendency of eyes to diverge for about 3–4 prism dioptres from point of fixation and this degree of deviation is considered as physiological.

Exophoria may be caused by

- *Insufficient convergence:* As we know that convergence insufficiency is generally associated with accommodation deficit.

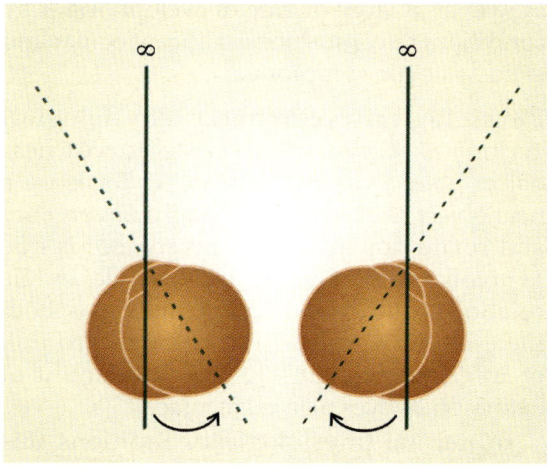

Fig. 9.2: Exophoria

Hence exophoria is common in those who utilize less accommodative effort for near vision, as seen in uncorrected myopes or first time corrected hypermetropes or presbyopes. Exophoria is more marked for near vision as compared to distance vision.

- *Excessive divergence:* Exophoria due to excess divergence is more marked for distance vision as compared to near vision.

- *Innervational:* Disturbances in central distribution of innervations of extraocular muscles may cause exophoria.

Hyperphoria

Hyperphoria is referred to a situation where visual axis of one eye is deviated at a higher level relative to visual axis of other eye, when fusion is broken. It means the deviation occurs in vertical direction (upwards or downwards). It may be left hyperphoria (left visual axis is higher than that on the right) or right hyperphoria (right visual axis is higher than that on the left). In other words, it can be termed left hypophoria (right visual axis is higher than that on the left) and vice versa. Hyperphoria is caused by either weakness in superior rectus and inferior oblique muscle or in inferior rectus and superior oblique muscle. As hyperphoria occurs due to involvement of more than one muscle, hence to maintain the correct position of visual axes, eyes have to adjust the activity of more than one muscle. Due to this, even a small deviation of this type leads to a great discomfort to person. Thus, the asthenopic symptoms are more pronounced in vertical phoria than horizontal phoria (esophoria or exophoria).

Depending on the associated inward or outward position of eyeball hyperphoria can be subclassified as

- Hyperesophoria
- Hyperexophoria

Hyperesophoria means where one eye is deviated in upward and inward direction or other eye in downward and inward direction. Hyperexophoria is a condition where visual axis of one eye is in upward and outward direction or in outward and downward direction for other eye.

Cyclophoria

Cyclophoria is referred to a condition where eyes are rotated around the anterior-posterior axis of eyeball when fusion is broken. Because of this clockwise or anticlockwise rotation of the eye the vertical meridian of cornea is deviated from its normal position. Depending upon the direction of rotation of eyes the cyclophoria can be incyclophoria (intorsion) or excyclophoria (extorsion).

When upper end of vertical meridian of cornea is deviated nasally, then the movement is called intorsion (Fig. 9.3) and it is due to involvement of superior oblique muscle. If upper end of vertical meridian is deviated temporally, then the movement is called extorsion (Fig. 9.4) and it is primarily due to involvement of inferior oblique muscle.

On the basis of clinical presentation, cyclophoria can be:

- Essential
- Physiological
- Pseudocyclophoria

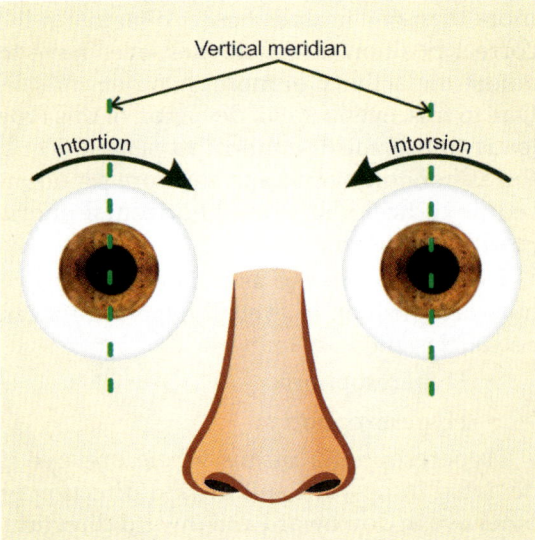

Fig. 9.3: Intorsion

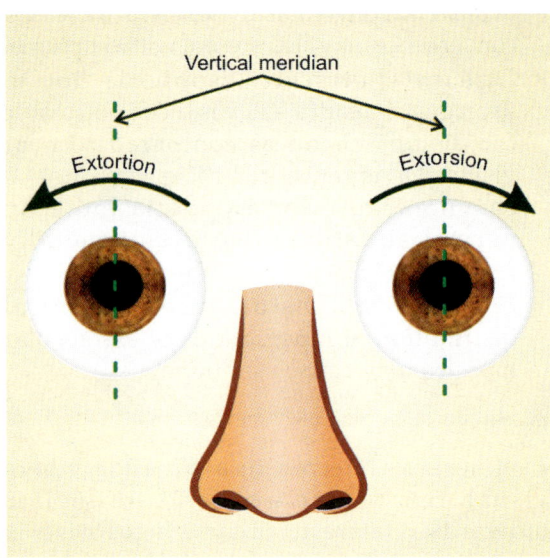

Fig. 9.4: Extorsion

Essential cyclophoria: The essential cyclophoria occurs mainly due to imbalance of superior and inferior oblique muscles. Muscular imbalance may arise due to muscular insufficiency or innervational disturbances. When there is insufficiency of inferior obliques or overaction of superior obliques, then intorsion will occur while with insufficiency of superior obliques and overaction of inferior obliques, extorsion will occur. Usually essential cyclophoria presents as low degree and in majority of cases remain asymptomatic. However, a large degree of cyclophoria (rare condition) may produce significant ocular and even systemic symptoms.

Physiological cyclophoria: Physiological cyclophoria occurs when eyes try to see a near object placed closely. When eyes focus on a near object, then eyes go through convergence and rotate downwards. Convergence is due to involvement of medial recti muscles, while rotation is due to inferior recti muscles of both the eyes. However, with the downward pull of inferior recti muscle certain amount of extorsion of eyes also takes place.

In normal physiological conditions this extorsion of eyes is neutralized by action of superior oblique muscle (cause intorsion). If this normal neutralizing action of oblique muscle is disturbed then some amount of cyclophoria can occur. This condition is usually asymptomatic and requires no treatment.

Pseudocyclophoria: Uncorrected oblique astigmatism persons (where principal meridia are not vertical and horizontal in nature) sometimes may imitate pseudocylophoria. In astigmatism the image formed on retina will incline towards the direction of maximal corneal meridian. Thus to bring this retinal image in appropriate alignment, the one or more oblique muscles of eye will act and lead to torsion. Patient may have distressing symptoms due to torsion, however, once correction of refractive error is done, then all these symptoms will disappear.

Clinical Presentation of Heterophoria

Symptoms

Horizontal phoria (esophoria or exophoria) of small degree usually does not produce any symptoms and remain compensated by the residual neuromuscular power of eyes. If deviation is of high degree (>6 Δ), then distressing symptoms may appear. As compared to horizontal phoria, hyperphoria even in small degrees can produce considerable amount of trouble. Furthermore, cyclophoria produces more significant symptoms than any other types of phoria.

- *Visual symptoms:* Blurring of vision is especially more marked after fatigue. Person experiences difficulty in gazing of any object continuously and this discomfort further increases if any attempt is made to follow a moving object. Patient may also not able to judge the exact location of objects in the space. The visual symptoms are usually improved after closing one eye.
- *Abnormal head posture:* Patient may have unusual head tilt to counteract the deviation along with associated blepharospasm and/or wrinkling of forehead.
- *Acute distress symptoms:* Acute distress symptoms are more common with high

degree of cyclophoria. Patient sees vertical lines as deviated lines and also feels difficulty to judge the positions and distance of objects especially of moving objects. There may be associated reflex labyrinthine disturbances leading to vertigo, nausea and occasionally even vomiting.

- *Reflex symptoms:* Headache is very common and may occur even after a short duration of near work, and make near work difficult or impossible to continue. Headache sometimes becomes severe and resemble with migraine. Occasionally, intermittent diplopia may occur due to fatigue.

Treatment of Heterophoria

Horizontal phoria of small degree is common but usually asymptomatic, hence do not require treatment. Heterophoria can be treated as follows

- *General health improvement:* As muscular imbalance is more evident during associated debility or excessive work or stress. So in majority of cases it is advised to take rest from work for sometimes, or change of occupation or improve general health along with some exercises, instead of prescribing for optical correction.
- *Correction of refractive errors:* Cycloplegic refraction preferably with atropine should be done to determine the degree of refractive error in all the age group patients presenting with heterophoria. Refractive errors are most common and easily treatable conditions associated with phoria, hence errors should be corrected fully and accurately by prescribing the glasses of appropriate power. Patients having heterophoria with refractive errors are advised to wear the glasses regularly and constantly, because any negligence in optical correction may lead to a more devastating condition of tropia.
- *Orthoptic exercises:* If patient shows poor response with abovementioned measures,

then the orthoptic exercises may be advised both for distance and near vision. In esophoria the aim of exercises is to improve the amplitude of fusional divergence and in exophoria is to improve the fusional convergence. Divergence exercises to improve fusional divergence can be done with help of prisms (placed base-in before eye), synoptophore, etc. Similarly, convergence exercises for exophoria to improve fusional convergence can be done with prisms (placed base-out before eye), synoptophore, stereograms, etc. For cyclophoria exercises are done by using two maddox rods which are placed vertically in front of each eye. Then a point light source is shown to patient. Cyclophoria patient will see two horizontal lines appearing at an angle to each other. One of the Maddox rods is rotated until two lines get fuse. Then light source is moved forward and backward and patient is asked to keep two lines fused during movement of light. Maddox rods should be rotated towards upper nasal quadrants to exercise superior oblique and towards upper temporal quadrants to exercise inferior oblique muscles, respectively.

- *Prism therapy:* Prism may also be used to relieve the symptoms of phoria if orthoptic exercises have failed. Both base-out or base-in prisms can be used to compensate the muscular balance for correction of phoria. The base of the prism should be positioned in the direction of the action of that muscle which need strengthening, whereas the apex should be towards the opponent muscle, which needs to be neutralized. Hence, for esophoria base-out prisms are prescribed because lateral rectus needs strengthening and medial rectus action needs to be neutralized as shown in Fig. 9.5A. Similarly, base-in prisms is prescribed for exophoria for similar reasons as shown in Fig. 9.5B.

In addition, prism therapy relieves strain and help in maintenance of binocular vision by stimulating fusion. Before prescribing prism therapy it is also necessary to rule out cause of phoria whether it is type of essential deviations (due to anatomical anomalies) or dynamic deviations. As prism therapy may worsen the symptoms in phoria occuring due to dynamic deviations. It is because of this reason full prismatic correction is prescribed in phoria

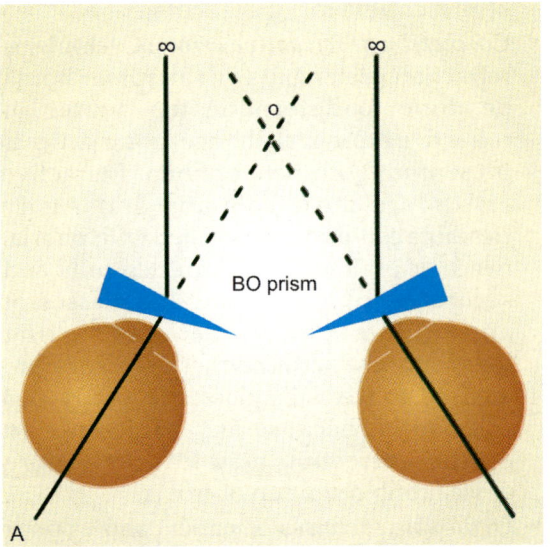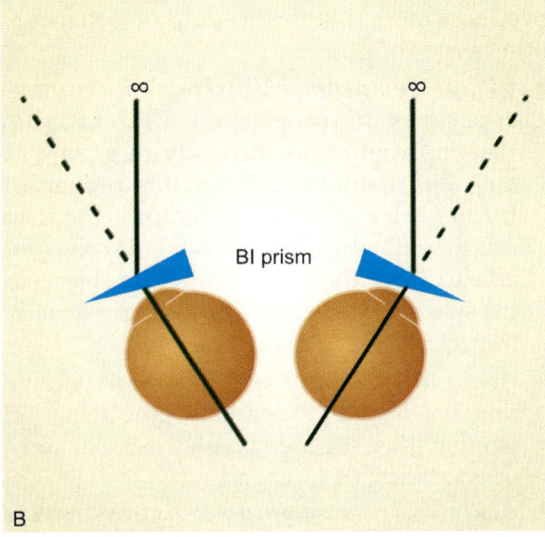

Fig. 9.5: Prismotherapy for phorias. A. Base-out prisms for esophoria; B. Base-in prisms for exophoria

due to anatomical factors while in horizontal phoria half correction is given.

In mixed deviation a vertical prismatic correction is effective for symptomatic relief. Usually, up to 6–8Δ prisms can be given to patient.

- *Surgical treatment:* Surgical treatment may be required in patients having high degree of heterophoria or where other treatment modalities had failed to relieve symptoms. Surgery on various muscles has been recommended to relieve the symptoms of heterophoria. Resection or recession of concerned muscle is advised to correct the deficiency or excessive power of muscle. Surgical correction of esophoria or exophoria is done by correction of one or more horizontal muscle. In hyperphoria muscle surgery done on either superior or inferior recti muscle while surgery on obliques is done in cyclophoria.

HETEROTROPIA (MANIFEST SQUINT)

Introduction

Heterotropia develops when deviation of eyes cannot be overcome by fusion reflex so that parallelism of visual axes is not maintained. As discussed before to achieve a perfect binocular single vision there must be

- Formation of two equal size images on the retina of both eyes
- Adequate muscular balance
- An adequately functioning cerebral mechanism to interpret and coordinate the two sets of images formed on both retina.

Disturbance in any of these three elements will affect the binocular single vision and lead to deviation of eye from their normal alignment. Formation of dissimilar images on retina may occur due to refractive errors, anisometropia, aniseikonia, etc. Muscular imbalance may occur during development period or due to paralysis.

Dissociation in accommodation-convergence mechanism as seen in some of hypermetropes is one of the important factors for development of convergent squint. This type of squint develops during early life due to loss of fusional reflexes. As a result the person uses excessive accommodation to correct hypermetropia and excessive accommodation causes stimulation of convergence leading to development of convergent squint. Presence of anisometropia, high astigmatism, general debility, etc. further aggravate the development of squint.

On contrary, divergent squint is more common in myopes due to dissociation of accommodation and convergence synergy. Myopes use less accommodation and use their convergence in excess as compared to accommodation. Hence, even if they develop a squint it will be divergent or outward in nature. In reality, myopes usually do not develop a manifest squint commonly; rather a latent strabismus or heterophoria is more common. Divergent strabismus is generally most commonly associated with emmetropia or an astigmatic refractive error.

The vision of other eye can be easily suppressed (to abolish diplopia) if there is any defect in that eye or fusion is not fully developed. However, in those persons where binocular vision had already developed, it will not be easy to suppress the vision of any one eye and as a result considerable amount of strain in dissociating accommodation from convergence will occur. These are the cases which are subject for heterophoria and due to lacking of stimulus will result into a case of heterotropia.

Note: In any type of squint it remains tendency of a person to use better eye than the affected eye so that vision of other eye is sacrificed in lieu to abolish diplopia and heterophoria will not manifest.

Clinical Presentations

- **Accommodative convergent squint:** This type of squint appears commonly during childhood (in the age group of 2–8 years) before full development of fusion. In this age group child develops interest in near objects like book, pictures or toys; hence the accommodation is first time used actively by the child. The squint appearance is more often preceded by debilitating illness (e.g. measles or whooping cough) in child, leading to reduction in tone of muscles.

- **Divergent squint:** It is usually associated with myopia but as the myopia is usually not present since birth, it usually develops with growth of child, hence divergent squint is not seen at early age. The squint is usually not seen in manifest form until the fusion is fully established, however, as the age advances and once near point is receded and convergence is still not much required, a tendency to diverge will increase and then become manifest squint. On contrary, if myopia is since birth (congenital or infantile myopia) although accommodation is not required but clear vision to see near object is attained by efforts of convergence. Due to presence of myopia the distance objects are permanently out of vision of child (hence are neglected by child), the efforts of convergence are continuously exercised. These efforts are rewarded in terms of good binocular vision. This excessive constant use of convergence gets established as esophoria for all distances and which may ultimately leads to a manifest convergent squint.

- In high degree astigmatism clarity of vision is not affected by the efforts of convergence rather there will be a relative blindness for both distant or near objects. In contrast to congenital myope, where clear vision can be attained by dissociating convergence from accommodation the congenital astigmatics fails to see clearly by any efforts. Hence they give up all efforts to see clear objects by development of divergence initially for near objects and then finally for distant objects also.

Effect on Vision in Concomitant Squint

Most cases of concomitant squint develop in early childhood are usually associated with diplopia. Occasionally, this diplopia persists because patient is being unable to either overcome it or avoid it, but in majority of patients disadvantages of diplopia are overcome either by suppression of images of deviating eye or by a mental reorientation of displaced image so that this image is projected in space at a position more near to the image of fixating eye (*false projection phenomenon*).

Suppression of the image of deviating eye is a psychological phenomenon. If this condition persists for some period then the visual function is impaired and vision gets deteriorated progressively. Cells present in visual cortex of occipital lobe receive impulses from both the eyes and if impulse from one eye excluded for binocular vision shortly after birth and is not reached on these cells, then the cells will completely loose their capability of binocularity.

In majority of cases having accommodative convergent squint (since very young age) this suppression of impulse from one eye will lead to a condition called amblyopia ex-anopia. The vision in this suppressed eye is very poor and if this condition persists for a long time, then it is difficult or impossible to recover the visual loss. To prevent the development of this type of blindness due to amblyopia of an untreatable degree it is important to start an early and effective treatment in every case of strabismus.

Heterotropia Classification

Heterotropia classification is based on the direction of deviated eye as shown in Table 9.2.

To understand easily and in convenient way the different hypertropia can be summarized as

- Esotropia means a convergent squint.
- Exotropia means a divergent squint.
- Hypertropia and hypotropia mean vertical squints. Because these terms are relative, they can further be differentiated as
    - Strabismus sursumvergence wherein eye is turned upwards
    - Strabismus deorsumvergence wherein eye is turned downwards

Table 9.2:	Classification of heterotropia	
Plane of deviation	Type of heterotropia	Direction of squinting eye
Horizontal	Esotropia	Inwards
	Exotropia	Outwards
Vertical	Hypertropia (strabismus sursumvergence)	Upward
	Hypotropia (strabismus deorsumvergence)	Downward

Treatment of Heterotropia

An ideal treatment approach in case of a strabismus is not only to correct the deviation, but also to establish a binocular vision. It is very important to start the treatment of squint as early as possible once squint is noticed because as child's age advances the reflex pathway which subserves the function of binocularity becomes difficult and at an adolescent age it becomes impossible. Preferably, a strabismus is considered cured only when with treatment person achieve good vision and both eyes are in a perfect alignment with binocular vision.

Two important steps of treatment which an ophthalmic expert can perform are

- Accurately determine and correct any refractive error, if present.
- Maintain and promote the vision in deviated eye.

Optical Correction

Determination of refractive error is done under full cycloplegia by atropine given for three consecutive days (preferably in an ointment form at bedtime) before examination. It is better to do retinoscopy for detection of refractive error and in cases of astigmatic errors (especially that of deviated eye), a special consideration is required.

It is possible to do retinoscopy in most of the cases including young child who can fixate a light and test lenses can be held in hand at an arm length. Sometimes difficulty can be faced in performing retinoscopy in high amblyopic eyes because central fixation is not present in these patients. In such cases retinoscopy is done by occluding the fixating eye so that amblyopic eye can centrally fixate and once the retinoscopy is done the fixating eye can also be refracted under atropine cycloplegia.

If significant refractive error is present then full correction should be given by just deducting plus one dioptre power (due to effect of atropine) from the retinoscopy values. If child is unable to tolerate the spectacles, then atropine is prescribed along with spectacles for a few weeks until child starts tolerating the spectacle corrections.

It is essential to wear spectacles constantly prescribed for refractive error, i.e. should be wear from morning and should be removed at night. If very young children resist wearing spectacles or remove them very often, then spectacles can be tied with the head of child as shown in Fig. 9.6.

As discussed above the accommodative squint usually develops between the age of 2–8 years and usually a 2–3 years old child can wear spectacles. If child is younger than

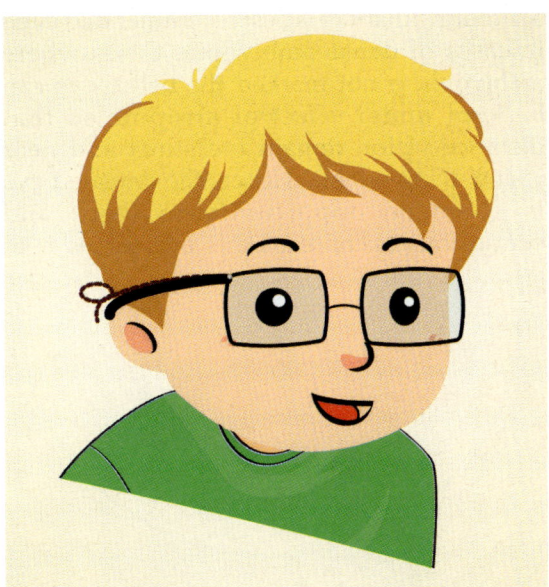

Fig. 9.6: Spectacle corrections for young child

this age or not accepting spectacles, then atropine can be given as daily or alternate day as ointment, until child is able to wear the spectacles. In some cases atropinisation rectifies the squint by abolishing the effect of accommodation and further deviation can be controlled by spectacles.

Maintenance of Vision in Squinted Eye

Once optical correction has been given, next step is to improve the vision of squinting eye. Vision is measured as routine and it is re-estimated after prescribing the glasses. If the deviated eye is amblyopic and its visual acuity is very poor, then the fixating eye should be occluded to encourage the vision of deviated eye. Best method to occlude fixating or better seeing eye is by applying the surgical plaster (e.g. opticlude) and spectacles can be worn over it. Alternative method for occlusion is use of spectacle having an occluder fixed inside the spectacle or a paper can be applied on one lens of spectacles. In cases of dense amblyopia this may not be effective and a total occlusion may be needed. However, total occlusion in order to improve vision in amblyopic eye may destroy remnants of binocular vision altogether. Hence, total occlusion of eyes in alternating manner is best recommended even in cases of dense amblyopia. Cases where amblyopia is not marked the better eye can be kept under effect of atropine so that distance vision remain indistinct and near vision is impossible. Hence, the deviated eye is given an opportunity to work and continuous exercise of this eye forces it to

improve its efficacy. A constant watch should be kept as sometimes the occluded eye gets deviated and vision gets deteriorate.

Result of such a treatment is variable and occlusion is tried for a month period and if no improvement occurs, then it can be tried for another month. In spite of this when no improvement occurs in deviation and visual acuity, then chances of correction are very less. Suppose there is improvement in visual acuity then the treatment is continued till there is further improvement in vision is obtained. The ideal duration of treatment is till the vision of both eyes become equal or until any further improvement in vision has stopped. In these cases a true equality of vision is maintained and squinting becomes alternate means a condition where one or other eye is used for fixation. If child is older, then the outcome is relatively very poor.

As soon as equality of vision is achieved an attempt should be made to develop a binocular vision by starting orthoptic exercises, in which habit of binocularity is practiced by training and facilitating a binocular vision of a degree sufficient enough to maintain alignment of two eyes.

Preferably once the desire for fusion is obtained by orthoptic exercises, surgical treatment is undertaken. However, in cases of accommodative squint operation is postponed until correcting spectacles has been worn for some months. For example, suppose the degree of deviation reduced from 25 to 15 degree by wearing spectacles, then only correction of 15 degree is required by surgery not of 25 degree.

Vision and Refraction

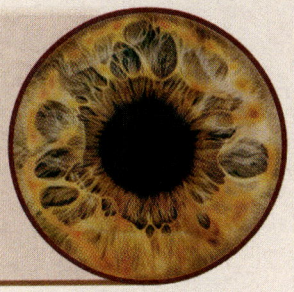

CHAPTER 10

Visual Perception

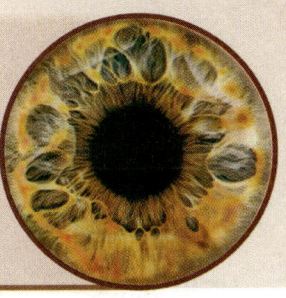

Learning Objectives

After studying this chapter the reader should be able to:
- Understand perception of light in terms of its all elements like light sense, form sense, contrast sense and color sense.
- Describe entoptic phenomenon and after images.
- Explain visual acuity in terms of various criteria and factors influencing visual acuity.
- Measure visual acuity for distance and near in infants, children and adults by various available methods.
- Describe the contrast sense, its types and methods of measurement.
- Understand color vision and theories of color vision.
- Explain color vision charts and color blindness.
- Understand potential vision and its methods of measurement.

Vision or perception of visual sense is a complex phenomenon and it involves:

- Light sense
- Form sense
- Contrast sense
- Color sense

LIGHT SENSE

Introduction

Light sense is the sensation of perception of light impulses by retina, nerve pathways and central nervous mechanism, not only as a whole but also in all its grades of intensity. Suppose intensity of light falling upon retina is progressively reduced, then after certain level of intensity a point will come when light is no longer perceived by the individual, this point is called light minimum. The light minimum is not constant at different portion of retina. For example, at foveal region it is significantly higher as compared to paracentral and peripheral region of retina. The normal human eye is exposed to a wide range of lighting environment, thus to function properly a very rapid adaptation to these changes in the range of lighting intensity is necessary to perform various activities in day-to-day life. This ability of human visual system which allows a person to see clear in different range of lighting intensity, is called light or dark adaptation. To understand this in better way, consider a situation when we suddenly enter from outside (bright sunlight) into movie theatre (dim lighted). Normally, we feel that objects inside the theatre are not visible for some time. Once our eyes become adapted to that dim illumination, we start seeing the objects in theatre. Hence, the interpretations about effectiveness of the process of light minimum can be judged once the retina is stimulated in the same illuminating conditions of dark adaptation, which can be achieved by eliminating light for at least 20–30 minutes duration.

In human eyes retina has two photoreceptors, i.e. cones and rods. In low illumination

Note: Diurnal animals like squirrel have very few or no rod whereas, nocturnal animals like bat have small numbers or no cones. Humans have sufficient number of both rods and cones.

conditions sensitivity of rods towards the light is much more as compared to cones, hence in dim illumination, as during early morning or during evening an individual sees with rods and this vision is termed scotopic vision, whereas in bright illumination as during daylight, person utilizes the cones to see the objects which is called as photopic vision.

Entoptic Phenomenon

The visual perceptions having their source inside the ocular structures of an observer's eye forms images which may or may not be perceived by the observer. These ocular structures which may cause formation of these images may be either normal anatomical components of the observer's eye or may be pathological components like opacities present in ocular media. As these images arise from "inside" they are called 'entoptic' phenomenon. Visual perceptions usually filter out these images, but if they appear suddenly or become annoying, patients may have symptoms. Several entoptic phenomena are the results of shadows falling on the retina, due to opaque portions inside the eye. Shadows on the retina from a collimated light are sharp irrespective of their position from the screen. For example, when a pinhole is placed near anterior focal point of eye, all the light rays falling on the eye becomes parallel and opacities present within the eye will produce sharp shadows on retina, irrespective of position of objects, i.e. either in anterior or posterior region of eye (as shown in Fig. 10.1). Though pinhole opacities present in anterior segment of the eye will appear as shadows at anterior focal point of eye. A small size pinhole, a large size pupil, and a very bright background will enhance the entoptic effect. Various shadows seen in cases of corneal and lenticular spots are shown in Fig. 10.2. Corneal

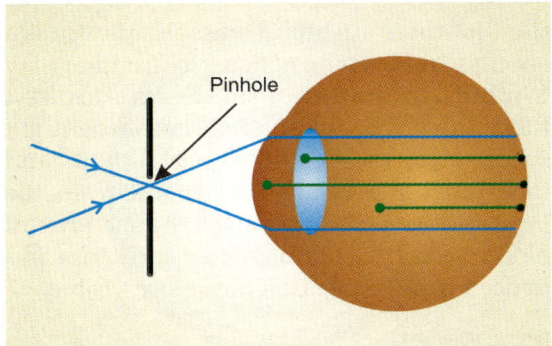

Fig. 10.1: Sharp shadows on retina

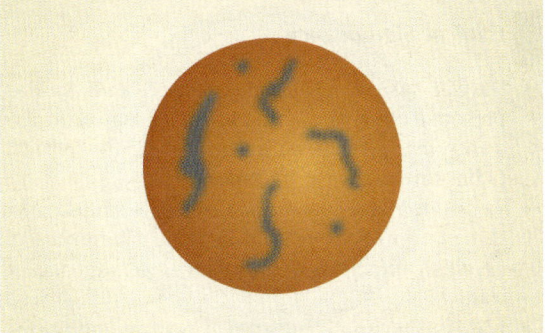

Fig. 10.3: Floaters

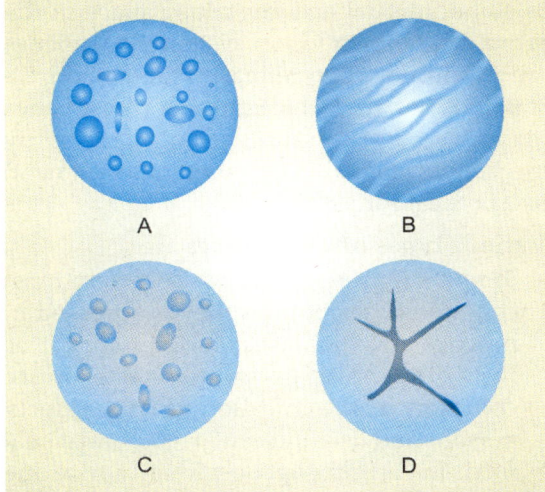

Fig. 10.2: Various entoptic appearances. A. Corneal spots; B. Corneal folds; C. Spots in crystalline lens; D. Star opacity in crystalline lens

spots or folds will appear as circular shadows of various sizes at anterior focal point of eye, whereas spots and star opacity in crystalline lens appears as shadows inside the eye which moves with ocular movement.

Floaters

Floaters [also known as 'muscae volitantes' (means flying bugs in Latin) or 'flying gnats'] are shadows which float like cobwebs or specks in the field of vision. These floaters appear as dark, shadowy shapes and may appear as spots, thread-like strands, or sometimes even curved lines as shown in Fig. 10.3.

They often move with the movements of eyeball but if someone tries to look them directly they float away. Floaters are characteristically found in the vitreous cavity as small opacities and they cast shadows on the retina.

Causes

- Most common cause is liquefaction and breaking of transparent vitreous gel occurring with age leading to shrinking of vitreous and results in detachment of vitreous from retina (posterior vitreous detachment). Consequently, the liquefied material gets chance to move between vitreous gel and the retina. Collagen fibers which were initially a part of vitreous now become loose clumps or debris and begin to float into vitreous cavity. The debris in vitreous cavity will cast shadow on the retina and moves around with the movement of eyeball.

Clinical Appearance

- Depending on the location from retina when floaters are present very close to retina, they cast sharp shadows or diffraction pattern (because of more obstruction of light) and when these floaters are located away from the retina they cast blurry and indistinct shadows.
- The shadows cast on the retina are visible only when they are moving. In resting position shadows are not seen. Clumps of different sizes moves with different speeds and appears as if an object is moving across our visual field.

- Foveal vision may get affected due to the presence of very dense floaters and may produce annoying symptoms in patients, for which patient may ask for treatment.
- Acute increase in amount of floaters indicates the presence of retinal tears, inflammation (uveitis), infection, hemorrhage, or any ocular injury.
- It is essential to exclude the important conditions like retinal detachment in every patient complaining of floaters; before assuring the patient that these floaters are usually common and not harmful.

- Sometimes remaining materials from break down of either hyaloid artery (during third trimester) or from the retina (during vitreous detachment) may cause floaters.

Treatment

- Mostly floaters are benign in nature so no treatment is required. Patients must be informed that these are due to natural process of aging and cannot be removed by simple uncomplicated procedures.
- A few severe cases may require vitrectomy which may be associated with complications like cataract or retinal detachment.

Note: To resolve floaters a partial vitrectomy can be done called "Floaterectomy".

Purkinje Tree

Purkinje tree are shadows or images which are produced due to superficial blood vessels of retina in the one's own eyes as vessels lies in front of photoreceptors. Normally these images are not visible because of adaptation mechanism in the retina and also they always remain in fixed position. The purkinje tree images can be seen when the light source moves at such frequency so that adaptation mechanism is failed and clear image of blood vessel can be seen. This can be accomplished by viewing through a pinhole pupil. As the pinhole pupil is moved across natural pupil, the shadows of blood vessels also move enough and become noticeable. Another way to induce shadows of blood vessels is to direct the bright light via sclera. Place a penlight source over the closed lid near limbus and then move the penlight in small circles, the light will penetrate and make the shadows of blood vessels to fall on visual receptors and hence Purkinje tree becomes more visible.

Phosphenes

These are vague visual sensations which are perceived as flashes of light, originating due to some internal activity taking place in the retina or at higher visual system. Phosphenes are produced when retina is stimulated by a source other than the light, i.e. phosphenes may arise due to stimulation of retina by mechanical forces (during vitreous detachment) or electrical forces.

Various types of phosphenes are:

- *Moore's lightning streaks:* These are most common types of phosphenes observed in practice and the flashes of light appear as lightning bolts or streaks. It is more common in the middle age and elderly persons and usually seen in temporal visual fields in vertical direction. Mainly arise due to posterior vitreous detachment which create more traction on the retina and hence will cause the retinal cells to discharge these lightening streaks.
- *Flick phosphenes:* These types of phosphenes appear when eyeballs are moved rapidly and in large and jerky manner. More commonly seen by older and dark adapted patients where probably the incompletely or fully detached vitreous might pull retina or bump on the retina.
- *Pressure or deformation phosphenes:* These are produced when eyeball is directly stimulated mechanically by applying pressure on the eyeball. To elicit these phosphenes, close the eyelids and move the eye toward the nose, now pressure is applied on the temporal side via eyelid. A bright spot will appear in nasal visual field.

- *Electrical phosphenes:* Electric current passing through neural network of retina or cortex will induce these types of phosphenes. The magnitude of stimulation of retina by electric current is decided by component of current density perpendicular to the surface of the retina. Electrical phosphenes are commonly observed by those patients who are undergoing electro-oculogram (EOG) test where retina is stimulated when examiners run a small amount of current through the electrodes to check the contact of electrodes.

- *Cortical phosphenes:* These are produced in a similar manner by electrical stimulation of cerebral cortex. It has been found that cortical phosphenes can be produced when there is direct electrical stimulation of cortical neurons as during brain surgery or during transcranial magnetic stimulation test.

Afterimages

Afterimages are produced due to the adaptation to light patterns. It means if we look at some object for a long time and then look away, then an afterimage will be noticed. As these images are localized to a particular retinal area so they move with eye movements. Normally, afterimages are not appreciated by person because eyes move constantly and change the local stimulation, as a result adaptation not occurs.

The Hermann grid or afterimage chart as shown in Fig. 10.4 illustrates about afterimage. When eyes are fixed on the tiny black dot at the center of chart for about a minute and then suddenly eyes are moved to focus on a white spot, then afterimage of the grid will be noticed means a dark grid floating over a white grid will be seen. The afterimages can be of various types like negative afterimage, positive afterimage or images on empty shapes. When photoreceptors, i.e. rods and cones, get overstimulated and loose their sensitivity they produce a negative afterimage in complementary color of the original stimulus color. Positive afterimages are produced

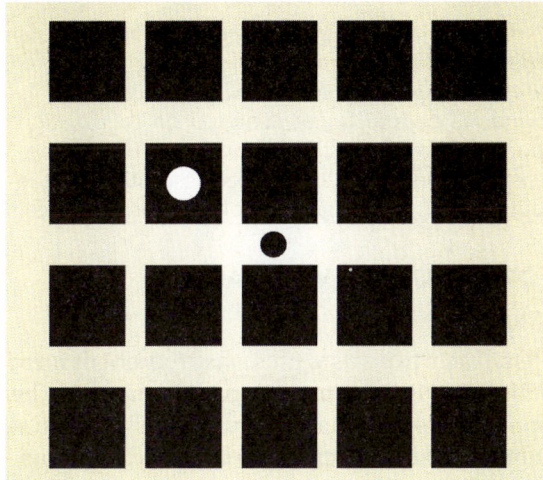

Fig. 10.4: Afterimage chart

only for a fraction of second in the same color as that of original stimulus color. However, their mechanism of formation is not clear.

> ### Clinical Application
>
> Afterimages can be used to test for presence of an anomalous retinal correspondence.

Maxwell's Spot

Macular pigment (zeaxanthin) present in the macular area selectively absorbs blue light and the retinal area covered by these macular pigments is roughly of the same size as foveal area. Before reaching the photoreceptors the light has to pass through these macular pigments. If a blue filter is placed before the eyes and an evenly illuminated surface is looked through it, then a circular dark disc is seen in macular area around the fovea (Maxwell's spot). Normally this dark spot is not noticed because person is adapted to the difference in color or brightness and also spot moves with the eye.

> ### Clinical Application
>
> Maxwell's spot can be used to diagnose eccentric fixation. As described in the above test, patients see the dark spot away from center of fixation point, means they are not using their central fovea for fixation.

Note: Similar technique was used in Haidinger's brushes, where a windmill pattern appears when viewed through a polarized blue light. If this windmill pattern is not centered on the fixation point, it shows an eccentric fixation. This phenomenon appears due to selective absorption of blue polarized light by pigment molecules in the fovea.

FORM SENSE AND VISUAL ACUITY

Visual Acuity

Visual acuity deals with measurement of form sense of visual perception. It measures the spatial discrimination function of visual threshold, i.e. it specifies the limit of discrimination of visual sense in space or it determines threshold of visual sense. Hence, acuity of vision is decided by the smallest retinal image formed by the smallest object which can be seen clearly from a certain distance. The visual angle is the most convenient standard to estimate the visual acuity.

Visual Angle

The angle formed at the nodal point of eye by joining the two lines drawn from the extremities of an object is called visual angle (v) as shown in Fig. 10.5. The visual angle is a suitable and valuable approach to make out the spatial extent of an object in the desired visual field.

To see an object clearly and for discrimination of size, it is necessary that two individual cones should be stimulated whereas, the one cone in between them remain unstimulated. The two adjacent points (for example, A' and B') can be seen distinctly only when they produce a visual angle (v) of at least one minute.

The size of visual angle is dependent on two factors:

- Size of the object
- Distance of the object from the eye

The average diameter of retinal photoreceptor cone is about 1.5 μ in the macular region, hence it is seen that these two points A' and B' will appear distinctly only when their retinal image size, i.e. AB is more than that of 4.5 μ, means two stimulated cones and one unstimulated cone in between them makes a total of $1.5 \times 3 = 4.5$ μ.

As shown in Fig. 10.6 the objects of same size are present at different distance will produce image of different sizes and farther away is the distance of object from the eye, smaller will be the image size on the retina. Hence, size of retinal image is inversely proportional to the distance of object from the eye, therefore, to see an object clearly either it should be of large size or should be situated near to the eye. If object AO is of same size as A'O' and the object AO is situated at one-half the distance of A'O', then the retinal image size (ax) is automatically will be double than that of image a'x, hence the retinal image size for a given visual angle can vary with the change in the viewing distance.

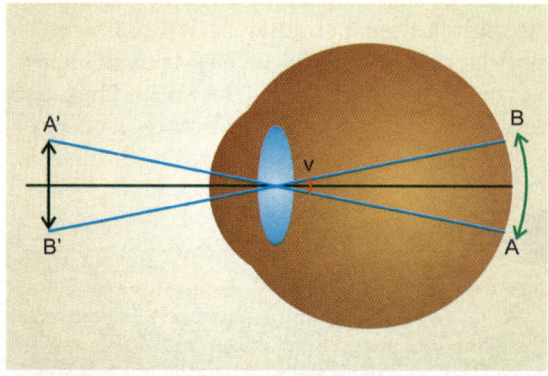

Fig. 10.5: Visual angle

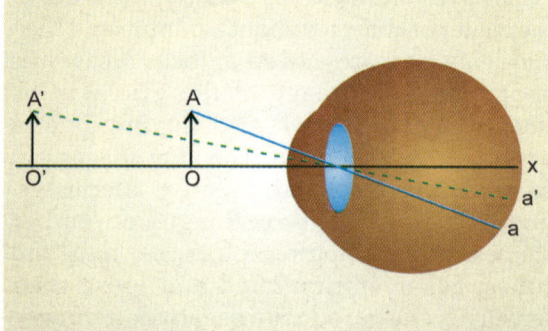

Fig. 10.6: Relation of object distance from eye, with retinal image size

Factors Influencing Visual Acuity

Ability to discriminate two spatially separated targets is termed resolution and it is equivalent to ordinary or normal visual acuity. To achieve this ordinary visual acuity all ocular elements (which are involved in vision) like anatomical, physiological and optical show their maximum performance. Various physical, physiological and psychological factors can influence the visual acuity.

Physical factors are the one which mainly influences the distribution of light characteristics like diffraction, aberrations, scattering, absorption and focus factors. Hence, these factors will affect the nature of formed retinal image. Illumination of the object and contrast sensitivity are important factors affecting visual acuity. Increase in the illumination causes increase in the visual acuity up to a point beyond which no improvement in visual acuity can be elicited. After this point increase in the illumination will cause glare. The usual range of illumination for optimal visual acuity should be 5–20 foot candles. Reduction in contrast will require more illumination for resolution of an object.

Physiological factors affect the processing of stimulus and are mainly related to the observer. These may be

Pupil size: Change in the size of pupil also affects visual acuity by altering illumination and diameter of circle of blur on the retina. In persons having pupil size less than 1 mm, visual acuity will decrease because of diffraction of light and reduction in illumination of retina. Similarly, large-sized pupil (> 6 mm) also decreases visual acuity because of more chances of scattering of light at the retina.

Accommodation: Accommodation is associated with decrease in the size of pupil (miosis), hence affects VA. Spasm of accommodation causes decrease in VA and induces myopia.

Age: With advancement of age changing in the integrity of eye and visual pathways may affect VA. It is because of these aging changes deterioration of vision is common after age of 40–45 years.

Retinal eccentricity: Centre of fovea shows maximal visual acuity. As the distance from fovea increases the visual acuity decreases.

Refractive errors: Presence of uncorrected refractive errors is generally common cause of reduced visual acuity.

Psychological factors: Altered mental status of person due to any disease or any intoxication may affect visual acuity.

Types of Visual Acuity

There are different criteria of visual acuity which are set for the responses of the observer. They are

- Minimal visible or detection acuity: criteria set for presence of a single feature
- Minimal resolvable or resolution or ordinary visual acuity: Criteria of presence of feature identification in a visible target
- Spatial minimal discriminable or hyperacuity: Criteria set for relative location of visible target.
- Recognition acuity

Minimal Visible

Minimal visibility means an ability to detect presence of a visual stimulus/object in an otherwise empty looking visual field. In other words, minimal visible criteria tell about the ability of a person to see a test object against the background. The maximum limit of detection acuity indicates absolute threshold of vision and it can be affected by factors like size, shape, illuminance and contrast of the stimulus.

For example:

- A black dot having diameter of 30 seconds of arc or more than that can be seen against a white background from a considerable distance.
- A thin telegraph wire having thickness of as little as 1 second of an arc can be detected against a uniform sky.

- A black square having diagonal length of 30 seconds of an arc or more can be detected against a white or light shade background from a reasonable distance.
- An illuminated object can be detected from a very long distance in dim light or dark not because of its size rather due to its illuminance intensity.

Thus we can say that minimal visual acuity tells about the brightness and detection discrimination, i.e. it is the ability of an observer to determine small differences in the brightness of two light sources so that presence or absence of a target can be determined.

Minimal Resolvable (Minimum Separable Acuity)

Commonly considered as an ordinary visual acuity and forms the basis for Snellen's letters or Landolt's C charts. A property of discrimination of two separated targets in space is called as resolution and a minimum amount of separation between these two separated targets which an observer can appreciate is called minimal resolvable. Thus minimal separable acuity tells about the resolution threshold or smallest visual angles at which two objects can be discriminated separately (Fig. 10.7).

In other words, we can say that measurement of resolution threshold is equivalent to assessment of function of the fovea centralis. In normal observers the angle subtended by two targets at the nodal point of eye gives an idea about the distance between them. Normal observer in his/her

best focus has a resolution limit between 30 seconds to 1 minute of an arc, which is called minimum angle of resolution (MAR).

Now consider minimum separation between two light bars present in a grid of alternate dark and light bars. As the width of these two light bars increases, the value of threshold decreases and at limit of nearly 1 second of arc the width of these light bars becomes so thick that observer sees only a thin black line against a white background as shown in Fig. 10.8.

Conversely, if the width of two black bars is increased, then the stimulus will appear as thin white line against a black background. Hence the minimal separation appreciated between the two black bars has reduced to a thin white line as shown in Fig. 10.9.

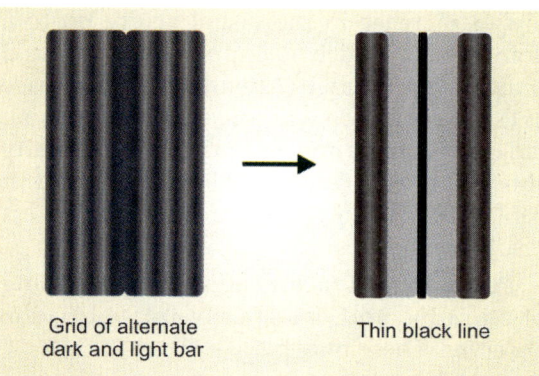

Grid of alternate dark and light bar   Thin black line

Fig. 10.8: Two light bars in a grid appearing as thin black line (minimal resolvable)

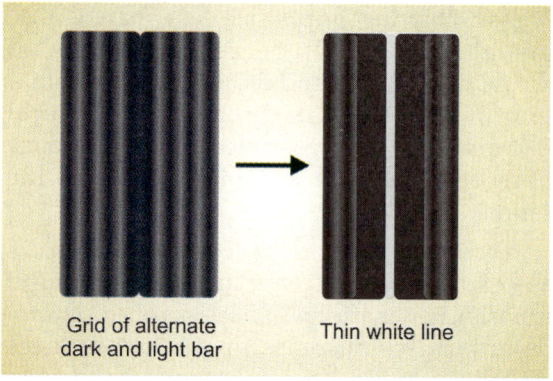

Grid of alternate dark and light bar   Thin white line

Fig. 10.9: Two black bars in a grid appearing as thin white line (minimal resolvable)

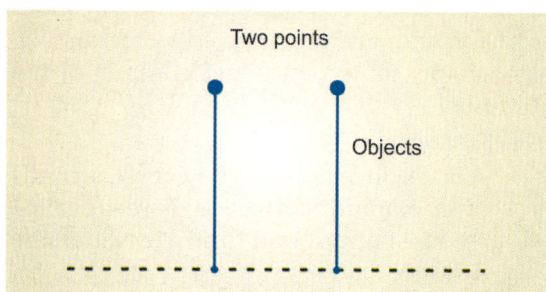

Two points

Objects

Fig. 10.7: Minimal resolvable between two-point objects

Hence, in practice visual acuity measures the minimal separation of target stimulus through form sense or reading ability of observer. To measure visual acuity the tests like Landolt's C (to detect the gap in a ring) and Snellen's optotypes (ability to read a letter) are used.

Minimal Discriminable

Normal observers are capable of making certain spatial distinctions of a stimulus even if the threshold level of stimulus is much lower than the level of an ordinary visual acuity. This state is also called hyperacuity and is best represented by an alignment or Vernier acuity. This simply means hyperacuity test or Vernier acuity task help to detect whether an observer is able to judge the alignment or location of two parallel straight lines in relation to each other (Fig. 10.10).

In hyperacuity the observer judges the location of an element of target in relation to another element of same target, and should not be confused with minimal visible

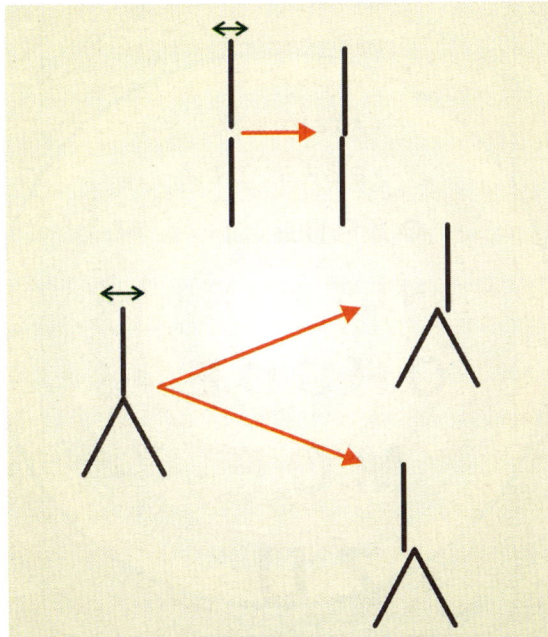

Fig. 10.10: Minimal discriminable showing Vernier's hyperacuity

threshold, where only presence or absence of a target is judged. In normal observers the threshold value of hyperacuity is between 2 and 10 seconds of arc.

Recognisation Acuity

An individual's ability is not only to discriminate the target in spatial characteristics but also to identify the pattern of target stimulus, if he/she is already familiar with that particular test pattern. This ability to identify a pattern or stimulus from a set of similar stimuli or patterns is called recognisation, hence it is a task which involves not only spatial resolution but also has an associated cognitive element. For recognisation an observer should be well known with the set of test figures with an additional ability to resolve these test figures.

Visual Acuity Measurement

Visual acuity per se is a complex ocular function and its components as discussed above are

- Ability to judge the presence or absence of a stimulus, i.e. minimal visible
- Relative judgment of location of one element of visual target with another element of same target, i.e. minimal discriminable.
- Ability to judge presence of feature identification in visual target, i.e. minimal resolvable (ordinary visual acuity).

In clinical scenario measurement of minimal angle of resolution (MAR) is considered equivalent to the measurement of visual acuity, although theoretically as we can see above, there is a lot of difference. Hence, various clinical patterns are established to measure the patient's threshold for a minimal resolvable angle.

Based on this principle various types of visual charts have been developed for clinical assessment of visual acuity or MAR.

To define visual acuity in terms of quantity several eye charts had been developed in early

19th century in Germany. In the year 1836, German ophthalmologist Küchler designed a chart using figures (for example, fire arms like guns, rifles, canons, farming equipments, animals, birds, and amphibians) cut from calendar, books, and newspapers and pasted them on the paper in rows of decreasing sizes. As these figures were selected vaguely thus, the visual design or style was not consistent, hence this system had its limitations. But Küchler refined his chart and in the year 1843, he published a newer version of his traditional chart. As shown in Fig. 10.11 this chart has 12 rows of black letters, which are gradually decreasing in the size. However, even this newer version of chart did not gain popularity and hence was published only once in the year 1843.

The term visual acuity was coined by Donders' in the year 1861 who defined it as "ratio between a subject's performance and a standard performance in distinguishing details of a test pattern". In the year 1862, Dutch scientist Harman Snellen published his famous eye chart, as a standardized measurement tool to check visual acuity. Till date only a few minor variations or improvement are made in the original Snellen's eye chart. In the year 1867, French ophthalmologist Ferdinand Monoyer invented an eye chart and introduces a decimal notation method to measure visual acuity (Fig. 10.12).

In the year 1868, scientist Green proposed an eye chart which has a geometric progression of letter size along with a proportional spacing in between these letters.

Later on in the year 1888, Landolt proposed an eye chart, where he used single symbol of broken ring in different orientations. This solved the problem faced by Snellen's chart optotypes, which were not equally recognizable by all subjects. In the year 1959, Louise Sloan designed a new set of 10 nonserif letters. Chart to be used at one meter distance and she also proposed the use of all 10 letters in each row to avoid any recognisation problems and crowding effects between letters.

Subsequently, Lea Hyvarinen of Finland, Taylor of Australia and Bailey and Lovie (1976) all of them designed their eye charts.

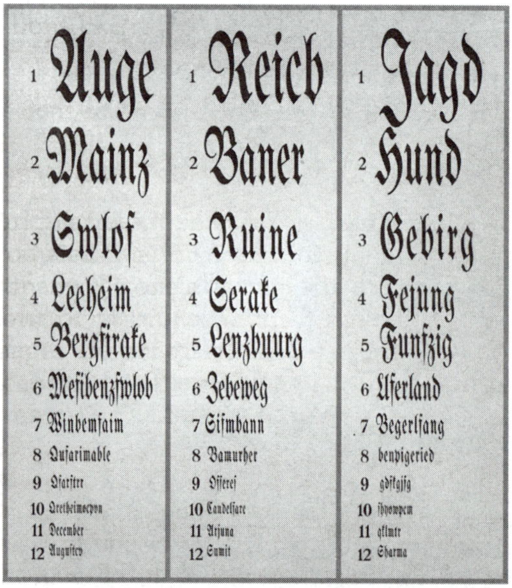

Fig. 10.11: Kuchler vision chart

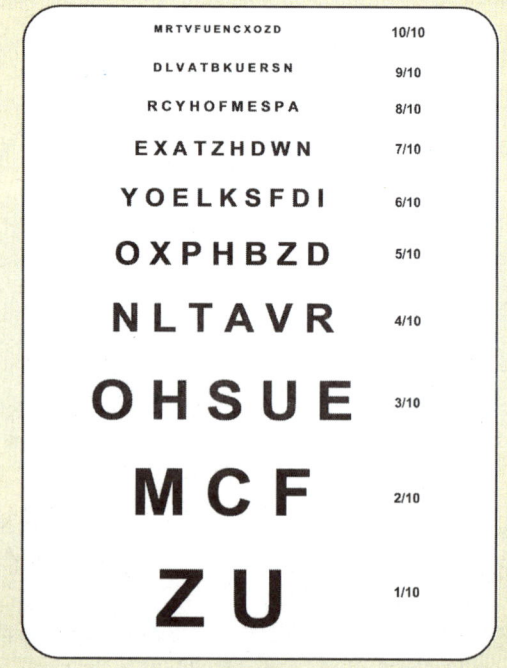

Fig. 10.12: Ferdinand Monoyer vision chart

Lea use pictorial optotypes like outlines of apple, house, square or a circle to test visual acuity for preschool children. Taylor created an eye chart using single optotype, letter E (like Landolt's broken ring) in various orientations. Bailey and Lovie re-invented the original Green's chart and used British letters as optotypes. In the year 1982, National Eye Institute combined the Bailey and Lovie layout with Sloan's optotype letters and created an eye chart called ETDRS chart. In recent years many new development has been done to create electronic type charts. An example is a British-designed Test Chart 2000, which became world's first Window based computerized test chart. This helps in solving many difficult issues like screen contrast and gives an opportunity to change the sequence of letter (so that patient cannot memorize letters).

Visual acuity can be measured by several tests based on the various methods of identification of targets as summarized in Table 10.1.

- Detection acuity, i.e. judgment of presence or absence of a target.
- Resolution acuity describes details of spatial characteristics present in a target in full resolution.
- Recognition acuity means an identification of a target.

Measurement of Ordinary Visual Acuity

Various tests for measurement of visual acuity in different age groups are summarized in Table 10.2.

Visual Acuity Measurement in Infants

Subjective Tests

Indirect assessment of vision can be done by following tests:
- Historical and observational tests
- Binocular fixation preference
- CSM method

Historical and observational tests: Newborn is responsive to sound and shows awareness for surroundings. Parents are usually asked whether child responses to a silent smile, light music or follow objects around the environment. Parental observation also includes presence or absence of deviation of eyes (squint). Suppose one eye is deviated, the visual acuity in that eye is likely to be poor, but in case of a constant alternating squint, visual acuity may be normal in both eyes. At an age of one month infants develop normal pupillary reflex, positive blink reflex and eye popping reflex; presence of these reflexes indicates a good visual acuity. Both pupillary reflex and blink reflex are learned by 30 weeks of gestation. Unique behavior in babies is eye popping, and if something else is not elicitable

Table 10.1: Tests for visual acuity measurement based on various acuity methods				
Detection acuity tests	Resolution acuity tests	Recognition acuity tests		
		Letter identification tests	Direction identification tests	Picture identification tests
Boek candy bead test	Preferential looking test	Snellen's letter chart	Arrow's test	Allen's picture card tests
Catford drum test	Optokinetic nystagmus test	HTOV chart	Snellen's E test	Pictorial vision charts
Dot visual acuity test	Visually evoked response (VER)	Sloan's chart	Landolt's C test	Miniature toy car test
Sty car graded ball's test		Sheridan's letter chart	Sjögren's hand test	Light house picture test
			Taylor's tumbling E test	

Table 10.2: Tests for measurement of visual acuity in various age groups for distance and near vision

In infant		Preschool going child		School going child and adults	For near vision
Subjective tests	Objective tests	1–3 years age	3–5 years age	Above 5 years age and adults	All age group
Historical and observational tests	Visual evoked potential (VEP) test	Marble game test	Tumbling E test	Snellen's visual acuity chart	Snellen's near vision chart
Binocular fixation preference	Optokinetic nystagmus (OKN) test	Worth ivory ball test	Landolt's C test	Landolt's 'C' chart	Jaeger's near vision chart
CSM method	Preferential looking technique (PLT)	Dot visual acuity test	Sheridan-Gardiner HTOV test	ETDRS chart	Roman near vision chart
		Coin test	Sjögren hand test	Modified ETDRS chart	
		Bock's candy bead test	Broken wheel test		
		Miniature toy test	Light house picture card test		

to evaluate visual acuity eye popping reflex can indicate that infant is able to detect the change in room illumination. When the light of room is dimmed suddenly, the upper eyelids of infant pops open wide for a moment and infant often closes the eyes once lights are brought back. This happens again when lights are dimmed.

Binocular fixation preference test: At an age of three months fovea gets fully developed and fixation behavior can be assessed accurately. Various examples of fixation behavior assessment are like identifying mother or fixing eyes on a moving toy. If child is trying to fixate with only one eye, means there is poor vision in non-fixing eye and child will resist violently, if we try to close the fixating/better eye (left eye in our example) as shown in Fig. 10.13A. However, when we close the non-fixating eye (right eye in our example), child continues to smile as shown in Fig. 10.13B.

Suppose visual acuity of child is poor in both the eyes or child is very irritated or not

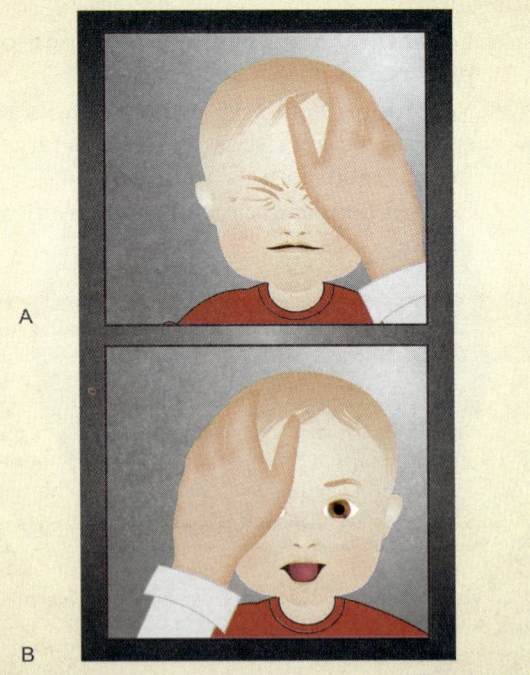

Fig. 10.13A and B: Binocular fixation preference test (*see* text): A. Closing fixating eye (left eye); B. Closing non-fixating eye (right eye)

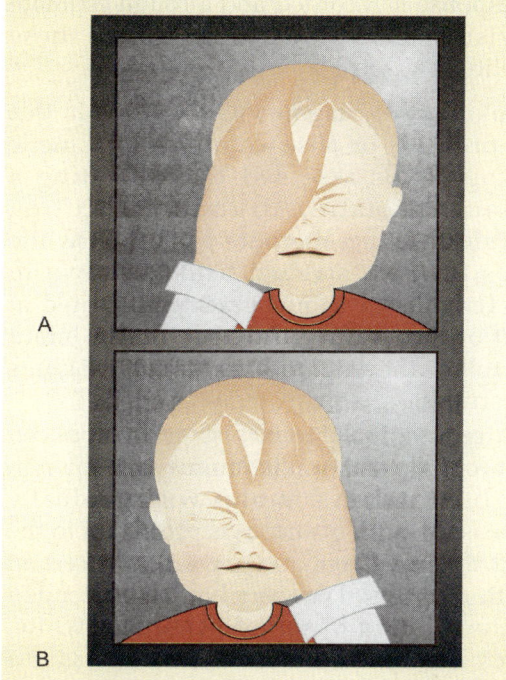

Fig. 10.14: Binocular fixation preference test (*see* text). A. Child resisting closure of right eye; B. Child resisting closure of left eye

liking the examiner's hand over face, then he/ she will resist closure of either eye and will starts crying or will try to remove the hand from eyes as shown in Fig. 10.14A and B.

CSM method: At 3–6 months of age an adequate amount of refixation reflex gets develop and a cover test or cover uncover test can be performed. Test is done with one eye of baby is fixed on an accommodating target held at 40 cm distance in front of the baby.

C refers to corneal reflex as the baby fixate the light held by examiner, normally light is reflected at center of cornea symmetrically.

S refers to steadiness of fixation by baby on the light held by the examiner.

M refers to the ability of child to maintain the alignment of light first by one eye, when other eye is covered and then by other eye when this eye is uncovered. Inability to fixate

Note: On clinical evaluation presence of all three elements, i.e. CSM indicates visual acuity of 6/9 to 6/6. Only presence of CS and no M indicates visual acuity of 6/36 to 6/60 and an unsteady central fixation indicates vision less than 6/60.

with either eye when other eye is uncovered is considered as an evidence of difference in visual acuity between two eyes.

This test will also help in diagnosing the underlying squint, if present. At an age of 6 months vergence response to base-in/base-out prism can be elicited. At this age vestibulo-ocular reflex induced nystagmus can also be elicited, which helps in differentiating normal seeing child from a blind child.

Note: Nystagmus persisting for 5 seconds or more than 5 seconds duration indicates blindness.

Between 6 and 12 months of age group if a response is tried to be elicited by giving forced choices of object, child will show optimal response, because by 9 months of age a habituation phenomenon is developed and an infant finds it difficult to sustain interest in any type of objects.

Objective tests: For assessment of detection/ resolution acuity in infants, various objective tests had been studied, among them most significant tests are:

- Visual evoked potential test
- Optokinetic nystagmus test
- Preferential looking technique
- Teller acuity cards test (TAC)
- Cardiff acuity test (CAT)

Visual evoked potentials: This technique is independent of behavioral response of the infant and is useful in assessing detection/ resolution acuity in preverbal infants. This is the only clinical objective test, which assesses the functional status of visual system from retinal ganglionic cells to occipital cortex. This test is performed in those infants or children who give unreliable results with other tests. Infant is presented with either flash or patterned stimuli and an electroencephalogram (EEG) is recorded from occipital lobe as shown in Fig. 10.15.

Visual potential responses (VER) recorded by flash stimuli tells only about the integrity of visual pathway from macula to occipital cortex. To record reversal VER, alternating black and white stripes or checks (like a checker board) patterns are positioned in front of the child and response of the brain is noticed. To record it, three metal electrodes are placed on the head of child which are connected to a computer. When the child sees the stripes, the signals are transferred from eyes to the visual cortex; these signals are then detected by metal electrodes. Mean amplitude of response is recorded and a rough estimate of visual acuity can be made by these amplitude values.

Optokinetic Nystagmus (OKN) Test: In this test presence or absence of an optokinetic nystagmus is assessed by presenting a patterned rotating drum or a drifting stimulus having alternate black and white strips to infant's visual field as shown in Fig. 10.16. The drum is gradually rotated in front of the infant and the eyes of an infant will follow the stripes with a jerky nystagmus pattern.

Interpretation of test: Nystagmus is noticed with rotation of drum (stimulus) as shown in Fig. 10.17. When stimulus with gradually decreased width of stripes is presented to the child, the movement of eyes will stop at certain width of strips. The visual angle subtended by the thinnest strips of black and white, which is able to elicit eye movements give a measurement of visual acuity. Positive nystagmus response indicate presence of counting finger vision between 3 and 5 feet in infant.

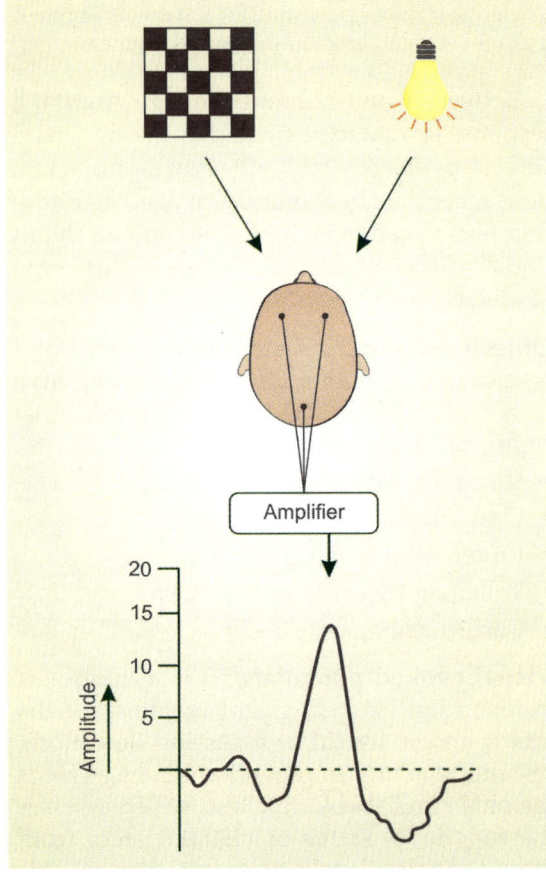

Fig. 10.15: Visual evoked potential

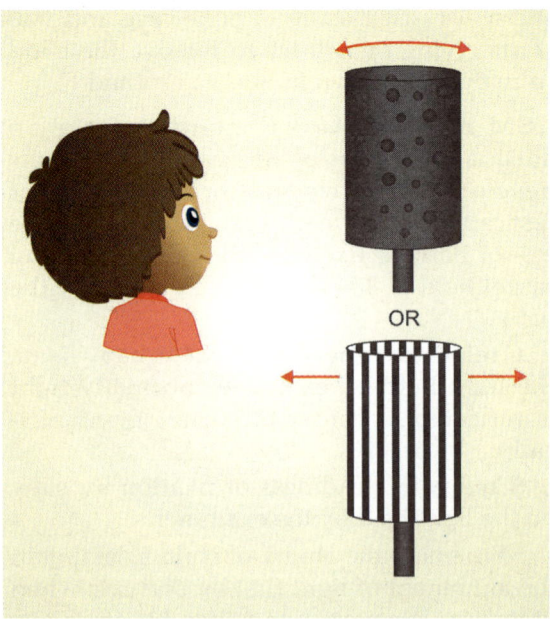

Fig. 10.16: Optokinetic nystagmus test (*see* text)

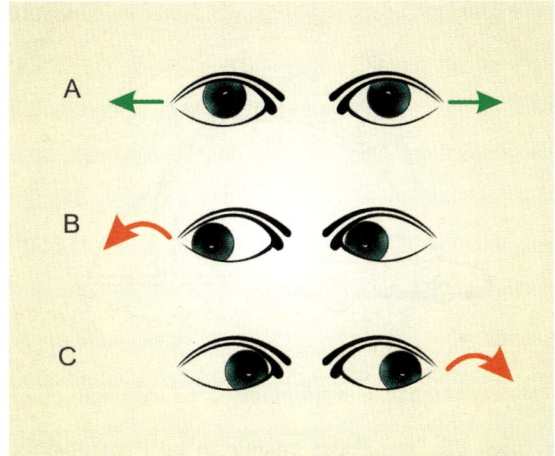

Fig. 10.17: Rotations of eyeballs causing nystagmus

Various studies reported that newborns have an optokinetic acuity of about 6/120, which rapidly improves to be about 6/6 at 2 years of age.

Preferentially looking test: For assessment of visual acuity in infants and toddlers the most commonly used clinical technique is preferentially looking test. Principle of this test is that when two different kinds of stimulus (one patterned and another blank) of equal brightness are presented to child, he/she prefers to look the stimulus with pattern as compared to the blank stimulus.

As shown in Fig. 10.18 examiner remains hidden behind a screen having two stimuli of equal brightness, one homogeneous or blank and other patterned with alternate black and white strips. Child is made to sit in front of this screen and these two stimuli are presented with random alterations. The pattern and position of these two stimuli are altered randomly so that child moves his/her head towards the patterned stimulus. Examiner will observe the head movement of the infant, through a peep hole present in the screen, although he is not aware of the position of patterned stimulus on screen. Examiner will record the head movement directions as right or left, in accordance with the presentation of patterned stimuli.

Thickness of strips in patterned stimuli is gradually reduced along with positional change from right to left, till infant stops moving his/her head; means infant is unable to resolve the stimulus and hence showing no preference to either a blank or patterned stimuli. This minimum thickness of strip, subtend a visual angle and gives an estimate of visual acuity.

As this technique employs square wave grating stimuli and estimate psychosocial resolution acuity, hence this test can be performed on newborn to 5 years of age group. This method gives best results up to 6 months of age because older child gets distracted by surrounding objects and hardly focuses on examination screen.

Teller acuity card test: Most commonly clinically used method among preferentially looking test is Teller's acuity card (TAC) test. Various test cards are presented to child and the preference of child to stimulus is examined.

Visual acuity is estimated by using TAC grating targets as shown in Fig. 10.19.

These cards consist of alternate black and white bars or stripes. The distance between bars varies ranging from widely spaced to narrow spaced in cards. Each card is presented to infant initiating from card with larger pattern and infant's eye is examined for fixation. The card with smallest pattern at

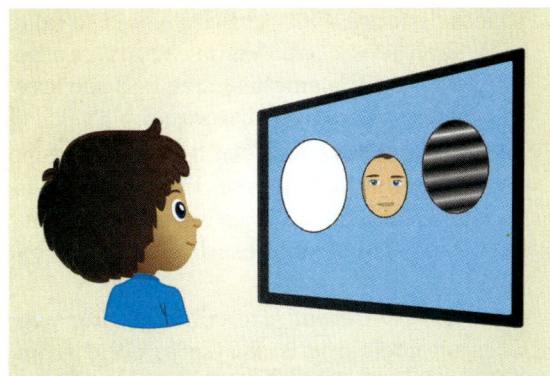

Fig. 10.18: Preferentially looking test (*see* text)

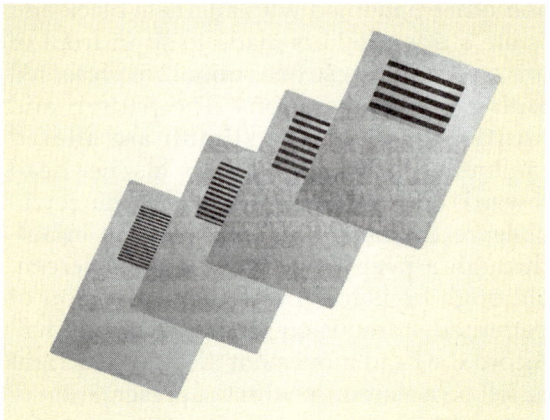

Fig. 10.19: Teller's acuity card (*see* text)

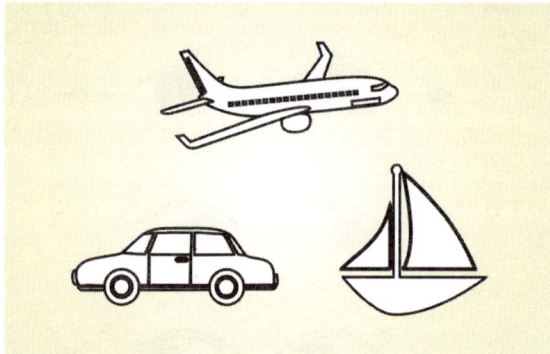

Fig. 10.20: Cardiff acuity card (*see* text)

which fixation achieved indicates the measure of visual acuity. In an infant development of visual acuity is rapid in initial months of age. For understanding at one month age visual acuity seen in infant is about 1 cycle per degree which increases to about 5 cycles per degree at 6 months of age, however, later on a gradual increase in visual acuity happens till 5 years of age; which equals to an adulthood acuity of 40 cycles per degree.

Cardiff acuity test: This test is based on preferentially looking and on vanishing optotypes where pictures are used as vanishing optotypes. Because infants/ toddlers often becomes bored with gratings, the pictures of fish, cow, car, train, boat, duck, house, etc. are presented as targets. These pictures are so designed that they are of the same size and have two black lines with a white space in between in such a manner that pictures can be seen only at a particular distance, i.e. get vanish at particular distance (Fig. 10.20). Examiner presents the various cards one by one to the child sitting at comfortable distance and notices the fixation of eyes by child on the cards.

Visual Acuity Measurement in Preschool Child

Children of age group 1–5 years are considered as preschool going and various tests are employed to assess the vision in this age group. Further these tests can be grouped as tests for age from 1 to 3 years and age from 3 to 5 years. In children the aim of measurement of visual acuity is to screen for high degree refractive errors and/or presence of amblyopia.

Various tests for age group 1–3 years are

- *Marble game test:* Child is encouraged to place the colorful marbles in holes of a card or in a box and examiner notices the eye function of child. This test is not to measure the visual acuity but is done to compare the function of eyes and vision is noted as useful or less useful. Function of one eye is compared with other eye by keeping one eye open and other eye closed and test is repeated vice versa.

- *Worth ivory ball test:* Ivory balls of sizes 0.5–2.5 inches diameter are rolled on the floor in front of the child nearly up to 10 feet distance. Now child is asked to take back each ivory ball. Visual acuity can be estimated by the smallest size ball retrieve by child at a prefixed distance.

- *Dot visual acuity test:* An illuminated box printed with black dots of different sizes is shown to the child. Visual acuity is estimated by the size of smallest dot identified by the child.

- *Coin test:* Different size coins having two faces on each side is shown to child from different distance and asked to identify the faces on the coin.

- *Bock's candy bead test:* Candy beads of 1.0 mm size are spread in front of the child. Child is asked to pick up the candy from a distance of 40 cm. Snellen visual acuity equivalent to 6/60 can be estimated by this test.
- *Miniature toy test:* Child is shown a miniature form of a toy from 10 feet distance and now child is asked to name or pick up the pair of that toy from collection of toys.

Some other tests commonly employed to test the visual acuity in preschool child in the age group of 1–3 years are

- Kay picture test
- Lea test
- Allen test

Various tests for the age group 3–5 years are:

- Tumbling E test
- Landolt's C test
- Sheridan-Gardiner HTOV test
- Sjögren hand test
- Broken wheel test
- Light house picture card test

Visual Acuity Measurement in School Going Children and Adults

Visual acuity in children above 5 years or in an adult can be assessed by Snellen's chart or Landolt's C chart.

Snellen's visual acuity chart: Most common and widely accepted method to test the distance visual acuity is by Snellen's chart. Prior to development of Snellen's chart most eye charts were using printed fonts, but Snellen's invented a new font and called them as optotypes.

Principle: Snellen laid out his optotypes on a grid of 5 × 5 (Fig. 10.21) and by using standard division of a degree into 60 minutes he defined standard vision. According to Snellen's definition "standard vision is the ability of an individual to recognize Snellen's optotypes from a standard distance of 20 feet; at which these optotypes subtend an angle of 5 minutes of arc".

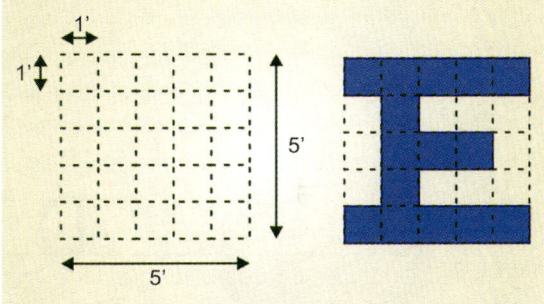

Fig. 10.21: Snellen's optotypes with 5 × 5 grid

For standard vision one grid element of his optotype was equal to 1 × 1 minute of arc, hence the visual acuity can also be considered as individual's capability to differentiate the smaller features of optotype separated by 1 minute of arc.

A ratio of individual's performance to standard performance in relation to vision is labeled as 20/20, 20/40, 20/100 and so on. Snellen arbitrarily choose 20 feet distance for the measurement of visual acuity. Snellen's used nine English letters [C, D, E, F, L, O, P, T, and Z] as optotypes, having serifs.

In the year 1875, Snellen's modified the vision charts that was used at 6 meters distance in place of older 20 feet distance and visual acuity is noted as 6/6, 6/12 and so on, instead of 20/20, 20/40 and so on.

The size of optotypes is designed in such a manner where for a given distance an angle of 5 minute is subtended by each letter at the nodal point of the eye as shown in Fig. 10.22. Hence, the patient should be able to read topmost letter clearly at 60 meter distance and the subsequent letters at 36, 24, 18, 12, 9, 6, 5, and 4 meters distances, respectively. The visual acuity is hence denoted as 6/60, 6/36, 6/24 and so on, where 6/6 is considered as normal limit of acuity.

These optotypes letters are series of black capital letters arranged in a line on a white board. Size of each letter is progressively decreasing from top line to bottom line. These lines comprising optotypes letters have such a width, that each letter subtends an angle of

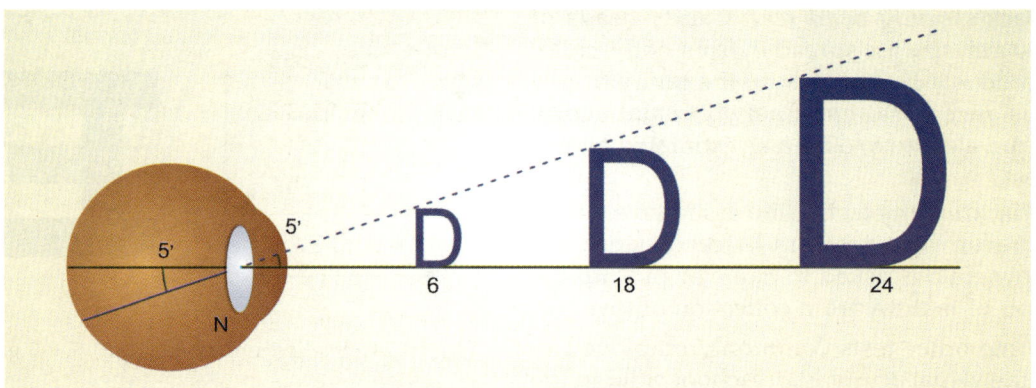

Fig. 10.22: Various size Snellen's optotypes subtend same angle at nodal point, kept at specified distance

5 minutes at nodal point of the eye. Snellen's chart commonly used to assess visual acuity is shown in Fig. 10.23.

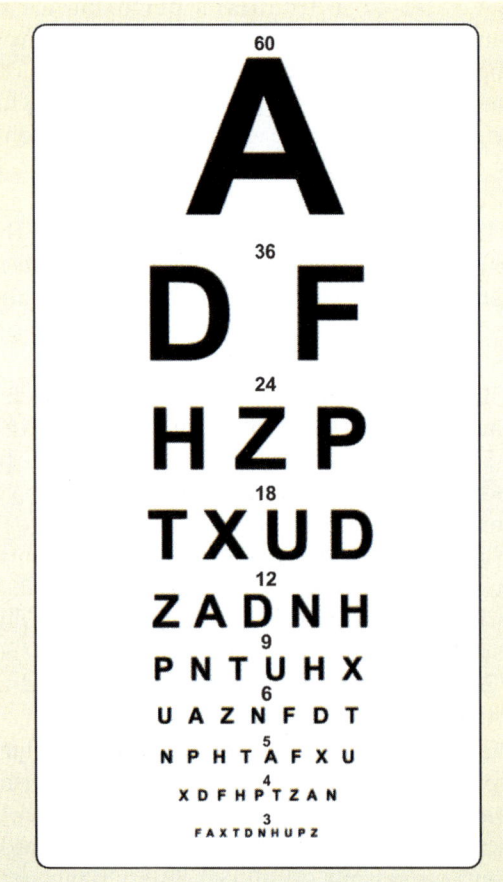

Fig. 10.23: Snellen's chart (*see* text)

Landolt's 'C' chart: As all optotypes in Snellen's chart were not equally recognizable, hence in the year 1888, Landolt proposed an eye chart which has only one prototype, i.e. symbol of a broken ring or circle. Landolt also used a grid of 5 × 5 to create the symbol and each broken circle subtended an angle of 5 minutes at the nodal point of the eye and the break in circle is representing 1 minute of arc, which is similar to Snellen's optotypes as shown in Fig. 10.24.

Size of symbol 'C' is constant of 0.35 inch with a gap of 0.07 inch, which subtend an angle of 5 minutes (or 1 minute arc at gap) when viewed from a 20 feet distance. Break in the ring was given at the top, bottom, right and left side of ring with 45 degree position in between them as shown in Fig. 10.25.

The size of broken circles varies in proportion to the distance of examination as shown in Fig. 10.26, similar to that of in Snellen's optotypes.

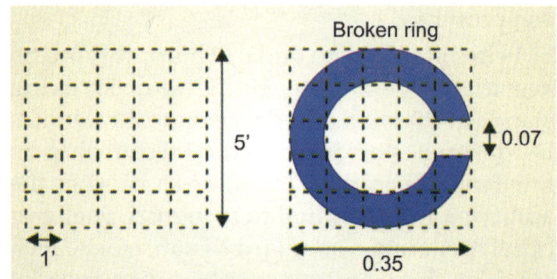

Fig. 10.24: Landolt's optotype (broken ring)

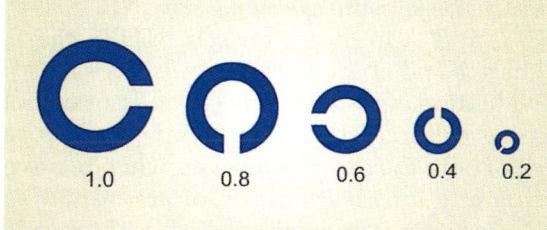

Fig. 10.25: Various orientations of Landolt's broken rings

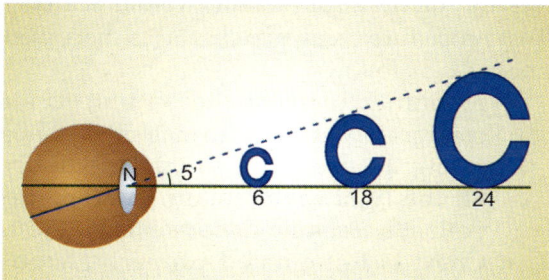

Fig. 10.26: Various size Landolt's optotypes subtend same angle at nodal point, kept at specified distance

Most commonly used design of Landolt's vision chart is as shown in Fig. 10.27.

Snellen's versus Landolt's vision chart

- In Snellen's chart the end point of test is recognition of letter, whereas in Landolt's chart test it is determination of the direction of the break in the circle, i.e. whether break is in top, bottom, right or left.
- Visual acuity is represented by the smallest letter read in the Snellen's chart, whereas visual acuity in Landolt's chart is represented by identification of direction of break in the smallest size circle and is represented as 6/6, 6/9 and so on.
- Although letter targets of Snellen's chart present a more practical visual test, but in identification of letters literacy along with experience with letters in past will influence the results; even if patient is seeing the letters blurred. Whereas Landolt's broken circles eliminate these factors and represent a more objective method of testing of visual acuity.

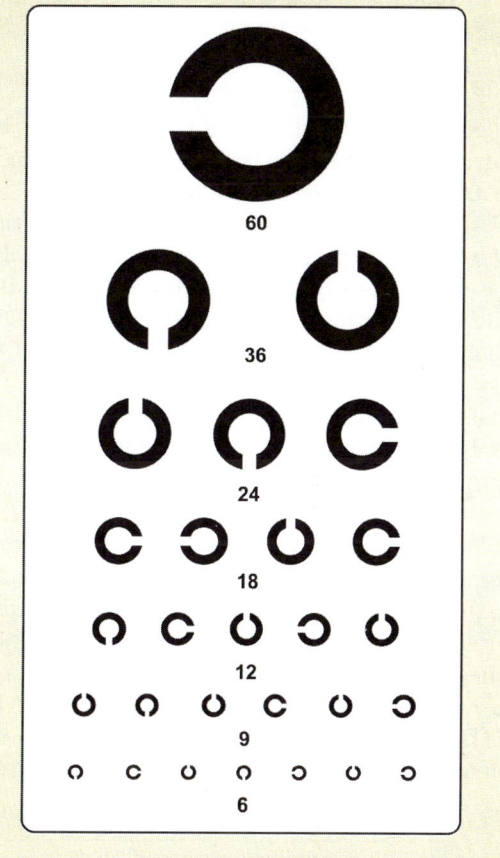

Fig. 10.27: Landolt's vision charts

- As circles in Landolt's chart can have break only in four directions, a possibility of guessing by patient is always there, whereas letter identification is immediate and clear in the Snellen's test, hence it remains less confusing for both the patient and the examiner.

ETDRS chart: ETDRS (Early Treatment Diabetic Retinopathy Study) charts are considered as gold standard for measurement of clinical acuity. ETDRS type charts have similar kind of layout and the prototypes in these charts can be modified according to convenience of examiner.

Essential features of ETDRS charts are

- Proportional layout: Letter or symbol spacing is proportionally designed so that it is equal to the width of letter and also the spacing of line is equal to the height of letters of the lower line.

• Logarithmic progression

In the year 1959, Bailey and Lovie introduced these two features simultaneously in the chart; these charts are also called "log MAR" charts. Original ETDRS chart consists of a set of optotypes having Roman alphabet based 10 letters designed on the basis of Bailey and Lovie principles. These original ETDRS charts were available in three test versions OD, OS and OU. Charts were designed for 4.0 m distance, hence can easily be used at 2.0 m or at 1.0 m distances. Charts were tested in a standard illumination (about 200 cd/m²) and had both front/back lit versions (Fig. 10.28).

Revised ETDRS charts were proposed to reduce the differences in reading occurred due to the relative difficulty of letter identification present in between two consecutive lines. These charts utilizes a new set of letters and are popularly called modified log MAR/ETDRS charts. In original ETDRS charts the Sloan letters C, D, N, R, S, V, and Z were used,

which are substituted by the letters E, P, X, B, T, Y, and A in theses revised ETDRS charts (chart 1 and chart 2 as shown in Fig. 10.29). Evaluation of visual acuity specially in school going children should be done with help of set of both the charts, however, when relative difficulty for identification of an individual Sloan letter is seen then the psychometric functions of the patient can be done for assessment.

Testing method for distance visual acuity

Test procedure using eye charts (as discussed above) is as follows

• Examiner instruct the patient to sit comfortably at 20 feet (6 meters) distance facing the eye chart, so that practically all the light rays remain parallel and patient's accommodation remain at rest.

• Chart is illuminated properly; about 200 Cd/m² and patient is asked to identify the optotypes or read the letters in vision chart with one eye while his/her fellow eye is closed; alternately a trial frame can be worn and one side is occluded by use of occluder.

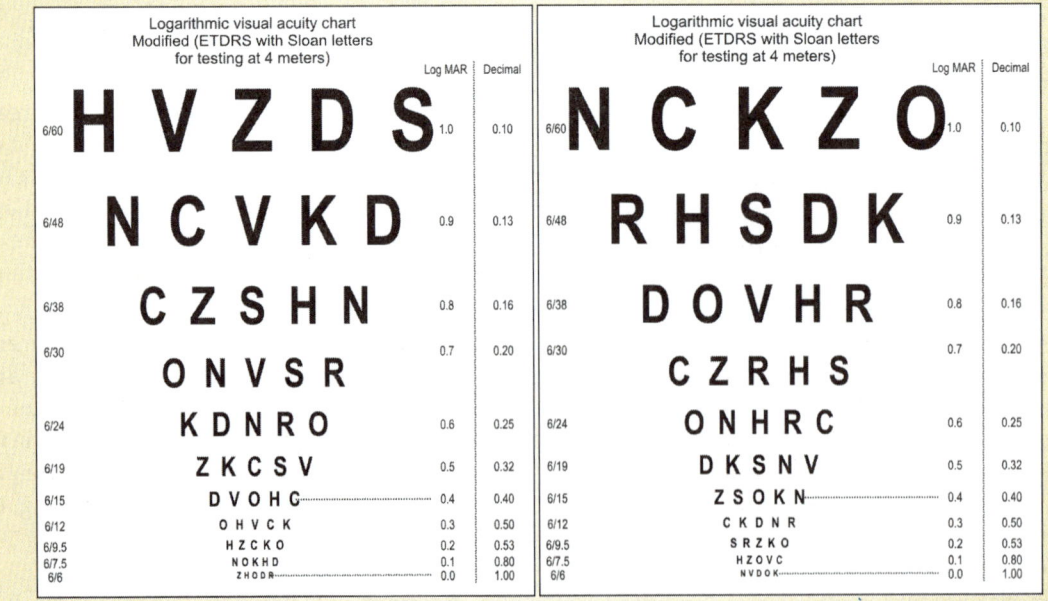

Fig. 10.28: ETDRS charts (*see* text)

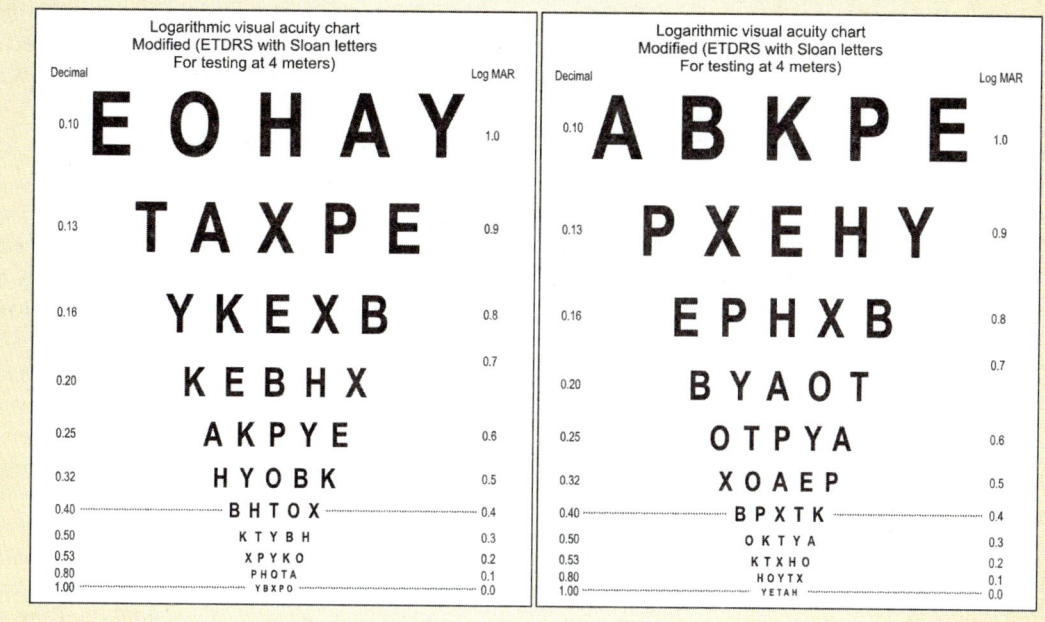

Fig. 10.29: Modified ETDRS charts

- Visual acuity is recorded by denoting the distance of letters/optotypes, from patient as numerator and accurately read smallest letter/optotype in the chart as denominator.
- Suppose patient sitting at 6 meters distance is able to read all the letters/ optotypes correctly up to the line representing 6 meters distance, then visual acuity is represented as 6/6, which is considered as normal.
- Similarly, depending upon the letters/ optotypes of smallest line read by patient from a 6 meters distance, vision is recorded as 6/9, 6/12 and so on. Patient can see up to 60 meters line from 6 meters distance and his/her vision can be recorded as 6/60.
- Suppose if patient is unable to see the 60 meters line optotype/letter from 6 meters distance, then to record his/her vision the patient is instructed to walk slowly toward the chart at 1 meter distance intervals, till he/she is able to see 60 meters line optotype/letter and

visual acuity is recorded as 5/60, 4/60, 3/60, 2/60 and 1/60 depending upon the distance at which the patient see the 60 meters line letter/optotype clearly.
- Suppose patient is not able to read the optotype/letter clearly even at 1 meter distance from chart, then vision is recorded as counting fingers (CF).
- Patient is shown fingers at various distances, i.e. 3, 2 and 1 meter, keeping one eye of patient closed; and patient is asked to count the number of raised fingers. Depending upon the examination distance at which patient is able to count the fingers accurately, vision can also be recorded as CF 1 meter, CF 2 meters and CF 3 meters.

Note: Examiner repeatedly changes the number of fingers at same distance to avoid any guess by the patient.

- Suppose patient is unable to count fingers very near to his/her face, then vision is recorded as hand movement (HM) close to face. Examiner moves his/

her hand with outstretched fingers repeatedly in good illumination in front of the patients eyes and asks whether he/she is able to perceive the movement of hand; if patient says yes then vision is recorded as HM positive (subjective method).

- Even if patient is unable to appreciate hand movement, then a bright beam of light is thrown over the eye of patient, while keeping fellow eye closed with palm of patient's hand and patient is asked whether he/she can perceive the light. Depending upon the response of patient vision is recorded as perception of light (PL) positive or as PL negative.

Note: Patient must be able to perceive the direction of light, not a feeling of heat from the light.

- If PL is positive, then to assess the integrity of retina, a test called projection of ray (PR) can be done. Patient is shown a bright beam of light from upper, lower, nasal and temporal quadrants and patient is asked to catch the light beam. If patient is able to catch the beam in all four quadrants, then a plus sign is used and when patient is unable to identify the direction of light in any one quadrant/all quadrants, then a negative sign is used to record the visual status.

Visual Acuity Measurement for Near Vision

Near vision test is done monocularly and also binocularly by using a trial frame. Near vision test is done by using near vision chart as follows:

- Full optical correction is done for distance vision if refractive error is present. One eye is occluded with the help of occluder and now with full distance correction in place patient is instructed to read the near vision chart from a normal reading distance (usually 30–40 cm).
- Additional convex lenses are given as per the requirement of patient or at power where he/she can comfortably read the smallest line of chart.

- Near vision chart consists of lines having different size fonts, which are arranged in a decreasing order and are marked with acuity values.
- Procedure is repeated for fellow eye and correction with convex lenses is done.
- Once both sides the correction for near vision is done, patient is instructed to read the entire near vision chart with both the eyes open with their respective additional convex lenses in frame.

Commonly used reading charts are:

- Snellen's near vision chart
- Jaeger's near vision chart
- Roman near vision chart

Snellen's Near Vision Chart

On the basis of his distance optotypes, Snellen introduced his Snellen's equivalent for near vision. He graded the thickness of near vision letters in different lines to be about 1/17th of his distance vision letters. Hence the near vision letters equivalent to 6/6 lines of distance vision were subtending an angle of 5 minutes at a distance of 35 cm (average reading distance).

Available printer's fonts were unable to construct the unusual configuration of these letters, hence it was produced only by doing a photographic reduction of standard distance vision chart to a 1/17th of their size as shown in Fig. 10.30.

Snellen's near vision chart lost the clinical interest, because graded size of charts containing pleasant literature phrases were available for commercial purposes to record the near vision.

Jaeger's Near Vision Chart

In the year 1867, Jaeger developed a near vision chart to measure the near acuity, for this he used the ordinary fonts from printers available in that era. These fonts were of various sizes and the fonts have changed considerably since then. In original near vision chart Jaeger marked these fonts from 1 to 7

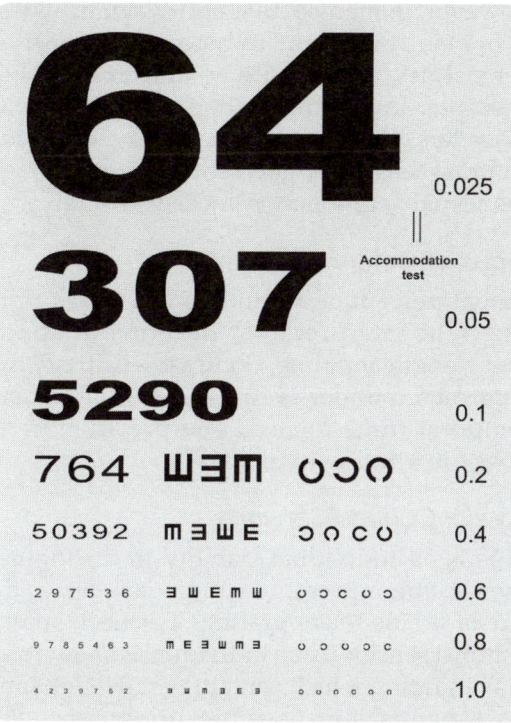

Fig. 10.30: Snellen's near vision chart

and accordingly the vision of patient was recorded as J1 to J7 (J goes by the name of Jaeger himself), which depend on the patient's ability to read the smallest print in chart (Fig. 10.31).

Roman Near Vision Chart

In the year 1952, Faculty of Ophthalmologists of Great Britain came up with a chart containing 'Times Roman' type fonts with standard spacing (Fig. 10.32). This helped in overcoming the problems faced to make the Jaeger's chart in modern fonts. When Jaeger's charts were tried to be made in modern day fonts they were getting significantly deviated from the original standards of Jaeger's chart although for practical purposes they were quite accurate.

The vision of patient is recorded as number represented above the smallest line, which he/she is able to read clearly from a distance of 30–35 cm. For example, suppose patient is comfortably reading the smallest line of near vision chart, then his/her near vision is recorded as N5.

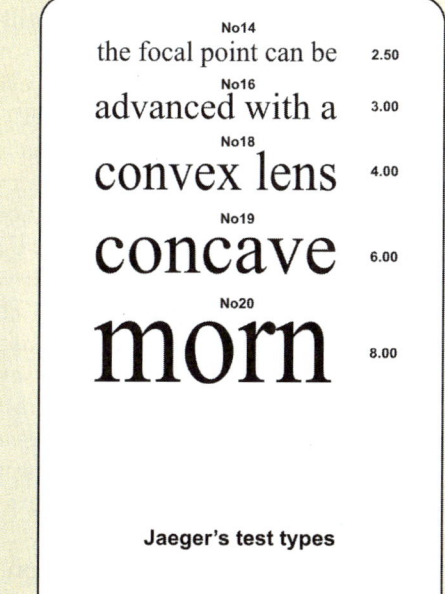

Fig. 10.31: Jaeger's near vision chart

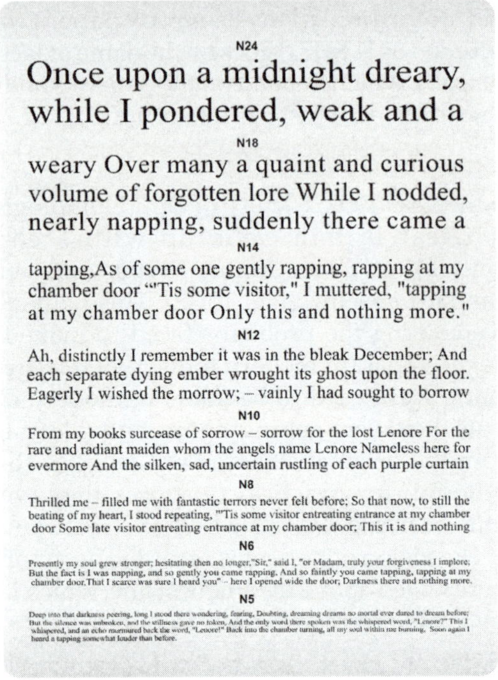

N24

Once upon a midnight dreary, while I pondered, weak and a

N18

weary Over many a quaint and curious volume of forgotten lore While I nodded, nearly napping, suddenly there came a

N14

tapping,As of some one gently rapping, rapping at my chamber door "'Tis some visitor," I muttered, "tapping at my chamber door Only this and nothing more."

N12

Ah, distinctly I remember it was in the bleak December; And each separate dying ember wrought its ghost upon the floor. Eagerly I wished the morrow; – vainly I had sought to borrow

N10

From my books surcease of sorrow – sorrow for the lost Lenore For the rare and radiant maiden whom the angels name Lenore Nameless here for evermore And the silken, sad, uncertain rustling of each purple curtain

N8

Thrilled me – filled me with fantastic terrors never felt before; So that now, to still the beating of my heart, I stood repeating, "'Tis some visitor entreating entrance at my chamber door Some late visitor entreating entrance at my chamber door; This it is and nothing

N6

Presently my soul grew stronger; hesitating then no longer,"Sir," said I, "or Madam, truly your forgiveness I implore. But the fact is I was napping, and so gently you came rapping. And so faintly you came tapping, tapping at my chamber door,That I scarce was sure I heard you" – here I opened wide the door; Darkness there and nothing more.

N5

Deep into that darkness peering, long I stood there wondering, fearing, Doubting, dreaming dreams no mortal ever dared to dream before; But the silence was unbroken, and the stillness gave no token, And the only word there spoken was the whispered word, "Lenore?" This I whispered, and an echo murmured back the word, "Lenore!" Back into the chamber turning, all my soul within me burning, Soon again I heard a tapping somewhat louder than before.

Fig. 10.32: Roman near vision chart

CONTRAST SENSE

Introduction

Contrast sense is more complex function of the retina. Normal sighted individuals are able to see an object and they can process the spatial characteristics of the object, if it differs from its surrounding in any one of these aspects:

- Luminance
- Color
- Texture
- Motion
- Binocular disparity

An individual's ability to perceive the spatial characteristics of an object (not separated by definite borders with its surroundings) with slightest change in luminance is called as contrast sensitivity. Hence in simpler words, contrast sensitivity can be defined as the threshold of an individual to differentiate between the visible and invisible.

Snellen's chart test measures the ability of an individual about his/her perception of the sharp outline of a small object (visual acuity), however, in many ocular and systemic illness it is also important to assess the contrast sensitivity along with visual acuity. For example, in conditions like visual pathway disorders, glaucoma and ocular hypertension contrast sensitivity gets reduced even though the visual acuity may be nearly normal.

Types of Contrast Sensitivity

Visual perception in human eye arises from the light interpretation in terms of space, wavelength and time. Contrast sensitivity can be grouped under spatial (space related) and temporal (time related) interpretation of an object in varying luminance.

Spatial Contrast Sensitivity

This is an individual's ability to distinguish the variations present in luminance across the bar of a sine wave grating. To check spatial contrast sensitivity an individual is shown sine wave grating which contain parallel light and dark bands with varying luminance. The individual is asked to inform at which minimal level of contrast he/she is able to detect the bars.

Spatial frequency defines the width of bars and is an expression of pairs of light and dark bands numbers, which subtend an angle of one minute at nodal point of the eye.

As shown in Fig. 10.33 periods (P) of grating is noted and if the grating has sufficient number of complete cycles (five cycles as a rule), then spatial frequency is denoted by P-1 cycles/degree. Hence, a high spatial frequency indicates narrow bars and low spatial frequency indicate wider bars. The spatial frequency of a grating, whose pattern can be just detected at 100% contrast luminance, is called grating acuity. Normally grating acuity at usual illumination levels is present in the range of 30–50 cycles/degree. For appreciation of Snellen's acuity a high grating acuity is definitely required.

Spatial frequency discrimination threshold is a minimal appreciable difference between spatial frequency of two gratings and at high contrast levels it remains almost constant.

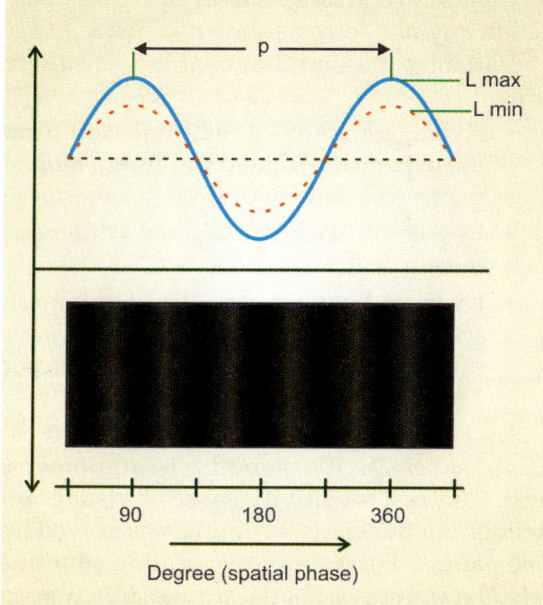

Fig. 10.33: Spatial frequency

Temporal Contrast Sensitivity

Detection of an object in visual world requires its presence for a finite time period. A single beam of light can evoke a neural response however, for a reliable visualization numerous quanta of light within a short period are prerequisite. This multiple quanta of light presented in a short period of time are termed as temporal summation.

Temporal sensitivity cannot be studied separately because following properties affect the ability of a person to detect temporal variations

- spatial properties
- chromaticity
- background characteristics
- surrounding characteristics

A uniform target field is presented to visual system for time related processing of modulated sinusoidal grating to generate contrast sensitivity function. In human visual system, a temporal summation occurs for about 40–100 milliseconds which depends on the spatial and temporal properties of the object and also on other factors such as background, adaptation and eccentricity of target stimulus.

Critical duration is the maximum time over which a temporal summation can occur. When a light is turned on and off for a finite time interval repeatedly in rapid sessions, this light appears as a flickering light. If these lights flickered fast enough, so that they appear as single light rather than flickering light, then it indicates that the limit of temporal resolving ability has reached. This transition from a flickered to fusion occur over a range of temporal frequencies and the boundaries between these two processes is termed critical flicker fusion (CFF) frequency. Hence, the upper limit of temporal sensitivity is defined by CFF frequency.

Testing of spatial and temporal sensitivity produces a systematic data which is significantly more complete for status of visual system as compared to data collected by conventional vision testing.

Measurement of Contrast Sensitivity

Historical Aspects

- French Scientist Pierre Bouguer attempted the measurement of contrast sensitivity first time. He used the ocular structures in the form of a null indicator to match the sensitivity and accuracy of the eye.
- In the year 1956, Schade made the first attempt to measure contrast sensitivity as a function of spatial frequency. He used a log scale which was uniformly spaced for contrast detection threshold at spatial frequencies (about five or so) to measure the contrast sensitivity function (CSF). Later on, in the year 1965, Green and Campbell documented that the CSF is an outcome of two important factors: Optical and neural.
- Modulation Transfer Function (MTF) is an optical function which serves to estimate the retinal image quality and is mainly dependent on size of pupil (simple measurable factor).
- Subsequently, in the year 1968 Campbell and Robson revealed that neurally multiple

channels are present in vision and each channel is selective for a different spatial frequency.

- Fechner reviewed his own work and also considered the measurements done in past especially by Mosson and then concluded that for a wide range of targets contrast threshold is about 1%. This threshold is not dependent on the size and/or luminance of target stimulus; which is an amazing and unexplainable finding till today.

- In the year 1993, Robson reviewed history of contrast sensitivity measurement and in the year 2003, Owsley reviewed importance of contrast sensitivity measurements for clinical assessment. Contrast sensitivity is impaired in several clinical conditions and peak contrast sensitivity is found to be reduced even when visual acuity was normal.

Note: Contrast level below which resolution of grating frequencies of the target is impossible, is termed contrast threshold.

In simpler words, contrast sensitivity is correlated with contrast threshold in reciprocal manner, means division of one by lowest contrast sense (at which gratings letters or lines present in stimulus can be recognized) is contrast sensitivity. It simply means that suppose a person is able to see details of a target at very low contrast, his/her contrast sensitivity is very high and when person is unable to see the target at higher contrast then his/her contrast sensitivity is very low. Contrast sensitivity of a person may vary depending on the structure of stimulus (different size gratings or symbols) used for measurement.

Clinically contrast sensitivity can be represented in any one form as shown in Table 10.3.

Variables measured in contrast sensitivity are

- Average amount of light reflected from the paper (determined by illumination of paper and density of ink).
- Degree of blackness against whiteness, means contrast.
- Distance between repetitions of pattern specified in terms of visual angle; means number of grating periods or cycles per degree of visual angle.

In clinical practice measurement of contrast sensitivity is similar to audiometry test. Contrast sensitivity curve or visuogram tells about the faintest contrasts perceived by the patient. For a sine wave grating stimulus visuogram curve shows similar function as pure tone audiogram does and for an optotype stimulus the visuogram resembles a speech audiogram. Similar to audiometry, in contrast sensitivity measurement also, the results are depicted as a figure (not as a single value).

Contrast Sensitivity Curve

A graph is plotted where X axis represents the visual acuity and Y axis represents the contrast sensitivity. Along horizontal direction of graph (X axis) the size of symbols gradually decreases, whereas along vertical direction (Y axis) the stimulus intensity gradually becomes paler. All points are drawn for the target symbols which are perceived by the patient as well as for the target symbols those

Table 10.3: Representations of contrast sensitivity		
Contrast sensitivity	Formula of calculation	Preferred stimulus
Weber contrast	$(\text{Luminance}_{maximum} - \text{Luminance}_{minimum}) / \text{Luminance}_{background}$	Letter type stimuli
Michelson contrast	$(\text{Luminance}_{maximum} - \text{Luminance}_{minimum}) / (\text{Luminance}_{maximum} + \text{Luminance}_{minimum})$	Grating type stimuli
RMS contrast	$\text{Luminance}_{\sigma} / \text{Luminance}_{\eta}$ Here, L_{η} = mean deviation, L_{σ} = standard deviation	Natural stimuli and efficiency calculations

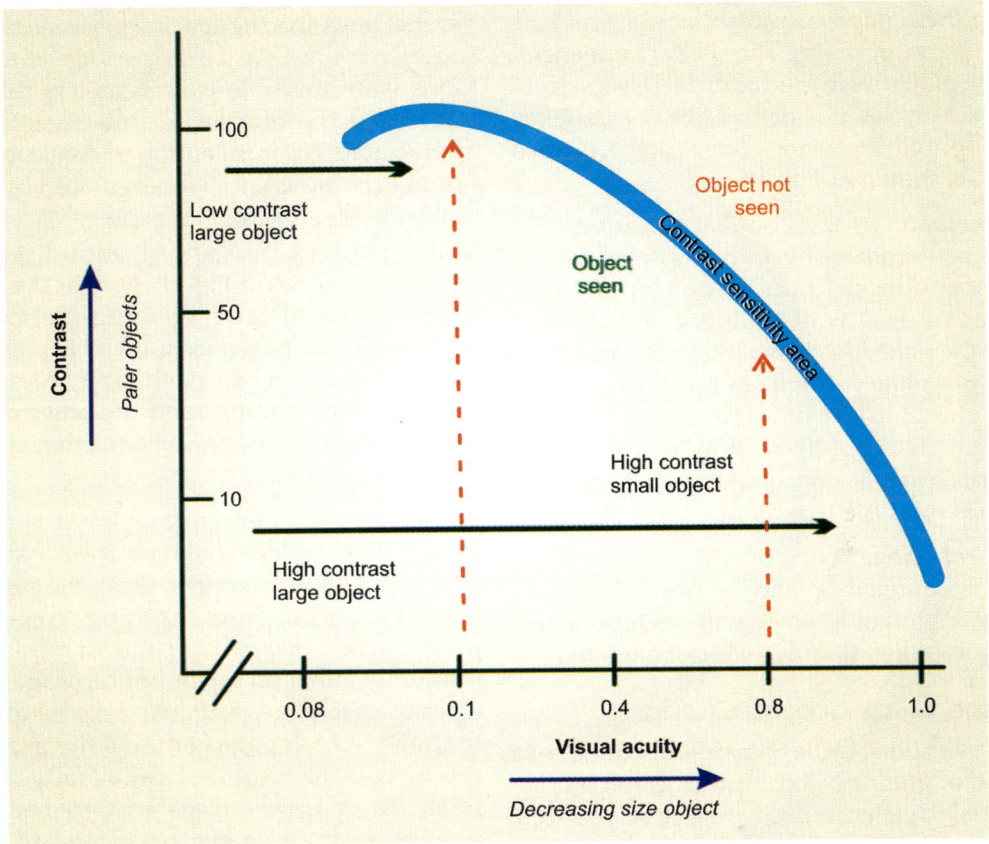

Fig. 10.34: Contrast sensitivity curve (Visuogram)

were too small in the size or too pale and are not seen by the patient. In normal conditions joining of these points form a curve which is popularly known as contrast sensitivity curve as shown in Fig. 10.34.

Various test methods available for the measurement of contrast sensitivity threshold can be grouped as shown in Table 10.4.

Arden's Gratings

In the year 1978, Arden developed a simple and economical technique to assess contrast sensitivity by sine-wave gratings. The gratings are oriented in vertical manner and contrast of grating varies from top (lowest contrast) to bottom (highest contrast). He introduced a booklet having seven photographic plates,

Table 10.4: Types of contrast sensitivity charts		
Grating charts	*Letter charts*	*Computer based charts*
• Arden's grating plates	• Regan charts	• Cathode rays tubes testing
• Cambridge gratings	• Pelli-Robson contrast chart	• Freiburg visual acuity and contrast test (FrACT)
• Ginsberg's chart	• Mars chart	
• Vistech chart		• Holladay automated contrast sensitivity system
• FACT chart		• Medmont AT-20
• Vector vision's CSV-1000		• Mentor B-VAT II

among them one was screening plate and six were diagnostic plates. The spatial frequencies of these plates were gradually increasing from 0.2 to 6.4 cycles per degree (next frequency being double of previous one; 0.2, 0.4, 0.8 and so on) as shown in Fig. 10.35.

Test method: To test contrast sensitivity the plates are studied by patients from 57 cm distance with an illumination of 100 foot candles or a 60 watt bulb about 14 inches above the plates. Each eye is tested separately. Scoring of plate varies from 1 to 20 depending upon the amount of plate uncovered by observer. Each plate is slowly withdrawn upwards from the grey holder until the grating becomes invisible to patient.

Interpretation: Score of all six diagnostic plates is summed up and for normal persons an upper limit of 82 score with an intraocular variation of less than 12 was documented.

Cambridge Low Contrast Gratings

In the year 1984, Della Sala described the first version of gratings. A computer graph plotter was used to generate fine ruling closely spaced parallel lines and the spacing between the two successive lines varied at periodic intervals. Lines were invisible from 6 meters distance but still a fluctuation in line density was appreciable. After invention of computerized dot matrix these lines were replaced by dots.

Cambridge gratings are set of 11 grating plates present in a spiral bound A4 size booklet as shown in Fig. 10.36. This booklet is hung on a wall at a viewing distance of 6 meters. These pages are showed in pairs, one above the other. In each pair, one page comprises the gratings and the other page is blank, although the mean reflection of both the pages is same.

Test method: Cambridge booklet is hanged on a wall at 6 meters distance from patient's sitting position. Examiner turns the pages of booklet one by one showing grating of progressively decreasing contrast, positioned randomly either on top or bottom page. After turning each page examiner asks the patient to choose which page contains the gratings, top or bottom. Gratings are usually shown with horizontal strips but to increase sensitivity booklet can be turned to other direction also.

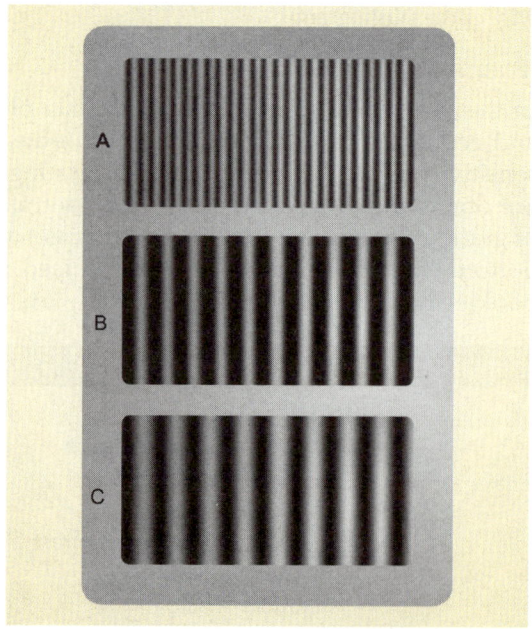

Fig. 10.35: Arden's gratings (*see* text)

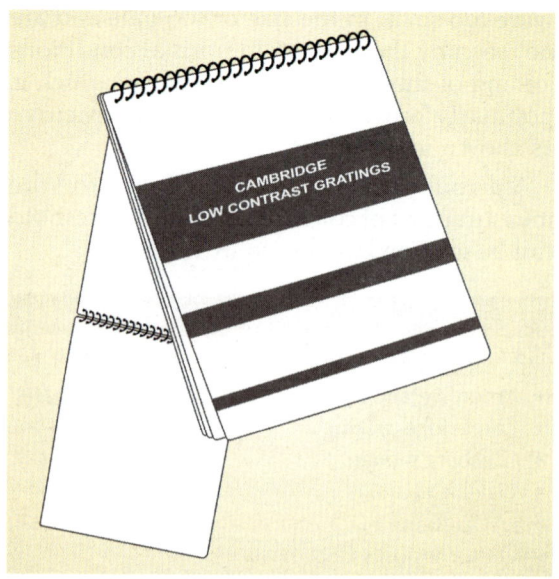

Fig. 10.36: Cambridge low contrast gratings (*see* text)

Original testing method was to present a set of plates three times to each eye and total number of errors made from weaker eye was recorded and compared with standard values obtained from age matched normal individuals. But this was time consuming, hence the recommended procedure is to show the pages in descending order of contrast but stop when first error by patient is made in identification of gratings.

Four descending series are shown separately to each eye and when first error is made or end of series is reached, a new series is started. Second or subsequent series are started not from the first grating page of that series; rather the next series is started from four pages previous to the one at which last error was made. For example, if a person does an error on 8th page in first series, then second series is started from 4th page, not from 1st page of second series and so on.

Interpretation: Sum of all four observations are added and is converted to contrast sensitivity by using a table provided with test.

> **Note:** The grating plate 11 has such a contrast threshold which is below to level of most of the normal individuals, thus in clinical practice this grating is excluded from testing and if no error is found in last grating (number 10), automatically a score of 11 is awarded.

Vistech Chart

Vistech chart for measurement of contrast sensitivity was presented in the year 1984. In this chart the sine wave gratings are present as circular photographic plates. There are five rows of sine wave gratings in total. These sine gratings show increase in spatial frequencies (as doubling at every step, i.e. 1.5, 3, 6, 12 and 24 cycles/degree) from top to bottom of chart. Vistech chart in total has nine columns and five rows and in each row the contrast of gratings decreases from left to right. These gratings are oriented in different directions such as in vertical direction or are tilted at 15° angle either right or left as shown in Fig. 10.37.

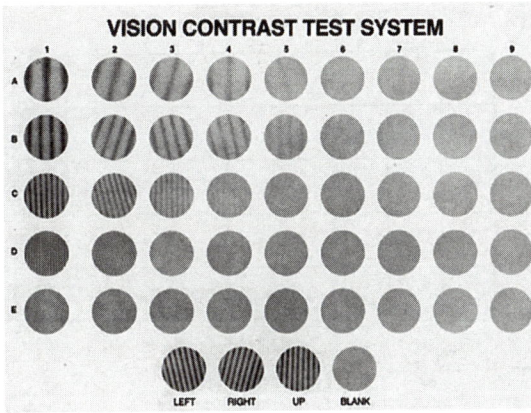

Fig. 10.37: Vistech chart (*see* text)

Test method

- The patient is instructed to recognize the orientations (vertical, right or left) of each sine grating.
- Suppose patient is unable to see the gratings, then he/she may respond the circle as blank.
- The lowest contrast grating recognized by patient will determine the sensitivity score for that spatial frequency.

This chart has a wide clinical application in the measurement of contrast sensitivity especially in cases of cataract and post-refractive surgery.

> **Note:** Step sizes in this chart are irregular; however, an average step size of nearly 0.25 log units having a range of 1.75 log units is present.

FACT Chart

Functional Acuity Contrast Test (FACT) is modified version of Vistech chart. Chart format is similar to Vistech chart in terms of orientations and spatial frequencies of sine gratings, however, average step size is smaller at 0.15 log units against 0.25 log units seen in Vistech chart.

For better test reproducibility, smaller step size of 0.15 log units and AFC method of calculation is used in FACT chart.

As shown in Fig. 10.38 chart also contains the blurred grating patch edges and a larger patch size. These gratings are smoothed into

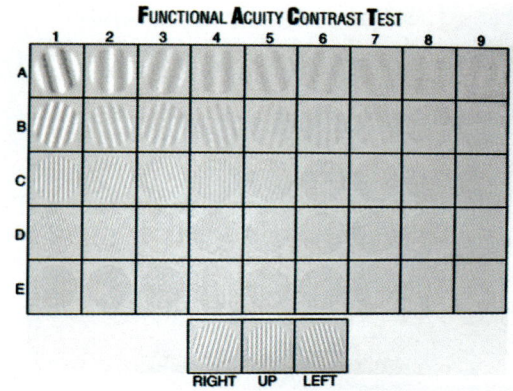

Fig. 10.38: FACT chart (*see* text)

PELLI-ROBSON CONTRAST SENSITIVITY TEST

0.00 **V R S**	**K D R** 0.15	
0.30 **N H C**	**S O K** 0.45	
0.60 **S C N**	**O Z V** 0.75	
0.90 **C N H**	**Z O K** 1.05	
1.20 **N O D**	**V H R** 1.35	
1.50 **C D N**	**Z S V** 1.65	
1.80 **K C H**	**O D K** 1.95	
2.10 **R S Z**	**H V R** 2.25	

Right Eye — Binocular — Left Eye

Log Contrast Sensitivity: _____   Log Contrast Sensitivity: _____   Log Contrast Sensitivity: _____

Acuity: _____   Acuity: _____   Acuity: _____

Correction: _____   Correction: _____

Pupil Diameter: _____ mm   Pupil Diameter: _____ mm

Name: _____   Comments: _____
Age, Sex: _____
Diagnosis: _____
Medications: _____
Date: _____
Examiner: _____

Fig. 10.40: Pelli-Robson contrast sensitivity scoring pad (*see* text)

a grey background which helps in representing a large number of cycles even at low spatial frequency.

Pelli-Robson Contrast Sensitivity Chart

Pelli-Robson chart is a letter identification chart and is used most commonly in clinical practice to evaluate the contrast sensitivity. This testing system consists of

- Two reading charts
- One scoring pad

As shown in Fig. 10.39 these two reading charts are identical but contain different sequences of letters. Whereas, the scoring pad as shown in Fig. 10.40 is a simple letter pad printed on both sides. Letter sets, similar to two Pelli-Robson reading charts, are printed on each side of the scoring pad to note down the correct letter read by the patient during examination. Pelli-Robson charts uses 10 Sloan letters of constant size and these letters are

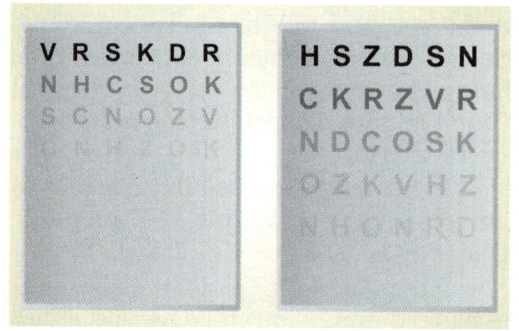

Fig. 10.39: Pelli-Robson contrast sensitivity chart

organized as triplets, there being two triplets per line (16 triplets over 8 lines). The amount of contrast seen among each triplet of letters is of same intensity, however, there is a gradual decrease in contrast intensity from one triplet to next triplet. Pelli-Robson chart is a wall mounted chart to be viewed from 1.0 meter or 40 inches distance.

Test method

- Patient is instructed to sit at 1 meter distance facing Pelli-Robson chart.
- Full amount of distance correction (if present) is placed in trial frame. If required, add +0.75 DS power lenses in front of both the eyes.
- Chart is uniformly illuminated say with nearly 85 cd/m² luminance of the white area and tries to avoid the glare as much as possible.
- Record all the information related to the patient on the scoring pad and then patient is asked to name/or read each letter in a single attempt present on the chart. Patient is instructed to read the chart lines horizontally starting from the darkest letter triplet present on upper left side of the chart.
- Do not allow the patient's to give up too soon, rather encourage patient to make guesses, when they start believing that letters are absent/or invisible. Give a few seconds for the faintest letters to appear until they had guessed correctly 2 out of 3 letters of triplet.

- Test is performed for one eye while the fellow eye is kept covered.
- Testing of contrast sensitivity is done for the fellow eye in similar manner keeping the first eye covered.
- In total the test is performed three times to measure the contrast sensitivity using Pelli-Robson chart. It means each eye is tested separately and then both the eyes are tested together.

Interpretation: On scoring pad mark each letter read correctly by underline or circling it and strike out if any letter read incorrectly. The faintest triplet in which patient identifies two out of three letters correctly represents the contrast sensitivity. Log contrast sensitivity value for the faintest triplet identified by the patient is represented as number written on the scoring pad which may be right or left of the triplet.

Mars Chart

This is designed in a similar way by using Sloan letters as that of Pelli-Robson chart. Only difference is that contrast levels decreases by 0.04 log units as compared to adjacent letter (not as triplet as in Pelli-Robson chart). Contrast range can be tested from 91% to 1.2%. As these charts are smaller in size they can be used for near testing also at 50 cm distance. Test is considered as completed once patient identifies two consecutive letters wrongly.

Regan Charts

These charts evaluate visual acuity at different levels of contrast, i.e. 96%, 25%, 11% and 4%. Each letter rows become gradually smaller in size, which enables different spatial frequencies to be tested. Disadvantage of test is that larger letters are easily seen without reaching the contrast threshold of the patient.

Medmont AT- 20 Test

This is a computer-based test unit used to measure contrast sensitivity by presenting variable contrast gratings and Bailey-Lovie visual acuity charts. This unit can test the visual acuity at eight contrast levels. A randomized display of stimulus can be done to avoid the memorization of chart by the patient. Along with different contrast sensitivity charts a staircase procedure can be used to determine the acuity. Other facilities included in the Medmont AT-20 system is binocular vision test, worth four dot test, Duochrome test, astigmatic fan and fixation targets for children.

Mentor B VAT II Chart

It is a commercially available computer-based video acuity system used to measure contrast sensitivity, visual acuity and grating acuity. Here optotypes are letters and visual acuity is tested at nine contrast levels.

Factors influencing contrast sensitivity

- *Ophthalmic conditions:* Contrast sensitivity can be impaired in ophthalmic conditions like glaucoma, crystalline lens changes in incipient cataract, ocular hypertension, amblyopia, age-related macular degeneration, retrobulbar optic neuritis, dry eye, diabetic retinopathy, etc.
- *Refractive errors:* Like myopia, glare can affect contrast sensitivity in higher frequencies.
- *Age:* With advancement of age there is decrease in contrast sensitivity, most likely due to change in spherical aberration of lens.
- *Systemic conditions:* Contrast sensitivity can also reduce in various neurological conditions like multiple sclerosis, Parkinson's disease, schizophrenia, pituitary adenoma, and cerebral lesions.
- *Drugs:* Contrast sensitivity may reduce side effect of some drugs, e.g. ibuprofen, vigabatrin, etc.

Note: Various available treatment modalities like optical, medical, surgical, or visual rehabilitation can produce reasonable improvement in selected contrast sensitivity deficits. Many a times mere accurate diagnosis of poor vision happening due to low contrast sensitivity may give satisfaction to a large number of low vision patients.

COLOR SENSE

Introduction

The ability of an individual to differentiate between various colors emitted by light of different wavelengths is referred as color sense. Although color vision is a complex process but for understanding purpose various salient features of color vision are

- The color appreciation in human eyes is entirely a function of photoreceptor, i.e. cones and as we discussed before that cones are related with daylight vision, so color vision can happen only in photopic conditions, i.e. color vision characterize the photopic vision.
- Color vision depends on the wavelength composition of light entering the eye, brightness (illumination/luminosity or light intensity) and saturation or calorimetric purity (i.e. ratio of mixing with white light).
- In the presence of moderate or high intensity illumination (where retina is fully adopted to light) an individual can appreciate colors, whereas in presence of very low intensity of illumination (where eyes are dark-adapted) person will not appreciate colors; rather he/she will see all objects as grey having some mild differentiation in their brightness. This phenomenon of shifting from color appreciation to grey appreciation in low illuminating condition is called *Purkinje shift phenomenon*.
- Color sensation is subjective in nature and initially all the individuals need to learn names of different color sensations. Thus, subsequently when the same sensation which individuals had learnt initially is felt by them then, they can name the color by their past experience.
- In retina of eye different types of cones are present. In these different cones there are three types of pigments, which preferentially absorb wavelengths of light in visible spectrum corresponding to three colors— red, green and blue. Hence, normal color vision is considered as trichromatic.

- Suppose these three colors or any three colors which are sufficiently far apart in spectrum of visible light are chosen, them all other colors including white can be made by mixing them in an appropriate proportion.
- For any given color there is always a complimentary color and when these two colors are mixed in appropriate proportions they will form white color.
- Color perception is dependent on the color of surrounding background. For example, if a green color object is placed in green illuminated background, then person will see the object as white. This green object will be appreciated as green if the background is illuminated with red or blue color.
- Three characteristics of color are: Hue, intensity and saturation. These attributes decide the nature of color appreciated by the person.
- Normally an individual can see all colors of visible light spectrum, i.e. violet to red. Wavelengths shorter than violet, i.e. ultraviolet or longer than red, i.e. infra red are not visible to an individual. However, some blue cones are sensitive to even ultraviolet range of wavelength, so an individual should have been able to see the UV light but normal crystalline lens has a property to block all UV wavelengths. Hence, persons undergone cataract surgery are able to see the UV rays, if UV protected IOLs are not implanted.

Theories of Color Vision

The two most popular theories of color vision are

- Young-Helmholtz theory (trichromatic or trireceptor theory)
- Hering theory (opponent process theory)

Trichromatic Theory

Originally, Young proposed the theory of trichromacy to explain the process of color vision. In subsequent years, Helmholtz did some modifications to explain various other factors of color vision. Although, the original form of this theory was unable to give an adequate explanation of all the phenomena associated with appreciation of color either by normal individuals or by individuals having color defects but none denied the existence of trichromatic stage in color visual process.

Young-Helmholtz theory presumes the presence of three types of color receptors however, each receptors is apparently responding to all wavelengths of light and they have various levels of spectral sensitivities for different light wavelengths. One receptor has more sensitivity for long wavelengths (red color), second for medium wavelengths (green color) and third for short wavelengths (blue color). All other colors are believed to be perceived by combinations of these three colors in various proportions. For example, perception of yellow color is a process which simultaneously stimulates red and green receptors and integrates these receptors with visual neural pathways and visual cortex.

The trichromatic theory was able to explain the various laws of color mixing but it was unable to explain some basic phenomena associated with color vision. For example, theory was not able to explain the phenomenon of color defect in dichromate patients (having confusion in identification of red and green color although these patients are able to see a mixture of these two colors, i.e. yellow color). This theory also had a difficulty in explaining the phenomenon of complementary color after-images.

Ewald Hering further expanded the process of color vision and put a hypothetical existence of three oppositional color pigment pairs. Trichromatic signals received by cones receptors are not combined at pigment level but are passed to the subsequent neural stages and reveal opponent pairs of color processing

- Spectrally opponent processes, which consist of pairs of red versus green and yellow versus blue.
- Spectrally non-opponent process, which consists of a pair of black versus white.

Opponent Process Theory

Hering hypothesis has been subsequently improvised by Hurvich and Jameson and is popularly known as opponent process theory. This theory is based on an assumption that there are three sets of receptor systems, viz red-green, blue-yellow and black-white. Each of these receptors is assumed to be working as antagonistic pair among themselves. It means that stimulation of one opponent pair will produce an excitation of one receptor system and will also produce an inhibitory effect on other receptor system; hence red light will stimulate the red receptors and also will simultaneously inhibit the green receptor.

Note: Opponent theory was successful in explaining nearly all phenomena of color vision and includes even color-contrast and color-blindness data which were difficult to be explained by trichromatic theory.

Both these theories helped enormously in understanding about the system governing color vision in human eye. The initial trichromatic theory works at the photoreceptor level and then these visual signals get recorded into the opponent process form; which is a higher level of neural system of color vision processing.

Another theoretical representation was proposed by Edwin Land to explain mechanism of color vision. His hypothesis explained the presence of three separate visual systems responding primarily to different wavelengths of light, are called *retinexes*. One retinex each among these three retinexes shows maximum response to long wavelength (red), middle wavelength (green) and short wavelength (blue) of light, respectively. Each of these visual systems is represented as an analogue, where black and white picture of an object is taken via a particular color filter.

Color Vision Charts

Majority of people think that color vision test means the test done by using dotted pictures or by chart named Ishihara.

Although in reality there are several other tests to detect the color defects. Ishihara test is used since long time and most of the time it is an incompatible test, however, till date it is the most commonly used test worldwide.

History: During 17th century, Turberville noticed that some individuals name the colors differently as compared to others and probably this was the first observation related to color blindness tests. Nearly hundred years later scientist John Dalton described the color vision in detail and he also examined several persons by using colored ribbons where color of ribbons has to be named by persons. During this era most of the color vision deficiency was simply explained by subjective means.

In the year 1837, August Seebeck tried various advanced technique to explain the color vision defects. He gave people some sample color and asked them to match these colors from the most closely related color in the set of more than 300 colored papers. This test removed the problem related to naming of color, which vary significantly in between persons. This test of Seebeck to identify color blindness resulted in identification of condition like red–green color deficiency.

In the year 1877, Holmgren developed similar type of test by using skeins of wool having various colors. This Holmgren wool test gained popularity worldwide, hence for more than hundred years it remained commercially available.

Around the same era these two developments took place which made the way for modern methods of testing of color defects.

- John William Strutt Rayleigh invented a test based on perfect matching of various colors. This test is popularly known as Rayleigh match which is the principle behind the development of instruments like anomaloscopes. This test also led to the discovery of conditions such as dichromatism and anomalous trichromatism.
- Dr J Stilling published his famous pseudoisochromatic plates first time to the world for testing color deficiencies. These plates were the antecessor of most popular Ishihara plates.

Color vision and color defects can be measured by methods shown in Table 10.5.

Pseudoisochromatic Plates

These plates are most widely and popular screening test used to assess the color vision. This test is also known as Ishihara plates test after the name of Dr Shinobu Ishihara who designed this plate test.

Principle used in the formation of these plates is co-punctual points. Color blind person is unable to distinguish colors along the line of confusion, so in these plates different patterns are used along the confusion lines, which are made of different colored dots or co-punctual points. Suppose if a person is color blind then he/she will be unable to identify the colored dots which are representing a pattern across these confusion lines.

Table 10.5: Color vision tests			
Pseudoisochromatic plates	Arrangement tests	Lantern tests	Anomaloscope
• Ishihara plates • HRR plates	• Farnsworth D-15 tests • Lanthony desaturated D-15 test • Farnsworth Munsell 100 hue test	• Holmes Wright lantern • Farnsworth lantern • Giles-Archer lantern • Edridge-Green lantern • Williams lantern	• Nagel anomaloscope • Neitz anomaloscope, • Heidelberg Multi Color (HMC) anomaloscope • Pickford-Nicolson anomaloscope.

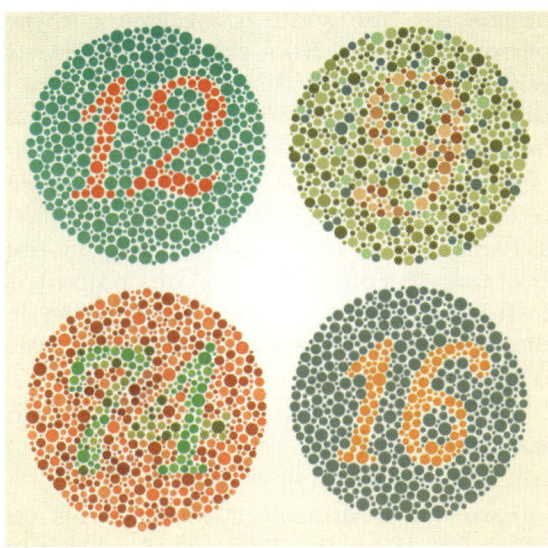

Fig. 10.41: Patterns of Ishihara plates

- *Hidden digit design:* These plates have hidden designs which can be seen only by people having color vision defects. Normal individuals are unable to see any designs in these plates.
- *Classification design:* These plates are specially designed to identify color blind persons. These plates have vanishing design on either side of plate, which helps in differentiation of person having red green color defects. One side of plate is used to identify red color defects and the other side for green color defects.

Standard version of these most popular Ishihara plates contain a set of 38 plates; although shorter versions containing 24 plates and 14 plates are also available (Fig. 10.42). These Ishihara plates can only identify red-green color deficiencies. Persons suffering from Tritan defects (blue color deficiency) cannot be identified by Ishihara test plates.

In the year 1954, other types of plates were produced which can be used to classify all three color deficiencies; they are called 24 HRR plates introduced by Hardy, Rand and Ritter (Fig. 10.43). There are several more of such pseudoisochromatic plate tests but none of them became popular and are not widely used.

Recently a few electronic color vision test equipment are also available which include certain types of pseudoisochromatic plates. Although these electronic devices can test color vision rapidly, however, none of these equipment provide very accurate and reliable results.

Various mathematical numerical, english letters, curved lines or any other pattern can be made invisible inside these dots patterns.

Four different types of plate designs are present in booklet as (Fig. 10.41)

- *Vanishing design:* These plates have designs which are seen only by the persons having good color vision. People with color vision defects are unable to see any design in these plates.
- *Transformation design:* Different types of design are seen by persons having color vision defects as compared to normal individuals.

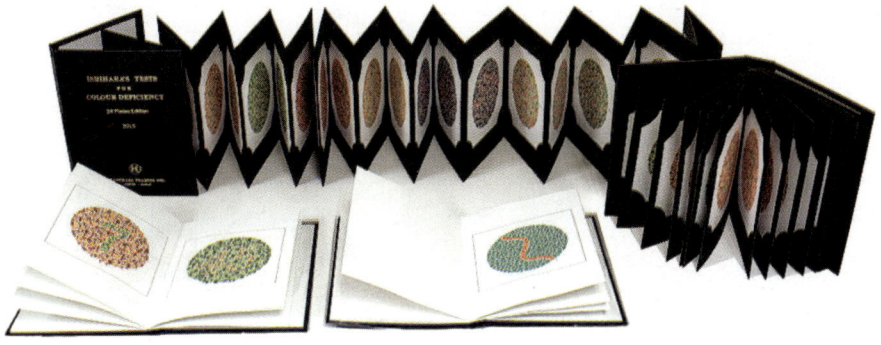

Fig. 10.42: Ishihara plates (*courtesy:* Bernell Corporation)

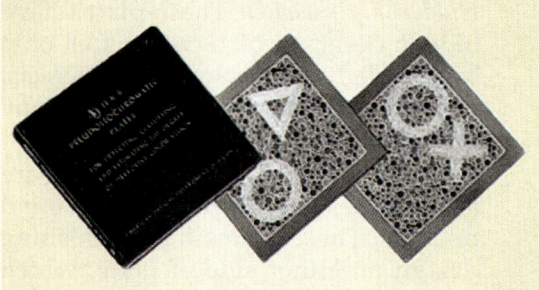

Fig. 10.43: Hardy, Rand and Ritter plates for color vision test

Arrangement Tests

Similar to pseudoisochromatic plate test the principle used in identification of color defect by arrangement test is also based on co-punctual points, however, as compared to pseudoisochromatic plates test, an arrangement test is dynamic in nature because here observer has to arrange a set of color discs or plates in order. Each of these test series contain a starting pilot plate having various colors and predefined number of color discs or plates. Patient is instructed to arrange the color discs or plates in the correct sequence as present in the pilot plate. Usually color of these discs is selected close to white color because majority of people having color vision defects are unable to differentiate colors along certain

lines across the white point. Hence, these persons suffering from color vision defects will arrange these discs completely in a different manner as compared to a normal individual.

In the year 1940 most popular arrangement test was introduced by Farnsworth and named as Farnsworth D-15 arrangement test. This test contains 15 colored plates and patient is instructed to arrange these colored plates in the correct sequence as compared to pilot plate (Fig. 10.44).

Lanthony desaturated D-15 test is similar kind of test and is helpful in identification of color blindness in milder cases.

Farnsworth-Munsell 100 hue test. This test comprises 100 plates arranged in a batch of 20 plates (Fig. 10.45). Patients need to arrange these plates in order as in D-15 arrangement test; results are very encouraging and are comparable to other arrangement tests.

Lanterns Tests

In Lantern test, colored signal lights are presented to observer for identification. These tests were primarily used as occupational or vocational tests especially for persons employed in railways, airlines, or in transport workers to identify their color recognition

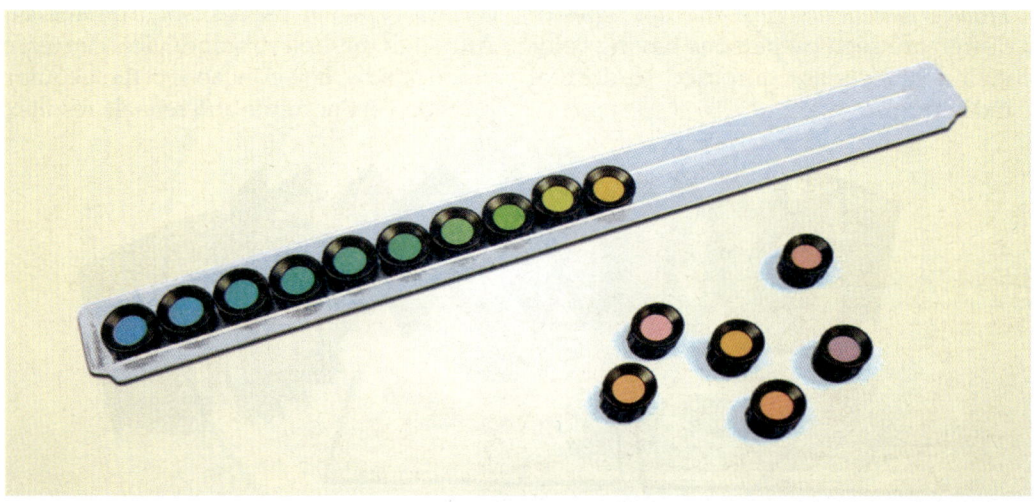

Fig. 10.44: Farnsworth D-15 arrangement tests for color vision (*courtesy:* Bernell Corporation)

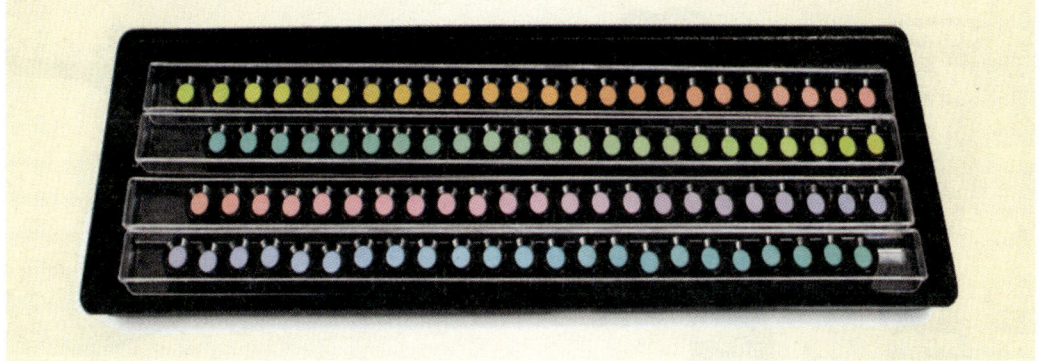

Fig. 10.45: Farnsworth-Munsell 100 hue test (*courtesy:* Bernell Corporation)

ability which helps them to identify and navigate signals. Lanterns tests were useful in detecting the ability of person regarding identification of various colors directly, hence practically it is a useful tool. However, these tests were unable to detect the type and severity of color deficiency, hence had limited value to classify type of color deficiency. In Lantern test the color signals are presented to observer either as single color or in pair and observer asked to identify and tell the name of color.

Various types of lanterns used to assess the color vision are

- **Holmes-Wright lanterns:** These lanterns have five lights (two green, two red and one white) which are arranged either vertically or horizontally. Patient needs to identify the color of lights when these lights are shown to him/her in pairs of low and high brightness (Fig. 10.46).
- **Farnsworth lantern:** These lanterns are specially designed to pass the people having milder form of color deficiency. Results of this test are comparable to Holmes-Wright lantern, although in severe deficiencies there are some differences in results (Fig. 10.47).

Various other types of lanterns were also popular in past, however, these lanterns were gradually replaced by newer techniques of color vision estimation. A few examples are shown in Fig. 10.48.

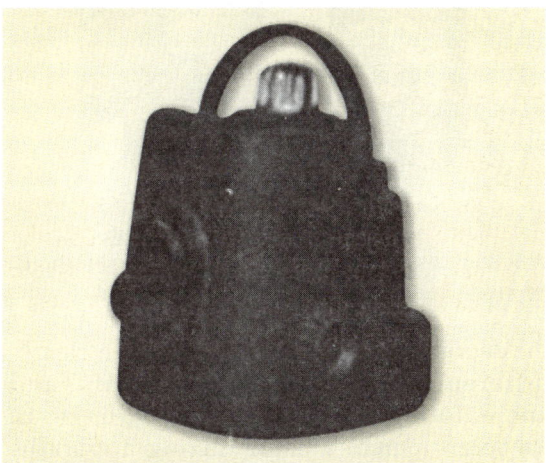

Fig. 10.46: Holmes-Wright lantern

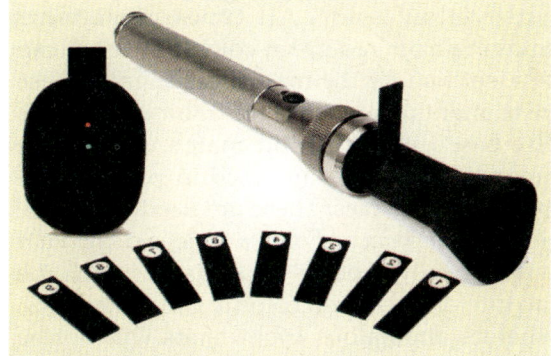

Fig. 10.47: Farnsworth lantern

Anomaloscope

These instruments are based on principle of either Rayleigh match or Moreland match system. Anomaloscope can be used to estimate

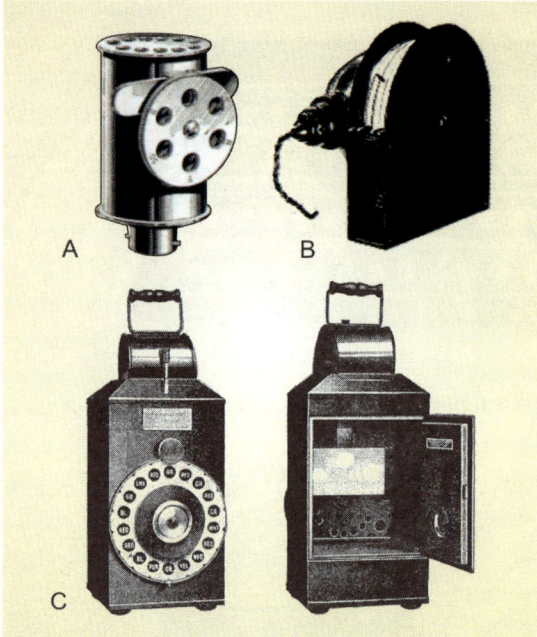

Fig. 10.48: Various lanterns used in past for color vision assessments. A. Giles-Archer lantern; B. Edridge-Green lantern; C. Williams lantern

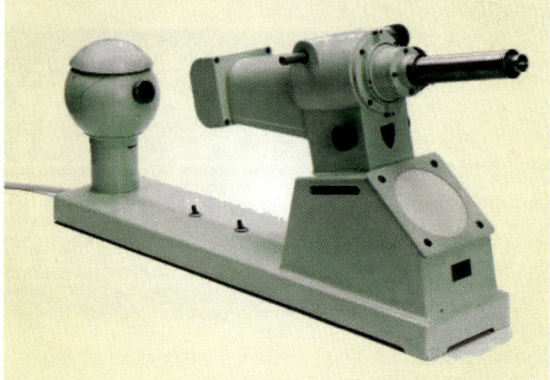

Fig. 10.49: Nagel anomaloscope

the degree of color blindness and also clearly differentiate between dichromats and anomalous trichromats individuals. In Rayleigh match, a color mixing apparatus consists of narrow spectral bands of red and green color and observer has to match these with yellow color. All types of patients suffering from red green color deficiency can be identified by the matching range of these instruments. A number of anomaloscope is also based on Moreland match where blue green light sources are used in place of red green light sources. These are used to test the tritan color defects. For example, a dichromat is specifically capable to precisely match the mixture of red–green color in different ratios, whereas anomalous trichromats will not be able to recognize normal color match. Difference in the distance of color match among them will indicate the severity of color deficiency. On contrary, to match the colors a person having protan type deficiency will utilize more red color and a person with

deutan type deficiency will utilize more green color. The main disadvantage with anomalscope is that it is expensive instrument and difficult to use. Examiner must be enough skilled and trained to do test with anomalscope.

In the year 1907, an eminent scientist Nagel invented an anomaloscope which is popularly called Nagel's anomaloscope (Fig. 10.49). This instrument is considered as the best instrument to detect color deficiency till date although it is not manufactured nowadays.

Some other types of widely used anomaloscope are

- Neitz anomaloscope
- Heidelberg Multi Color (HMC) anomaloscope
- Pickford-Nicolson anomaloscope

Color Blindness

Color blindness is also called achromatopsia and may be

- Congenital
- Acquired

Congenital Color Blindness

This is an inherited condition and transmitted as X-linked recessive disorder, females are usually unaffected and act as carrier. Color blindness is probably due to the absence of one or more photo pigments like red, green, etc. which are normally found in the foveal cones.

Congenital color blindness may present as
- Total blindness
- Partial blindness.

Total color blindness is very rare and generally it is associated with nystagmus and/or central scotoma. Probably a central defect is responsible for causing the total color blindness. Patient suffering from total color blindness sees all colors as grey color having different levels of brightness. The entire light spectrum appears as a grey band, similar to those patients' having normal scotopic spectrum.

Partial color blindness is more common condition than total color blindness and affects about 3–4% of male population (common) and 0.4% female population (rare). Milder cases suffering from partial color blindness are more common in males. Clinically, majority of patients remain asymptomatic, because they compensate for their color defect by improving their attention for shade and texture of object and combine it with their experience. It is difficult to diagnose partial color defects, unless and until several special color vision tests are performed to detect it.

Usually most of these patients have good visual acuity but has confusion in identification of red and green color, hence this defect of color identification is a serious problem in certain occupations like rail engine drivers or ship sailors. These red–green color defective cases are grouped as protanopes and deuteranopes. Patients suffering from red color defects or protanopes have defective sensation for red wavelength range of light spectrum; red color appears much less brighter than that seen by a normal individual. In deuteranopes or green color defective patients, the sensation for green wavelength range of light spectrum is defective. These groups have a dichromatic vision; means they see only two out of three basic color with maximum brightness. Although the color defects in both these groups may not be complete, therefore, these cases are also called protanomalous and deuteranomalous for red color defect and green color defect, respectively.

Note: Theoretically there might be few other cases having color blindness due to defective or absence of blue sensation, i.e. tritanopes, although these cases are very rare.

Acquired Color Blindness

It can be presented as partial or as complete color defect. Partial defect is seen in cases having relative scotoma while complete color defect is associated with disease of the optic nerve. Usually most of diseases that affect retina and choroid influence the color perception, mainly in the blue wavelength range of light spectrum. Although, a slight diminution in perception of rays with blue wavelength is normal because of an increased physical absorption of blue light. An increase of amber pigmentation in the nucleus of crystalline lens causes increase physical absorption of blue range wavelengths and this condition is commonly called blue blindness.

POTENTIAL VISION

Introduction

Potential vision means a preoperative assessment of visual outcome in cases of media opacity. In patients having a poor visual acuity due to cataract, various tests are employed to know the potential visual outcome after the removal of the cataractous lens. Before cataract surgery, it is important to know the potential vision to rule out the fact that the cause of obvious diminished vision is either purely cataractous lens or any other retinal pathology is also contributing in diminution of vision.

Various subjective and objective methods are used for assessment of potential vision in a patient having media opacity, although all of them have some limitations but still are very useful to predict the potential visual outcome after surgery. These methods are summarized in Table 10.6.

Subjective Methods of Measurement

Basic clinical tests were the earliest attempts to investigate retinal/neural function behind

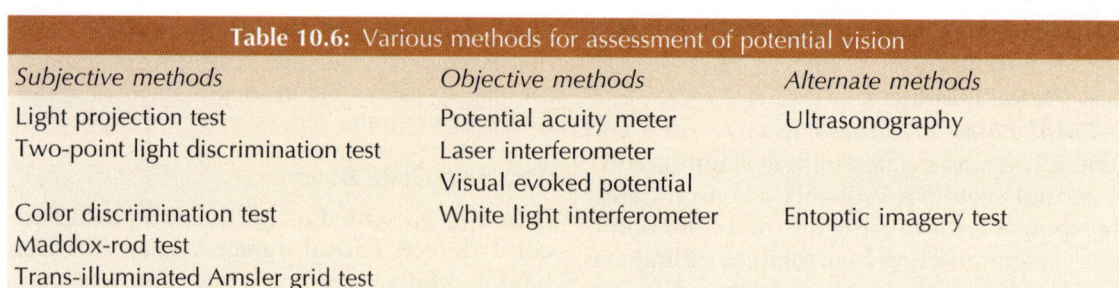

Table 10.6: Various methods for assessment of potential vision

Subjective methods	Objective methods	Alternate methods
Light projection test	Potential acuity meter	Ultrasonography
Two-point light discrimination test	Laser interferometer	
	Visual evoked potential	
Color discrimination test	White light interferometer	Entoptic imagery test
Maddox-rod test		
Trans-illuminated Amsler grid test		

ocular media opacities. Various subjective tests done to assess the potential vision are

- Light projection test
- Two-point light discrimination test
- Color discrimination test
- Maddox rod test
- Trans-illuminated Amsler grid test

These tests are simple and can be performed quickly; but all of them have several limitations and moderate predictive value. However, these tests are very useful in remote locations, where newer modern instruments are unavailable.

Light Projection Test

If surgical removal of cataractous lens has been decided for visual improvement in an elderly patient, then before planning the surgery, it is necessary to check the presence of light perception to execute the cataract surgery. A gross and accurate assessment of retinal function can be done by simply evaluating the presence of light perception in the patient eye. This can be tested by confirming the ability of patient to perceive the projected light. Directional quality of projected light can get diffuse by opaque media but still light perception test gives a practical clue whether gross retinal and/or optic nerve pathologies like giant retinal detachment or advanced visual field defects are present or not. Retina is bleached for nearly 20–30 seconds by using an indirect ophthalmoscope, if patient is unable to perceive the light it implies a significant abnormal retinal pathology.

Two-Point Light Discrimination Test

Another simple and useful clinical method to assess potential vision and retinal integrity is the 'two-point discrimination' test. Two bright pointed light sources of 2 mm size are kept 2 inches away from each other and are shown to patient from 2 feet distance, keeping one eye closed. If patient is able to identify two distinct lights correctly, then grossly his/her retinal function is presumed to be intact. However, this method is unable to give any significant idea regarding macular function of patient, so it is not widely used in clinical practice.

Color Discrimination Test

Similar to light discrimination test general retinal integrity can be assessed by testing the gross perception of color. However, this test also gives some information about the macular function. This test can easily be performed with the help of slit lamp in clinic. Patient is instructed to discriminate the color (cobalt blue or red- free green filters) of lights shown to him/her by slit lamp.

Maddox Rod Test

A clinically reliable and simple method to assess macular function is Maddox rod test. A Maddox rod can be held in front of the eye under examination or can be placed in the trial frame. With help of occluder one eye of the patient is occluded and with fellow eye the patient is instructed to fixate on a bright light source held by examiner at one and a half feet distance as shown in Fig. 10.50.

If the patient sees a continuous red line (Fig. 10.50A) it means that the macular integrity is present. If, patient sees a broken red line (Fig. 10.50B) it means that a macular lesion is present. To identify retinal detachment or glaucomatous visual field defects, the

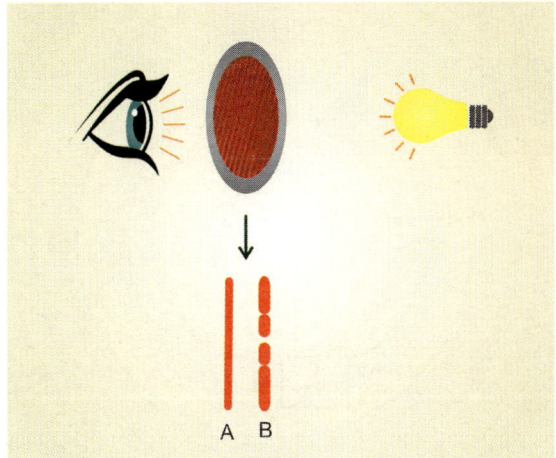

Fig. 10.50: Macular function test using Maddox rod

Maddox rods are placed in various meridians and test is repeated. This test also helps in the evaluation of patient's color sensitivity. Sometimes it becomes difficult to perform this test due to presence of dense media opacities.

Trans-illuminated Amsler Grid

In the year 1978 Miller, Lanberts and Perry depicted a modified form of the standard Amsler test. Instead of standard Amsler grid, a trans-illuminated grid is used to test the potential vision in patients having media opacities. Trans-illuminated Amsler grid is similar in size as standard Amsler grid but it has 1 mm holes at every intersection of horizontal and vertical grid lines with a 4 mm fixation hole at its centre. This grid is mounted on an illuminated light box fitted with 15 W neon tubes.

Interpretation: Patients having media opacities (e.g. cataract) are unable to see the lines on the standard Amsler grids, however, if they can perceive all the lines joining the retro-illuminated holes, then the person has normal macular function. Suppose the patient sees distortion of illuminated lines (metamorphopsia) or dark area (scotoma), it implies an abnormal macular function. However, a significant disadvantage of this test is that majority of patients having dense media opacities are unable to see the grid.

Objective Methods of Measurement

Commercially available instruments to predict the post-operative visual outcome or to determine the potential vision are mainly of two types

- Potential acuity meter (PAM)
- Interferometer

Guyton-Minkowski PAM is an instrument which projects a miniature Snellen's chart on the retina of patient via a pinhole. This Snellen's chart is seen through the clear areas in between the opaque crystalline lens and is projected over the macular region.

Lotmar and Rodenstock interferometers are laser-based instruments and utilizes two coherent beam of helium-neon laser which generates interference patterns and are projected on patient's retina through pupil. Width of the interference fringes corresponds to the visual acuity of the patient.

White light interferometers are similar to laser interferometers but they use polychromatic white incandescent light source instead of laser beam, which produces a large depth of field grating image in the eye.

Potential Acuity Meter

In the year 1980, Guyton and Minkowski designed this potential acuity meter (PAM) which can be mounted on slit lamp. This device projects a miniature form of Snellen's visual acuity chart via a pinhole of 0.15 mm diameter, using coherent white light through the clear areas present in opaque crystalline lens on patient's retina (Fig. 10.51A).

Optics of PAM device: As shown in Fig. 10.51B, a white coherent light from a point source passes through an aperture and focuses on Snellen's chart via a prism. These images are focused on patient's retina via a condensing lens and a focusing prism. Knob of PAM helps in rapid focusing of Snellen's optotypes by adjusting the lens (+12 D power) and focusing prism. These black optotypes on a white chart can estimate a visual acuity ranging from 20/20 to 20/400.

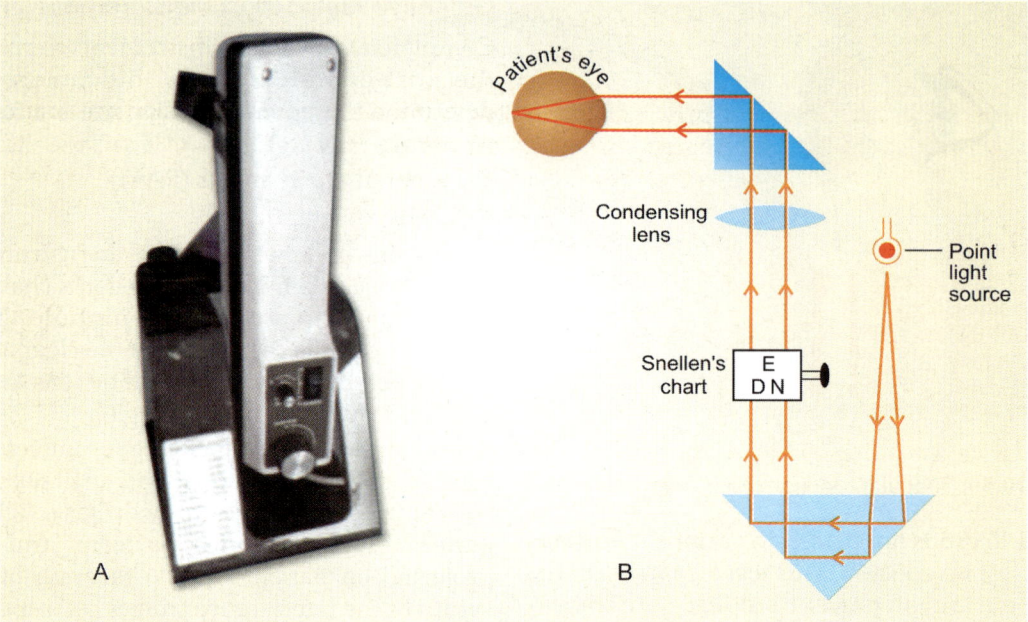

Fig. 10.51A and B: A. PAM device; B. Optics of potential acuity meter (*see* text)

Test procedure

- Test should be done in dimly lighted room and eyes of patient should not be exposed to bright lights before test.
- Dilate the pupil by mydriatics for better and accurate testing.
- Full optical correction is worn by patient or can be fitted in instrument with the help of trial lenses.
- Light beam is now projected via clear area of cataractous lens (window) and patient is instructed to identify the letters on the Snellen's chart.
- Letters on chart will appear and disappear with the movement of patient's eye or while he/she spell the letters.
- Patient may see some disturbing entoptic images in between letters but slowly he/she will adjust to it.
- Patient is instructed to read the lines of Snellen's chart until he/she is not able to read other smaller legible lines.
- Macular function is considered normal if patient is able to read an entire line correctly from the Snellen's chart (Fig. 10.52).

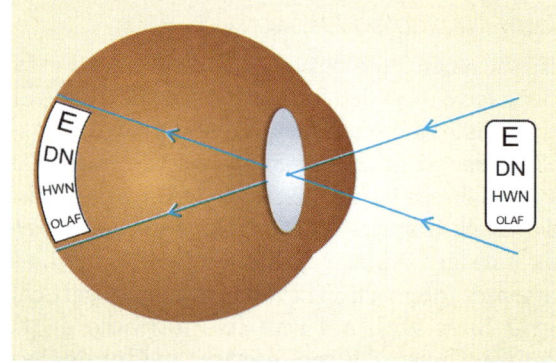

Fig. 10.52: Retinal image of chart in potential acuity meter (*see* text)

- Test chart should be adjusted several times before confirming the poor macular function.

Interferometry: Interferometry is a method to predict the potential vision in eyes having mild to moderate media opacities either due to cataract or corneal pathology. Devices designed on the principle of interferometry are called interferometers.

Principle: As we discussed in previous chapter these instruments are designed on the

Clinical Inference

- In mild to moderate degree cataracts having visual acuity 20/200 or better; post operative visual acuity can be correctly predicted by the PAM in range within 3 Snellen's line in 100% cases and within 2 Snellen's line in 90% cases.
- In cases having cystoid macular edema, recent postoperative reattached retina, serous detachments of neurosensory retina, macular hole or cyst, very dense cataract, advance glaucoma, geographical atrophy of macula or dense opacities, PAM can falsely predict an improved or poor visual outcome. However, amblyopia does not interfere in accurate prediction by PAM, unlike laser interferometer.

Note: In cases having very dense sub capsular or diffuse cortical cataract it is difficult to find a clear window for projection of light beam; means least information is achieved in cases where we need it the most.

property of interference of light. DG Green and co-workers thought of projecting a resolution target directly on the retina after bypassing the media opacities for the assessment of visual acuity. A set of light interference fringes having alternate light and dark bands were considered ideal.

As shown in Fig. 10.53 a fringe pattern is produced on the retina by interference of light waves generated from two coherent light sources, less than 0.1 mm in diameter. These

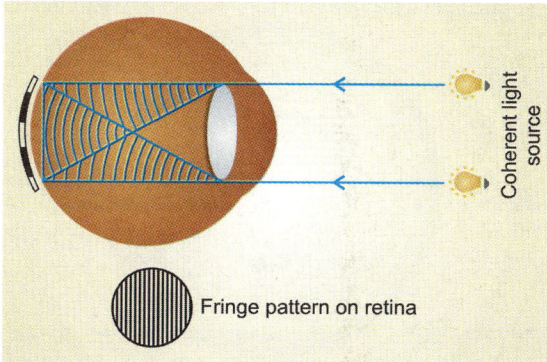

Fig. 10.53: Principle of interferometry (fringe pattern on retina)

are not the usual images, hence are not affected by optical defects, focus defects, mild to moderate media opacities or imperfect refracting ocular system. Observer can see these fringes purely on the ability of his/her retina to conduct signals from photoreceptors to visual cortex. Hence, these interference fringes become an important tool in distinguishing media opacity from retinal and/or neurological factors.

Commercially two types of interferometers are available: Laser interferometer and white light interferometer.

Laser Interferometer

These devices use laser beam to produce interference fringe patterns. These devices can be attached with slit lamp for examination purposes.

Instrument design: Light source used for laser is Helium-Neon, which produces a laser of 632.8 nm wavelength. This laser beam is splitted into two beams having the same coherent property of laser. Each splitted beam of laser is pulsed with the help of an acousto-optic modulator; which produces 1 msec duration rectangular pulses with frequency of 400 Hz. When these pulses were alternated there was no overlap and hence no interference was possible. However, when pulses arrived simultaneously, the two beams overlapped and interference occurred. This overlapping can be controlled by computer and finer fringe pattern can be produced.

Optics of laser interferometer: Laser interferometer can be attached to a slit lamp for examination purpose. Laser is produced and directed towards the slit lamp mirror via rotating glass plates and a rotating prism which allows the axis of gratings to be changed as per requirement (Fig. 10.54).

Laser devices use low frequency patterns by using two periodic waves, which produce interference fringes by moving in-phase and out-of-phase with each other. These waves

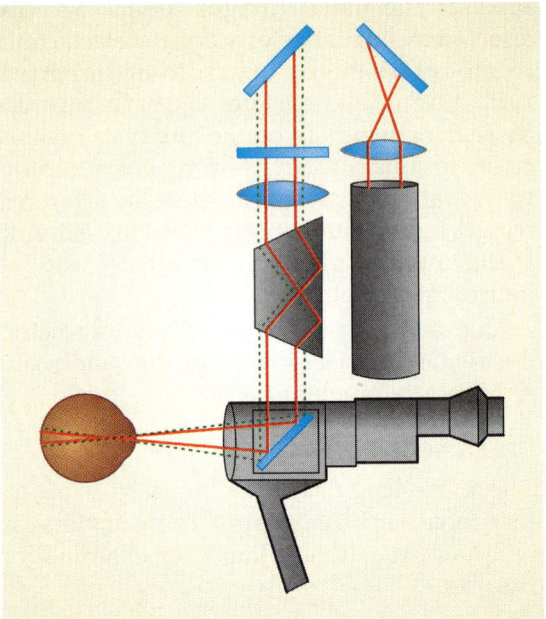

Fig. 10.54: Optics of LASER interferometry (*see* text)

pass through the glass plates and rotating prisms to produce fringe pattern on patient's retina via mirror of slit lamp. When both these waves are in phase with each other, they are seen as white bar and are called maxima. On contrary, when out of phase then are seen as dark bar and are called minima. The spatial frequency (space between black and white bars) of inter-ference pattern can be adjusted by changing the spacing between two beams. Separation between two pin-point beams (i.e. grating angle) decides the fringe pattern (i.e. fringe pitch), increase in grating angle will produce finer interference pattern or fringe pitch which requires a greater macular resolution to identify it.

The grating angle is constantly adjusted till patient is unable to identify the fringe pattern. The last perceived grating value is recorded in decimal system present on the instrument and an equivalent in Snellen's visual acuity can be done by conversion table. Snellen's equivalent to 6/6 corresponds to a 33 maxima/ degree of visual angle.

Electromagnetic wave amplitude decides the production of fringe pitch not the light intensity, hence only 20% transmission of each laser beam is required for reading. Interference fringe field size varies from 1.5 to 8 degrees and test is independent of presence of refractive error.

Test procedure

* Patient education is most important before performing the interferometry procedure. Various possible fringe patterns are demonstrated to patient by showing pattern display cards (Fig. 10.55A). Patient should also be explained about partial pattern possibilities due to scotoma in these fringe patterns as shown in Fig. 10.55B. If scotoma are seen, then patient is advised to ignore them and look only at the fringe pattern direction and orientation.
* Once patient has been explained about patterns, then laser interferometer is mounted on slit lamp and patient is asked to sit in front of the slit lamp by putting his/ her chin on chin rest and forehead against the forehead strip.
* For better and accurate examination patient's pupil is widely dilated by mydriatics and examination room should be dark.
* Highest transparency area of patient's crystalline lens is identified by using retroillumination method and laser beam is targeted in this area of lens.
* Scan the pupil until patient starts identifying the fringe patterns, now an entrance

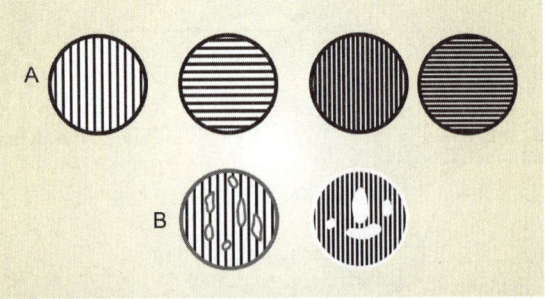

Fig. 10.55: Various fringe pattern seen during interferometry. A. Normal patterns; B. Pattern with scotoma

pupillary area of 1.5 mm is made by adjusting the knob on instrument.

- Testing is continued by increasing fringe pitch at a step of 0.1 using another knob on instrument. Patient is asked about the orientation (i.e. vertical, horizontal or oblique) of fringe pattern at every interval of increasing steps.
- By adjusting another knob on instrument orientation of fringe can be changed at every increasing steps and patient needs to identify them.
- Initially, large grating should be used and then grating should be reduced gradually until the patient is not able to detect their correct direction.
- Four consecutive correct patterns identification by patient is needed to finalize the acuity reading; a slower patient response indicates an end point of test.
- End point fringe pitch reading is recorded from the markings on one of the knobs on instrument in decimals and is converted to Snellen's acuity with help of a conversion table supplied with instrument.
- In dense media opacity cases, voltage of instrument can be increased from 5 to 7.5 volts for a convenient examination.

Note: Prolonged exposure of high intensity light like indirect ophthalmoscopic examination should be avoided prior conduction of interferometry test.

Clinical Inference

In normal individuals
- Normal individuals having no media opacities will see a circular fringe pitch having alternate light and dark bands as shown in display cards.
- With breathe of an individual, these patterns move because laser spots move, disordered pattern gets replaced by new ordered patterns when settled.

In mild to moderate media opacity cases
- Patients having mild to moderate media opacities will initially report that they are seeing only disordered, moving array of shooting stars or jumbled up moving worms, (an effect on interference fringe produced by media opacities).

- Spatial structure of these moving arrays will give an idea about the transparent areas in crystalline lens, i.e. in relatively clear areas there will be an increase in the size of shooting stars or jumbling worms. Perfect clear area is the one, where star increases in size to cover this entire clear area.
- Once this clear area is identified now patient is advised to look inside this area to identify the fringe direction and orientation, while ignoring the other surrounding area.
- Finest strip pattern identified by the patient decides the end point and acuity is recorded as discussed above.
- Sometimes patient is able to identify the strips but is unable to identify their pattern and orientation correctly; then examiner should encourage the patient to pursue further for identification of the fringe pattern.

In dense media opacities cases
- Patients are unable to see the fringe pattern because the opacities are very dense and do not allow even laser beams to penetrate them.
- In these cases any amount of perseverance is not going to help and potential vision cannot be assessed, where it is the most important to know the status of potential vision of patient.

False positive results may be seen in following cases:
- Patients of cystoid macular edema having healthy photoreceptors.
- Patients with viable tilted retinal receptors usually give poor Snellen's visual acuity results, but can give normal reading in laser interferometry test.
- Patients having macular hole or cyst, cystoid macular edema and geographical macular atrophy with viable para foveal tissue stimulation can give readings in laser interferometry test.

False negative results may be seen in following cases:
- Dense cataract
- Dense vitreous hemorrhage
- Insufficient pupillary dilatation

White Light Interferometer

White light interferometers use polychromatic white light produced by an incandescent bulb as source of light beam instead of a laser beam.

Working optics and test procedure of these white light interferometers is similar to laser interferometers, however, contrast of gratings may be reduced by chromatic aberrations in white light interferometers against that of laser interferometers (Fig. 10.56).

Factors affecting accuracy of test results: Many factors can influence the outcome of vision when tested by either PAM or interferometer. Hence, it is important to consider these factors during preoperative counseling of patient, while explaining the predicted visual outcome.

Various factors affecting test results are as follows:

- *Density of cataract:* Both PAM and interferometers predict visual outcome in mild to moderate type cataracts (according to lens opacity classification system II). In severe cataracts the accuracy of potential vision assessment by these tests is poor.

- *Type of cataract:* Both PAM and interferometer underestimate the visual outcome in cases of dense posterior capsular opacification as compared to cortical cataract or diffuse nuclear cataract because posterior sub-capsular cataract is dense and centrally located,

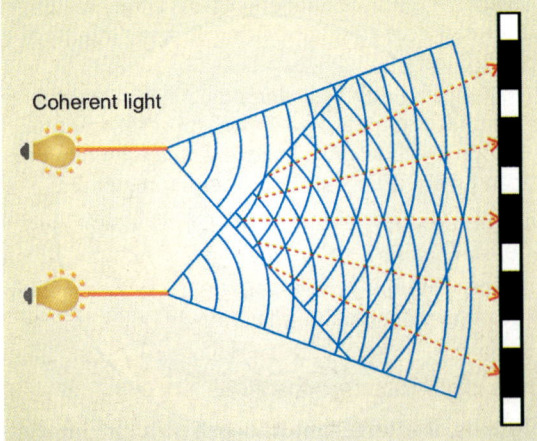

Fig. 10.56: White light interferometers showing fringe pattern

whereas cortical cataracts are peripherally located and nuclear cataracts are diffuse in nature.

- *Preoperative poor visual acuity:* In patients having preoperative VA lower than 6/60; both PAM and interferometers are less effective in predicting visual outcome postoperatively.

- *Ocular diseases:* Interferometers overestimates the visual outcome as compared to PAM in patients having poor retinal functions due to conditions like macular degenerations, retinal degenerations and retinitis pigmentosa.

Alternate Methods

When the abovementioned tests have a questionable response or it is impossible to perform any test, other alternate methods can be employed to assess the visual outcome in media opacities such as

- Ultrasonography
- Visual evoked potential
- Entoptic imagery test

Ultrasonography

Evaluation of ocular structures can be done using ultrasonography, i.e. B-scan or A-scan. Brightness scan or B-scan gives a gross but accurate assessment of ocular anatomical status and also rules out pathological conditions like vitreous hemorrhage, retinal detachment, and optic disc anomalies. When B scan is unavailable, then A-scan (amplitude scan) can be used for assessment of ocular anatomy.

Test method:

- Entire eyeball is scanned by ultrasonography in eight meridians which are divided longitudinally.
- Examiner keeps the ultrasound probe on the limbal area while patient is instructed to look into the direction of probe tip.
- Then examiner slowly moves the probe towards fornix covering all eight meridians and patient simultaneously looks in the

direction of respective meridians under examination.

- To obtain detail information about ocular structures the ultrasound scanning is performed in lower and higher tissue sensitivity settings as compared to normal.

Note: Ultrasonography gives information about anatomical status of macula, not the functional status of macula.

Visual Evoked Potential

The visual evoked potential (VEP) test is considered as more specific because the prerequisites for this test is an intact macula, optic nerve and visual cortical centre. This is a very helpful method to predict potential visual acuity in patients especially in total media opacities, where other available tests are not useful to assess visual acuity.

Entoptic Imagery Test

Entoptic images are visual perceptions that arise from optical structures within the eye. Many types of entoptic phenomenon are Maxwell spot, Purkinje vascular shadow, blue-field entoptic phenomenon, etc. These entoptic images are sufficiently reliable and their accurate description by a patient gives presumptive evidence that a significant level of macular function exists. Usually the Purkinje vascular shadow and blue-field entoptic phenomenon are considered most accurate test to check functional status of retina behind ocular media opacities. It is recommended that an entoptic imagery test should be performed first in cataractous eye, and then in the normal fellow eye (if applicable). If patient perceives entoptic images by normal eye but not by cataractous eye, then it indicates poor visual prognosis in cataractous eye.

Retinoscope and Retinoscopy

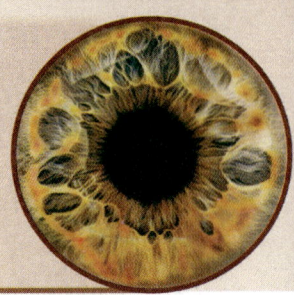

HISTORY OF RETINOSCOPY

Introduction

History of retinoscopy goes back to 1859, when initial observations about the images were made by Sir William Bowman which finally led to the basis of present day clinical retinoscopy. Sir William Bowman observed a linear shadow (linear fundus reflex) while he was doing examination of the fundus of a patient who had an astigmatic refractive error. He used a plane mirror ophthalmoscope for examination of astigmatic eye and illuminated this plane mirror ophthalmoscope with the help of a burning candle and this light was then focused on the patient's eye. Thus, it was Bowman who first described this method to detect astigmatic error in a patient of keratoconus and he established the basis for assessment of refractive status by objective means. Because prior to this observation made by Bowman, refractive status of patients was corrected by subjective methods only. Finally, H. Parent in 1880 established the quantitative refraction test by measuring refractive error using lenses and coined the term retinoscopie.

Retinoscope used in earlier times had simple mirrors either plane or concave to reflect the light coming from of a candle. The candle light created a "spot of light" which in turn produced shadows instead of linear reflection from eye of the patient. Gradually it was tried and understood by various scientists working on this, that a linear streak of reflected light can be produced by utilizing slit-shaped mirrors as shown in Fig. 11.1.

Pioneers of Retinoscopy

In the year 1873, French ophthalmologist Ferdinand Cuignet compared various reflexes in the eyes by using a simple mirror ophthalmoscope. When he observed through the peephole of his plane mirror he noticed that the reflexes varied in different patients. He thought that this phenomenon might be happening because every person has different refractive status. This became the basis for a *qualitative* test.

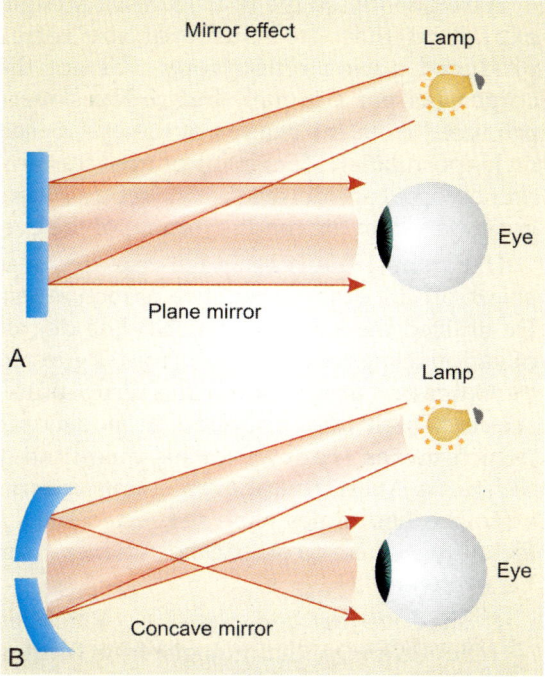

Fig. 11.1: Mirror effects on light. A. Plane mirror emits parallel, uncrossed rays; B. Concave mirror converge rays at a point, from which light rays cross and diverge hence produces an opposite reflex or reversed motion.

Cuignet observed that when the light from the plane mirror is moved across the pupil then the reflexes from the fundus also move with light movement. Occasionally, the movements of fundus reflex was in the same direction as that of mirror light, but most of the time it was in the opposite direction. He thought that the cornea was responsible for the production of these reflexes in the eyes and hence coined the term for his method as keratoscopie ('kerato' means cornea).

He further observed these reflexes in details in terms of the reflex sizes, brightness of reflex, speed and direction of the reflexes in relation to the movement of projected light. On the basis of his observations Cuignet classified these patients with various refractive errors as myopia, hyperopia or astigmatism. Because of this contribution in field of retinoscopy, he is known as Father of retinoscopy.

Subsequently, in the year 1878, M. Mengin explained that the source of the reflex produced during retinoscopy was not the cornea (as per Cuignet) but reflexes were produced from the fundus of the eye. Based on his postulation Mengin introduced the term retinoscopie considering that the reflexes were generated from the fundus (retina) of the eye.

H. Parent (1849–1924) in the year 1880 was able to produce the quantitative refraction test. He utilized the lenses to quantify the degree of various types of refractive errors suggested by Cuignet. Parent coined the term retinoscopie which later changed to skiascopie (which means shadow) for his quantitative technique. Apart from abovementioned terms various other names were suggested for the techniques done to study the reflexes from the eye were

- Shadow test (proposed by Priestley Smith, an Ophthalmologist from Birmingham)
- Skiaskopie (Egger translated the word shadow in Greek and coined this term)
- Pupilloskopie (korescopy)
- Umbrascopy
- Scotoscopy
- Dioptroscopy

The electric retinoscopes commonly used in the beginning of 20th century had spiral filament bulb with a rotating sleeve. These spiral filaments used to give the spot of light which was not in line or very sharp. Later on, Jacob Copeland introduced a bulb in retinoscope which had linear filament. The light produced by this bulb was sharp, bright and linear. This change in bulb became the basis for the discovery of Copeland's streak retinoscope which passed many phases of development to reach the present day retinoscopes.

Over the last 100 years many improvement and modifications in the design and functioning of retinoscope in terms of viewing system of retinoscope, meridians of bulb filament and control of light vergence, etc. had been done. During this period of development the Retinoscope handles and sleeve design were made handy, compact, more comfortable and user friendly, with better battery power.

Various Theories of Retinoscopy

Though the technique of retinoscopy was put to an effective clinical use during the 19th and 20th centuries, however, the principle of retinoscopy was still a debatable issue among scientists. The most popular theories regarding the principle of retinoscopy emerged during this period were:

- The far point theory (proposed by Landolt)
- The observer pupil theory (proposed by Wolff)
- The photokinetic theory (proposed by Haass)

Out of these theories the far point theory proposed by Landolt is most widely accepted theory and forms the basis for understanding the principle of retinoscopy till date. Eminent scientists like Priestly-Smith, Donder, Gullstrand, Wolff, Haass and others also put theories for optics and mechanism of retinoscopy.

In the year 1903, scientist Duane started use of cylindrical lenses in cases of astigmatism. He developed method to use cylindrical lenses while performing retinoscopy to neutralize the reflexes. Most widely accepted far point theory of Landolt which still forms the basis for understanding the principle of retinoscopy was challenged by theories proposed by Wolff (observer pupil theory) and Haass (photo kinetic theory).

In initial phases, for illumination of retina gaslight was used as a light source. This light source was later on replaced with an incandescent lamp. Examiner used a mirror retinoscope to reflect the rays from the gaslight into the patient's eye, while studying the fundus reflex through the peephole of mirror retinoscope.

Gradually, a miniature bulb was developed which could be placed inside the instrument. This was the model of an early luminous retinoscope. These small electric bulbs projected a spot of light to illuminate the retina much similar to present day's Ophthalmoscope. Later on, various designs of retinoscope came with variable vergence. These vergences were produced by the use of either plane or concave mirror. These mirrors were also fitted in the same instrument.

Over a period of nearly 100 years the initially designed spot retinoscopes have not changed much in their design. There were several limitations in function and handling of these instruments but still they remain in use till recently. However, streak retinoscopy in reality is more accurate, much simpler and faster than other techniques of retinoscopy. With time the importance of a linear fundus reflex as compared to spot reflex especially, in the patients having astigmatism was recognized. Many researchers stressed on the importance of linear reflex and by using various types of slit-shaped mirrors they tried to create a linear beam (or streak) of light, which lead to development of streak retinoscope. This streak retinoscope simplified the procedure of refraction in astigmatism. With further advancement an electric retinoscope which consisted of a rotating slit was produced which allowed the examiner to compare various ocular meridians simultaneously.

RETINOSCOPE: AN OVERVIEW

Retinoscope as a Tool

Retinoscopy is also known as skiascopie. This terminology is more accurate because it indicates that the shadows (reflexes) from the fundus are being observed by use of an instrument.

Retina by itself is a thin and transparent structures, hence it cannot casts a shadow. So the structures get illuminated by the light are retinal pigment epithelium and choroid. These structures reflect the light and shadows or reflexes of this reflected light are seen by the instrument called retinoscope. Previously, spot retinoscopes were used which are now replaced by streak retinoscope in modern era and designed by many manufactures commercially. All these brands of retinoscopes have slight difference in their appearance and design of instrument but the basic principles remains more or less similar in all commercially available instruments.

Parts of Retinoscope

Though from external appearance the retinoscope looks like a simple instrument with head and handle. It has several smaller units which are compiled to perform various functions.

To know the retinoscope in better way we can broadly divide this instrument into two parts as shown in Fig. 11.2.
- Head piece
- Handle piece

Head piece: It is the upper portion of retinoscope which consists of
- A peephole, through which examiner looks the retinal reflex.
- A sleeve which rotates the projected streak of light, hence increases or decreases the width of projected beam.

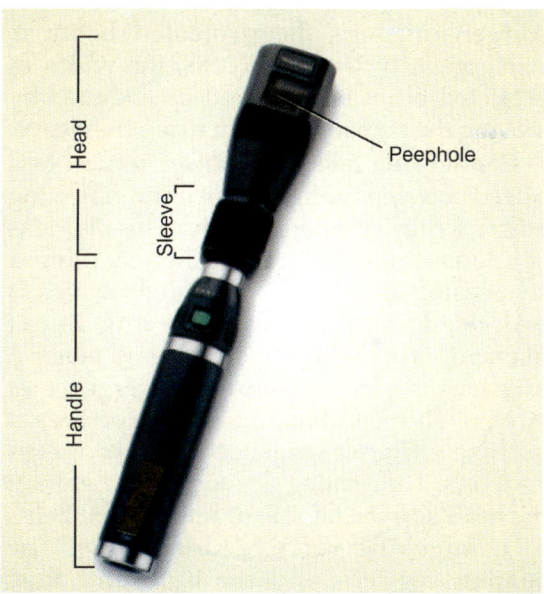

Fig. 11.2: Retinoscope

- A socket for source of illumination, i.e. bulb at its terminal end.

   This head piece is fixed by the socket system into the handle.

Handle piece: It is the lower portion of retinoscope and has an elongated hollow tube where battery is inserted inside. This battery may be rechargeable or non-rechargeable. This handle is fixed with head piece by socket locking system.

Internal Components of Streak Retinoscopes

Various commercially designed streak retinoscopes basically have two main components:
- Light projection system
- Examiner observation system

Light projection system: The projection system is the one which provides illumination to the retina and involve the following major components

Light source: In majority of designs a small bulb having a linear filament is used as light source. This filament produces a line or streak of light because the design of this filament is linear or straight. This bulb is fixed with sleeve in such a manner that by turning sleeve up or down the bulb also moves up and down and as it comes near to the lens the light is divergent and as it goes away from the condensing lens the projected beam is convergent. In simpler words, the width of projected beam is narrowed or widened by moving the bulb up or down using the sleeve.

Condensing lens: Plus power convex lens placed between the light source and reflecting mirror is called condensing lens. This plus lens condenses the light ray, hence named condensing lens. Streak of the light which is produced from the bulb (having linear filament) is a highly diverging ray, hence a plus lens is used to control the vergence of streak. This condensing lens produces a positive effect on vergence of the projected light rays. The rotating sleeve present between the head and the handle of retinoscope helps to change the relative position of the condensing lens and the bulb and thus vergence of emitted light streak can be altered

by either raising or lowering the sleeve according to the convenience of the examiner. As this condensing lens lies in the path of light streak, hence it focuses the rays from the bulb onto the mirror.

Mirror: The mirror (mostly plane mirror) causes bending of the light rays which emerges from the bulb, so that it is projected inside the patient's eye. The light from bulb filament emerges in upward direction towards the ceiling and has an axis parallel to the floor, which is then bended and reflected by the mirror. Although 100% of the emerged light from the bulb filament is not reflected by the mirror but to a certain extent some of light rays pass via the mirror. These bypassed light rays give an opportunity to the examiner to view inside the patient's pupil. These light rays are coaxial to the path of the reflex streak. As this reflecting mirror is placed at prefixed angle inside the head of retinoscope, the path of emerging light is at right angle to the axis of the retinoscope handle.

Focusing sleeve: Sleeve is a hollow cylinder, can be mounted in the head or over the handle of retinoscope. Function of sleeve is to narrow or widen the width of light streak and it also changes the direction of the light streak by rotation movement. This is used to control the amount of light projected inside the eye and also controls the direction of eye examination. The sleeve when moved up or down, the distance between the bulb and lens varies, hence it allows the retinoscope to project the rays which are either divergent (plane mirror effect) or convergent (concave mirror effect). Because of this function it is also called the vergence control of retinoscope.

In most of the commercially available retinoscopes, the sleeve changes the focus (vergence) by moving the bulb up or down keeping the lens at a fixed place. But in some commercially available retinoscopes, the condensing lens (rather than the bulb) is moved up or down to change the vergence. The movement of lens can also be done by raising or lowering the sleeve.

As discussed later in this chapter, that instruments which use a fixed bulb system and movable condensing lens, they work just the opposite way as compared to those retinoscopes which use a fixed lens and movable bulb in up or downward direction.

In present day retinoscopes, the sleeve controls both the factors, i.e. rotation of the light streak in different axes and vergence of light focused by the streak. In all types of retinoscopes, we progressively increase the vergence of the light beam from diverging rays (plane mirror effect) through parallel rays to converging rays (concave mirror effect), as we move the sleeve from top to bottom or vice versa.

Electric current source: This is provided by a battery in the handle (e.g. rechargeable single battery or replaceable small batteries). There are a few models of retinoscope, which use electric connections for providing the current source to the bulb.

> **Note:** In a nutshell, the projection system is simple to understand. The retinoscope emits rays of light to illuminate the retina. By rotating the sleeve the projected streak is rotated and by moving the sleeve up or down the projected ray can be made divergent or convergent.

Examiner observation system: The observation system enables examiner to see the reflex from the retina. The illuminated retina reflect back some of the light rays and these few rays then go into retinoscope and pass through a small hole in the mirror and later on they reach at the back end of the head of retinoscope. This small hole in the mirror is called the peephole. Thus, examiner can see the retinal reflex through this peephole. When examiner move the retinoscope up or down, while still looking through the peephole, he/she can observe the up and down movement of the light streak.

Generally, these rays when emerge from the patient's retina, they pass through various optical components of the eye and thus get affected by the various eye components of the patient. The manner in which these reflected rays get affected tells the examiner about the optics of the patient's eye.

Optics of Peephole

Usually people think the peephole of retinoscope as the hole which is present on the examiner's side of the retinoscope (we see the emerging reflected light through it). But in reality, peephole is the "hole" present in the center of the reflecting mirror inside the retinoscope. As examiner peep (see) through this hole it is called peephole. This peephole can be manufactured in the following ways

- One way is that a small circular portion of the mirror can be left unsilvered and the remaining area is silvered so that the light is not reflected from this small unsilvered area.
- Other way is that the mirror is partially silvered, so that this mirror will act as a beam splitter.

Size of peephole is a major contributing factor in designing of retinoscope because a very large size peephole will reduce the amount of valuable light reflecting into the patient's eye. To decrease the chances of these internal reflections producing glare and polarization, some manufactures of retinoscope have introduce various types of filters which are fixed in between the peephole of the retinoscope and the true peephole.

This true peephole is the one which allows the observer to see inside the patient's eye by maintaining a coaxial relationship between his eye and the light emerging from the peephole of retinoscope. This coaxial (having same axis) relationship among the observer's eye and emitted light streak from patient's eye is very important and prerequisite to view a red reflex inside the eye of patient as shown in Fig. 11.3.

> **Note:** If this coaxial relationship of light is not maintained, then examiner will see only a black pupillary area inside the patient eye, instead of a red reflex.

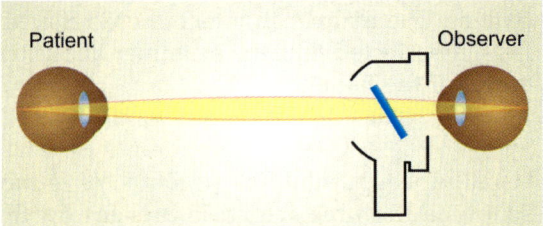

Fig. 11.3: Observation system illustrating the path of light through mirror from patient's retina to observer's retina.

Tilting of the retinoscope in sideways will allow the examiner to see some area of the red reflex of retina present in alignment with retinoscope peephole, whereas a few area of red reflex which are not in line, get cut off. These cut-off areas will be seen as a dark shadows inside the patient's pupil, whereas remaining area which are coaxial will be seen as red glow.

Note: In a nutshell, the observation system of retinoscope is simply to observe the reflected light ray from illuminated retina through a peephole in mirror.

Optics of Retinoscope

Figure 11.4 is a diagrammatic cross-sectional representation of streak retinoscope. Bulb emits light from its filament, which passes through a convex lens (condensing lens) and then this light hits the plane mirror. From the mirror light rays get reflected outside the retinoscope toward the patient's eye. The examiner observes a portion of these reflected light rays via an aperture in mirror called peephole.

The arrows shown in Fig. 11.4 on sides of retinoscope are representing two types of movements done by the sleeve of retinoscope, i.e. up or down and rotation. The straight arrow represents the vertical movement of sleeve where upward or downward movement will change the vergence of the emitting light rays by altering the distance between filament of bulb and convex lens. The curved arrow represents the bulb, which can be rotated both clockwise and anticlockwise; to move the orientation of reflex either vertical or horizontal, as per requirement.

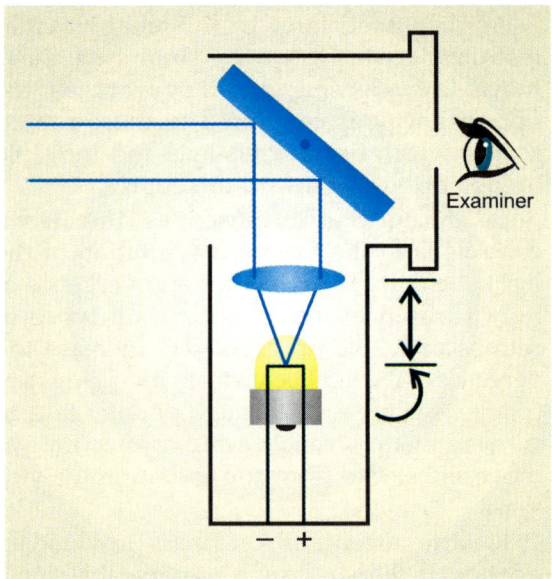

Fig. 11.4: Optics of retinoscope showing positions of bulb, condensing lens and mirror.

In our diagrammatic illustration the filament of bulb is considered to be present at the focal point of convex lens, hence the light rays emerging after reflecting from the mirror are parallel in nature.

Two types of retinoscope are available
- Type I: In this type of retinoscope, the bulb is moved up or down with the movement of sleeve, whereas convex lens remain fixed.
- Type II: In this type of retinoscope, the convex lens is moved up or down with the movement of sleeve, whereas bulb remains fixed.

Type I retinoscope

Optics and cross section view of the first type of retinoscope in which the bulb moves up or down and convex lens remains fixed is as follows:

As shown in Fig. 11.5A, when sleeve of retinoscope is moved in downward direction, the bulb moves downward (away from lens) and the effect produced is similar to a concave mirror which means emerging light rays will be convergent in nature.

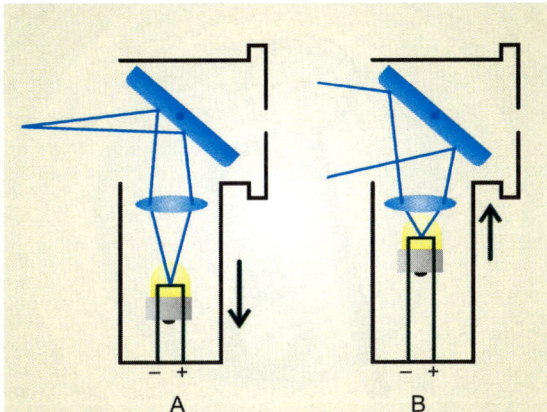

Fig. 11.5A and B: Optical effects by the movement of retinoscope bulb. A. Bulb moving downwards; B. Bulb moving upwards

As shown in Fig. 11.5B, opposite will happen when sleeve is moved up, i.e. the bulb will move up (nearer to lens) and produces plane mirror effect, hence emerging light rays will be divergent in nature.

Type II retinoscope

Optics and cross section view of the second type of retinoscope in which the lens moves upward or downward and bulb remains fixed.

As shown in Fig. 11.6A, when lens is moved up (away from bulb), an effect similar to a concave mirror is produced and hence emerging light rays are convergent when

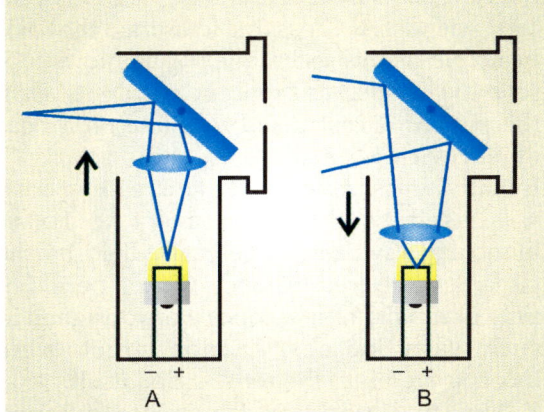

Fig. 11.6A and B: Optical effects by the movement of retinoscope lens. A. Lens moving upwards; B. Lens moving downwards

sleeve of retinoscope is moved in upward direction.

Opposite effect happens as shown in Fig. 11.6B, when sleeve is moved down, the lens moves downward (nearer to bulb) and produces plane mirror effect and hence emerging light rays are divergent in nature.

Various Types of Retinoscopes

Retinoscopes took a long revolutionary path to reach present day's sleek retinoscope models. Various types of retinoscopes are

- Simple retinoscopes
- MacNab retinoscope
- Dynamic retinoscopes
- Spot retinoscopes
- Streak retinoscopes

Simple retinoscopes: These were the earliest and oldest instruments used to perform retinoscopy. Initially, these were nothing but simple circular mirrors which had a central perforation or a hole. These mirrors were mounted on a metallic handle. Initially practitioners worked really hard to train themselves to use these simple plane mirrors along with a source of illumination (present either on a wall or over the patient's head by a light mounted on patient's chair). The practitioners observed the red reflex from patient's eye and tried to neutralize these reflexes with the help of various concave or convex lenses.

In Fig. 11.7A, three types of simple retinoscopes are shown, which are collectively called 'Orthops' retinoscope. In Fig. 11.7B the two reflecting retinoscopes are Lister plain mirror retinoscope and Priestley- Smith Bright double mirror. Lister reflecting retinoscope has a plane mirror, which is mounted on a handle with central peephole, whereas Priestley retinoscope has plane mirror on one side and concave mirror on the other side. These retinoscopes were manufactured in mid 20th century and the bright double mirror retinoscope is used till date by various institutions for teaching and learning purposes.

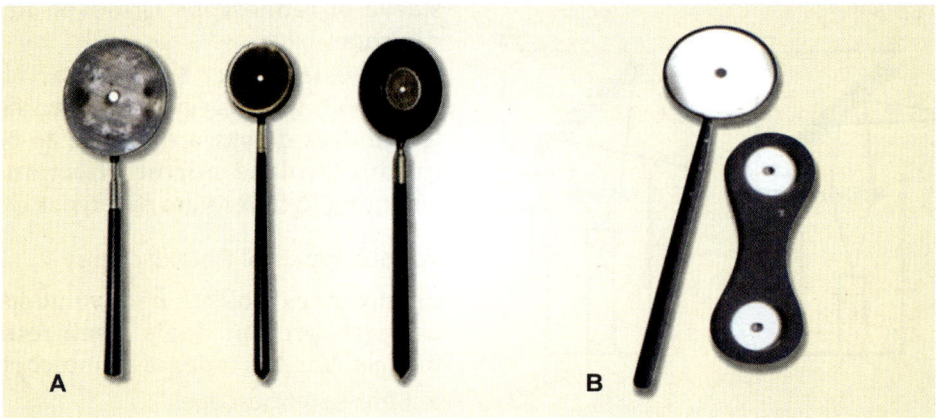

Fig. 11.7A and B: A. Orthops retinoscope; B. Reflecting retinoscopes

MacNab retinoscope: In year 1909, an Ophthalmologist Angus MacNab (1876–1914) had designed a retinoscope for study purposes. MacNab's retinoscope was a unique kind of retinoscope. It has an ivory handle with a gilt screw to fix. This retinoscope had an axis indicator wheel (marked from 0 till 180 degrees) with gear underneath the peephole of retinoscope. This axis wheel was operated by use of gears and had a central peephole as shown in Fig. 11.8.

Once the red reflex is neutralized in one meridian and if there is a movement in other meridian, then this meridian was neutralized by use of the axis wheel. This was a sophisticated retinoscope and needed continuous practice to master this instrument. Actually, this retinoscope was an improvement over the existing simple retinoscope because an astigmatism error can also be neutralized by use of this retinoscope.

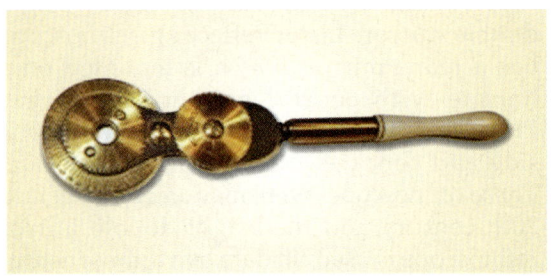

Fig. 11.8: MacNab retinoscope

Dynamic retinoscopes: In earlier days, when performing retinoscopy with simple retinoscopes patients were instructed to fixate on a target situated at far distance and their accommodation was kept relaxed. This method of retinoscopy was called static retinoscopy because accommodation is at rest and no change of refractive status can occur due to accommodation during retinoscopy. Usually, to relax the accommodation of patient various mydriatics or cycloplegics drugs were used sometimes, even high convex lenses in the fellow eye were used to relax the accommodation.

Dynamic retinoscopy was a revolutionary thought in the field of retinoscopy. In the year 1902 scientist AJ Cross first identified the basic principle of this technique. Dynamic retinoscopy is defined as "retinoscopy done when the patient is instructed to fixate on a near object with both the eyes (binocularly)". Initially, any simple object like a reading book was used as the near object to fixate binocularly which can be easily held by the patients at desired distance. Over a period of time gradually retinoscopes were designed in such ways that near fixation targets were incorporated into the retinoscope itself.

The two popular types of dynamic retinoscopes were present in the era of 1930s. These were Margaret Dobson retinoscope and Turville-Pascal Dynascope.

Margaret Dobson retinoscope: As shown in Fig. 11.9A the Margaret Dobson dynamic retinoscope had a spiral filament fitted inside the retinoscope bulb to produce a spot of light and emerging rays were made slightly divergent by using a plane mirror before they were reflected into the eye of the patient. This instrument was specially designed so that when patient try to compensate for achieving the binocular fixation, the working distance of retinoscope is compensated automatically.

A revolving disc present on the retinoscope had eight targets; out of these seven targets were near fixation charts which were designed to be examined from a reading distance of 30–35 cm. The eighth target designed for patient was a simple blank chart. This blank slot of target was designed to decrease the illumination from all other near targets and hence will convert this dynamic retinoscope into an old traditional static type of retinoscope. The fixation target shown in above retinoscope picture is that of a horse. These kinds of pictures were used to perform retinoscopy in children so that while doing the retinoscopy the examiner can ask simple questions to child such as whether this horse has a tail or can you see the beautiful eyes of the horse. These simple questions will help child as well as examiner in fixating the object and relax their accommodation.

Turville-Pascal dynascope: The Turville-Pascal retinoscope or 'Dynascope' (Dynamic retinoscope) (Fig. 11.9B) was introduced in the year 1931. It was designed by the collective efforts of both scientists, who worked together with an aim to remove different errors supposedly introduced by the retinoscope itself in the process of dynamic retinoscopy.

Spot retinoscopes: In the year 1901, first electric retinoscope was introduced by Wolff (Fig. 11.10). This newly designed self-illuminated retinoscope was fitted with a small bulb which emitted a spot of light inside the patient's eye. In the subsequent years various other vergence models of retinoscopes were introduced which were capable of

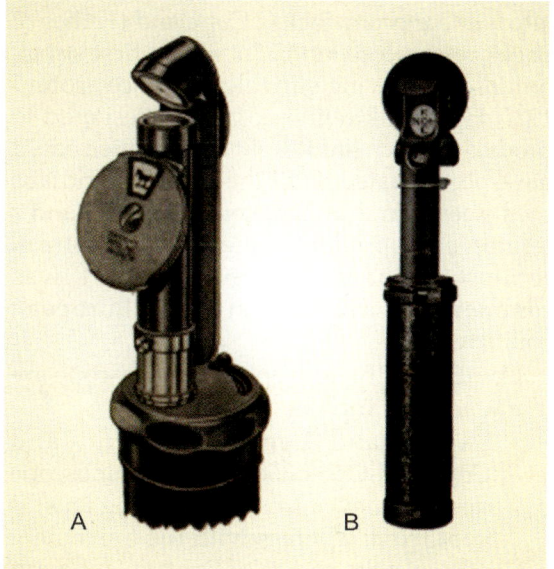

Fig. 11.9A and B: Dynamic retinoscopes. A. Margaret Dobson retinoscope; B. Turville-Pascal dynascope

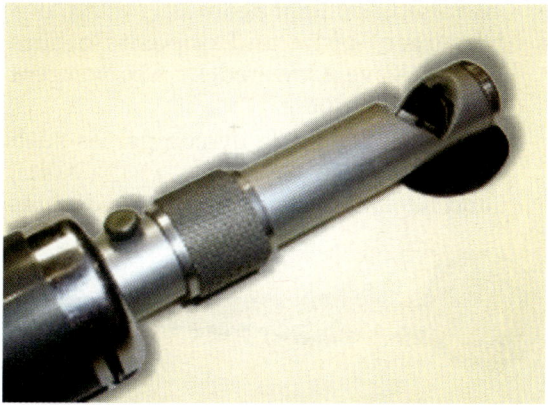

Fig. 11.10: Spot retinoscope

producing the vergence to spot light, either getting reflected from a plane mirror (more common) or a concave mirror (less common).

Streak retinoscopes: The fundus reflexes produced in an astigmatic eye are linear, thus for accurate detection of astigmatism it was better to use a rectangular streak of light than a spot light. To produce this type of streak early researchers tried to produce their own reflecting mirrors having a slit in the middle and this helped in conversion of a spot light into a linear beam. Jack C Copeland (Father of streak retinoscopy) introduced the first streak retinoscope having variable vergence around 1920. His streak retinoscope was designed to produce its own linear light beam which could have been rotated in all the ocular meridians by a sleeve. In mid 20th century, Copeland's retinoscope popularly called Pulzone streak retinoscope as shown in Fig. 11.11 was commercially available in entire European countries.

Commercially two types of retinoscope are manufactured such as

- Bausch and Lomb, Copeland and Copeland-Optec 360: In these retinoscope designs convex lens (condensing lens) is kept fixed, whereas with the movement of sleeve the source of light, i.e. bulb can be moved upwards (towards the lens) or downwards (away from the lens). When sleeve present on the retinoscope handle is raised, the light beam is emitted as a divergent beam and opposite occurs when sleeve is lowered, i.e. a convergent beam is produced.
- Retinoscopes made by companies such as Welch Allen, Heine (Fig. 11.12), Neitz, and Keeler: In these retinoscope designs

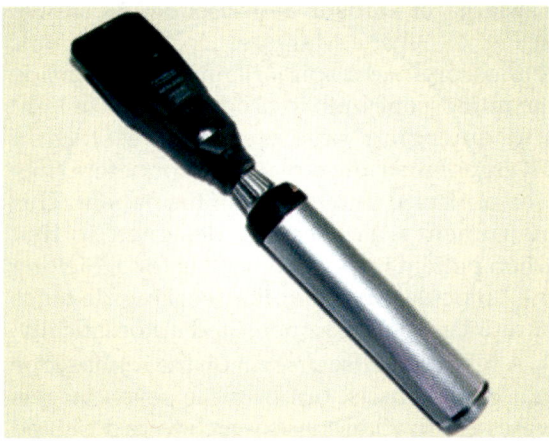

Fig. 11.12: Heine streak retinoscope

the source of light, i.e. bulb is kept fixed, whereas the convex lens (condensing lens) can be moved upwards (towards mirror) or downwards (towards bulb) by raising or lowering the sleeve. When sleeve present on the retinoscope handle is raised, the light beam is emitted as a convergent beam and a divergent beam is produced by lowering of sleeve.

Note: As these types of retinoscopes need to control two different functions such as moving the condensing lens upwards/downwards and also rotate the filament of bulb, their mechanism and linkage design is quite complex as compared to retinoscopes manufactured by Bausch and Lomb Copeland.

RETINOSCOPY

Principles and Techniques of Retinoscopy

The principle is to observe the different kind of retinal reflections (reflex) obtained from patient's eye when light beam produced from retinoscope illuminates the internal portion of patient's eye. The examiner observes the relative movement of the retinal reflexes when he/she moves the streak or spot of light beam either in vertical or horizontal meridians from corner to corner of patient's pupil. Then examiner tries to neutralize these retinal reflexes manually by placing trial lenses of different power in front of the eye in a trial frame.

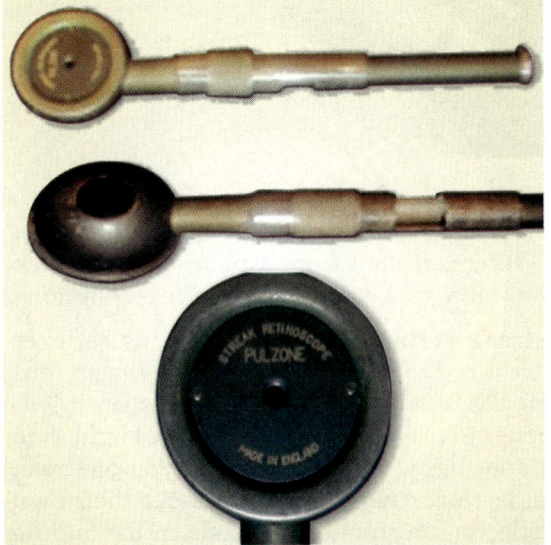

Fig. 11.11: Pulzone streak retinoscope

Retinoscopy is a technique used to calculate the amount of refractive error by an objective means. Objective refraction test is done by performing retinoscopy under the effect of mydriasis. Retinoscopes' light source is utilized to illuminate the fundus of patient's eye while examiner will observe and measure the reflected rays of light from the retina. Retinoscopy may be followed by various subjective tests to calculate an accurate amount of refractive correction required for the patient.

Over many decades retinoscopy has proved to be an excellent method to evaluate the refractive status of an eye and is considered as a clinically effective method to assess an accurate refractive correction needed by patient in very less time without compromising the quality of result.

Retinoscopy Reflex

Various images obtained while performing retinoscopy need evaluation for the calculation and estimation of refractive status of the eye. As discussed above, when fundus is illuminated with the retinoscope light source and examiner observes the emerging rays coming from the retina (as if retina is luminous), the optical system of eye exerts various types of vergence to these emitting rays. For example, when retina is illuminated with parallel rays (by plane mirror), the rays reflected from the retina will emerge from the eye according to the refractive status of eye as follows

- Reflected light rays will emerge from the eye as parallel rays in case of emmetropia.
- Reflected light rays will emerge from the eye as divergent rays in case of hypermetropia.
- Reflected light rays will emerge from the eye as convergent rays in case of myopia.

The emitting rays will behave differently if we illuminate the retina with rays which are not parallel.

The optics of retina in different ocular status, i.e. emmetropia, hypermetropia and

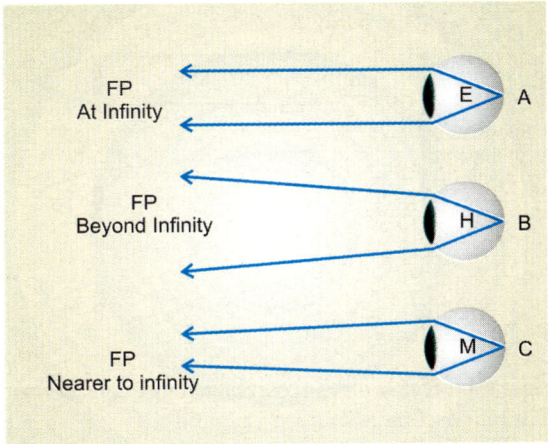

Fig. 11.13: Emerging rays pattern and focal point (FP) for emmetropic (E), hypermetropic (H) and myopic (M) eyes.

myopia, assuming that the entering light rays were parallel in all three ocular states, can be understood by graphic representation as shown in Fig. 11.13. In an emmetrope, the focal point is at infinity, in hypermetrope it is beyond infinity, whereas in myope the focal point is at lesser distance than infinity.

Consider that examiner is sitting at infinity distance and looking through the peephole of retinoscope. Various observations in three basic conditions as mentioned above will be as follows

- Retinal reflex moves along with the movement of retinoscope streak (WITH motion reflex) in case of emmetrope and hypermetrope because emerging light rays are not converging to a focal point as shown in Fig. 11.14.
- Against movement of retinal reflex along with the movement of retinoscope streak (AGAINST motion reflex) will be seen in case of myope because emerging light rays are converging to a focal point (FP) and then diverging as shown in Fig. 11.14.

Similarly, when examiner is looking through the peephole of retinoscope from a finite distance, then the emerging light rays will appear as red reflex inside the patient's pupil (Fig. 11.15A). When examiner moves

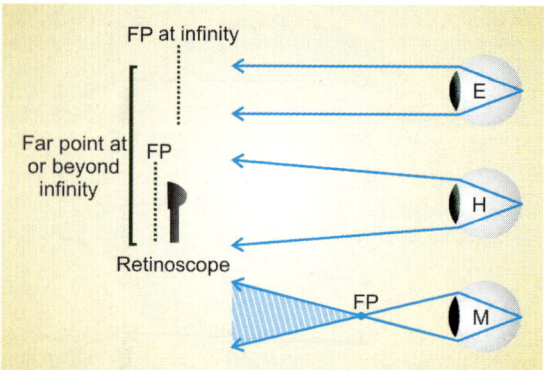

Fig. 11.14: Different types of retinal reflex considering that retinoscope is situated at infinity

retinoscope across the eye, the red reflex will also move with retinoscope movement. Suppose the emerging light rays are parallel or diverging, then the red retinal reflex will move in the same direction as of the retinoscope streak (intercept), this is called with movement (Fig. 11.15B). In contrast, if emerging light rays meet at focal point and are diverging, then the retinal reflex will move in opposite direction, as that of retinoscope streak; this is called against movement (Fig. 11.15C).

Note: An interesting way to interpret this condition is that, if we observe against movement we are beyond the focal point and if we see with movement, then focal point is beyond us.

Practically, optical infinity is considered beyond 20 feet or 6 meters distance but it is impossible for an examiner to sit at this far distance and then observe the retinal reflex or add the correcting lenses in trial frame. For practical convenience either one meter or 66 cm distance is advocated to observe the retinal reflex, from where reflex appears brighter and examiner can easily add or remove lenses in/from the trial frame.

When examiner observes from 1 meter distance, then in case of emmetrope and hyperopes still the examiner will observe with movement reflex (Fig. 11.16) because focal point in both these cases is beyond the examiner. However, in case of myope (for example, having one dioptre refractive error) following typical reflexes are observed with various positions such as

- Suppose examiner leans forward with retinoscope: With movement of reflex is seen
- When examiner goes backward: Against movement reflex will be seen
- However, with retinoscope exactly at one meter distance no movement of reflex or a neutrality reflex will be seen because focal point in our example is at one meter distance.

A neutrality of red (retinal) reflex is seen when peephole of retinoscope coincides with focal point. This reflex is the one which fills the entire pupil with light (Fig. 11.17). At this point there is no streak of light and also there is no movement of retinal reflex either with or against. At this point the retina of eye is in conjugate with the peephole of retinoscope. As retinal reflex reverses its direction from with movement to against movement, this focal point is also called reversal point in retinoscopy.

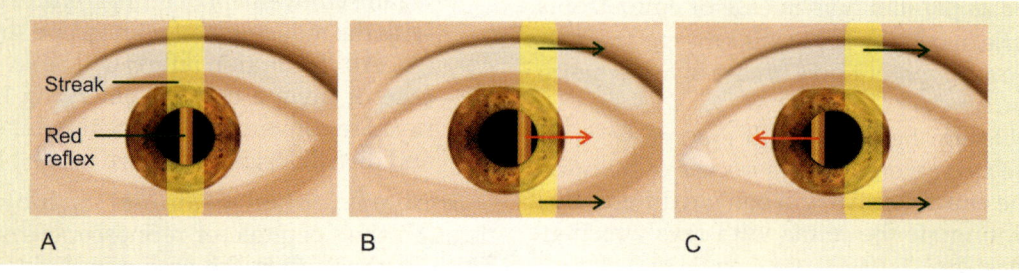

Fig. 11.15A to C: Red reflex motion with retinoscope streak (intercept). A. In center with streak; B. With movement; C. Against movement

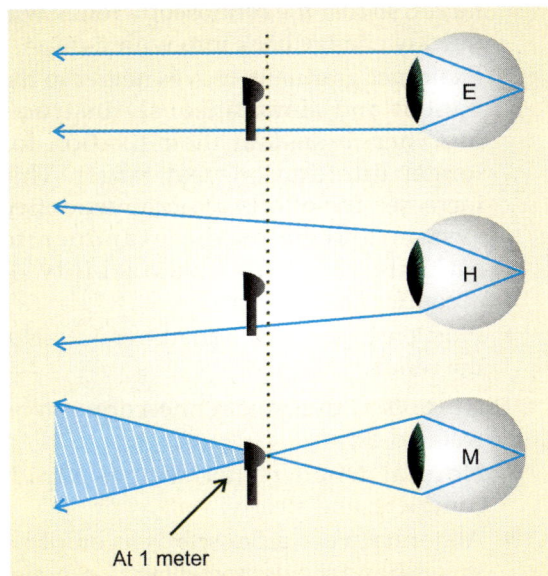

Fig. 11.16: Different types of retinal reflex considering that retinoscope is situated at one meter distance.

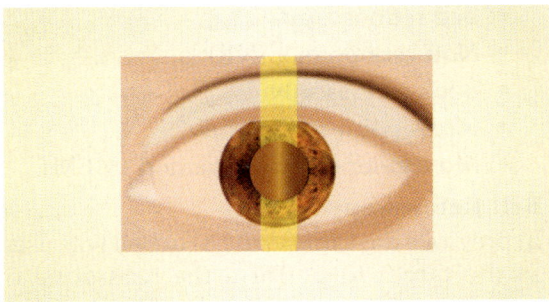

Fig. 11.17: Neutrality of red reflex

Methods of Retinoscopy

Retinoscopy methods can be grouped mainly as

- Static retinoscopy
- Mohindra near retinoscopy
- Dynamic retinoscopy

Static retinoscopy: This is the most widely and routinely performed retinoscopy technique to estimate the accurate amount of distance refractive error. Static retinoscopy is based on Foucault's principle, which states that "the exact refractive status of patient is achieved when the observer create an optical

infinity". In this technique the patient is advised to relax his/her accommodation completely. This state of fully relaxed accommodation can be achieved either by providing a distant fixation target to the patient or by using cycloplegics in cases of hypermetropes and children.

To obtain the patient's exact refractive status, the dioptric power equivalent to cycloplegic (if used) and also working distance are mathematically subtracted from the total amount of retinoscopy. The working distance lens has power equivalent to the focal length equal to distance between examiner and patient. For example, +1.00 dioptre lens equates for one meter of working distance.

Mohindra near retinoscopy: This technique is also used to measure distance refractive error in a non-accommodative state, however, this technique differs from dynamic retinoscopy. This is a very useful technique to assess refractive state of eye in infants.

Steps of retinoscopy technique are

- The examination room must be dark as much as possible. Underlying principle is simple that the dim light emitting from retinoscope will act as a fixation target for the child so that accommodation will not get stimulate.
- Sometimes this technique can be performed over the shoulder of parents while parent is holding the infant or feeding the infant. The examiner performs retinoscopy from 50 cm distance and two principal meridians of retinal reflexes, i.e. horizontal and vertical are neutralized separately by using spherical or a combination of spherical and cylindrical trial lenses.
- Originally, Mohindra used a –1.25 D lenses for adjustment; this dioptric value of –1.25 D was mathematically added with the total neutrality dioptric value to get a final result. For example, if neutrality is achieved with +4.50 /–1.75 × 90°, then the final result would be + 3.25/–1.75 × 90°.

- In infants having high degree hyper-metropic refractive error, Mohindra retinoscopy showed less accurate results when compared with cycloplegic retino-scopy. Although Mohindra technique remained a unique child-friendly method as not much cooperation is required with the child.

Dynamic retinoscopy: Difference between static and dynamic retinoscopy is that working distance and accommodation are not only equated with lens power rather convergence and information processing are also considered in the dynamic retinoscopy. No cycloplegia is required to perform this retinoscopy.

Simple method to perform a dynamic retinoscopy is by using retinoscope and a near fixation target, say reading chart.

Method of dynamic retinoscopy

- Fixation target is held by the examiner at the nearest possible distance to peephole of retinoscope, without blocking the aperture of peephole.
- Darken the examination room and a light is directed towards the reading chart so that patient is able to read this chart. Examiner holds the reading chart and retinoscope at the normal reading distance.
- If distant vision correction is present, then patient is instructed to wear the distance vision glasses. Then patient is instructed to fixate on a distant target wearing distance correction (if present) and fundus reflexes are observed in both the eyes, usually with motion is seen.
- Now the patient is instructed to suddenly fixate on the reading chart from the distance target, while examiner continues the retinoscopy. Usually the previously observed with motion will either swiftly converts into the state of neutralization or may appear as against motion.
- Suppose neutralization of reflex is incomplete, then patient is instructed again to fixate on the previous distant

target, so that the retinoscopy reflex will quickly change back into with motion.

- Examiner gradually moves nearer to the patient and simultaneously instructs him/her to sustain their fixation for longer duration on near target. This increases the efforts of accommodative system and helps the examiner to estimate about the sustainability of accommodative efforts.
- Plus lenses are now added to neutralize the reflex.

The results of dynamic retinoscopy can be interpretated as:

- Normal when reflex seen is rapid, complete, and steady.
- Abnormal when reflex seen is incomplete, sluggish and shows momentary accommo-dation and/or accommodative lag.

Various techniques to execute dynamic retinoscopy are:

- Bell retinoscopy
- Nott retinoscopy (NR)
- Book retinoscopy
- Stress point retinoscopy
- Monocular estimate method (MEM)

Bell Retinoscopy

In previous days originally a cat bell was used as the target to perform the technique of dynamic retinoscopy, hence was named as Bell retinoscopy. Although nowadays Wolff wand is used as target to perform this technique. As shown in Fig. 11.18, Wolff wand target has a gold or silver metal ball of ½ inch diameter mounted on one or both ends of a rod.

Procedure of retinoscopy

- Examiner holds the retinoscope at 50 cm distance from the patient and observes the fundus reflex. Now examiner gradually moves the ball towards the patient, while patient is instructed to look at the ball continuously. Simultaneously, examiner continues to perform the retinoscopy and observe the movements of reflex in relation with the movement of ball target.

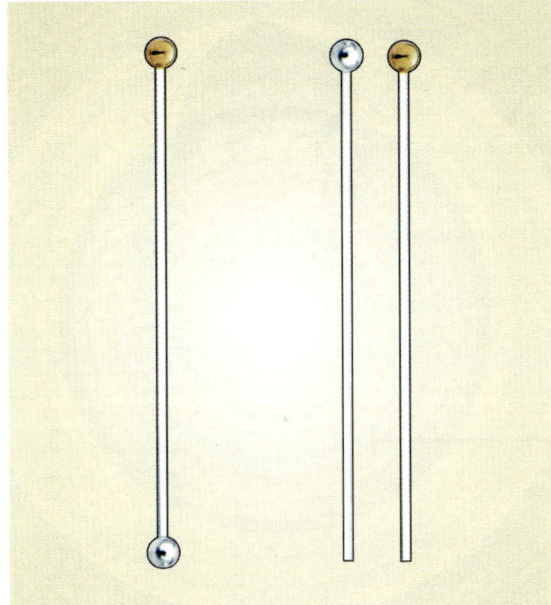

Fig. 11.18: Wolff wand target for bell retinoscopy (*courtesy:* Bernell Corporation)

- As the ball moves closer, usually a fast with motion is observed, gradually reflex changes to neutral and then against.
- Now when examiner gradually moves the ball away from the patient a reverse order of changes in reflex, i.e. from against to neutral and then with motion will be observed by the examiner.
- Firstly record the distance between ball and the patient's nose at which a change from with motion to against motion had occurred while ball was moved towards the patient.
- Secondly, record the distance between ball and the patient's nose at which a change from against motion to with motion had occurred while ball was moved away from the patient.
- These two distances are recorded as fraction in centimeters. For example, 36/42 which means first recording with motion to against motion had occurred at 36 cm distance and change from against motion to with motion had occurred at 42 cm distance.

- Normal values for bell retinoscopy are an inward shift, i.e. from with motion to against motion is in the range of 35–42.5 cm and an outward shift, i.e. from against motion to with motion is in the range of 37.5–45 cm.

Note: Suppose lag of accommodation is not observed within these ranges, then procedure is repeated by using plus lenses. Lenses which bring the recordings within these ranges are acknowledged as near vision prescription.

Nott Retinoscopy

Nott retinoscopy (NR) is a unique method of retinoscopy. Here an internally-illuminated cube is used as a target which contains high contrast cartoon images (usually in black and white color). This cube is attached on a retractable tape measure and is viewed from a 40 cm distance in a dim illumination as shown in Fig. 11.19.

The target is kept stationary (D1) and examiner moves in backward direction holding retinoscope, while observing the reflex till it becomes neutralized. This distance between the examiner and the child (D2) is recorded and accommodative response is equal to the inverse of this final distance.

Book Retinoscopy

In book retinoscopy various changes in retinoscopic reflex are observed depending upon the involvement level or interaction of child, who continuously read a book as target. These changes in retinoscopic reflexes could be

- A bright, sharp edged pinkish colored reflex with motion is seen, while child is reading freely and easily.
- A bright, sharp and dark pink colored reflex having fast against motion is seen, while child is reading on instructions of examiner, means maintain the reading task in spite of being stressed.
- A dull brick red colored reflex having slow against motion is observed, while child is reading with frustration.

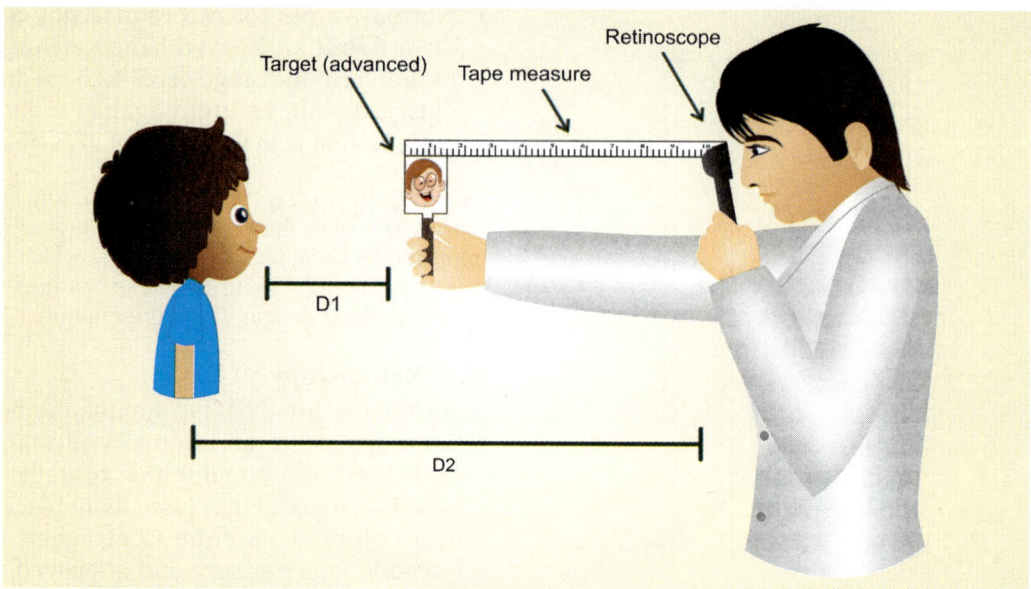

Fig. 11.19: Method of Nott retinoscopy. D1—fixed distance; D2—final distance

Stress point retinoscopy

Harmon and Kraskin described stress point retinoscopy. As discussed above, in Bell retinoscopy a change in motion of reflex was observed, whereas in stress-point retinoscopy a change in reflex quality is observed. Following three types of observations can be seen when near point stress is observed

- A change in radial pulse of subject
- An inner canthal twitch
- A color change in retinal reflex

Harmon distance: It is measured from the elbow to the knuckle of middle finger as shown in Fig. 11.20.

Test procedure

- Examiner initially observes the fundus reflex, then patient is instructed to focus on a Wolff ball as near target.
- Now examiner slowly moves Wolff's ball closer to the patient and simultaneously observes that at what distance the patient's fundus reflex pops.

Note: A retinoscopy reflex is called popping reflex when reflex initially brightens, then becomes dull and again becomes bright.

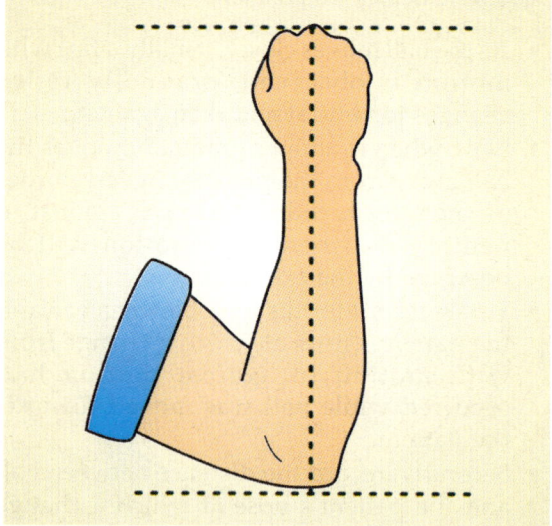

Fig. 11.20: Harmon distance

Interpretation: Normally, in children the stress point should be 10 cm nearer than Harmon distance of that subject, whereas normally in adults the stress point is 20–22.5 cm away from the face. For example, suppose in a 10 years old child, Harmon distance is 22 cm and a stress point is 18 cm. When stress point is measured again with add of + 1.0 DS lens, the stress point becomes 14 cm, whereas with add of +1.5 DS lens, it becomes 24 cm. In this case + 1.0 DS lens is serving as counterstress lens, whereas +1.5 DS lens is inducing a new stress pattern. Hence, we will prescribe + 1.0 DS lens for near work to this child.

Monocular estimate method
Monocular estimate method (MEM) is performed in an entirely different way than that from other methods of dynamic retinoscopy. Most of the near dynamic retinoscopy methods are performed by inserting a lens and its effect on the performance is observed.

MEM is a distinctive method where lenses are principally used to confirm the observations done by the examiner. A fixation card is attached to the retinoscope and under normal illumination conditions examiner views retinal reflexes through a central aperture from a distance of 40 cm.

Techniques of Retinoscopy

- Dry retinoscopy
- Wet retinoscopy

Dry retinoscopy: Most widely used technique to perform the retinoscopy is dry retinoscopy. Dry simply means that no mydriatic is used while performing the retinoscopy. Hence, a correction from total refraction is done only for distance, for example, if we are doing retinoscopy from 66 cm distance, then simply +1.5 D is deducted from the total refractive

---

Clinical Inference

- In low degree hypermetropes dynamic retinoscopy may show a rapid, complete but unsteady or discontinuous accommodation which confirms a diagnosis of an accommodative insufficiency and should be treated by prescribing glasses.
- In non-ocular causes a brisk normal dynamic retinoscopy response is present but if symptoms persist then an addition of reading glasses (small power) can be used in cases of a fallaciously normal dynamic retinoscopy.

amount obtained at neutralization and if doing from 50 cm, then +2 D is deducted from total refractive error.

Wet retinoscopy: When mydriatic is used to perform retinoscopy, it is called as wet retinoscopy or cycloplegic refraction. Normally in clinical practice tropicamide with phenylepherine drops are used to perform retinoscopy. These drugs produce pupillary dilatation but are weak cycloplegics, hence when strong cycloplegic effect is needed as in cases of very young child or high degree hypermetropes, then atropine, homatropine or cyclopentolate is used. Here a correction is done for both distance and mydriasis, for example, if retinoscopy is done from 66 cm distance by using atropine, then +1.5 D for distance and +1 D for atropine is deducted from total refractive value obtained by neutralization. For homatropine +0.75 D and for cyclopentolate +0.5 D is deducted.

Note: No correction for cycloplegic is needed when tropicamide is used for retinoscopy.

Retinoscopy Working Distance
If retinoscopy is performed at 25 cm distance; the retinal reflex will be bright and it is easy to reach the patient, but at the same time chances of the distance error is very high. If it is performed at 100 cm distance, the retinal reflex will be dim and it is difficult to reach the patient for changing trial lenses, however, the distance error is very low.

As shown in Fig. 11.21 space (X) of 8 cm width at 25 cm retinoscopy distance is representing 1 D difference, whereas same 8 cm space (Y) is representing only 0.09 D difference near 100 cm distance. So when retinoscopy is done at 25 cm distance then an error of few centimeters in distance estimation can bring a large change in results (by 0.50–1.0 D), whereas a distance error of equal magnitude gives negligible change in results (by 0.05–0.1 D) at 100 cm distance.

Considering these advantages and disadvantages of near and far working distances,

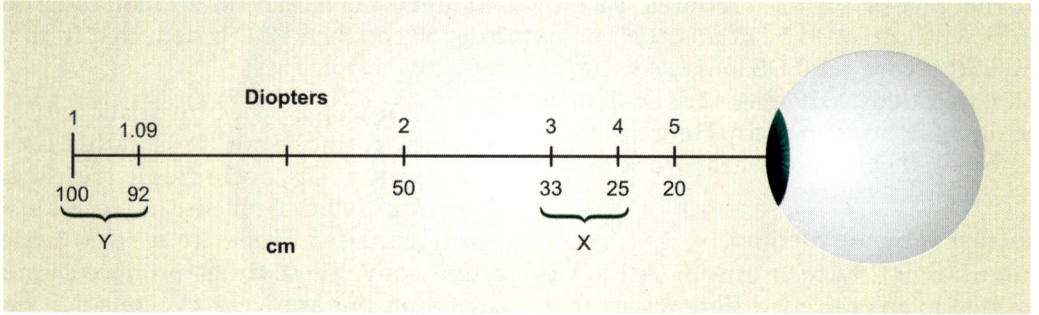

Fig. 11.21: Retinoscopy distance (cm) with corresponding dioptric power (D)

most of the examiners compromise for a working distance of either 66 cm or 50 cm. These are practically convenient distances with a suitably bright retinal reflex. 66 cm is nearly an arm's length and the dioptric value deducted is +1.5 D, whereas 50 cm is a distance roughly equal to a bend arm's length and dioptric value deducted is +2 D.

Routine Retinoscopy Reflexes

Reflexes in Emmetropes

Normally when retinoscopy is performed from 66 cm distance, an emmetrope will produce "with movement" in both vertical and horizontal meridians. These reflexes can be neutralized by small power plus lenses as shown in Fig. 11.22. For example, with +1.5 DS lens because retinoscopy was done from 66 cm.

Reflexes in Hypermetropes

Various reflexes seen in hypermetrope depend upon the degree of hypermetropia (Fig. 11.23). In low degree hypermetrope the retinal reflex is of small width and fast moving "with motion", however, as the degree of hyperopia increases the width of reflex increases and speed of reflex decreases.

This 'with motion' can easily be neutralized by using a plus lens whose power depends upon the degree of hypermetropia. For example, as shown in Fig. 11.24, a hypermetrope of +1 DS will get neutralize by adding a +2.5 DS lens when retinoscopy is done from 66 cm distance (without cycloplegic drug).

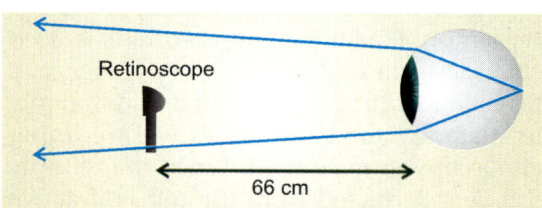

Fig. 11.23: With motion

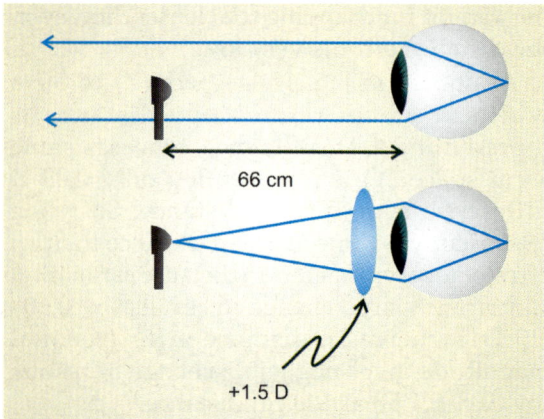

Fig. 11.22: With motion getting neutralize with small power plus lens in emmetropia

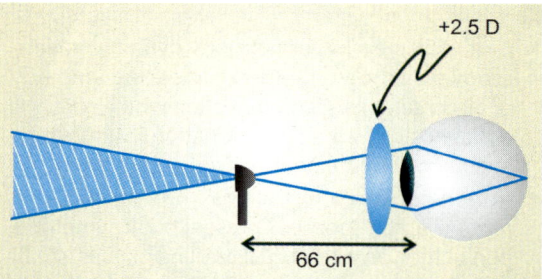

Fig. 11.24: Neutralization with +2.5 DS lens, in case of +1 DS hypermetropia

Reflexes in Myopia

Similar to hypermetropia various reflexes are seen in myopes depending upon the degree of myopia. In low degree myopia the retinal reflex is small width and fast moving 'against motion', however, as the degree of myopia increases the width of reflex increases and speed of reflex decreases, although it still remains an against motion as shown in Fig. 11.25.

This against motion can be neutralized by using a minus power lens whose power depends upon the degree of myopia. For example, as shown in Fig. 11.26, a myope of –3 DS will get neutralize by adding a –1.5 DS lens when retinoscopy is done from 66 cm distance (without cycloplegic drug).

Reflexes in Astigmatism

Astigmatism is a state of refractive error where a few rays of incident light focus on the retina and a few behind or in front of the retina. Hence, when retinoscopy is done we get different kind of movement of retinal reflexes in different meridians. For example, in case of simple hyperopic astigmatism the retinal reflex may be neutral in 90° meridian and will be 'with motion' in 180° meridian as shown in Fig. 11.27.

Here the light rays emerging from retina are refracted in a different way by the principal meridians of the cornea, hence reflexes behave as if there are two eyes instead of one eye and each of these principal meridians is acting like a separate eye. Once the retinoscopy has been performed on the eye with one principal meridian, then simply repeat the retinoscopy second time on the same eye.

Several phenomena observed while performing retinoscopy in case of astigmatism are

- Eye will show two types of reflexes one in each principal meridian as shown in Fig. 11.27.
- Retinal reflexes will have different speed, width and brightness in both principal meridians.
- Movement of retinal reflex will not be parallel to the movement of retinoscope intercept; unless scoping along the principal meridian.
- Both principal meridians cannot be neutralized by a single correcting lens. This simply means that there are two focal points.

Various types of astigmatic error will show following reflexes when retinoscopy is done

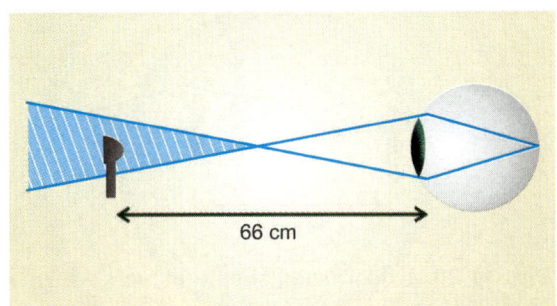

Fig. 11.25: An against motion in myopia

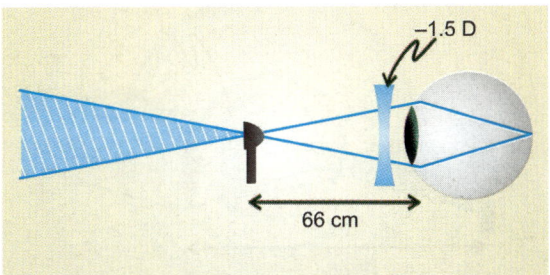

Fig. 11.26: Neutralization with –1.5 DS lens, in case of –3 DS myopia

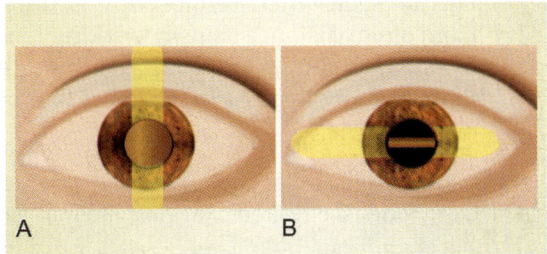

Fig. 11.27: Astigmatic reflex. A. Neutral reflex at 90° meridian; B. With motion reflex at 180° meridian

using working lens of +1.5 DS (compensating for a retinoscopy distance of 66 cm) in the trial frame.

- In case of an uncorrected simple hypermetropic astigmatism, one focal point lies at peephole of retinoscope and other is behind it. For example, a neutral reflex at 90° meridian and with motion in 180° meridian will be seen when retinoscopy is done from 66 cm distance using a working lens of +1.5 D as shown in Fig. 11.28.

- In case of an uncorrected compound hypermetropic astigmatism both focal points are behind retinoscope, so 'with motion' in both meridians will be seen when retinoscopy is done from 66 cm distance using a working lens of +1.5 D as shown in Fig. 11.29. However, in our example, the reflex will be more with motion at 180° meridian.

- Uncorrected simple myopic astigmatism cases are similar to simple hyperopic astigmatism, except that in these cases one focal point is in the front and another point is at peephole. Hence, for example, in these cases 'against motion' at 90° meridian and neutral reflex at 180° meridian will be seen when retinoscopy is done from 66 cm distance using a working lens of +1.5 D as shown in Fig. 11.30.

- Uncorrected compound myopic astigmatism is a state of eye where both focal points are in front of the retinoscope peephole. Hence, in these cases 'against motion' in both 90° and 180° meridians will be seen when retinoscopy is done from 66 cm distance using a working lens of +1.5 D as shown in Fig. 11.31, although there is more against in 90° meridian in our example.

Note: Practically during retinoscopy it is very difficult to judge the degree of against motion.

- In case of an uncorrected mixed astigmatic one focal point is in front and other point is behind the peephole of

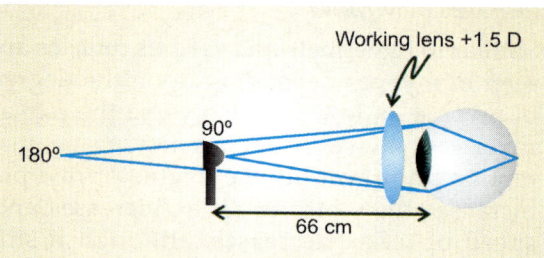

Fig. 11.28: Uncorrected simple hyperopic astigmatism

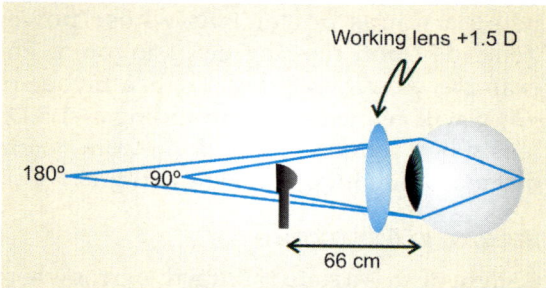

Fig. 11.29: Uncorrected compound hyperopic astigmatism

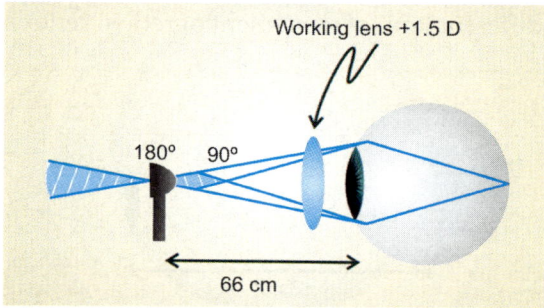

Fig. 11.30: Uncorrected simple myopic astigmatism

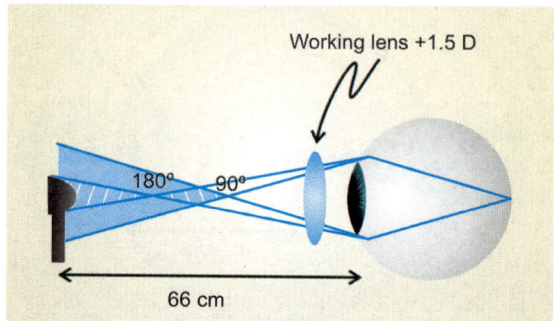

Fig. 11.31: Uncorrected compound myopic astigmatism

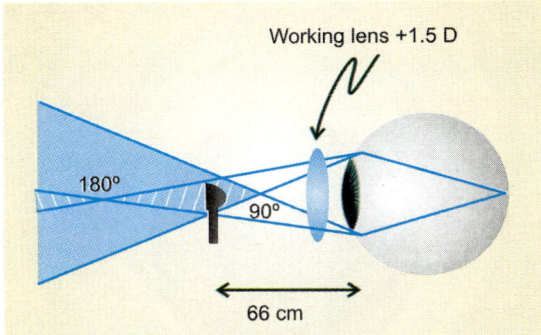

Fig. 11.32: Uncorrected mixed astigmatism

retinoscope. On retinoscopy 'against motion' in one meridian and 'with motion' in other meridian, i.e. 90 degree and 180 degree meridians, respectively (in our example) will be seen when retinoscopy is done from 66 cm distance using a working lens of +1.5 D as shown in Fig. 11.32.

Rare Retinoscopy Reflexes

Reflexes in Pseudophakia

Pseudophakia is a state of eye where an intraocular lens is implanted inside the eye after cataractous lens has been removed surgically. The retinoscopy images seen in these cases are of different types. There may be 'with motion' or 'against motion' or may have mixed movements of retinal reflex. Examiner needs to closely observe these reflexes to neutralize them, a wet retinoscopy is preferred over dry retinoscopy in these cases.

Reflexes in Aphakia

Aphakia is a state of eye where cataractous lens is removed surgically without implantation of an intraocular lens. The retinal reflexes seen in these cases are similar to those seen in high hypermetropic cases. In aphakia very slow moving, wide width and dull image is seen, when high plus lenses, say +6–7 D are added then the speed, brightness of reflex increases and width decreases (similar to a hypermetropic case).

Reflexes of Rare Types

- Scissor movement on retinoscopy means when one arm of retinal image is moving in opposite direction to that of other arm of retinal reflex, like the blades of scissor. Most of the time these images are difficult to assess, but on careful examination one can see that there are two arms of retinal reflex as shown in Fig. 11.33. Usually one arm is thicker and show 'with movement', whereas other arm will be thin and have 'against motion'.

- Oblique movement on retinoscopy means movement of reflex is not in coordination with our retinoscope intercept. In these cases when intercept of retinoscope is moved either horizontally or vertically the retinal reflex moves oblique to the movement of intercept either in 'with' or 'against' motion. Retinal reflex in these cases will appear as shown in Fig. 11.34.

- No movement on retinoscopy examination is considered when practically almost entire pupillary area is filled with reflex and examiner cannot see the boundary of retinal reflex easily. When observer try to move the streak of retinoscope in any meridian, say horizontal or vertical, no appreciable movement of retinal reflex will be seen. Clinically, these reflexes are very confusing and appear as shown in Fig. 11.35.

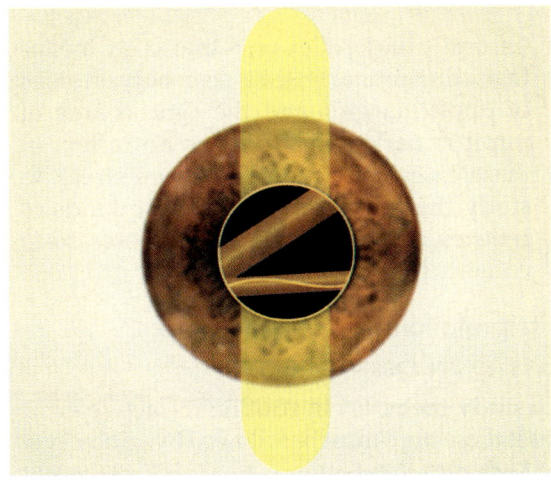

Fig. 11.33: Scissor reflex

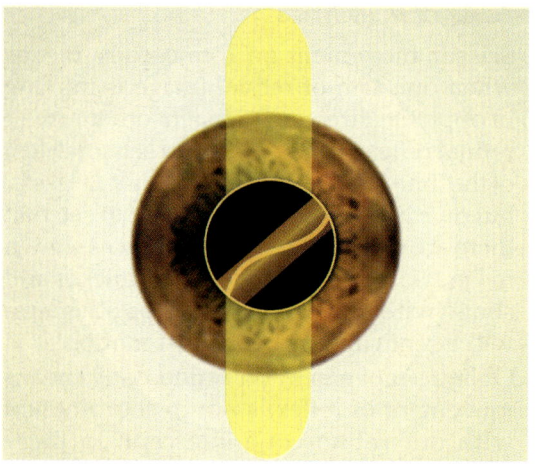

Fig. 11.34: Oblique retinal reflex

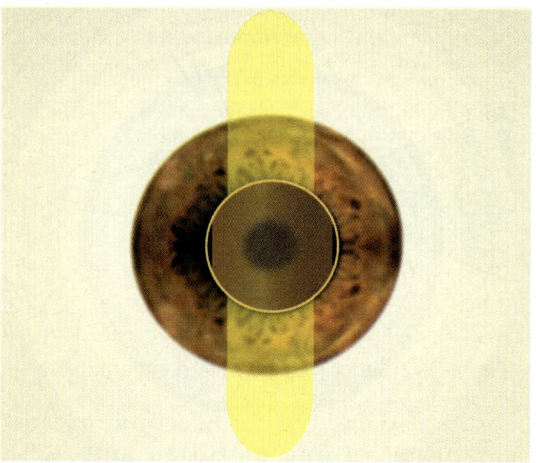

Fig. 11.36: Centrally dark retinal reflex

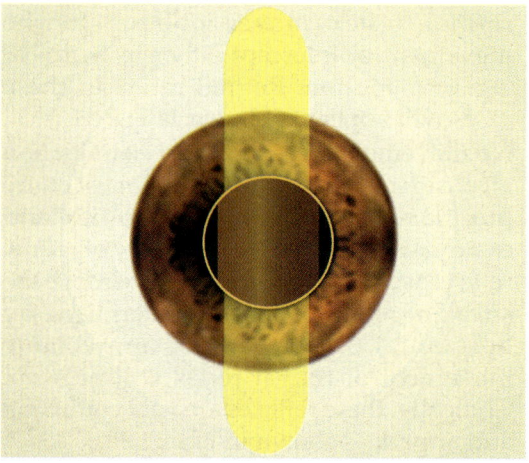

Fig. 11.35: Dim retinal reflex

- Centrally dark reflex on retinoscopy means that a dim retinal reflex is seen only on sides of pupil margins and the central area of pupil is dark, which shows no reflex. In these cases bend the retinoscope streak to study the characteristics of these kinds of reflexes, also examiner can lean forward to enhance the brightness of reflex (Fig. 11.36).

Interpretation of Retinal Reflexes

Routine Images

To study the reflex in routine refractive error cases these steps must be followed by an observer

- First decide whether retinal reflex is 'with' or 'against' movement which is decided by

the location of focal point relative to the observer's eyes, i.e. it is in front or behind the observer.

- Then it is important to judge the amount of 'with' or 'against' movement to decide how far the observer is from neutrality point. Certain identifiable characteristics of moving reflex will help in the estimation of distance from neutrality.
- Indirectly this will help to decide how much correcting lens power will be needed to move the focal point in conjugate to our retina.

Note: This experience in rough estimation of lens power will save much trial and error, and will shorten the time to reach at neutrality.

The moving retinal reflex can be characterized by three main features

Speed: Depending on the distance from focal point, the retinal reflex moves very slowly when retinoscope is situated far from the focal point and it becomes more rapid as retinoscope gets closer to focal point. When neutrality point is reached, the pupil fills with light reflex and no movement of retinoscope streak is seen. In simpler words, large degree refractive errors will have a slow moving retinal reflex and small degree refractive errors will have a fast moving retinal reflex (Fig. 11.37).

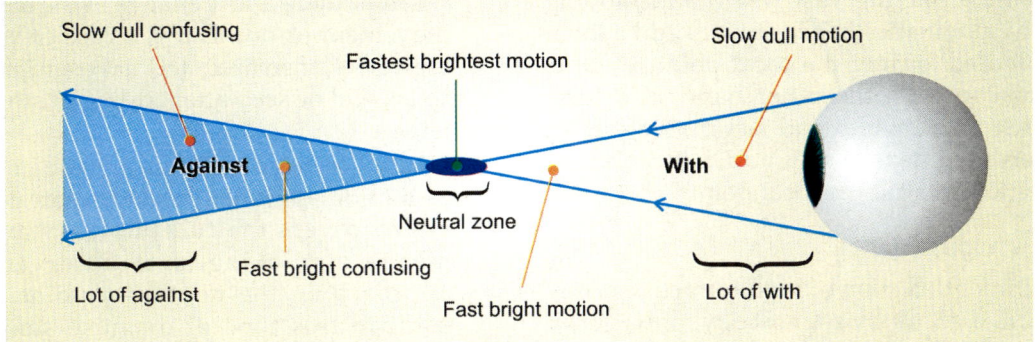

Fig. 11.37: Speed and brightness of reflex at various intervals in relation to position of retinoscope

Brightness: The retinal reflex will appear dull when retinoscope is situated far from the focal point and it will become brighter as examiner approaches at the neutrality point. Hence, refractive errors of large degree will have a dull reflex and small degree refractive errors will have a brighter reflex (Fig. 11.37).

Note: In Fig. 11.37 against portion is shown as cross-hatched because against retinal reflex is dimmer as compared to with reflex at any comparable distance from the focal point.

Width: The width band of retinal reflex in the pupillary area is narrow when retinoscope is situated at a far distance from the focal point, width of the band broadens as the observer approaches near the focal point and ultimately reflex width will fill the entire pupil when the refractive error gets neutralized as shown in Fig.11.38.

However, in clinical practice these characteristic of reflex may be sometimes misleading in nature. For example, when retinoscope is situated very far away from neutrality point then the retinal reflex appears to become widen as if approaching the neutrality as discussed above. This state is termed pseudoneutrality and is commonly seen in very high degree of refractive errors, means when position of the retinoscope is a long way from the focal point.

However, with continuous practice of retinoscopy it becomes easy for examiner to find out the distance of focal point as observer becomes able to judge speed, brilliance and width of retinal reflex simultaneously. For example, when examiner notices enough 'with

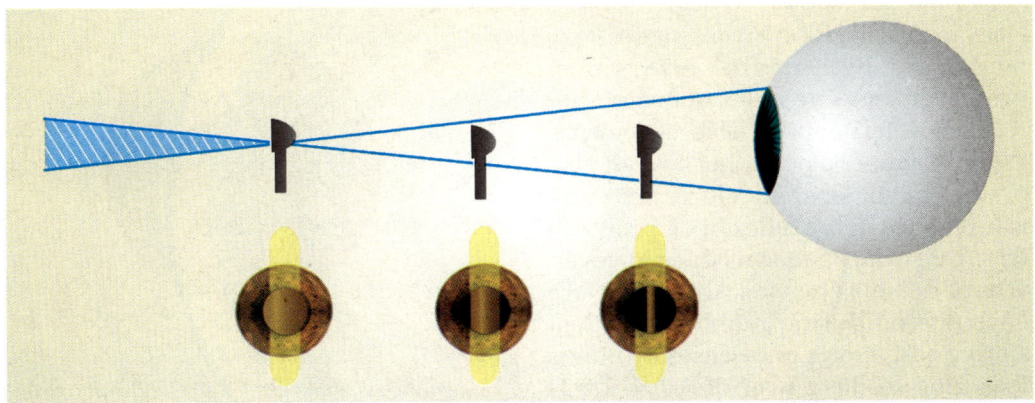

Fig. 11.38: Change in width of retinal reflex with distance of retinoscope

movement' having vast width and moving slowly, automatically he/she will add a lot of plus lenses to drag the focal point towards retinoscope. On the other hand, if a little 'against' small width and fast moving reflex is seen then he/she will add a little minus lenses to push out the focal point.

Rare Images

Sometimes detection of high refractive errors appears difficult by retinoscopy, however, it is not so difficult. Once the examiner is able to identify the type of error and does retinoscopy after partially correcting them, then these error starts appearing as routine small refractive errors and examiner can easily neutralize these errors as routine reflexes. For example, suppose if an aphakic patient is presented to clinic for retinoscopy. Patient is already wearing a +11 DS power spectacles and still is not able to see clearly. On retinoscopic examination, the retinal reflex seen in this patient is peculiar and it is little difficult to assess the movement or margins of reflex. Simply, add + 8 or +9 D spherical lens in the trial frame (as the patient is aphakic) and again observe the retinal reflex. Now it will be a nice smooth with reflex which can easily be neutralize by adding more plus power lenses gradually.

It is very important to recognize presence of high spheric error because sometimes they may remain unrecognizable due to presence of

- Hazy media disguise: In presence of hazy media, the high degree errors may present either as no reflex or a very dull reflex showing no appreciable movements. When examiner place either a weak plus or weak minus lens and notices that there is no change in the reflex, then probably it is a case of an opaque media. However, when these types of situation are encountered during retinoscopy, then simply add strong plus lenses or minus lenses up to the power of 5.0 to 7.0 D directly. Reassess the retinal reflex whether there is any change in the reflex movement or not. If it is a case of very high error, then definitely a recognizable reflex will be seen after adding of strong lenses.

- Neutrality disguise. These are also called as motionless reflex (pseudoneutrality) which covers the full pupillary area, means mimicking as if observer is approaching the neutrality point. To confirm this type of disguise simply move forward about 15–20 cm and now again assess the movement. If the characteristics of reflex do not change, means we are not near to neutrality, now add the strong plus or minus lenses to check whether there is any movement. If high refractive error is present, then there will be a definite reflex movement after adding the strong power lenses (Fig. 11.39).

Various retinal reflexes encountered during regular retinoscopy examination and their interpretation is shown in Table 11.1.

Neutralization of Various Reflexes

Neutralization State

Neutralization state is defined as the state achieved when the focal point of the emerging light lies at the peephole of retinoscope. At this

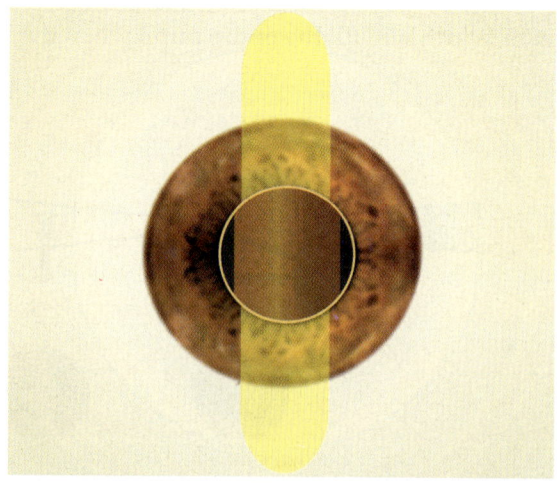

Fig. 11.39: Retinal reflex showing neutrality disguise

Table 11.1: Routine retinal reflexes and their interpretations

Retinal reflex	Characteristics	Interpretation
	Small width fast moving bright with reflex	Emmetropia or Hypermetropia/Myopia (less than 1D)
	Small width fast moving very bright against reflex	Myopia
	Medium width medium speed bright with reflex	Hypermetropia
	Medium width medium speed bright against reflex	Moderate degree myopia
	Large width slow moving dim with reflex	High degree hypermetropia
	Large width slow moving dim against reflex	High degree myopia
	Medium width medium speed dim reflex oblique to retinoscope streak	High degree astigmatism usually regular type
	Very large width no appreciable movement very dim reflex	High degree hypermetropia or myopia/ Aphakia
	Two reflexes moving against each other like blades of scissor one bright with and one dim against reflex	High degree irregular astigmatism, e.g. keratoconus

point the movement of reflex is not seen and is called neutral reflex. Trial correcting lens which is applied by the examiner to achieve this state of neutralization is the measurement of error of refraction. Hence, to achieve the state of neutrality the aim of the examiner is to bring the focal point to the peephole of retinoscope while simultaneously remains at the working distance.

Figure 11.40 tells about the approach which should be followed by the examiner to achieve this point of neutralization, while maintaining the working distance. If the examiner with retinoscope is situated in the cone of emerging

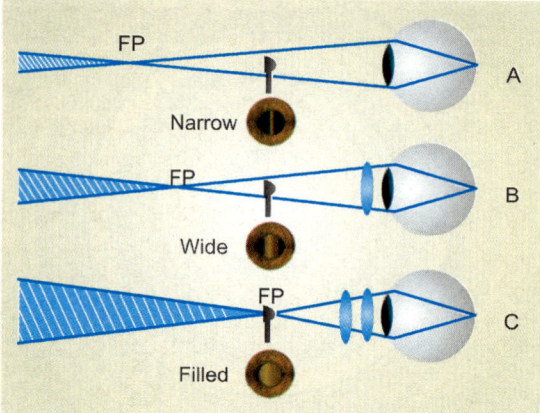

Fig. 11.40: Achieving neutralization state

light **(Fig. 11.40)** and the focal point is behind the examiner **(Fig. 11.40A)**. Now as the examiner adds the convex lens, the focal point starts moving towards retinoscope and the retinal reflex gradually gets widened **(Fig. 11.40B)**. After adding another plus power lens as the focal point reaches to the peephole of retinoscope, then the retinal reflex will fill the entire pupillary area and no movement can be appreciated. This is called the neutralization state of reflex **(Fig. 11.40C)**.

Note: In case of 'with motion' plus lenses are added; because the focal point lies behind the retinoscope and we need to pull it towards the peephole of retinoscope. On the other hand, in case of 'against motion' minus lenses are added, because the focal point lies in front of the retinoscope and we need to push it towards the peephole of retinoscope.

Although in routine practice of retinoscopy especially for beginners it is difficult to approach the neutralization state from 'against motion'. To simplify this, one can overcorrect 'against motion' by adding extra minus lenses so that the retinal reflex gets converted into 'with motion'. Now this 'with motion' can be neutralized by adding plus (means reducing minus) lenses, in smaller steps, say 0.25 D power. This approach to achieve neutralization is superior and easier as compared to neutrality achieved by gradually increasing the power of minus lenses.

Avoid against movement: Practically while neutralizing any retinal reflex, 'against motion' creates more difficulty than 'with motion' so always try to avoid these against motions.

Study these following reflexes carefully:

As shown in **Fig. 11.41B** that 'against motion' appears first at the side of pupil opposite to the streak of retinoscope. When streak is moved across the pupil, this reflex moves in a reverse direction across the entire pupil and finally get disappear on the opposite side of the retinoscope streak. Because of this opposite, fast and disappearing property of 'against motion', it is difficult to quantify the three basic characteristics (speed, brilliance and width) of reflex with 'against motion'. For example, speed of the reflex cannot be assessed easily when it moves in a reverse direction. Similarly, as the 'against motion' moves always away from the illuminated retina, its brightness is reduced and hence reflex margins become hazy. Because of these blurry reflex margins, the width of the reflex is also difficult to appreciate clearly.

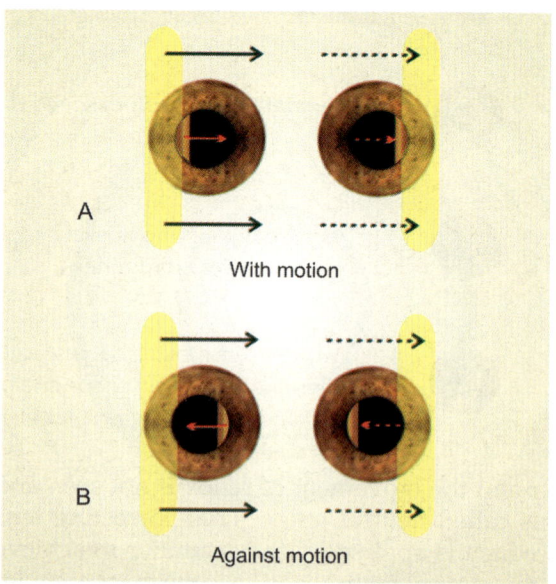

Fig. 11.41: Reflex movement. Compare retinoscope streak with retinal reflex and notice both types of movements: A. With motion; B. Against motion

Another problem with 'against reflex motion' is that it also poses difficulties during neutralization. The movement of 'against motion' opposite to streak of the retinoscope appears highly irregular especially, near neutrality state. 'Against motion' is usually dull, confusing, difficult to evaluate and measure, hence a general concept is that "when observer is unable to identify the type of reflex, then it is taken for granted that it is against reflex".

On the other hand, as shown in Fig. 11.41A 'with motion' reflex can be identified easily and is more feasible. The 'with reflex' is bright, crispy, rarely confusing and can be assessed without difficulty. A 'with motion' is highly dependable, easily agreeable and never contrary, hence one can quickly learn to recognize its degree, width and speed which helps to neutralize it faster and accurately. Therefore, whenever performing retinoscopy always first recognize 'with movement' if by chance 'against motion' is seen, then immediately convert it into 'with motion' by adding minus lenses.

"Always work with a WITH and against an AGAINST"

Rules to be followed to Achieve Neutralization

Rule 1: Suppose if 'with motion' is observed, then add plus lenses or reduce minus lenses until neutralization is attained.

Rule 2: Suppose if 'against motion' is observed, then add minus lenses or reduce plus lenses until 'with motion' is seen and then follow the rule 1 for neutralization.

Rule 3: For neutralization, always use plane mirror or keep sleeve up at working distance.

In the abovementioned rules the terms add plus (or minus) lenses or reduce minus (plus) lenses have been used. Remember the fact that "adding plus power is the same as that of reducing minus power or vice versa". By doing this basically we are changing the vergence of the emerging light rays which depend on the starting point. This concept can be understood by phenomenon of dioptric continuity which

can be elucidated with the help of a lens power wheel (Fig. 11.42) used in a lensometer. Rotation of this wheel in clockwise direction from any point will result in increase of minus power or decrease of plus power, while opposite occurs when rotated in counterclockwise direction, i.e. increase of plus or decrease of minus power. The signs and numbers mentioned on this wheel are irrelevant, only the direction of rotation of wheel has value.

Thus, either neutralizing case of myopia or a hypermetropia, the basic principle of neutralization remains the same. In case of 'with motion' the plus power lenses are added to increase the convergence of emitting light rays until there is no movement of reflex. Similarly, in 'against motion' minus power lenses are added to increase the divergence of emitting rays until 'with movement' is seen (then reduce the divergence of rays until neutralization state is reached).

"With motion is key to the neutrality or endpoint of retinoscopy and the power of lens with which it is achieved is the measure of refractive error".

Interpretation of Neutrality

In reality, neutrality is not a point rather it is area or zone created as a result of spherical aberrations and many other factors. Size of this zone varies with the size of pupil and working distance.

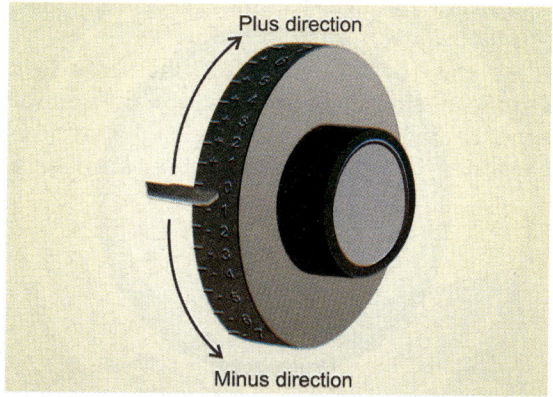

Fig. 11.42: Lens power wheel showing dioptric continuity

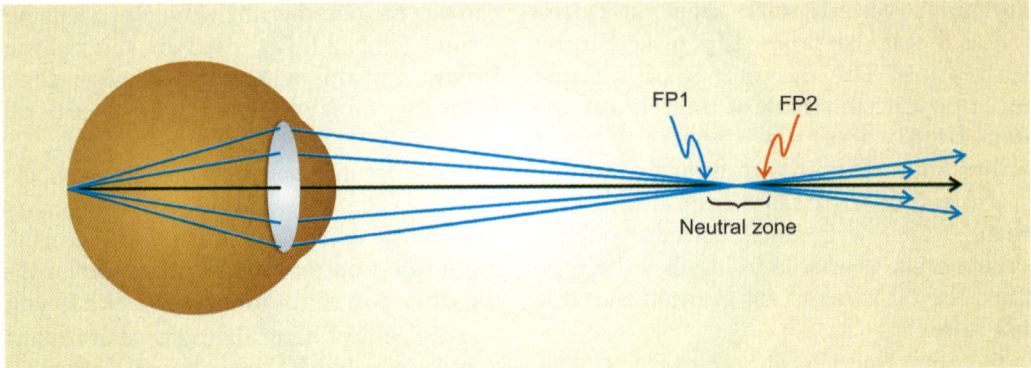

Fig. 11.43: Neutral zone; spherical aberration causes nearer focal point FP1 for axial rays, and a distant focal point FP2 for peripheral rays

Size of pupil: The width of neutral zone is directly proportional to the size of pupil. As the size of pupil increases, the width of this neutral zone also increases. In Fig. 11.43, we can see that there is no pupil in the eye thus the zone of neutrality is magnified due to spherical aberration. Axial rays are focused in nearest focal point (FP1) and peripheral rays on distant focal point (FP2). While doing retinoscopy on a dilated pupil, always concentrate only on the central pupillary reflex and avoid the peripheral aberrations.

Working distance: Width of neutral zone is narrowest when the working distance is closer, however, if the neutral zone is very narrow, then an accurate estimation of retinal reflex and working distance becomes so significant that even a minor inaccuracy may produce a major error in evaluation.

As shown in Fig. 11.44, that there is a significant amount of doubt within the neutral zone. Examiner remains indecisive about the presence or absence of reflex, similarly examiner is unable to assess the movement and position of the reflex within this neutral zone. Easiest way to avoid this confusion and stay in a safe (with) zone is to make a judgment of neutrality just before the doubt of movement begins as shown in Fig. 11.45.

In a nutshell accurate judgment of a neutrality state is a skill and basically it is to judge a point just before the zone of doubt appears, means there is still a weak 'with movement'. At this point when observer leans forward with retinoscope a definite and clear 'with motion' will be seen and if bend backwards then in the beginning an uncertain type of reflex movement and on further leaning backwards a confusing reflex suggestive of an early 'against motion' will be seen.

Various Neutralization Methods

Retinal reflex can be neutralized by either only spherical lenses (in cases of spherical and/or astigmatic errors) or by a combination of spherical and cylindrical lenses (in case of astigmatic error).

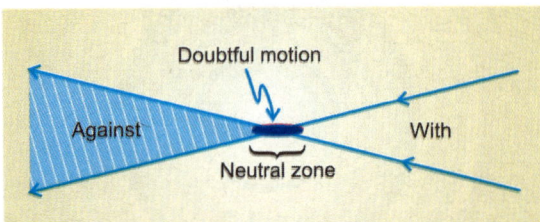

Fig. 11.44: Doubtful motion within neutral zone

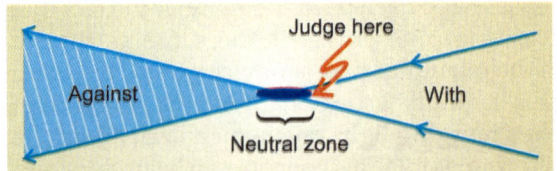

Fig. 11.45: Point of judgment for neutrality

Neutralizing with Only Spherical Lenses

To understand the neutralization with use of only spherical lenses, consider an example where on retinoscopy at 66 cm 'with motion' at 90° and a larger width slower moving 'with motion' at 180° is seen as shown in **Fig. 11.46**.

Now place a plus spherical lens (say +4 DS) at the 90° meridian (having lesser 'with motion') to neutralize this meridian. Now, on doing retinoscopy having +4 DS lenses in vertical meridian (90°) no reflex movement is seen, whereas horizontal meridian (180°) will still show 'with motion'. Continue to add plus spheres till this horizontal meridian becomes neutral. Suppose after adding an additional +2 D sphere (above +4 DS) 180° meridian also gets neutralized. These retinoscopy values will be recorded in the form of a retinoscopy cross as shown in **Fig. 11.47**.

This can also be represented as gross sphere + 4 Dsph × 90° + 6 Dsph × 180°

Deduction for the working distance (66 cm or +1.5 DS in our example) from this gross refraction will give +2.5 D × 90° +4.5 D × 180° net refraction value.

Note: Always reduce the working distance from gross sphere in both the meridian spheres.

It is important to understand that when neutralization is done using only spheres, it is necessary to measure and record the spherical value of the first meridian before performing retinoscopy for the second meridian. Hence, in the above example, when 90° meridian is reexamined after completing the neutralization in 180° meridian, this 90° meridian will show 'against motion' because now it is overcorrected by +2 DS. In cases of compound refractive errors when neutralization is done with only spheres both the meridians will not be seen as neutral at the same time.

Neutralization with only spheres is a good technique for children, as they resist wearing trial frame and it is practically very difficult to hold the cylindrical lens on its axis or hold two lenses for a longer duration. A lens rack as shown in **Fig. 11.48** is particularly useful while performing this retinoscopy method in clinic or when doing refraction under anesthesia.

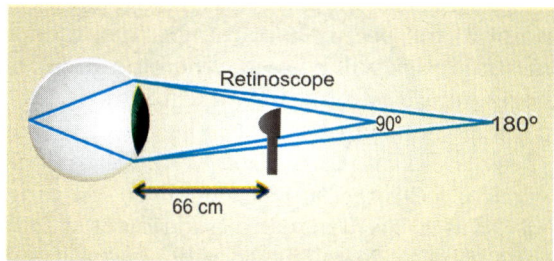

Fig. 11.46: Retinoscopy showing with motion at 90° and more with motion at 180°

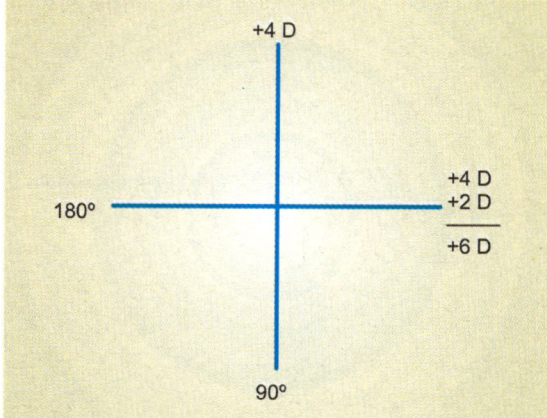

Fig. 11.47: Diagrammatic representation of neutralization with spheres

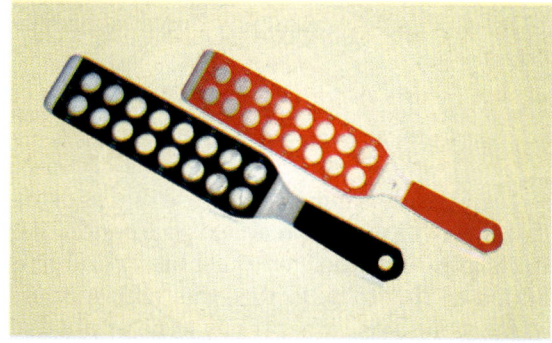

Fig. 11.48: Lens racks. Red color racks have minus lenses and black color has plus lenses. (*courtesy: Bernell Corporation*)

Neutralization with Spheres and Cylinders

Consider the same example as discussed above, where 90° meridian gets neutralized with +4D sphere, which is considered as spherical meridian. As per our previous discussion, spherical lenses produce power in all meridians, hence this +4 DS power (in our example) is also working in 180° meridian (which is still having 'with movement'). Add a +2 D cylinder at 180° axis to neutralize this 'with movement'. By adding + 2 D cylinder at 180° axis (horizontal meridian) there is no change in the reflex movement at 90° meridian because cylindrical lenses exert power only in one particular axis. This 180° meridian is considered as cylindrical meridian.

After neutralizing the principal meridians independently when the streak of retinoscope is rotated, both the meridians now appear neutral and show no movement of retinal reflex. This is more accurate method to neutralize compound refractive errors because both the meridians can be seen neutral at the same time.

In our example the gross refraction or lenses in front of eye are +4 DS/+2 DC × 180°.

Always write the spherical power first and then the cylindrical power with axis. As this is the gross refraction deduct the working distance of 66 cm, i.e. +1.5 D from spheres only to get the net refraction +2.5 DS/+2 DC × 180°.

Universally the spherical and cylindrical powers are written in this order hence this net refraction can also be conveniently written as +2.5/+2 × 180° (without any power abbreviations).

Note: No correction for working distance or cycloplegic is done from the cylindrical power.

Many readers may get confuse that as cylindrical power works on an axis perpendicular to its position, then why a plus cylinder is added at 180° to neutralize the 'with motion' at the same axis rather it has to be applied at 90° so that cylindrical power will be applicable at 180°. To understand this study the streak meridians and corneal meridians are discussed below.

Streak Meridian Versus Corneal Meridian

In reality, the orientation of retinoscopic reflexes does not correspond to corneal meridians. For example, the reflexes seen at 180° or horizontally on retinoscopy in reality are produced by the 90° corneal meridians and vice versa. In other words, retinoscope streak actually tests the power of corresponding corneal meridian. If retinoscope is scooped vertically, i.e. retinoscope streak is at 90° and examiner is moving the retinoscope sideways to judge the movement of reflex, then actually examiner is evaluating the refractive power of the eye at horizontal or 180° corneal meridian. Hence, when a cylinder is placed vertically or at 90°, it is going to neutralize the power of eye at 180°, i.e. perpendicular to the cylinder axis which in reality is the corneal meridian needed to be corrected in this example.

If 90° corneal meridian (say +47 D) has focal point at the peephole of retinoscope, then a neutral reflex will be seen, when the streak is horizontal (testing for 90 meridian). If 180° corneal meridian has only +44 D, so it will show a 3 D with motion when streak is vertical (testing for 180 meridian). Adding +3 DC at 90°, will in reality add power at 180° thus it will neutralize the reflex seen at 90° (Fig. 11.49).

Although it all looks a little confusing, a simple rule to remember is that "simply place

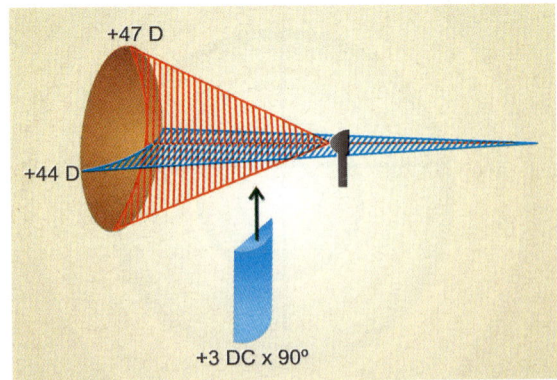

Fig. 11.49: Effect of corneal meridians on emerging rays.

a plus cylinder in the same axis where there is with movement". Hence it is very comfortable to neutralize compound refractive errors with a plus cylinder system. Once spherical meridian is neutralized, place the cylindrical axis of trial cylindrical lens on the same axis as that of remaining with reflex axis, this will correct the corneal cylindrical axis properly.

Ocular Meridians

Ocular meridians universally are defined from 1 to 180 degrees in both the eyes as shown in Fig. 11.50, there is no meridian labeled as 'zero' and there is nor any angle larger than 180°. Traditionally, right eye is abbreviated as OD (oculus dexter) and left eye as OS (oculus sinister).

Neutralization in Astigmatic Errors

As discussed before astigmatism is a phenomenon when the entire light rays do not refract to a single focal point. In aspheric eye all the ocular meridians refract the light differently because corneal surface is toric in nature. Ocular meridians which refract the light maximum and minimum are called 'Principal meridians'. Each of these principal meridians focuses the arriving light rays to a different point of focus at the back of the eye, which are called principal foci. These principal foci may be in front of the retina, on the retina or behind the retina; but for retinoscopy it is immaterial.

Neutralization of various types of astigmatic errors is done as

- In regular astigmatism the principal meridians are perpendicular or 90° to

each other, i.e. 90° and 180° and so on. These can be corrected by cylindrical lenses because they also have their principal meridian perpendicular to each other. For example, if a plus cylinder is placed with its axis in alignment with that of most refracting or stronger meridian, then it will add power to the weaker meridian. Hence, when the correcting cylindrical lens placed in proper axis, which equals the corneal cylinder, then the meridians gets balance and astigmatism gets neutralized, as a spherical condition of eye had been created by balancing the corneal cylinder with cylindrical lens power.

- In an irregular astigmatism principal meridians are not perpendicular to each other; hence they cannot be neutralized with cylinders alone. These conditions are usually caused due to corneal irregularities.

- An oblique astigmatism is simply a regular astigmatism, where principal meridians are perpendicular to each other, but are not usual (90°/180°) and it should not be confused with irregular astigmatism. The principal meridians are tilted, for example, at 45°/135°. These can be neutralized with cylinders similar to a regular astigmatism.

- 'With the rule' astigmatism is referred to a condition where correcting plus cylindrical axis is more or less vertical, i.e. between 75° and 105°. 'Against the rule' astigmatism refers to a condition where the correcting plus cylindrical axis is more or less horizontal, i.e. 15° to 165°. These conditions generally describe the location of most refracting corneal meridians and hence the axis of its accompanying plus cylindrical lenses.

- Symmetrical astigmatism is a condition where the total axis of correcting cylinders of both the eyes equals to 180°; means, for example, OD 70° and OS 110°. These can be corrected by cylindrical lenses easily as in regular astigmatism.

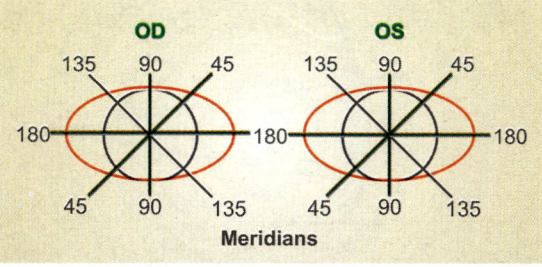

Fig. 11.50: Ocular meridians

- Asymmetrical astigmatism is a condition where the axis of cylinders of both the eyes has no rule, means, for example, OD 75° and OS 25°. These conditions are not abnormal but are rare, hence whenever such conditions are encountered try to reevaluate the retinoscopy.

Note: Usually in younger people the most refracting corneal meridian is vertical and in older people it is horizontal, means over the years of age a young person having 'with the rule' astigmatism will develop an 'against the rule' astigmatic in older age.

Simple astigmatism whether it is simple hypermetropic or simple myopic are in fact simple to neutralize because one of the principal meridians is already neutral at working distance and second meridian can easily be neutralized by either plus or minus cylinder.

Figure 11.51 represents example of simple hypermetropic astigmatism where one principal meridian, say 90°, is neutral and other principal meridian, i.e. 180°, is showing 'with motion' at working distance of 66 cm (keeping working lens in the position). We simply need to add a plus cylinder at 180° with gradual increasing in power until with motion gets neutralize.

Figure 11.52 represents an example of simple myopic astigmatism where 180° meridian is 'neutral' and 90° meridian is showing 'against motion' at working distance of 66 cm (keeping working lens in the position). Neutralization in this case is a little complicated, first add minus spheres to push

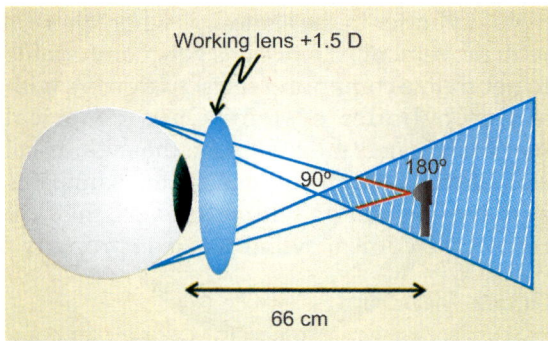

Fig. 11.52: Simple myopic astigmatism

out the focal point of myopic meridian (90°) and neutralize it. This minus sphere has also pushed out the focal point at 180° meridian and converted it into 'with motion' which was initially neutral. Now add plus cylinders at 180° meridian to neutralize this with movement.

Compound astigmatism is a condition where neither meridian is neutral at working distance of 66 cm (keeping working lens in position). This could be of following types

- Compound hypermetropic astigmatism
- Compound myopic astigmatism
- Compound mixed astigmatism

These conditions seem difficult to neutralize, but simply the rules of neutralization are followed to convert these three conditions first into simple hypermetropic astigmatism and then neutralize them accordingly.

Compound hypermetropic astigmatism **(Fig. 11.53)** can easily be neutralized because

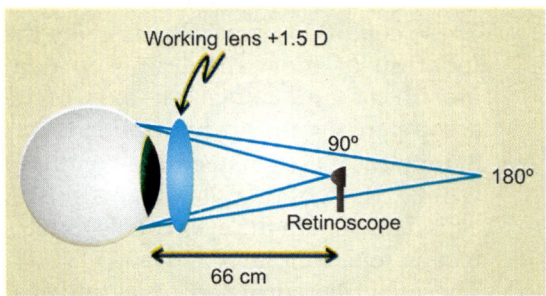

Fig. 11.51: Simple hypermetropic astigmatism

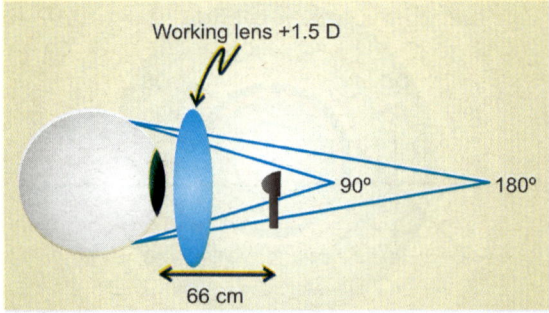

Fig. 11.53: Compound hypermetropic astigmatism

both the principal meridians are having a 'with motion' although of different amount. First add plus spheres until the weaker or least with meridian (spherical meridian) becomes neutralized. Now add plus cylinder to neutralize the stronger with meridian (cylindrical meridian). Now rotate the streak of retinoscope in both the directions to confirm that both the meridians are neutral.

In compound myopic astigmatism (Fig. 11.54) both the principal meridians show 'against motion', and it is difficult to assess which meridian is more against or stronger. First add strong minus spheres to push out the focal points beyond retinoscope, this gives a friendly 'with motion' in both the meridians. Now simply proceed as in the case of a compound hypermetropic astigmatism. Slowly reduce the minus spherical powers or add plus spherical powers, until first meridian (more myopic) gets neutralize, add plus cylinders in the opposite meridian (least myopic) to neutralize the remaining 'with motion'.

Mixed astigmatism (Fig. 11.55) is a condition where both 'with and against movement' are seen in different meridians. First add minus spheres until 'against movement' becomes 'with movement', then slowly reduce the minus spherical power or add plus spherical power to neutralize this meridian. Once this is done, then the opposite meridian having 'with movement' can easily be neutralize by using plus cylinders.

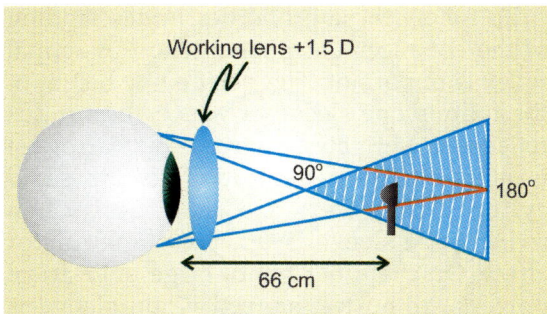

Fig. 11.55: Mixed astigmatism

To summarise the principles of neutralization

- First neutralize the least hypermetropic or most myopic meridian with appropriate spheres, means first neutralize the meridian having focal point closer to patient's eye.
- Now neutralize remaining most hypermetropic or least myopic meridian by using plus cylinders, because this meridian will always show 'with movement' means fill the remaining astigmatic interval by using plus cylinders in the opposite meridian which has a focal point farthest from patient's eye.

Note: However, in these illustrations the actual amount of refractive error is not mentioned, because while performing the retinoscopy amount of refractive error is immaterial. Simply neutralize the reflexes in all the meridians and get the gross refraction, then deduct the values of working distance and cycloplegic (if used) from gross refraction and one can get the actual amount of refractive error.

Estimation of Cylindrical Axis and Power

Estimation of Cylindrical Axis

To understand the direction of cylindrical axis four properties of retinal reflexes are needed to be studied such as

- Break
- Width
- Intensity
- Skew

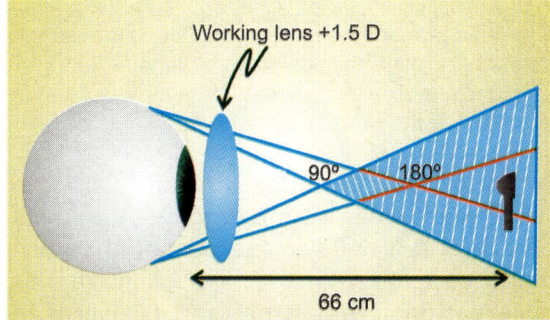

Fig. 11.54: Compound myopic astigmatism

To follow these properties understanding of the enhancement phenomenon of retinal reflex is important. The position or height of the retinoscope sleeve at which the fundus reflex seen is brightest, sharpest and narrowest is called enhancement position. Usually small cylindrical powers are seen well when retinoscope sleeve is up, i.e. plane mirror effect. On the other hand, large cylindrical powers are best enhanced when sleeve is down, i.e. concave mirror effect.

Image of retinoscope streak on the surface of eye is called intercept. In low cylindrical powers the retinal reflex is narrowest when intercept is wide, while in high cylindrical powers the reflex is narrowest when intercept is narrow as shown in Fig. 11.56.

Break: When retinoscopy streak is off axis, i.e. not on the correct astigmatic axis (XX' in our example), then a break is seen. Here, intercept and streak are not parallel, hence a broken line is formed which can easily be observed by rotating the retinoscopy streak on either sides of astigmatic fundus reflex as shown in Fig. 11.57A.

This break will disappear when intercept and retinal reflex become parallel, means retinoscope streak is on the correct astigmatic

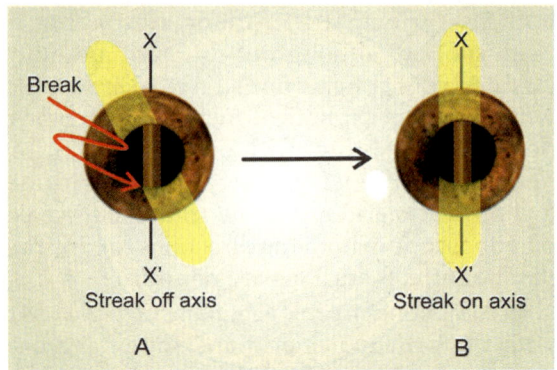

Fig. 11.57: Phenomenon of break

axis, i.e. on XX' axis (at 90° in our example) in Fig. 11.57B. We will place the correcting cylindrical lens on this axis for neutralization in trial fame. To practice, adjust the retinoscopy sleeve at enhancement position and rotate the sleeve about 15° on either side of XX' axis, i.e. at 75° and 105°. A break which will be more clear at the extremes of this arc (i.e. 75° and 105°) will be seen and it will be less appreciable when examiner approaches near XX' axis, i.e. 90°; and no break in intercept will be seen exactly at 90°.

Thickness: Thickness of retinal reflex modifies when examiner rotates the streak on either sides of the correct astigmatic axis. The reflex is narrowest when the streak of retinoscope is on the correct axis and becomes wide as it moves away from the correct axis. For example, if astigmatic axis is 115° (XX in Fig. 11.58), then the width of retinal reflex will change as retinoscope move on either sides of correct axis or will be narrowest at correct axis.

Note: To practice retinoscopy, enhance the retinal reflex and rotate the streak on either side of 115° (in our example for correct astigmatic axis) observe the change in width of retinal reflex.

Intensity: Retinal reflex intensity varies to some extent when examiner rotates the streak off-axis and it will become very bright when on the correct astigmatic axis. Although, this observation is indistinct and is useful in patients having low degree astigmatism,

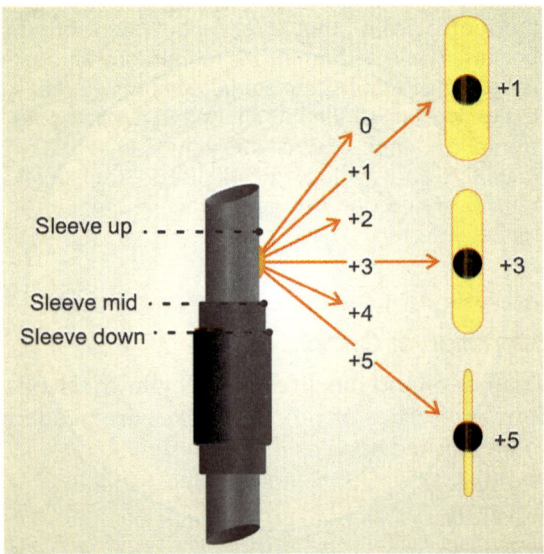

Fig. 11.56: Enhancement and midpoint position

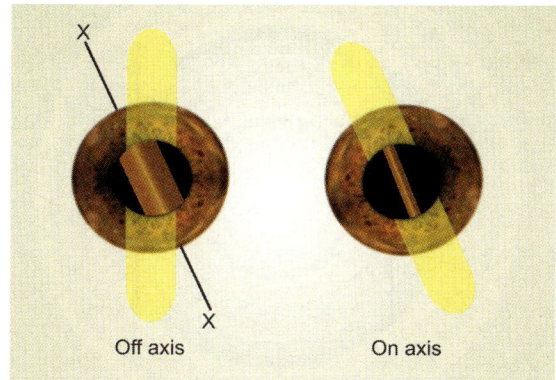

Fig. 11.58: Change in thickness of reflex

because small cylinders cannot be enhanced, whereas larger cylinders can be enhanced to high brightness.

Skew: Skew is also called oblique motion and is used to refine the cylindrical axis in small power cylinders. In this case examiner does not rotate the retinoscope streak rather moves his/her head or wiggle the retinoscope streak in a 30° zone. Notice the movement of retinal reflex in comparison of intercept. Retinal reflex will move parallel to intercept if streak is on the correct axis and when the streak is off axis, the retinal reflex and intercept will move in different directions.

As shown in Fig. 11.59, consider that the correct axis of astigmatism is XX (90 degree), but retinoscope streak is at somewhere X'X'

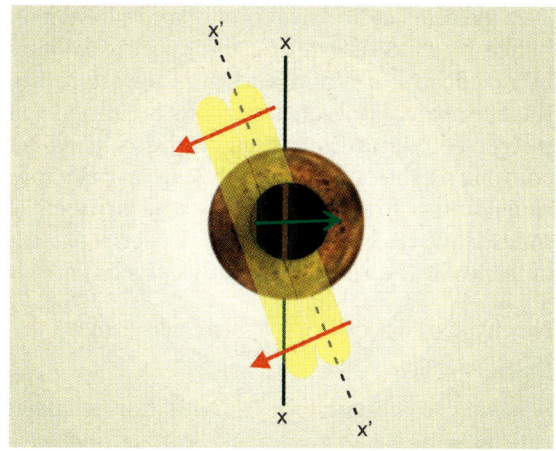

Fig. 11.59: Skewed motion

(say 110 degree). Now when examiner moves his/her head 'against motion' of retinal reflex in comparison to retinoscope intercept will be seen. This movement of retinal reflex in comparison to movement of intercept is called as skewed motion.

> **Note:** All these four characteristics help in determination of correct cylindrical axis. Break and thickness of retinal reflex help in high degree astigmatic errors, whereas intensity and skew motion help in low degree astigmatic errors.

Estimation of Cylindrical Power

As discussed before, gradually widening of pupillary reflex indicates that the point of neutralization is approaching. To estimate the cylindrical power, first neutralization of spherical power is done and then the width of retinal reflex in the astigmatic axis will give a rough estimate of the amount of astigmatism and hence the power of cylinder requires for neutralizing. As a general rule width of astigmatic reflex is inversely proportional to degree of astigmatism; i.e. thinner the astigmatic reflex, larger will be the degree of astigmatism.

Low degree astigmatism cannot be enhanced, hence width of retinal reflex in astigmatic axis gives an estimate of amount of cylindrical power require to neutralize it. Whereas high degree astigmatic errors can be enhanced, hence width of retinal reflex shows a gradual narrowing along with decrease width of intercept (Fig. 11.60). In these cases the width of intercept required to enhance the

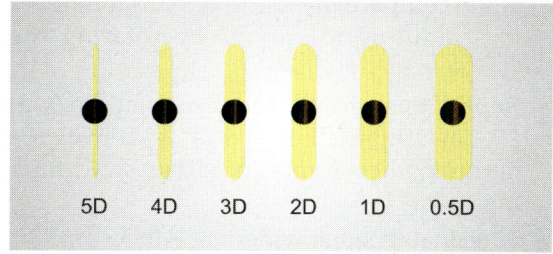

5D   4D   3D   2D   1D   0.5D

Fig. 11.60: Narrowing of retinal reflex width with decreasing intercept width in cases of high cylindrical power

retinal reflex gives an estimate of amount of cylinder which is required to neutralize the reflex.

Note: Once a rough estimate of amount of cylindrical power is obtained, then astigmatic errors can be neutralized with routine technique with keeping sleeve up. "An accurate location of cylindrical axis cannot be achieved with an incorrect cylindrical power; an accurate cylindrical power cannot be achieved with an incorrect cylindrical axis".

Refining Cylindrical Axis and Power

Refining Cylindrical Axis

The method used to refine the cylindrical axis is called straddling. In this technique the correcting cylinder is placed in the axis obtained by neutralization methods as discussed above. Straddling meridians are situated at 45° away on either sides of the astigmatic axis at which the examiner had placed the correcting cylinders and needs to be compared at sleeve up position. For example, if correct axis of astigmatism is at 90° and examiner had placed the correcting cylindrical lens axis at 100°, then the straddling meridians will be 55° and 145° as shown in Fig. 11.61.

Refining Method

- Place the entire correction of cylindrical power in the position and perform retinoscopy while comparing the width of retinal reflexes in each straddling meridian.
- Slowly move back to about 10 cm distance keeping retinoscope in the position and again compare the width of retinal reflexes in straddling meridians by rotating the sleeve.
- Repeat this procedure by moving back at 10 cm steps till there is widening or neutralization in one of either straddling meridians is seen.
- Note that whether widening is in 55° or 145° axis. Because there is difference in width of reflex at the same distance, it means there is an axis error.

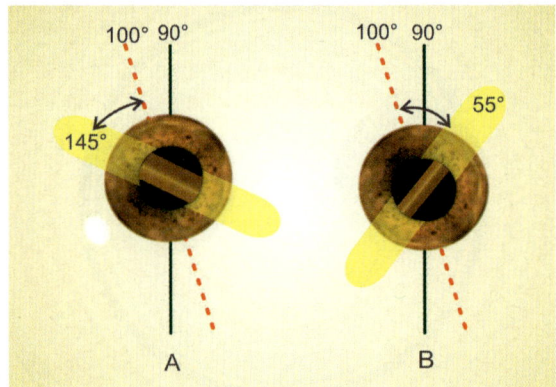

Fig. 11.61: Straddling meridians and respective retinal reflex width

- In our example as shown in Fig. 11.61 widening of reflex is occurring at 145° axis and retinal reflex remains narrow at 55° meridian, then this 55° axis is called guide. Now to correct the axis error, turn the correcting plus cylinder axis towards 55° (initially in 5° steps) means make 100° as 95°.
- Again check the straddling meridians and see if there is any axis error or not.
- If still there is an axis error, then slowly turn the correcting plus cylinder axis towards the narrow reflex axis (guide) in 2° steps (means from 95° to 93°) and so on till there is no difference in width of reflexes.

Refining Cylindrical Power

As a rule an incorrect cylindrical axis will not give a correct cylindrical power and vice versa, hence by rule first refine the cylindrical axis by straddling method and then before refine the cylindrical power. Once axis is refined the power of cylinders can easily be refined by comparing the neutralization state in principal meridians. First neutralize the spherical meridian and then refine the correcting cylinder at the refined cylindrical axis.

Neutralization of Rare Refractive Errors

Scissor Reflex

Scissor movement will be considered when retinal reflex has two arms joined one side (usually nasally) and open on other side (usually temporally). These two arms move in opposite directions to each other when examiner moves retinoscope streak in either vertical or horizontal meridians.

- To neutralize this scissor reflex as shown in Fig. 11.62, first see which arm is moving in 'with direction'.
- Then neutralize the movement of the arm which is moving in 'with motion' of scope by using plus spherical power lenses.
- Now focus on the remaining arm and observe its movement, whether it moves 'with or against' the scope and what is the meridian.
- If 'with movement' is seen then add plus cylinder in the meridian where motion is seen till there is no movement of reflex is observed.
- If 'against movement' is seen, then add minus cylinder in that particular meridian of motion till there is no movement of reflex is noticed.
- Note down the power of spherical lens and cylindrical lens along with axis.
- Recheck both the arms of reflex for any kind of movement.

Oblique Reflex

Oblique movement is seen when there is astigmatism or compound refractive errors. The reflex will move oblique to the scope.

- To neutralize this oblique retinal reflex (Fig. 11.63) change the direction of retinoscope intercept parallel to the oblique meridian in which the retinal reflex is moving.
- Notice the movement of retinal reflex with retinoscope movement.
- If movement of reflex is 'with' streak, then add plus cylinder in that particular meridian, till no movement of reflex is seen.
- If movement of retinal reflex is 'against' the retinoscope streak, then add minus cylinder in the same meridian till no further movement of reflex is noticed.
- Sometimes when we scope horizontally the reflex movement is 'with' and in vertical

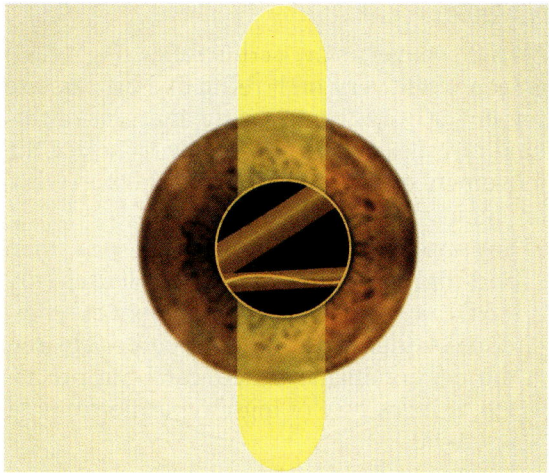

Fig. 11.62: Scissor reflex

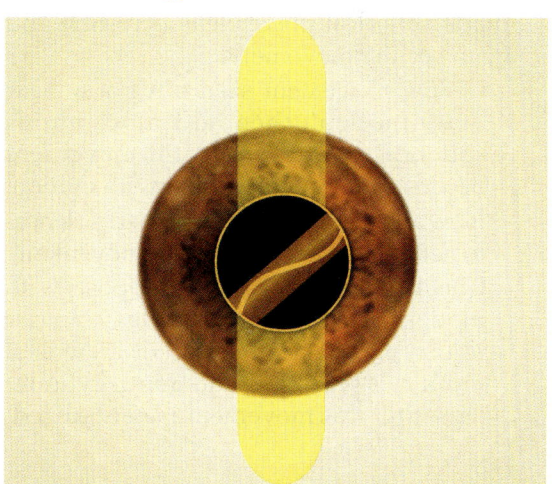

Fig. 11.63: Oblique retinal reflex

meridian the movement becomes oblique. In these cases first neutralize the horizontal meridian by plus spheres and change the scope parallel to other meridian and see whether 'with or against' movement. If see 'with motion' in oblique meridian, then add plus cylinders and if 'against motion', then add minus cylinders to neutralize this remaining oblique retinal reflex.

- Note the spherical and cylindrical power of lenses with axis.
- Recheck all meridians whether there is any residual movement present or not.

No Reflex

No reflex or very slow or dim reflex (Fig. 11.64) is seen when very high refractive powers are present. Always try to see the margins of this kind of reflexes, and if seen try to notice the movement of reflex with streak whether 'with' or 'against'.

- Suppose slow 'with motion' is seen, then add high plus spherical power lenses (say +6 D) and again see the movement of reflex. Usually the retinal reflex becomes clearer, thinner and its movement can be appreciated, if it is a case of high hypermetropia or aphakia.
- Suppose very dim retinal reflex is present and no margins are seen, then try high minus spherical power lens (say–6D) and again see the movement.
  - If slow movement seen but not a clear 'with motion', then add more minus spherical power lenses, till movement becomes clearer and crisper with motion.
  - Now add small power plus spherical lenses to neutralize this clearer 'with movement'.
  - Check other meridian and suppose 'with motion' is seen, then add plus cylinder in that particular meridian or if 'against motion' is seen, then add minus cylinder lenses till this movement is neutralized.

Note: Sometimes dim reflex can be neutralized by starting with addition of high plus spherical lenses, especially in cases where adding quite high power minus spherical lenses are unable to produce a clearer with motion.

Centrally Dark Reflex

Centrally dark reflex (Fig. 11.65) is seen in media opacity cases like cataract or corneal opacities. Always dilate these patients for retinoscopy, because it is very difficult to appreciate any kind of reflex centrally, however, after dilatation one can see some peripheral retinal reflexes.

- Try to see the sides of reflex motion, which is seen on the periphery of reflex and notice the movement.
- Suppose if 'with motion' is seen in periphery, add plus spherical power lenses and if 'against motion' (rarely appreciable) is seen, add minus spherical power lenses.
- Neutralize all meridians by rotating scope in vertical, horizontal and other meridians by basic principal of neutralization.
- Note the power of neutralizing lenses and recheck the movement.

Note: In majority of these cases even after dilatation, retinoscopy is not easy and results are variable even in an expert's hand.

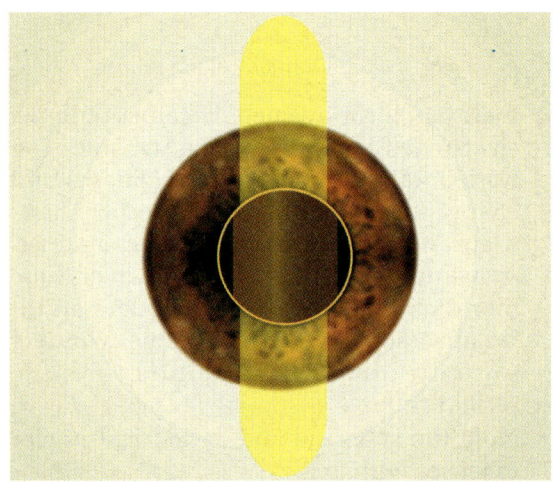

Fig. 11.64: No reflex or very slow or dim retinal reflex

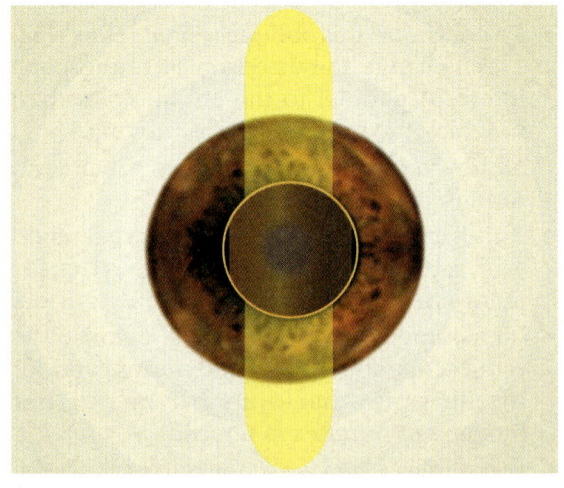

Fig. 11.65: Centrally dark retinal reflex

Retinoscopy After Refractive Surgery

Retinoscopy method remained constant since day of its origin, however; important advances have been achieved in refractive surgery field. These new techniques have resulted in new challenges by producing various kinds of new retinal reflexes postoperatively. Development of newer corneal procedures generated the possible need to re-evaluate the routine retinoscopy techniques. Many a times, after corneal refractive surgery, ambiguous retinoscopic reflexes are seen depending on the patient selection, type of procedure, and complications arising after surgery (radial keratotomy, photorefractive keratotomy, penetrating keratoplasty, etc.)

Nowadays, LASIK surgery is the most commonly performed procedure for correction of refractive errors. Depending on various factors like use of different types of lasers, surgical techniques and instruments and patient's cornea, LASIK surgery can produce its own set of unique reflexes.

The optical zone of cornea (laser treated area) may differ in the geographic location and size. Moreover, the position of optical zone may not align with the visual axis of eyes. Due to all these variations, a number of possible reflexes may be seen in postoperative period. In early postoperative period (say first week) all these variables vary in nature. Continuous change of variables gives challenges to ophthalmologist and makes their job much more exciting as well as frustrating.

Refraction in post-LASIK patients is mainly discussed, however, these principles can be applied on other refractive surgery also done on the cornea.

- Usually in first few days after procedure, the good retinoscopic reflex of any type is not seen and also no directional indications are seen.
- Moving the retinoscope forward or backward will give no result, however, sometimes examiner may see two or three distinct areas of retinal reflexes. Out of these reflexes which one to be used

for neutralization will be a dilemma for the examiner.

- By experience one will know that whenever in doubt always concentrate on the reflex in the center of the pupil; a principal specifically used after corneal surgery.
- When central reflex is identified and point of neutralization is reached in the center of pupil, examiner may get confused by seeing 'with or against' reflexes in the surrounding cornea.
- Make sure to concentrate on the point of neutralization or neutrality reflex in the pupillary center because if examiner over refract this point an odd reflex will be seen which differs from "scissors" movement.
- This odd reflex becomes wider in one meridian and becomes narrower in the other meridian; and to some observers will appear as a "Guillotine effect".
- Hence observe very carefully in the center and judge neutrality when central retinal reflex is still having a little 'with motion'.

Rarely, surface reflections or glare from the flat treated cornea may interfere in the interpretation of fundus reflex and produces difficulty in assessing the type of reflex. When this becomes problematic, just move the streak of retinoscope to sideways. This method will decentre the retinal reflections from the centre of pupil as shown in Fig. 11.66.

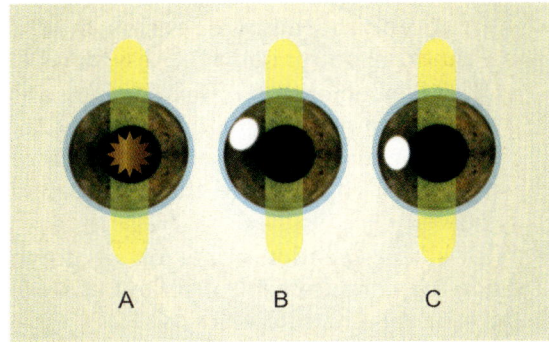

Fig. 11.66: Refractor reflections (A) Glare seen when centered on axis. (B) High reflex on lens indicates that too high. (C) Ideal situation in which reflex is beside pupil.

First post-operative month after LASIK appears to be most challenging and it is better to wait till this situation subsides because as the corneal edema disappears, the retinal reflexes become sharper and one can easily interpret them.

> **Note:** Always be sure to concentrate only on the central and treated areas of cornea, while ignore the reflexes from the peripheral rim of cornea, as they vary considerably. Never get confused by these extra or contra-movements from corneal periphery, simply focus on the central cornea.

Summary of Retinoscopy

Any type of refractive error can be neutralized via these six cardinal steps of neutralization.

Step 1: Use spheres
- Keep sleeve of retinoscope in up position, i.e. plane mirror effect, and observe reflexes in all the meridians to find 'with motion'.
- Then place appropriate power spheres to get 'with motion' in all meridians at your working distance.
- Now neutralize the spherical meridian or meridians (first, weakest or least with motion) by adding plus spheres or reducing minus spheres.

Step 2: Estimation of cylindrical axis and power
- Observe the remaining with meridian by making retinoscope sleeve down, which causes enhancement:
  - If no enhancement of reflex means cylindrical power is low, i.e. less than 1 D
  - If enhancement of reflex seen means cylindrical power is high, i.e. more than 1 D, means need to see the width of intercept to estimate the cylindrical power.
- With sleeve position either up or down (showing enhancement of reflex) observe the four axis characteristics as
  - Break
  - Thickness in high cylindrical powers
  - Intensity
  - Skew in low cylindrical powers

- Pin point the axis on the trial frame marking by moving sleeve down for enhancing the retinal reflex.

Step 3: Place cylinder on axis
An estimated power cylinder is placed at an approximate axis (the remaining with meridian).

Step 4: Refining of cylindrical axis
Cylindrical axis is refined by straddling method, i.e. move the sleeve up and then lean forward, now gradually recede in straddling meridians. Turn the cylindrical axis as per guidelines.

Step 5: Refining cylindrical power
Move the retinoscope sleeve in up position and lean forward; now recede gradually comparing the reflex in principal meridians. Gradually adjust the plus cylindrical powers until these meridians appear equally filled at same distance.

Step 6: Refine spheres
Check the working distance and gradually adjust the spherical powers (if needed) to get neutralization at 66 cm distance.

> **Note:** Once the retinal reflexes are neutralized, a subjective verification of retinoscopy findings are necessary and a subjective refraction is performed.

OBJECTIVE AND SUBJECTIVE REFRACTION

Objective Refraction

With this enormous theoretical knowledge of retinoscopy one can start retinoscopy on the patient practically as follows
- A fixation target is presented to the patient and a trial frame is placed, keeping both the eyes open.
- Advice the patient to fixate on the target with his/her right eye, while examiner scope the left eye of patient as shown in **Fig. 11.67A**.
- Study the reflexes and make them 'with motion'.
- Neutralize the retinal reflexes by using six cardinal steps.

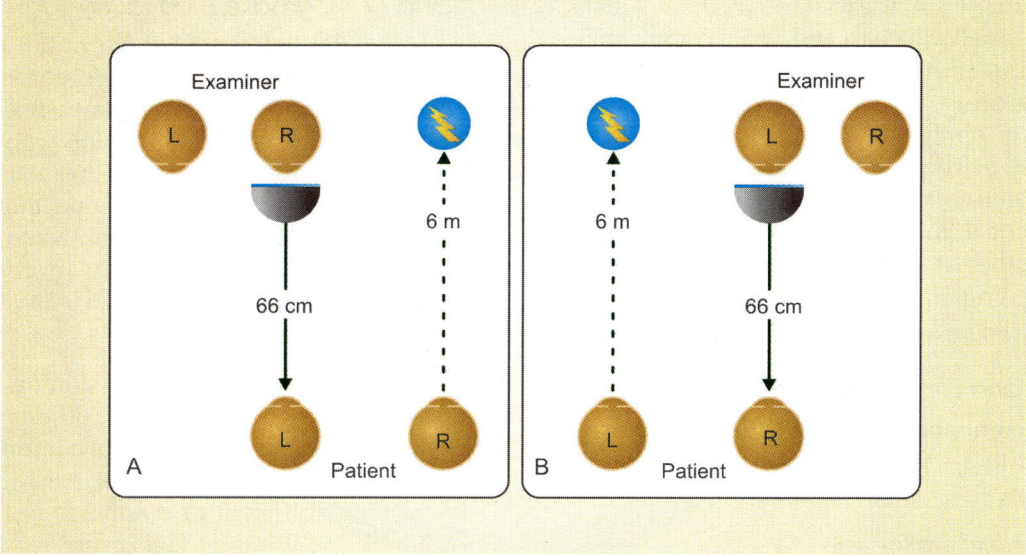

Fig. 11.67: Retinoscopy method: A. For patient's left eye; B. For patient's right eye

- Now scope the right eye while patient is fixating the target with his/her left eye as shown in Fig. 11.67B.
- Repeat the same procedure to neutralize, as in right eye.
- Note the gross retinoscopy values in both the meridians.

Subjective Refraction

Once an estimate of refractive error is obtained by objective retinoscopy as described above, a subjective verification is done. This is less time consuming and not very cumbersome, however, when objective refraction is impossible in conditions like media opacities or dense hazy media, examiners are dependent only on this subjective refraction for improvement in visual acuity.

Here, the patient is asked that which lens help him/her to see the visual acuity chart best. In subjective refraction, more complex phenomenon involved like quality of retinal image, photoreceptors integrity, visual pathway up to hindbrain and lastly the occipital cortex response. All these factors decide the response of the patient about the better visualization of the target. Along with these factors intelligence, emotions, and fatigues of patient will also influence the test result. Hence in young children and incoherent patients it is difficult to perform a subjective refraction so in these cases glasses are prescribed only on the basis of objective retinoscopy values.

If a cycloplegic drug had been used to perform retinoscopy, then post-mydriatic test (PMT) or a subjective refraction should be done after some interval, e.g. if homatropine or cyclopentolate has been used for refraction, then post-mydriatic test is done 4–5 days later, whereas if atropine has been used, then PMT is done 2–3 weeks later.

Subjective refraction is performed on the following guidelines
- Adjustment of refraction
- Refinement of refraction
- Binocular balancing

Adjustment of Refraction

Although one can perform a totally subjective refraction but it is always better to do an objective refraction prior to subjective refraction which not only saves the time but also gives an idea where to start.

Patient is made to sit at six meters distance from Snellen's chart and a trial frame is placed, visual acuity of both the eyes is tested separately and noted. Place the lenses of power obtained from objective refraction in front of the each eye accordingly. Now a subjective verification and adjustment of spherical and cylindrical lenses can be done by either of two techniques

- Trial and error technique
- Fogging or astigmatic dial technique

Trial and Error Technique

Different spherical and cylindrical lenses are tried to get the best corrected visual acuity as follows

Spherical lenses

- Spherical lenses are adjusted first and the patient is asked that with the help of which lens he/she is able to see clearly and comfortably. Strongest plus lens and weakest minus lens which provides the best corrected visual acuity is noted in case of a hypermetrope and myope, respectively.
- In myopic patients record the power of that weakest minus lens which makes the letters of Snellen's chart clear not that one which make them darker and smaller.

Cylindrical lenses

Cylinders need adjustment both in terms of axis and power and by the rule axis must be adjusted first followed by the power.

- *Axis verification:* Simply rotate the axis of cylinder at a step of 5° in either direction and ask the patient whether visual acuity improves or detoriate. Although, with small cylindrical powers patient may not be able to appreciate the difference in visual acuity, then high power cylinders can be used to verify the axis.
- *Cylindrical power verification:* Once axis is confirmed power of cylinder can be adjusted simply by changing the cylindrical lenses of various powers in the trial frame and asking patient at every step about the improvement in clarity of visual acuity.

Fogging or Astigmatic Dials Technique

Astigmatic dial is a chart having radial lines drawn at 30 degree intervals. Before starting test it is necessary to make the patient artificially myopic (fogged) by adding a plus (convex) sphere (+0.50 D) before the eye so that all meridians are focused in front of the retina, thus the fogging of the eye eliminates the natural accommodation response and artificially increases blurring of vision as naturally seen in myopia.

Test method

- The spherical powers are placed in front of test eye (e.g. right eye) and the other eye is occluded, i.e. to obtain a state of compound myopic astigmatism the right eye is fogged by placing sufficient plus spheres in front of it in the trial frame. This brings forward all hyperopic meridians, i.e. simple, compound or mixed to get focused in front of the retina as shown in Fig. 11.68.
- Because of fogging the accommodation will blur the lines more than normal, hence patient tries to relax his/her accommodation to prevent the further blurring of lines. In Fig. 11.68 vertical line (V) on dial (appearing darkest), is focusing in front of the horizontal line (H) on dial (appearing broken) inside the eye.
- After fogging the eye, now patient is instructed to look at the astigmatic dial. He/she is asked to identify the darkest and sharpest line (V) seen on the dial say at 6–12 o' clock position or at 90° axis in our example as seen in Fig. 11.69.

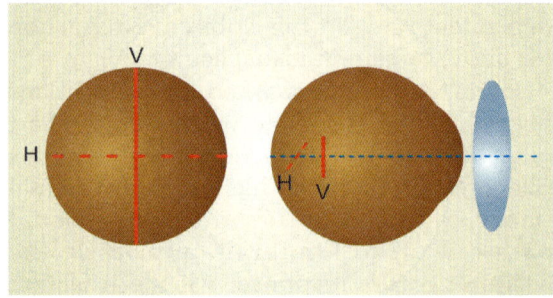

Fig. 11.68: State of compound myopic astigmatism induced by high plus spherical lens

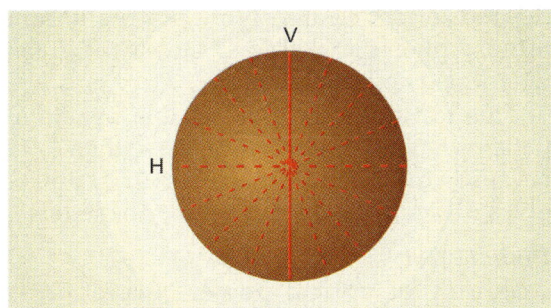

Fig. 11.69: Astigmatic dial showing darkest line V

- Once patient identifies the axis showing darkest line, i.e. 90° (V) in our example, now gradually add increasing power minus cylinders at an axis perpendicular to it (i.e. 180° in our example) till all the lines appear equally dark or blur to the patient as shown in Fig. 11.70.
- As shown in Fig. 11.70 addition of minus cylinder moves the vertical focal line (V) to a backward position where horizontal line (H) is present, hence the interval of Strum's conoid collapsed and a focal line becomes a point focus (C).
- To calculate the axis of correcting minus cylinder a 'rule of 30' can be applied. Multiply 30 to the lower number of clock hour showing the darkest line, i.e. 6–12 o' clock in our example. Hence in our example the axis of minus cylinder is 6 × 30 = 180°. If darkest line is at 3–9 o' clock position, then minus cylinders will be applied at 3 × 30 = 90° axis. Similarly if this darkest line is seen between one clock hour, say 2 and 3 o' clock;

then to get axis of minus cylinder, multiplication is done with lower number plus half, i.e. 2.5 × 30 = 75°.
- Now all the lines on astigmatic dial appear equally dark but none of them are clearly focused, because of the fogging of the eye.
- Change the fixation of patient to a Snellen's chart and gradually reduce the plus spherical power either by removing the plus or adding minus spheres until patient is able to read the chart clearly (Fig. 11.71).

Note: After performing a subjective verification of refraction either by trial and error method or by fogging or astigmatic dial method; always refine the refraction subjectively. Like retinoscopy first refine the spheres and then cylindrical axis and power.

Refinement of Refraction

Refining spheres
Snellen's distance vision chart is used to refine the spherical powers along with help of Duo chrome test and/or pinhole test.

Snellen's chart for refining of spheres
- Simple method to refine the spherical power is that once the cylindrical axis and power had been established by fogging method, then gradually defog by decreasing the spherical power at steps of 0.25 D and ask the patient to read the Snellen's chart after every step.
- Once patient reads 6/6 line comfortably, stop the changing of spherical power,

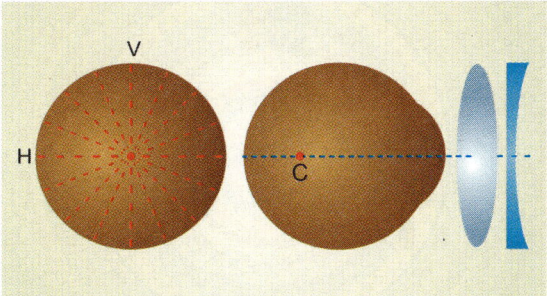

Fig. 11.70: Addition of minus cylinder focuses both line V and H at point C

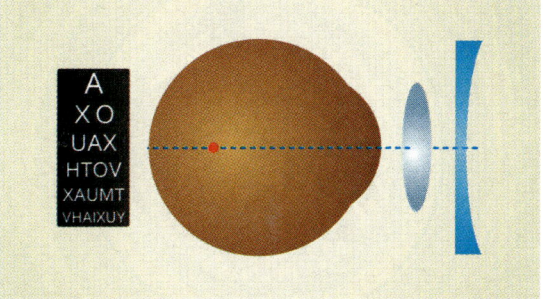

Fig. 11.71: Final adjustments done in astigmatic dial technique

however, near the end point there may be some confusion because patient will comfortably read at certain point even if examiner defog for another 0.25 D power.

- Accurate assessment of end point is a little difficult because patient may not be able to read 6/5 line with increasing or decreasing spherical power to 0.25 D range, this can best be assessed by help of duo chrome test.

Duo chrome test

Principle: Basic principle of test depends on the phenomenon of chromatic aberration. When a target of letters having red and green background are presented to an emmetropic person then he/she sees these letters equally sharp and bright because green light rays focuses slight anteriorly to the retina, whereas red light rays focuses slight posteriorly to the retina (wavelength of green light is shorter than red light thus green light waves are refracted more than red light waves).

For example, if during subjective refraction more minus power lenses are added, then patient will see the green portion clearer (Fig. 11.72A) while if too much plus power lenses are added then patient will see red letters more clear as shown in Fig. 11.72B.

This test is simple and reproducible, but the only disadvantage is that it does not relaxes the accommodation of patient, hence to relax accommodation slight fogging is done with plus spheres until patient is able to see only the red letters clearly. Now gradually add minus spheres in a 0.25 D steps, till green letters also becomes clearer.

This test does not give reliable results in patients having visual acuity worse than 6/12 because a difference of more than 0.5 D power gives difficulty in distinguishing the letters.

Pinhole test

Accuracy of optical power correction is confirmed by pinhole testing (Fig. 11.73).

Test method: After placing the entire optical correction in the trial frame the patient is instructed to look through the pinhole, if he/she reports no improvement in the visual acuity, it means the total correction given is correct.

Suppose if, the patient reports further improvement in the visual acuity with pinhole, then it means that total correction given is incorrect. So reconsider the refraction and try to improve the optical correction till the patient gives no improvement with pinhole testing.

Refining the cylinders

Most common employed methods to refine the cylinders are

- Astigmatic fan and block method
- Jackson's cross cylinder method

Astigmatic fan and block method

This is an old method to assess the axis of astigmatic error and is also called Maddox V test.

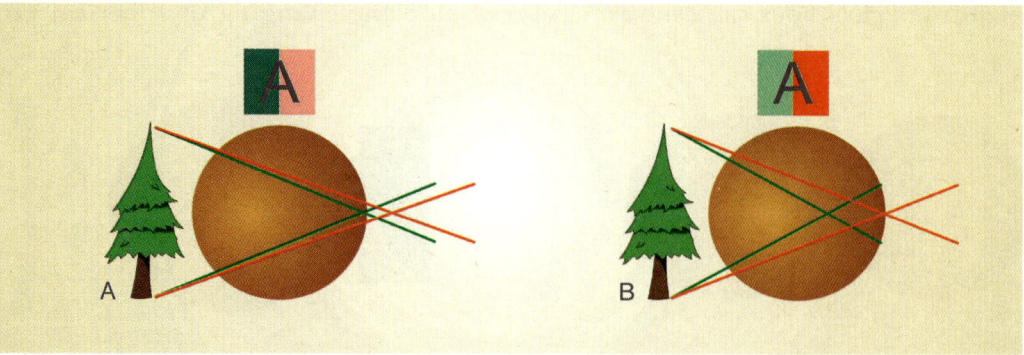

Fig. 11.72: Duo chrome test. A. Too much minus power green is clearer; B. Too much plus power red is clearer

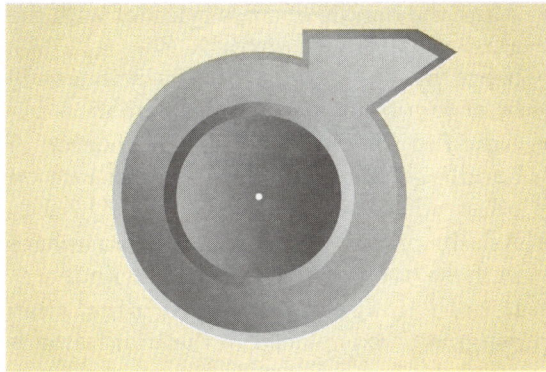

Fig. 11.73: Pinhole

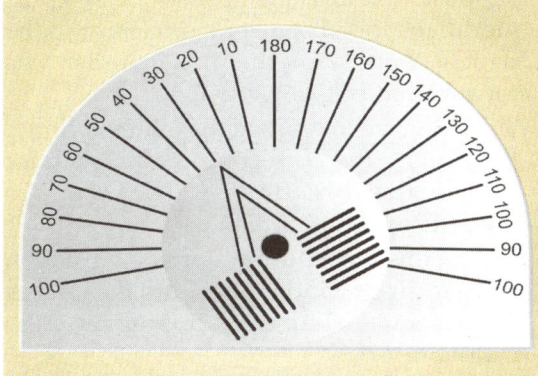

Fig. 11.74: Astigmatic fan

This consists of two components; a fan and a block. Fan is nothing but a series of 100 angled radiating lines appears as the rays from a rising sun. Whereas block is a centrally placed panel having a letter 'V' along with two sets of mutually perpendicular lines. For testing purposes this central panel having V and block lines can be rotated up to 100° on either side against the dialing fan (Fig. 11.74).

Test procedure
- Best corrected visual acuity is obtained by using only spheres; considering the fact that best corrected spherical powers brings the circle of least confusion on the retina.
- Then add plus spherical equivalent of estimated cylindrical power (spherical power half of cylindrical power is called as spherical equivalent to cylinder); this will make the eye in a simple myopic astigmatic state.

- Instruct the patient to look at the lines on the fan and ask him/her whether all lines are equally dark and distinct. If all the lines appears equally dark or equally blur; then either there is no astigmatic error or the eye is fogged in the excess.
- For confirmation of simple myopic state at this juncture add 0.5 D plus sphere and again ask the patient whether there is any change in the darkness on group of lines. If yes, then state of simple myopic astigmatism is present and if answer is no, then add another plus sphere at 0.5 D steps, till patient sees a change in the darkness of lines.
- If patient sees some lines darker than other, ask him/her which group of lines is clearer or darker.
- Now instruct the patient to focus on the Maddox V and ask which limb of V is blurring. Then examiner slowly rotates the central panel towards the blurred limb of V, until both the limbs of V becomes equally blur to the patient. The tip of V indicates the axis of astigmatism.
- Once patient observes equal blurring of limbs of Maddox V then ask him/her to focus on the blocks of lines and ask him/her which set of lines or block is darker. Now add minus cylinders in 0.25 D steps at the direction of axis determined as above; until lines in both the blocks appear equally dark.
- To confirm this, add plus 0.5 D sphere and patient should see the lines in both the blocks equally blur. If dark lines are changed to other block which was originally blur, then we had overcorrected the cylinders and if the originally darker block lines become more darker then initially added spherical power was not correct.

Jackson's cross cylinder method
Jackson's cross cylinder
In the year 1887, Dr Edward Jackson discovered the cross cylinder which is essentially a spherocylindrical lens having plus power in one meridian and an equal minus power in

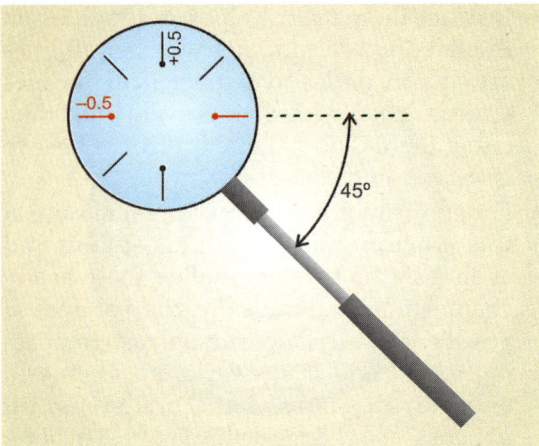

Fig. 11.75: Jackson cross cylinder

the other meridian. This is used to refine both the axis and power of cylindrical lens and also can be used to check the accuracy of spherical power.

Jackson's cross cylinder is effectively a lens having two cylinders of equal power with opposite signs placed 90° to each other, which is mounted on a handle at 45° angles to these meridians as shown in Fig. 11.75. In routine ophthalmic practice cross cylinders of power 0.25 D or 0.5 D are most commonly used. Plus meridian is marked by black/white line and minus meridian by red line. This cylinder is flipped by rotation of handle, which shows two blur images to the patient, then ask the patient to compare on which side the image is more blurred. When both the images become equally blur that is the endpoint of testing.

Test procedure
This test is performed for refinement of cylindrical axis and power, and it is recommended that always refine the axis of cylinder before the power, because correct power cannot be found in the absence of correct axis.

Refining the cylindrical axis
After placing the entire optical correction in the trial frame cylindrical axis is verified uniocularly.

- Align the handle of cross cylinder with the axis of astigmatic error X (Fig. 11.76A); hence the plus meridian of cross cylinder will lie at 45° off on one side of astigmatic axis.
- Now flip the cross cylinder by rotation of handle so that plus meridian will lie on other side of astigmatic axis (Fig. 11.76B).
- Ask the patient to compare the two images in these two positions of cross cylinder.
- If both images are equally blur, then astigmatic axis placed in the trial frame is accurate.
- When refining the plus cylinder and suppose if in any one position of two plus meridians the image appears clearer to the patient then rotate the plus cylinder axis toward that plus direction.
- Similarly, when refining the minus cylinder then rotate the correcting minus cylinder axis in the direction of clearer image towards minus meridian.
- Repeat this procedure at steps of 5° rotation of correcting cylinder until both the images appear equally blur after flipping the cross cylinder.

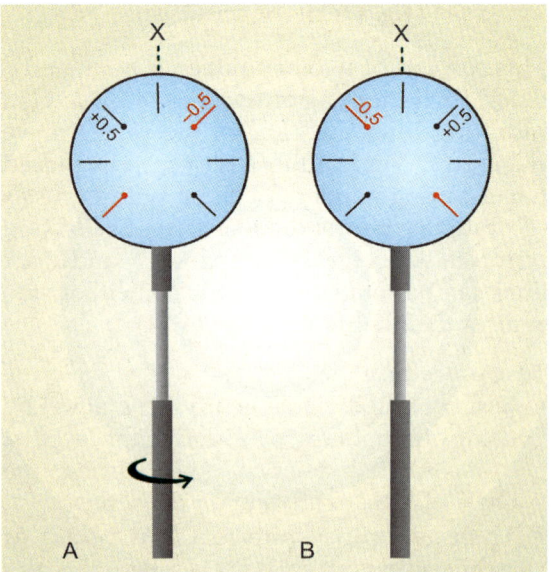

Fig. 11.76: Refining the cylindrical axis. A. Alignment of cross cylinder handle with astigmatic axis X; B. Flip position of cross cylinder

Refining cylindrical power

After placing the entire optical correction in the trial frame and verifying cylindrical axis, verify the power of correcting cylinder uniocularly.

- Align the handle of cross cylinder so that it lies at 45° angles with the astigmatic axis 'X' and plus meridian of cross cylinder align with the astigmatic axis as shown in Fig. 11.77A.
- Now when examiner flips the cross cylinder, there is an alternate alignment of plus and minus power with the astigmatic axis of correcting cylinder as shown in Fig. 11.77B.
- Ask the patient in which position of cross cylinder the image is clearer.
- Suppose if the image is clearer with alignment of plus meridian, then we increase the power of plus correcting cylinder, because when we place plus meridian over the astigmatic axis we are increasing its power.
- On contrary, if image is getting clearer with alignment of minus meridian, then we decrease the power of plus correcting cylinder or increase the power of minus correcting cylinder, because when we place minus meridian over the astigmatic axis we are decreasing its power.
- End point of test is when both the images get equally blur.

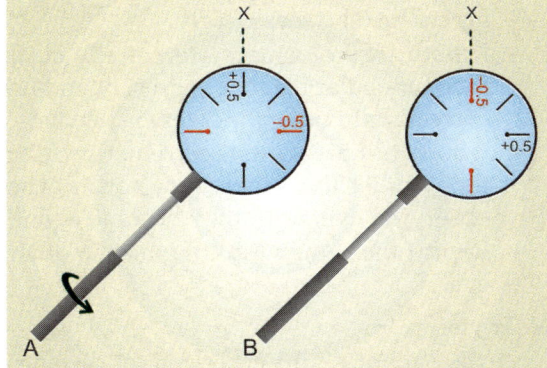

Fig. 11.77: Refining power of cylinder. A. Alignment of cross cylinder handle at 45° with astigmatic axis X; B. Flip position of cross cylinder

Binocular Balancing

Once the refractive status and best visual acuity has been confirmed uniocularly, then to confirm the optical correction or balance of vision under binocular conditions, a binocular balancing is needed. This can also be termed an equalization of visual or accommodative efforts. Binocular balancing provides a ground to focus a simultaneous retinal image in both the eyes because an imbalance in images will give rise to asthenopic symptoms.

Binocular balancing is done for both distance and near vision and many studies were done in past to achieve the accommodation balance for distance and near vision after refraction. Basic mechanism require to perform balancing is done by masking certain portions of the visual stimulus from either eye and this can be achieved by

- Alternate occlusion with fogging
- Complementary colors
- Prismatic doubling
- Polarization
- Haploscopic presentation

Balancing for distance vision

This can be done by several methods. Most commonly used methods are explained here

- *Alternate occlusion with fogging:* Place the best corrected optical lenses in the trial frame and add + 1D sphere in front of both the eyes. Alternately, occlude one eye and ask the patient to compare the images from each eye. If both are equally blur, then add –0.25 D sphere in front of one eye and again alternately occlude one eye. Now ask patient to compare the images from each eye. He/she will report a clear image from the eye in front of which a –0.25 D sphere was added. Suppose patient says no, then add or subtract spherical power in a 0.25 D steps till balancing or image clarity becomes equal in both eyes.
- *Turville binocular balance technique:* In the year 1930, Turville proposed an infinity balance technique for binocular balance of refraction. Principle of this method is that

a septum is positioned at the junction point of two diagonals from each eyes, which were connecting the nodal points and foveal targets. Various foveal targets or test objects shown in original test method are shown in Fig. 11.78A. This septum occludes one of the two foveal targets and hence only one retinal image from either eye is formed when both the eyes remain open. In case of binocular balancing the images will be seen as shown in Fig. 11.78B.

- *Bichromatic binocular technique:* Cowen modified binocular unit in an instrument which projects the ring targets (Verhoeff) in opposition to two halves of red and green duchrome background, which are cross polarized. After placing the best correcting lenses in the trial frame, the ring targets are viewed through appropriate polarized filters. Alternately, the eyes are occluded and patient is asked to compare the ring targets. By adjustment of optical correction we can achieve binocular balancing using these duchrome charts.

- *Prism dissociation method:* It is most commonly used and is the most sensitive method to test binocular balancing. Minimum amount of binocularity is a prerequisite to perform this method. This method is not useful in presence of severe amblyopia or high anisometropia.

Test method
- Place the best corrected optical lenses in the trial frame and perform uniocular acuity.

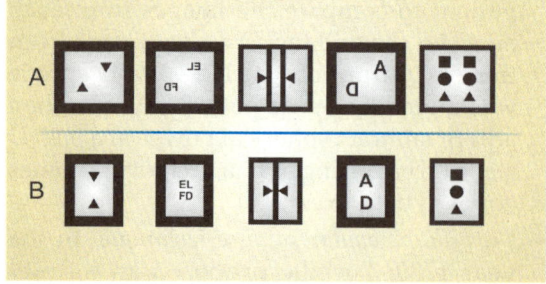

Fig. 11.78: Turville infinity binocular balance test. A. Test objects; B. Normal results

- Project a single row of letters on Snellen's chart of 6/9 (preferably a line better than weaker eye). Now place a vertical prism of 4–5Δ in front of one eye in the trial fame. (This will dissociate the images of two eyes).
- With both the eyes open ask the patient to read the letters of Snellen's chart. Now add plus 0.25 D sphere in front of one eye and then alternate it with other eye.
- If refractive correction in both the eyes is balanced, then patient will see blurring of letters from the eye having additional plus 0.25 D sphere.
- Once balance is achieved in both the eyes prism is removed and the patient is defogged until maximum acuity is reached, either with a maximum plus power or with minimum minus power.

- *Fogging with Duo chrome test:* In this method of binocular balancing of refraction, testing of corrective power by duo chrome chart is done along with fogging of one eye.

Test method
- Best corrected optical power lenses are placed in the trial frame and patient is asked to see the red green bars present on a vision chart.
- Fog one eye with a plus 2 D sphere and ask the patient to observe the red green bar with the other unfogged eye.
- Patient is asked which bar either red or green, he/she sees clearly.
- If both the color bars are equally clear then binocular balance is present and no correction in optical powers is needed.
- If both the bars are not seen equally clear, then adjust the spheres in front of the observing eye, until they become equal.
- Repeat the same with fogging the other eye.

Near vision

Once the patient is fully corrected for distance vision then test for near vision may also be required if patient age is over 40 years, or hyperopic, or has any difficulty in reading. In appropriate illumination in room, ask the patient to read the near vision chart preferably at 35–40 cm distance after wearing of full optical correction for distance vision. Always check with both the eyes open, do not occlude either eye.

Examiner asks the patient whether he/she can read the smallest line with ease or not. If not, then add plus spherical powers in front of both eyes together, according to the age or by assuming till which line patient can read comfortably as shown in Table 11.2.

If patient is unable to read the smallest letter line, then add the power as per chart and increase gradually in 0.25 D steps till patient is able to read comfortably. Difference in spherical powers for near and distance is calculated and recorded as 'Add' for near vision.

For example, if power of distance vision is plus 1.0 D and near vision is plus 2.5 D then 'Add' for both the eyes is plus 1.5 D. Similarly, in myopes if distance power is minus 1.0 D and near power is plus 2.0 D then 'Add' in both eyes will be plus 3.0 D.

Binocular balancing for near vision refraction is done by several methods such as

- Near vision balance with Bisurface reflectors
- Freeman near vision unit
- Rodenstock near vision unit
- Osterberg-Bino near vision unit

Near vision testing by bisurface reflectors
In this instrument an angled bisurface mirror is used to separate the right and left eye fields, whereas in original Turville method a septum

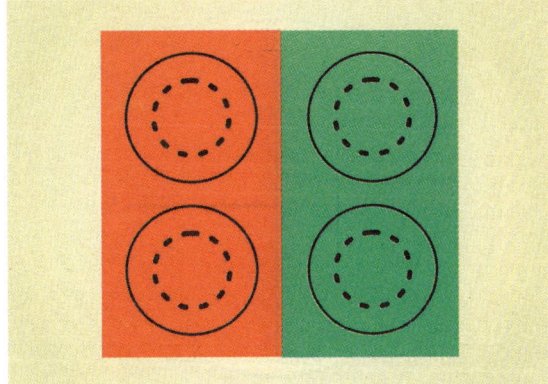

Fig. 11.79: Freeman bichromatic polarized modified ring targets

was used. One area has figured target and other area has undifferentiated targets, however, patient can compare both images by rapid alteration of bifixation of either views.

Freeman near vision unit
This unit consists of bichromatic polarized modified ring targets (Verhoeff types) along with two cross-polarized letter charts (Fig. 11.79).

Rodenstock near vision unit
Here balancing of accommodation is done by presenting a duo chrome target having letters and double Verhoeff rings. For balancing of near vision two cross-polarized letter charts are also present in testing unit.

Osterberg-Bino near vision unit
This consists of a non-polarized duo chrome reducing number chart along with two cross-polarized charts, which are separated vertically.

Note: These near vision units have similar kind of purpose. Binocular bichromatic balancing method is better than simple duo chromatic principle as it assesses the balancing of monocular accommodation efforts.

PRESCRIBING POWER FOR GLASSES

Retinoscopy Representation

Universal method of representation of retinoscopy values are in the form of a cross as shown in Fig. 11.80.

Table 11.2: Average addition required by emmetropes at 35–40 cm reading distance	
Age in years	Plus addition in dioptres
40–45	0.75
46–50	1.25
51–55	1.75
56–60	2.00
60–70	2.50
71 and above	3.00

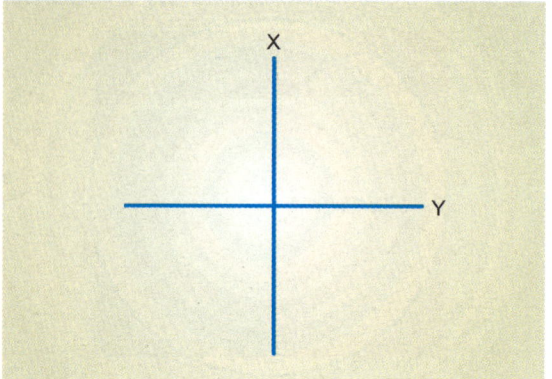

Fig. 11.80: Retinoscopy representation (*see* text)

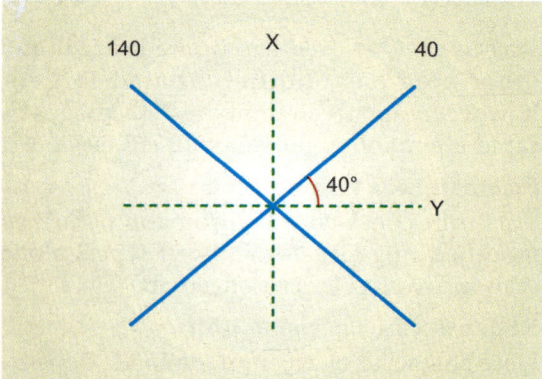

Fig. 11.81: Retinoscopy representation (*see* text)

Here, X and Y represent the two principal meridians, i.e. 90° and 180°, respectively. If the neutralization meridians are not at these angles then they can be represented accordingly, for example a 40° meridian and 140° meridian, which will be represented as shown in Fig. 11.81.

Similarly, the gross retinoscopy values are represented along the axis of neutralization.

For example,

- If both vertical and horizontal meridians get neutralized by plus 5 D power, when retinoscopy is done at 66 cm distance with atropine as cycloplegic drug, then value of 1.5 D for distance and 1 D for atropine drug is reduced from gross retinoscopy and net value of retinoscopy will be represented as shown in Fig. 11.82.

- If vertical meridian is neutralized by plus 5 D power and horizontal meridian by plus 7 D when retinoscopy is done at 66 cm distance with atropine drug then the gross and net retinoscopy will be represented as shown in Fig. 11.83.

- Similarly if neutralization occurs by –4 D power in both the principal meridians when retinoscopy is done at 66 cm distance with atropine, then gross and net retinoscopy is represented as in Fig. 11.84.

- Suppose vertical meridian is neutralized by –3 D power and horizontal meridian by minus 5 D, when retinoscopy done at 66 cm distance with atropine drug then gross and net retinoscopy will be represented as shown in Fig. 11.85.

- In case of oblique astigmatism when neutralization is at 30° meridian and 120° meridian say with +2 D power and +4 D power, respectively and retinoscopy is

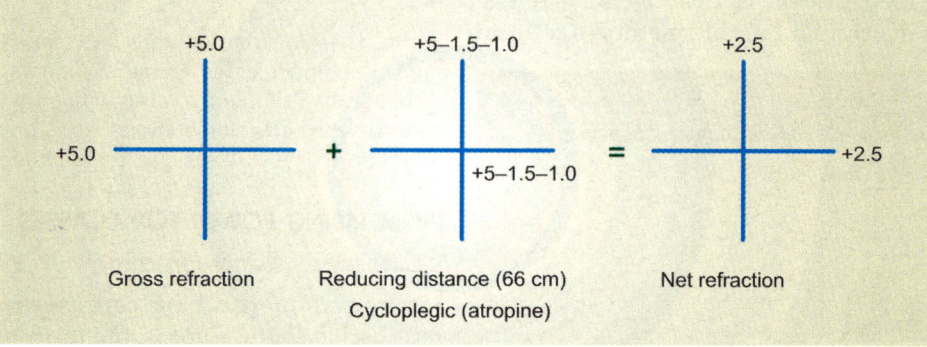

Fig. 11.82: Optical cross in simple hypermetropia

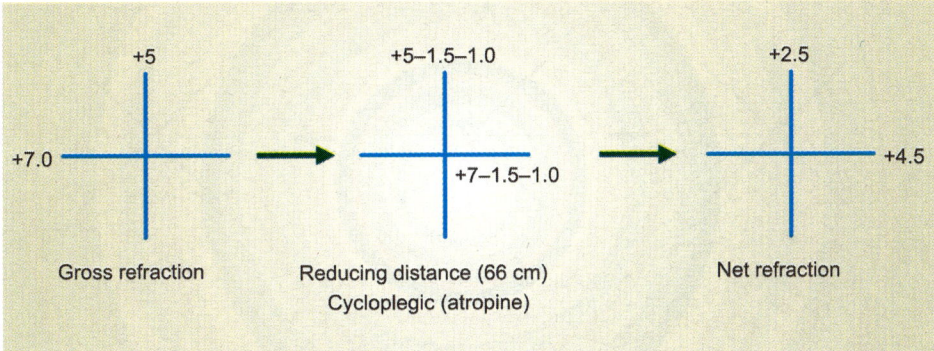

Fig. 11.83: Optical cross in compound hypermetropia

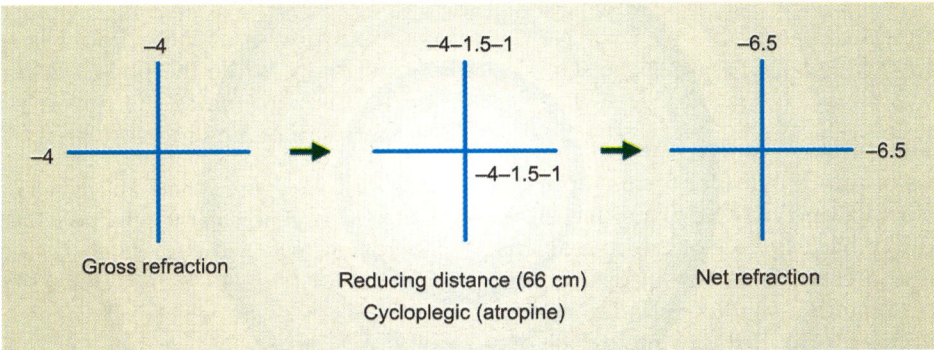

Fig. 11.84: Optical cross in simple myopia

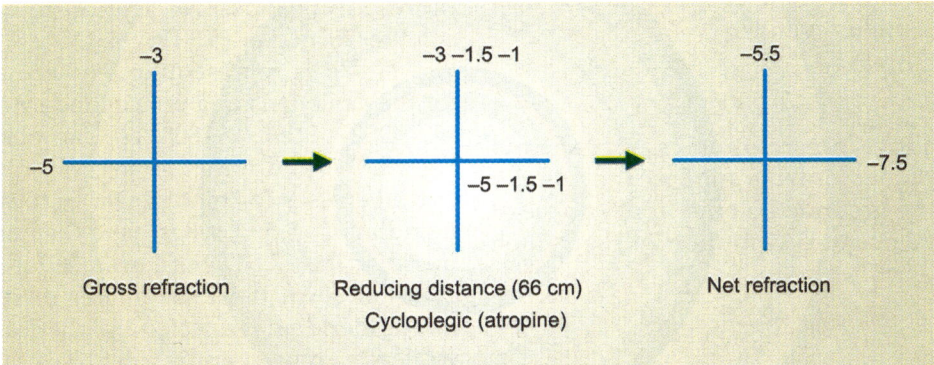

Fig. 11.85: Optical cross in compound myopia

done at 66 cm distance with atropine then gross and net retinoscopy will be represented as shown in Fig. 11.86.

Prescription Writing

In an ophthalmic lens prescription, spherical lens power is written first, followed by cylindrical lens power and then cylindrical lens axis. These values are represented with the help of net retinoscopy representation.

For example, the above net retinoscopy findings will be written as

- Figure 11.82: + 2.5 DS
- Figure 11.83: + 2.5 DS/+ 2 DC × 90°

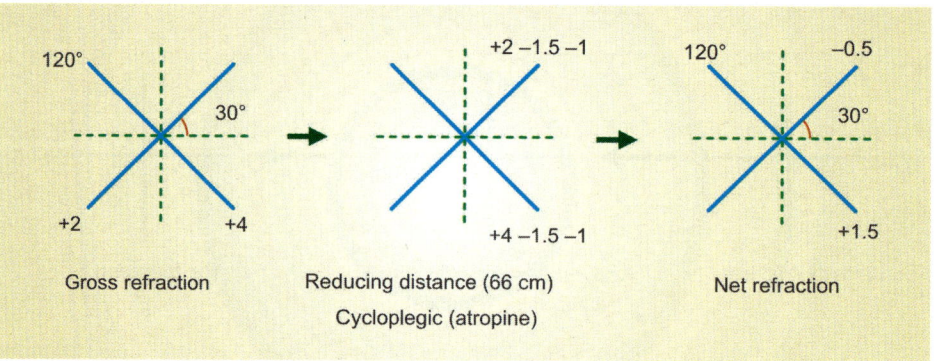

Fig. 11.86: Optical cross in oblique astigmatism

- Figure 11.84: – 6.5 DS
- Figure 11.85: – 5.5 DS/–2 DC × 90°
- Figure 11.86: – 0.5 DS/+2 DC × 30°

Plus versus minus cylinder form

These plus or minus cylinder forms represent the toric surface and may be grounded either on the front or back surface of the optical lens, hence these prescriptions for an optical lens can be written either as plus-cylinder form or minus-cylinder form. If the front surface of a lens is grounded it forms a plus cylinder and if the back surface of a lens is grounded then it forms a minus cylinder.

For example,

$$- 5.5 \text{ DS}/-2 \text{ DC} \times 90°$$

This above prescription is written in a minus cylinder form but suppose the cylinder needs to be grounded on the front surface of lens then the same prescription will be written as

$$-7.5 \text{ DS}/+2 \text{ DC} \times 180°$$

THE OPTICAL CROSS

Optical cross is a graphical representation which explains the relationship between spherical and cylindrical components of an ophthalmic lens, also known as power diagrams. To understand power diagrams three crosses are drawn; one will represent the spherical component where power is same in both the principal meridians. Second cross will represent the cylindrical component where

maximum power of the cylinder is specified in a meridian, while the power in remaining meridians is zero (since the power is zero in axis meridian of a cylindrical lens).

Note: The power of cylindrical lens is represented at an axis perpendicular to the one written in net prescription, means when cylindrical axis is written as 90° in the prescription, then the power in the optical cross will be taken at horizontal or 180° and vice versa.

The optical crosses shown in Fig. 11.87A is representing lens prescription in a minus cylinder form, i.e. –5.5 DS/–2 DC × 90° while Fig. 11.87B is representing lens prescription for the same lens in a plus cylinder form, i.e. –7.5 DS/+ 2 DC × 180°. We can observe in Fig. 11.87A and B that in both examples, the optical crosses for total power in the vertical meridian is –5.5 D, whereas in the horizontal meridian it is –7.5 D. Furthermore, for a minus cylinder form the total power of the least minus meridian is selected as spherical power while for a plus-cylinder form the total power in most minus meridian is selected as spherical power.

There is another way to write a net power figure in a prescription form as follows: Consider any meridian power as spherical power, say vertical or horizontal. Now just subtract the spherical meridian power from the other meridian power mathematically and get the cylindrical power with spherical meridian axis as cylindrical axis.

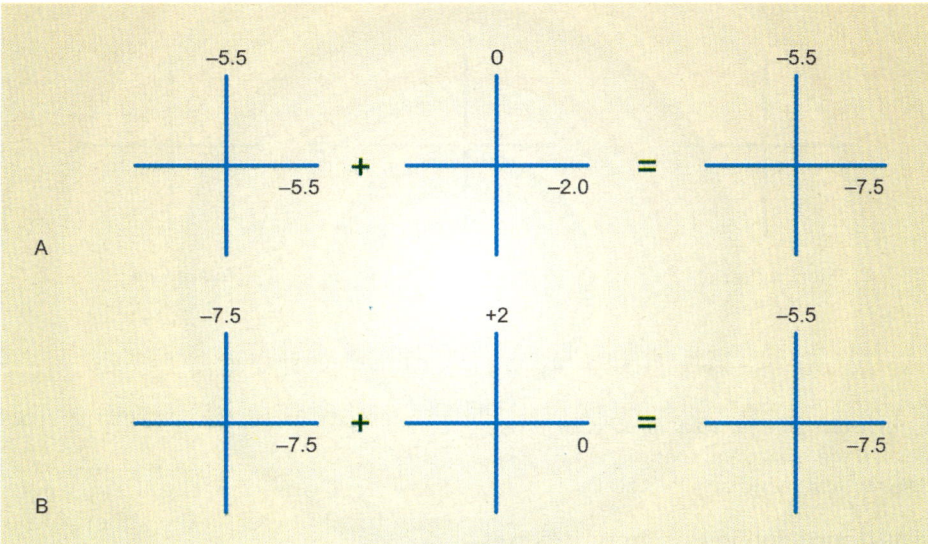

Fig. 11.87: Optical cross representations of same prescription in various cylindrical forms. A. Minus cylinder form; B. Plus cylinder form

If we consider above discussed example:

If horizontal meridian is considered as spherical power (–7.5 D), then subtract the horizontal meridian power, i.e. –7.5 D from the vertical meridian power, i.e. –5.5 D and resultant is –5.5 – (–7.5) = +2.0, i.e. plus cylinder at 180° (horizontal/spherical power meridian)

Hence, the final prescription will be –7.5 DS × +2 DC × 180°

Alternately, when vertical meridian is considered as spherical power (–5.5 D), then subtract the vertical meridian power, i.e. –5.5 D from the horizontal meridian power, i.e. –7.5 D and resultant is –7.5 – (–5.5) = –2.0, i.e. minus cylinder at 90° (vertical/spherical power meridian)

Hence, the final prescription will be –5.5 DS × –2 DC × 90°

So in a nutshell we can consider any meridian power as spherical power and to get final prescription just follow this simple rule:

"Always spherical powers are deducted from cylindrical powers mathematically and the resultant power becomes cylindrical power, whereas for cylindrical axis use the same axis of spherical power".

Transposition of Prescription

Transposition of a spherocylindrical perception is necessary for a laboratory when they need to manufacture a specific form of lens, i.e. either the front surface cylinder or back surface cylinder lens.

Three steps rule for transposition of prescription

This simple 3 steps rule is applied for transposition of a spherocylindrical prescription to convert plus (+) cylinder form into a minus (–) cylinder form or vice versa.

Step 1: Mathematically, add spherical power and cylinder power to get new spherical power.

Step 2: Reverse the sign of cylinder, i.e. from plus to minus and vice versa.

Step 3: Rotate the cylindrical axis by 90°.

Cross cylinder form: When a lens is grounded as plus cylinder on its front surface and as minus cylinder on its back surface, having axes of these two cylinders at 90° apart, is called as cross cylinder.

An example of a cross cylindrical lens is + 0.50 DC × 180° combined with –0.5 DC × 90°.

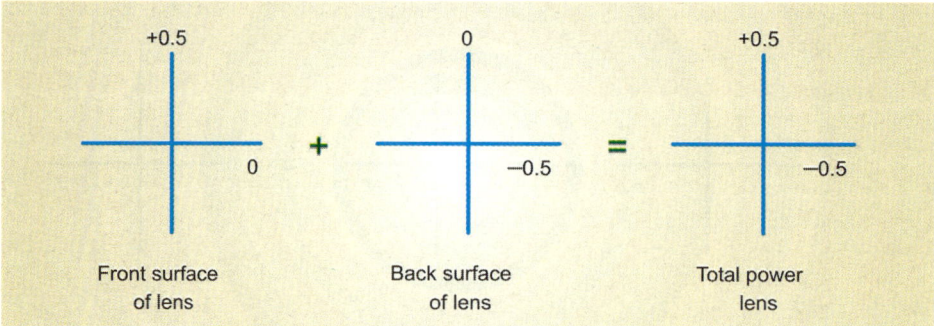

Fig. 11.88: Cross cylinder form representation

Note: In our example the total power of cross cylinder lens in the horizontal meridian is –0.5 D, while in the vertical meridian is +0.50 D.

Optical cross representing this prescription is shown in Fig. 11.88.

In routine ophthalmic practice these cross cylinders are used to refine axis and power of patient's best cylindrical correction (Jackson's cross cylinder) and also can be used for near point testing (e.g. in determination of power of a bifocal addition).

A spherocylindrical prescription can be formed into a cross cylinder prescription by this simple two steps rule:

Step 1: First obtain both the plus cylinder and minus cylinder forms of the prescription.

Step 2: Now combine the two powers mathematically (connect extremes)

For example, if a spherocylindrical lens prescription is written in a plus cylinder form and then in a minus cylinder form, i.e. –0.5 DS/+1.0 DC × 90° and +0.5 DS/–1.0 DC × 180°, now if we connect the powers, the resultant prescription will be +0.50 DC × 90° combined with –0.5 DC × 180°.

Similarly, a crossed-cylinder prescription can be converted into a spherocylindrical

prescription by this simple three steps rule

Step 1: Consider the first encountered cylindrical power as the spherical power.

Step 2: To get cylindrical power, reverse the sign of this new spherical power and then mathematically add it with second cylinder power.

Step 3: To get the cylinder axis use the same axis that of second cylinder.

Continuing to the same example of cross cylinder as above mentioned, the lens prescription is + 0.50 DC × 90° combined with –0.5 DC × 180° and by applying this three step rule to get a spherocylindrical prescription, + 0.50 DC × 90° will become as

+0.50 DS/–1.0 DC × 180°

Now on applying the original three steps rule and this minus cylinder prescription can be transposed into a plus-cylinder prescription as follows:

–0.5 DS/+1.0 DC × 90°

Note: Spherocylindrical prescriptions are same in both the methods of transposition of cross cylinder. Since routinely in our ophthalmic practice we encounter transposition between minus cylinder and plus cylinder forms, hence readers are advised to memorize the original three steps rule for conversion of spherocylindrical powers.

Visual Rehabilitation

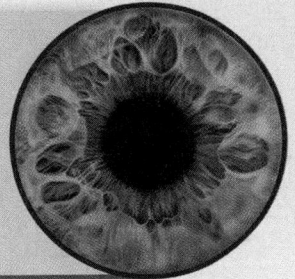

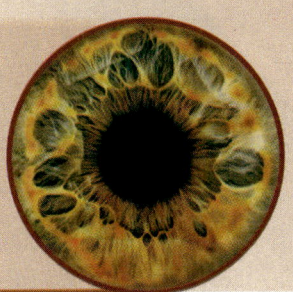

CHAPTER 12

Spectacles, Spectacle Lenses and Spectacle Lens Fitting

Learning Objectives

After studying this chapter the reader should be able to:

- Record the historical events of progress during development of spectacle frames and glasses.
- Understand various designs of spectacle frames and mountings.
- Describe the different types of optical material used in spectacle lenses with their special features.
- Explain the terminologies in relation to spectacle lenses and classify the spectacle lenses.
- Understand various types of spectacle lenses and their fitting requirements.
- Describes principles and steps of fitting lenses in spectacle frames.
- Verify and dispense an accurately fitted spectacle glasses.

Chapter Outline

- Spectacles
  - History and events of progress
  - Frames and mountings
  - Materials of frames and mountings
    - Metals
    - Plastic frame materials
  - Bridges and temples
- Optical Materials
  - Optical glasses
  - Optical plastics
  - Spectacle lens materials
    - Glass lenses
    - Plastic lenses
    - Absorptive lenses
- Spectacle Lenses
  - Spectacle lens design
    - Spherical lens design
    - Spherocylindrical lens design
    - Design of high plus lenses
  - Terminologies in spectacle lenses

- Classification of spectacle lenses
- Trifocal lenses
- Progressive lenses
- Spectacle Lens Fitting
  - Interpupillary distance
  - Frame dimensions
  - Datum system
  - Boxing system
  - Frame specification
  - Spectacle frame selection
  - Principles of fitting
    - Pantoscopic tilt
    - Temple angle
    - Fitting triangle
  - Lens decentration
  - Glazing of lens
  - Verification of spectacles
    - Surface defects
    - Lens power measurement
    - Frame alignment

SPECTACLES

History and Events of Progress

Introduction

Art of glass making is much older than invention of spectacles. Glasses were used since ages for various purposes, however first time glass were used as a visual aid in the form of a simple magnifying glass called eyeglass. These eyeglasses were mounted on various materials like wood, metals, leather, animal horn, bone, etc. and with the help of a handle these mounted eyeglasses were held in front of eye to visualize the objects.

An optical device used for visual purpose by only one eye is known as an eyeglass, however, when two such devices are used for both the eyes together, are called a pair of eyeglasses or spectacles. Initially, only eyeglass was invented and used in front of one eye but with trial and error two such devices were hinged in a manner that one of eyeglasses lies in front of each eye together and this leads to a primitive pair of spectacles as shown in Fig. 12.1.

It is not exactly known who invented the spectacles, but several people had contributed in the process of invention to produce the present form of spectacles.

Events of progress

- Roger Bacon, a monk in his famous Opus Magnus (1267) first described that small letters or objects can be magnified with help of a strong plano convex lens and he suggested that such device can be used in those people having poor vision. However, it is not exactly known whether he mounted these lenses in any frame or not.
- The first evidence about invention of spectacles has been found in a sermon (1305) written by the monk Giordano da Rivalto.
- Furthermore, other evidence about invention of glasses were found in a manuscript and an epitaph written by Alexandria de Spina and Salvino d'Armati of Florence.
- Primitive forms of spectacles because of their weight and assembly were difficult to mount steadily in front of the eyes and thus were clamped to the nose which was uncomfortable for patient and often interfered with breathing. Subsequently, spectacle devices in the form of head bands were produced for better comfort.
- Around 17th century Spanish spectacle makers used loops of silk or cord which were attached with the outer edges of frames and then loop were extended to the ears.
- In the year 1730, Edward Scarlett (English optician) developed rigid side pieces (temples) of eyeglasses.

Frames and Mountings

The devices which act as support for spectacle lenses can be classified as

- Frames
- Mountings

These two terms are commonly interchangeable, though have different meanings.

Frames: Frames can be prepared using metals, plastics or combination of both metal and plastic. Usually, metal or a combination frame consists of an adjustable nose pads for better comfort, whereas plastic frames has fixed nose pads or no pads for adjustments as shown in Fig. 12.2.

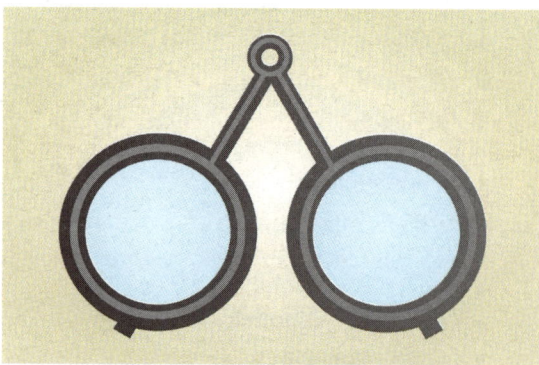

Fig. 12.1: Primitive spectacles

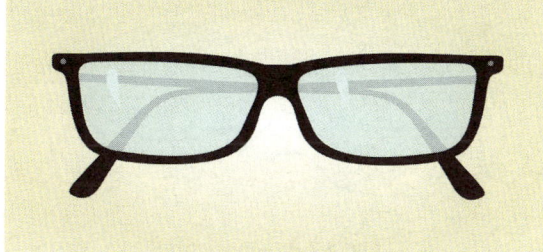

Fig. 12.2: Plastic frame

Frame mainly consists of three parts
- Front: Encircles the lenses and hold them
- Bridge: Keeps the entire front together and rests on the nose
- Pair of temples: Rests on the ears and hold the front in alignment with eyes.

Mounting: A device which holds the two optical lenses in front of eyes without encircling them completely is called mountings as shown in Fig. 12.3. These mountings were classically manufactured with gold filled materials in past and were classified as either rimless or semi-rimless.

A typical rimless mounting has three parts
- Single bridge or center piece: Helps to hold the two spectacle lenses together towards nose (nasally).
- End pieces: Two in number which hinges the spectacle lenses with temples.
- Temples: Two in number, one on each side.

To fit lenses in a rimless frame, two holes are drilled in each lens, i.e. one hole nasally to fix the center piece and second hole temporally to fix the end piece. Center piece consists of two adjustable nose pads to be placed on the sides of nose, which carry the weight of entire

mounting and lenses. Two temples are fixed with end pieces so that a rimless frame can be worn comfortably.

A typical semi-rimless frame also has three portions
- A front: Which has both bridge and two arms
- Two temples

In past, two commercial versions of semi-rimless mountings were manufactured
- American Optical Numount was the first version which attaches only to the nasal side of spectacle lens and requires only one hole per lens. Numount is a light weighted mounting and a tri-flex spring is present in mounting at the location where spectacle lens is attached with the mounting. Although in look, Numount mounting appears very delicate but presence of tri-flex spring prevents breaking of spectacle lenses during pressure and shocks (Fig. 12.4).
- Similarly, American Optical Rimway was second version of semi-rimless mountings which attaches to both the nasal and temporal sides of each spectacle lenses, thus require two holes per lens for fitting (Fig. 12.5). Although

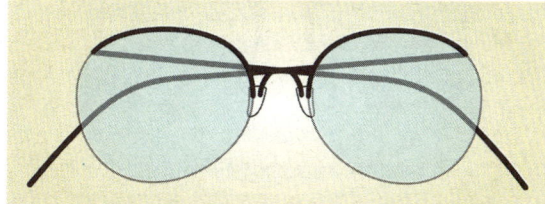

Fig. 12.4: Numount mounting

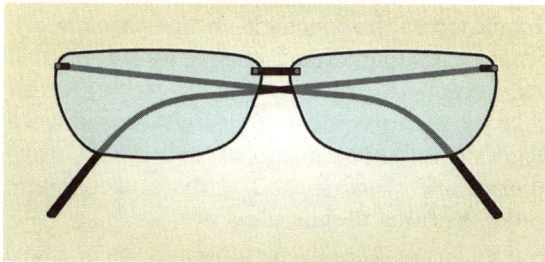

Fig. 12.3: Mounting

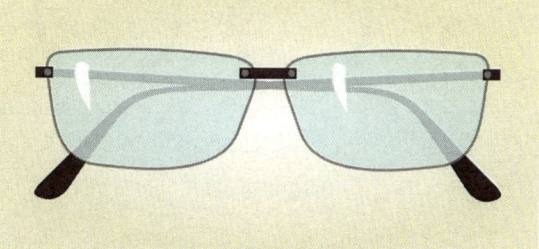

Fig. 12.5: Rimway mounting

Rimway mountings were appearing tougher than Numount mounting but in reality temporal corner of this spectacle lens get easily breaks away on pressure application.

In addition to these abovementioned conventional frames or mountings which contain bridges and temples, the other devices were also available which hold either a pair of spectacle lenses or a single lens in front of the eye.

Pincenez or eyeglass was a term used for a pair of spectacle lenses, which were held in front of eyes by pinching the nose. These eyeglasses have no temples and lenses are fixed in a circular frame like structure as shown in Fig. 12.6.

Similarly, Lorgnette was spectacle which indicates that either a pair of spectacle lenses (usually) or a single spectacle lens (rarely), held in front of the eyes with the help of a handle as shown in Fig. 12.7.

Monocle which means a single lens, it appears similar to a trial case lens and was

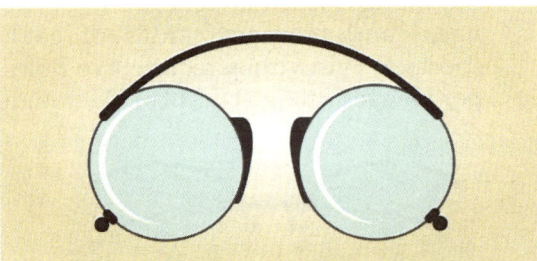

Fig. 12.6: Pincenez

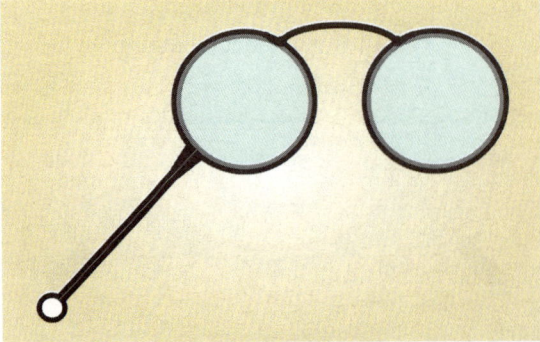

Fig. 12.7: Lorgnette

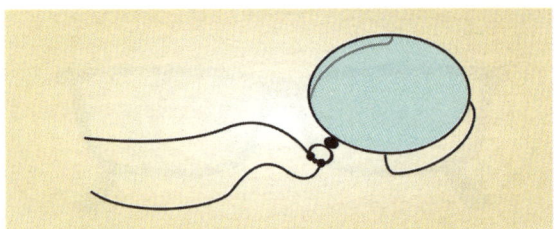

Fig. 12.8: Monocle

worn very often for special motive. The muscular pressure of facial and brow muscles hold this Monocle in front of one eye as shown in Fig. 12.8.

Materials of Frames and Mountings

Spectacle frames and mountings can be prepared by using various materials like natural substances or synthetics substances. Materials having following properties are considered ideal for manufacturing spectacles frames

- Non-corrosiveness
- Adjustability
- Light weighted
- Non-allergic
- Sturdiness
- Low cost

In older times, naturally available materials like wood, animal horns, tortoise shell and leather, etc. were used to make the spectacle frames for holding the lenses. Nowadays the commonly used materials are

- Metals
- Plastics
- Nylon

Metals

Most commonly and widely used material to manufacture the spectacles frames are metals; because use of metal was convenient and inexpensive to produce the spectacle frames in large quantity. Most of the metals used were highly moldable, non-corrosive and non-allergic and were durable with good cosmetic looks. Various metals used are

Gold and silver: Initially gold was extensively used for frames and mountings in western countries because it meets all the properties of an ideal material except cost. These frames were marked with content of gold percentage in terms of Karat. Pure gold was too soft, hence other metals were added to increase its hardness and durability. Similarly, silver was also tried because of its similar properties like gold, but it was also too soft and needed other metals to increase its utilization.

Silver when mixed with nickel forms a metal, commonly called German silver which became popular for making of frames because of its anti-corrosive property, however, the high percentage of contact allergy due to these metals discouraged its wide usage in population.

Later on, gold was layered over this German silver by electroplating process, which not only eliminated its allergic nature but also maintained the properties like adjustability and durability. These gold frames remain popular till date because of their cosmetic reasons, non-allergic nature and anti-corrosiveness; still the only hurdle is cost.

Stainless steel: This came as an inexpensive alternative to gold and silver in large-scale manufacturing of frames. Steel meet nearly all the qualities of an ideal material being very stable, adjustable, non-corrosiveness, non-allergic and light in weight, and can easily be manufactured in mass productions.

Aluminium: Like steel, aluminium is also inexpensive, noncorrosive, light-weighted material and thus can also be easily used in large-scale frame manufacturing. Aluminium metal also has an advantage over steel that the frames of aluminium can be dyed easily with different colors which improved its cosmetic appearance and sale value.

Plastic Frame Materials

A constant search for a better, inexpensive material for huge production of spectacle frames lead to the discovery of plastic material. Initially, these plastics were either the derivatives of natural occurring cotton or petroleum, but with the time various synthetic materials were developed in laboratories to produce plastics.

Mainly two types of plastics are used for frames

Thermosetting: These materials convert from a liquid state into a solid state during the process of manufacturing by application of heat and pressure. Once the manufacturing had occurred, then even high temperatures or pressure application cannot soften these materials and in these circumstances they basically decompose. For example, melanines used for Melmac dishes, phenolics (Bakelite), polyesters used for clothing and allyls used in CR-39 material (very popular as plastic lens material, however, rarely used for manufacturing spectacle frames).

Optyl: Optyl is an epoxy resin containing thermosetting plastic material. To manufacture frames from optyl, the liquid of it at high temperature is poured into a mould followed by a curing process. After moulding different parts of the formed frame can easily be dyed using different colors. The optyl material on heating becomes soft and flexible and thus can be shaped in any desired form easily.

Advantages of optyl frames are
- Hardness
- Dimensional stability
- Good shine
- Non-inflammability
- Light in weight.

Disadvantages of optyl frames are that they need higher temperatures compare to their counterpart materials to work on; and if any attempt is made to adjust them in cold, frames will break.

Thermoplastic: These materials get soft on heating and hard on cooling and even basic structure of these material is not altered even on repeated exposure to this process.

Hence, these materials are widely used for large-scale production of inexpensive and durable spectacle frames. Various thermoplastics commonly used to manufacture spectacle frames are

Acrylics: Acrylics are the most common name for the family of thermoplastic materials, which include polymethyl methacrylate (mainly used in the manufacturing of hard contact lenses and occasionally used for spectacle frames). Various acrylics used commercially for spectacle frame manufacturing are

- PMMA
- Plexiglas
- Perspex
- Lucite

Most advantageous features of acrylics are dimensional stability, surface hardness, good wear resistance, clarity, color fastness, light weight, and non-flammable. Disadvantages of acrylics are brittleness and low impact resistance; due to which these materials are not preferably used for spectacle frames.

Polycarbonate: This thermoplastic material was used widely in past for manufacturing of spectacle frames. Only disadvantage was that it was too hard to work on, so gradually its use declined over a period of time.

Presently, mainly two materials are used for the mass manufacture of spectacle frames, cellulose nitrate and cellulose acetate. Although both are similar in appearance, but when used for spectacle frames they exhibit different properties.

Cellulose nitrate: This is also called xylonite and is commonly known as celluloid in the film industry. Camphor is added as a plasticizer during manufacturing of cellulose nitrate, hence when a cellulose nitrate frame is rubbed vigorously with a cloth, an odour of camphor may be noticed. Due to its hard nature it retains its shape even in hot climate.

Cellulose acetate: Most commonly used plastic material to manufacture spectacle frames is cellulose acetate because of its less inflammable nature and hardness.

Both cellulose nitrate and cellulose acetate are produced by cotton lint and are soluble in various ketones such as acetone; although neither of them is soluble in alcohol. Hence, acetone is often used as a polishing or repairing substance for the frames made up of cellulose material.

Comparison of cellulose nitrate and cellulose acetate

Cellulose nitrate is superior to cellulose acetate because

- Cellulose nitrate can be easily stretched by heat and also shrinks minimally when cooled, so moulding of these frames is comparatively easier than acetate frames.
- Harder surface of nitrate frames is an advantage for better polish and trouble-free maintenance.
- Much thinner frames can be made by nitrate because it is tougher than cellulose acetate.
- Nitrates softening point is higher than that of cellulose acetate; and its water absorption is lower, hence better dimensional stability is seen in warm and clammy environments.

Conversely, cellulose acetate is superior to cellulose nitrate because

- Less production time as compared to cellulose nitrate.
- Frames made are more colorfast compared to cellulose nitrate.
- Cellulose acetate frames are much less flammable compared to cellulose nitrate.

Cellulose propionate: It is also an ester of cellulose family. Several properties of propionate resembled the optyl material including the manufacturing by moulding process. Frames prepared by cellulose propionate are quite tough and light in weight, so can easily be made into various styles and sculpturing effects. However, use of cellulose propionate frames has decreased in recent years.

Nylon: Polyamides are a generic class of thermoplastic polymers which are commonly known as nylon. Nylon material is very costly when manufactured in the form of sheet, hence an injection moulding technique is used to decrease the cost of manufacturing. Nylon is very tough and hard in nature but its brittleness, poor color acceptance, high water absorption and less transparency has limited its usefulness in competitive spectacle frame market. Nylon spectacle frames are currently available in market, but are less preferred as compared to the cellulose material frames.

Note: Although several materials have been used for the manufacture of plastic frames; but great majority spectacle frames are currently made of thermoplastic material, cellulose acetate.

Bridges and Temples

Following types of bridges and temples can be used in plastic spectacle frames

Bridges: Usually in metallic frames and/or rimless or semi-rimless mounting, bridges make no direct contact with nose; rather contact is made with the help of adjustable nose pads (Fig. 12.9).

However, in plastic frame there is a direct contact of bridge with the sides of nose. Plastic frame's bridges are either saddle type bridges or keyhole type bridges or occasionally modifications of either type.

A saddle bridge directly rests on the crest of nose like a horse back and distributes the weight of spectacles evenly on the top and sides of the nose (Fig. 12.10). It has no nose pads for contact to the sides of nose, hence suitable for those persons who compliant of sensitivity due to nose pads. For proper fitting

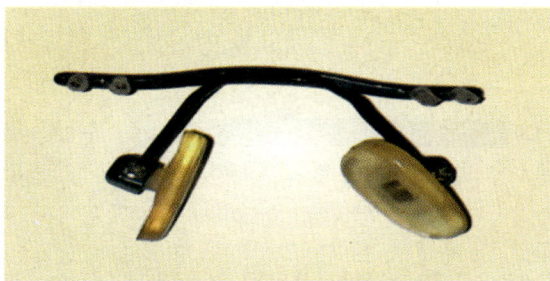

Fig. 12.9: Adjustable nose pad

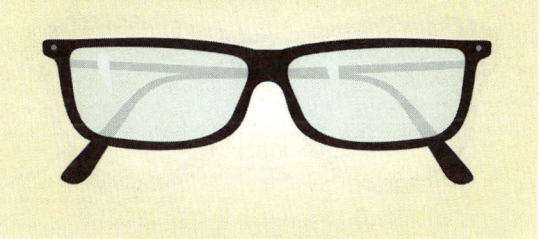

Fig. 12.10: Saddle bridge

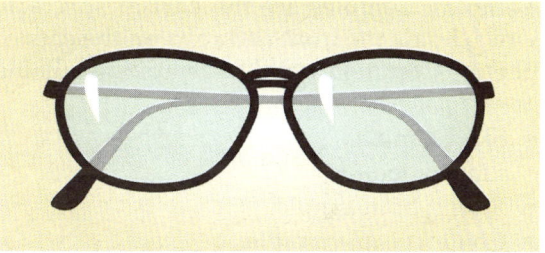

Fig. 12.11: Keyhole bridge

of this kind of bridge, the saddle shape must be a perfect fit with contour of the nose. Various modified saddle bridges have also been developed which include built-up areas on either side of bridge in such a way that the apparent length of nose looks short.

The keyhole bridges are useful for those persons who cannot tolerate pressure on the top of the nose because these types of bridges make direct contact only with the sides of nose, not the top (Fig. 12.11). Fixed, nonadjustable pads are made with the frame which make the contact with nose and are usually of the same material as that of frame. As compared to saddle bridge, wearing of keyhole bridge frames usually accentuate the length of the nose.

Some plastic spectacle frames also contain other type of bridges which compromise features between saddle and keyhole types and are effective in better nose fitting.

Bridge width: For all types of spectacle frames bridge width remain specified and it defines as the shortest distance between the two lenses or in a simpler term, as DBL, i.e. distance between the lenses, measured in millimeter unit (Fig. 12.12).

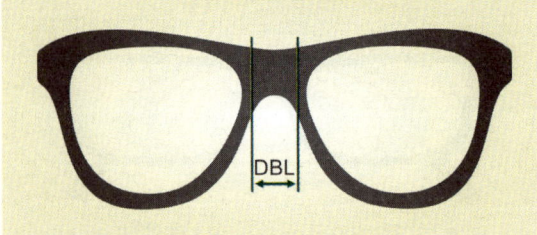

Fig. 12.12: Bridge width specification showing DBL

Temples: Temples are the part of spectacle which holds the front and rests on the ears of person. Common types of temples available are

- Skull temple
- Library temple
- Riding bow temple
- Comfort cable temple.

Skull temple is most commonly used temple designs for plastic spectacle frames. These types of temples remain bent downward behind the ear and follow the curve of the ear of person and shape of skull (hence are called skull temple). Advantage with skull temples is that they do not create excessive pressure on the mastoid process or ear lobe so are more comfortable for wearer. (Fig. 12.13A). Several modifications of skull temple have been done in terms of width which may vary in different frames from standard form of skull temple. Most of these modified skull temples, particular the thinner styles, contain a wire core to provide added strength.

Library or spatula temple does not have any curve like skull temple rather it lays straight back over the ear (Fig. 12.13D). Spectacle glasses remains in the position on the head due to pressure of temples which is exerted on the sides of skull by temple and this pressure is not seen with library temple, hence the fitting of these types of temples is difficult. The straight back design of temple helps the wearer to position the frame on and off the face very rapidly thus these temples are convenient for those who wear glasses irregularly and usually for a brief period of time.

Riding bow temple is the one which encloses the back and lower part of ear (Fig. 12.13B). Usually these are made up of plastic material having a central metallic core, mainly indicated for frames used in children and safety frames.

Comfort cable type of temple appears similar to riding bow temple; but the difference is that all and/or part of this type temple (specifically the part encircling the ear) is made up of a coiled metal cable instead of plastic (Fig. 12.13C).

Because of their identical appearance riding bow and comfort cable temples are used synonymously where a comfort cable temple

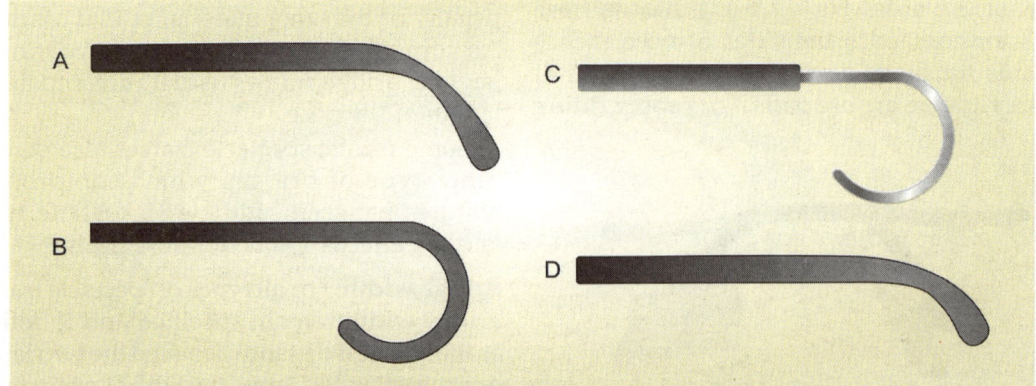

Fig. 12.13: Showing various types of temples. A. Skull type; B. Riding bow type; C. Comfort cable type; D. Library type

is considered as a type of riding bow temple. Metal spectacle frames and mountings usually have comfort cable/riding bow temples. These types of temples because of their structure can hold a frame securely in place and thus commonly used for children's spectacles and in some occupation like by mechanics and electricians.

Temple length: Previously, temple length was calculated by either measurement from length to bend or overall length from front to tip of temple. Now usually temples are specified as overall length only. Previously it was measured in inches but now represented in millimeter unit.

Bridge Fitting

The bridge fitting is an important step during spectacle fitting because usually most of the weight of spectacles is carried on the nose of person holding head in erect position. However, different styles of frame and positions of head may affect the percentage amount of total weight of the spectacles which is carried by the nose. Ideally, bridge fitting should be in such a way that weight of the spectacle frame remains distributed over a large area on the nose so that the irritation on the nose is reduced. It is essential to check bony angular configuration (i.e. frontal angle and transverse angle) of the nose by palpation of nose.

As shown in Fig. 12.14A frontal angle of the nose is an angle formed between midline of nose and a vertical line passing through each sides of nose, whereas transverse or splay

angle of nose is an angle formed between median sagital plane, i.e. an anterio-posterior plane passing through the midline of nose and line passing by the side of nose as shown in Fig. 12.14B.

> **Note:** Nose pads are selected in such a way that they closely match both the frontal angle and transverse angle of nose.

Temple Fitting

Normally, majority of spectacle's weight is borne by the nose but if a person tilt head in forward direction, then spectacle weight gets transfer from the nose to the ears. This weight shift will possess difficulty when patient is wearing library or skull types of temples, because pressure of the sides of temples against the patient's head on an area behind the ears maintain the position of the glasses in these types of temple designs. On contrary, riding bow temples encircle the ears and hence secures the position of frame by making contact at the lower arc of the external ear.

Important features to remember while fitting the temples of spectacle frames are

* Relation of angle of external ear to sides of patient's head.
* Shape of mastoid process

Hence, it is important for ophthalmic personnel to inspect the top and back of ear along with mastoid process; before deciding upon the type of temple he/she is planning to dispense to the patient.

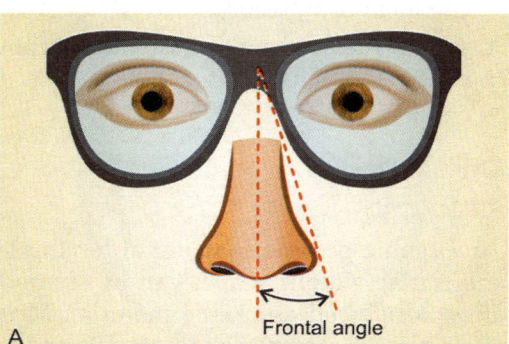
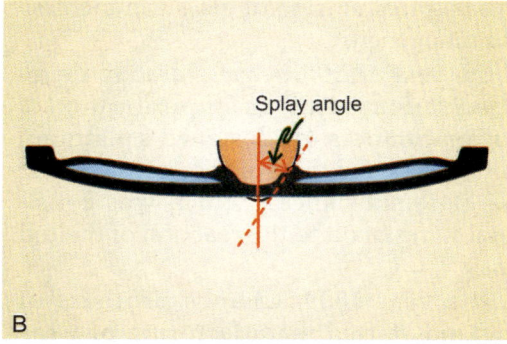

Fig. 12.14: Bridge fitting method. A. Frontal angle; B. Transverse or splay angle

OPTICAL MATERIALS

Optical Glasses

History

- In the year 423 BC Aristophanes, a Greek play writer, mentioned the use of a convex lens as a burning glass in his play 'Comedy of the Cloud'.
- However, early forms of spectacles were invented in late 13th century and these primary lenses were utilized mainly for correction of presbyopia.
- With the invention of telescope in the year 1608 by Galileo, demand of high quality optical glasses rose abruptly.
- English scientist John Dolland developed an achromatic lens in the year 1757. These achromatic lenses were made up of compounds crown and flint.

Crown glass: Originally window glasses were called crown glass, pieces for these glasses were used to make lenses and were called crown lenses. Nowadays crown glasses are the one which have silica, soda or potash and lime as basic components.

Flint glass: In the year 1676, George Ravenscroft used ground flint as silica source and added lead as basic component to form brighter, clearer, softer and heavier glass which was called flint glass. Nowadays flint glass contains lead oxide primary component along with other crown glass components.

Events of progress

- In the year 1814 PL Guinand of Switzerland revealed that stirring of glass can increase its homogeneity.
- In the year 1827, Michael Faraday developed various methods for purification of glass substances. He designed a platinum melting pot for the purpose of purifying the glass substances, which was considerably resistant to the reaction of melted glass.
- In the year 1839, Chance brothers of England started manufacturing of wide range of optical glasses.

- Later on in the year 1876 Ernst Abbe and Otto Schott of Germany extended the use of chemical oxides in manufacturing of glass and produced an extensive range of all new glasses for optical purposes.
- Until 1880, optical glasses quality available was either crown or flint. In the year 1880, Abbe introduced a glass of high refractive index without any noticeable rise in its dispersive power.
- In the year 1915 Bausch and Lomb Optical Co. started producing an extensive quantity of glasses having very good optical quality. Nowadays Bausch and Lomb, Corning Glass Works, and Pittsburgh Plate Glass Company contribute as major optical glass manufacturers in the world.

Optical glasses have vital properties like

- Refraction index: This is identified at the wavelength (589 nm) for Fraunhofer D line and is denoted by symbol η.
- Dispersion: This is defined as the variation in refraction index with wavelength. This is quantified by Abbe number (v) and is called nu value.

Following characteristics in an optical glass are required to make them useful for ophthalmic purposes

- Physical and chemical stability of high grade
- Transparency of high degree
- Homogenecity in both physical state and chemical composition.
- Appropriate refraction index and chromatic dispersion values.
- Colorless

Optical Plastics

Introduction

An organic polymeric material having large molecular weight which can be shaped by flow is referred as plastic material. Most of these plastics are synthetic materials produced by combination of organic and inorganic materials such as carbon, oxygen, nitrogen, hydrogen, chlorine, and sulphur. Commonly, plastic raw materials are derived from fossil-formed products such as oil, coal, and natural gas. Plastics used for optical purposes are very small fraction of total plastics. Materials used in fusion of bifocals should be physically stable; so that no stress occurs along the line of fusion.

Development of optical plastics: Different types of plastic materials were available since many years but use of plastics for production of lens increased primarily during and after World War II. Polymethyl methacrylate (PMMA), also known as Lucite or Plexiglas or Perspex, was one of the major plastic materials developed during World War II. It is a synthetic thermoplastic resin used for production of aircraft windshields. It is more durable than a non-tempered glass but also has a disadvantage of easy scratchability.

Another plastic material developed during World War II was allyl diglycol carbonate commonly called Columbian Resin 39 (CR- 39). A large series of 170 clear allylic materials were compounded when concentrated on a thermosetting in place of a thermoplastic material. The thirty-ninth compound among 170 were designated as CR-39, which was an allyl diglycol carbonate monomer. CR-39 was much more scratch resistant than PMMA.

- Robert Graham in 1947 made first ophthalmic lenses from CR-39.
- In the year 1957 GE Company developed a new plastic material, a polycarbonate resin called Lexan. This material has a great mechanical strength and high service temperature. In the year 1978, first ophthalmic lenses were produced from this material.
- In the year 1982, Corning Glass Works came up with a lens called Corlon. This was a two-layered glass lens where a very thin layer of polyurethane is bonded to the back surface of glass lens.

Spectacle Lens Materials

Glass Lenses

As discussed above glass had been used since old ages to form a spectacle lens for correction of refractive anomalies. Main varieties of optical glasses are

- Crown glass
- Flint glass
- Barium crown glass

Crown glass: Glasses having nu value greater than 50 are called crown glasses. Basic components of an ophthalmic crown glass are 70% silica (sand), 14–15% sodium oxide (soda), 11–12% calcium oxide (lime), and small percentages of potassium, antimony, borax, and arsenic. These glasses are mainly used in single vision glass lenses, and also as distance portion in most of the glass bifocal and trifocal lenses. Its refraction index is 1.52 and nu value is 59.

Flint glass: Glasses having nu value less than 50 are called flint glasses. Basic components are 45–65% lead oxide, 25–45% silica, and nearly 10% mixture of soda and potassium oxide. These glasses have more refraction index from 1.58 (light flint) to 1.69 (dense flint) and higher chromatic dispersion with a nu value of 30–40. They are mainly used for near segments in bifocal and also as single vision lenses where thinner lenses are required due to high degree of refractive error.

Barium crown glass: Its basic components are 25–40% barium oxide, along with other crown glass compositions. These glasses have refraction index 1.54 to 1.61 with nu values from 59 to 55. Barium crown glasses are mainly used in near segments of fused bifocals (Nochrome series).

Plastic Lenses

PMMA lenses: Polymethyl methacrylate is a thermosetting plastic material mainly used to manufacture contact lenses, although spectacle lenses such as Igard lens were made in Great Britain by using PMMA material.

Lens properties
- Refraction index: 1.49
- nu value: 57.2
- Specific gravity: 1.19

Advantages of PMMA lenses are
- High order transparency
- Shatter proof
- Light weight
- Tintability
- Optical design versatility

Disadvantages of PMMA lenses are
- Easily scratchability
- Damage due to glazing
- Unsuitable in extremely hot environment

CR-39 Lenses: Ophthalmic lenses prepared from material allyl diglycol carbonate monomer, popularly called CR-39 (Columbia resin 39) were supplied as a yellowish viscous liquid from a single western manufacturer. Initially this manufacturer produced CR-39 lenses in a variety of forms, powers and sizes. Some manufacturers added substances like UV absorbers, anti-yellowing agents and mould releasers to change the properties of lenses for better clinical usage.

Lens properties
- Refraction index: 1.498
- nu value: 58
- Specific gravity: 1.32

Advantages of CR-39 lenses are
- CR-39 lenses are chemically inert to majority of commonly used solvents such as benzene, acetone and gasoline.
- These lenses are highly resistant to impact.
- CR-39 lenses resist pitting from scatter particles especially from welding or grinding machines.
- Fogging due to sudden change in temperatures is less common than glass lenses because of lower thermal conductivity of CR-39 material.
- Other properties like tintability, light weightedness and optical design versatility are similar to PMMA lenses.

Disadvantages of CR-39 lenses are
- Increased lens thickness compared to glass lens due to lower refraction index.
- CR-39 lenses have relative lower resistance than glass lenses for surface aberrations.
- Significant damage to lens surface due to glazing.
- CR-39 lenses loses its photochromatic property in very less duration, hence are not used widely as photochromic lenses.

Polycarbonate Lenses: Polycarbonate is a thermoplastic material exist in solid state which is melted at about 320°C temperature and then injected in a mould to form a lens. A device then squeezes the lens to prevent shrinkage and to ensure the optical accuracy of surfaces. Polycarbonate lenses need a hard coating of surface to increase scratch resistance and chemical protection.

Lens properties
- Refraction index: 1.586
- nu value: 30
- Specific gravity: 1.20

Main advantages are high resistance to impact and higher refraction index, so very thin durable non-breakable lenses can be formed from polycarbonate material. Disadvantages are difficulty in surface molding, lens glazing/fitting and easily scratchability.

Absorptive Lenses

Absorptive lenses have been developed with the purpose to decrease the amount of light transmission or radiant energy, i.e. lens works as a filter. The light absorption may be uniform (absorbs all wavelengths of light) or selective (absorbs some wavelengths). These lenses are not colorless, so they are also called tinted lenses.

Mainly following types of absorptive lenses are routinely manufactured for optical purposes
- Tinted glass lenses
- Tinted plastic lenses
- Glass lenses with surface coatings

- Photochromic lenses
- Younger PLS filter lenses
- Polaroid lenses

Tinted glass lenses: Tinted glass lenses can be produced during manufacturing of crown glass (mixture of silica, soda, lime with small amounts of potassium, aluminium and/or barium oxides) by adding one or more metals or their oxides which results in the formation of different types of tinted color lenses as shown in Table 12.1.

Absorptive lenses have several advantages and disadvantages.

Advantages
- Low cost of manufacturing
- Little surface scratching
- Absence of reflection
- No special equipment needed for surfacing and lens finishing

Disadvantages
- Color tint of lenses is permanent in nature.
- High power tinted lenses had variations in transmission of light from central portion to peripheral portion of lens.
- Similarly, in patients having high degree of anisometropia the transmission of light in one eye is variable from fellow eye.

Tinted plastic lenses: Surface of plastic lenses cannot be coated by method of evaporation as there are chances of distortion of lens due to exposure to high temperature. Thus, these lenses are tinted by dropping them in a solution having desired organic dye. Resulting color density of tinted lens depends on two factors: Organic nature of the dye and immersion time.

To achieve a particular type of tint and/or light transmission; these plastic lens may be immersed into several kinds of tinted solutions. The variation in thickness of lens from center to periphery does not affect the density of tinted lens as penetration of dye in the surface of lens is up to a uniform depth. Hence, lenses of uniform density are formed. For any reason, if required, the tint color of lens can be changed by dipping the lens in bleaching solution.

Glass lenses with surface coatings: Surface of a glass lens can be tinted by coating it with a layer of metallic oxide by evaporation process under high temperatures in vacuum conditions. As discussed above plastic lenses are unsuitable for this process due to high temperatures. Refraction index of metallic oxide is higher than the glass, hence the amount of light reflecting from absorptive surface is more than that of uncoated surface of glass lens. To prevent this phenomenon of higher light reflection an anti-reflection coating of magnesium fluoride is done over and above the metallic oxide coating.

Photochromic glass lenses: In the year 1964, Corning Glass Works company begins the manufacturing of glass lenses having photochromatic properties, means these lenses become dark in sunlight and converts back to clarity when sunlight exposure is seized.

These lenses are composed with silver halide microscopic crystals. Sunlight (ultraviolet radiation) decomposes these microscopic crystals into silver and halide ions. These ions cluster together and when these clusters get larger they become darker. Hence the lens

Table 12.1: Metallic oxides and respective tinted color lenses

Metallic oxides	Lens color
Iron	Green
Cobalt	Blue
Manganese	Pink
Cerium	Pinkish brown
Uranium	Yellow
Chromium	Green
Nickel	Brown
Gold	Red
Silver	Yellow
Vanadium	Pale green
Didymium	Pink

color appears darker in the presence of sunlight, whereas in the absence of sunlight these silver and halide ions again converted into crystal form. Lens color fades and becomes clear in the absence of sunlight.

Rate of darkening of lens depends on the temperature, faster and deeper degree of darkening occurs in low temperature.

Degree of darkening of lens depends on
- Intensity of the radiation
- Length of exposure
- Surrounding temperature

Similarly, rate of fading of photochromic lenses depends on
- Glass composition
- Thermal bleaching (higher temperature, faster fading)
- Optical bleaching means exposure to a longer wavelength than that used for darkening

Photochromic plastic lenses: Photosensitive plastic for formation of ophthalmic lenses was introduced by American Optical Company (1982) and named the plastic photochromic lens as Photolite. These lenses were manufactured by the process of chemical impregnation rather than a usual dye pot process.

Properties of Photolite lenses are
- It shows about 90% transmittance of light in the faded state and about 45% transmission in dark state.
- Within 2 minutes time lens become darker to 45% out of total darkened state.
- Similar to other photochromic materials, less is the temperature of surrounding more will be the darkening of lens.

- Normally Photolite (fully activated) lens turns into blue color however, it can also be tinted to different colors.
- Life expectancy of Photolite lenses is nearly 2 years.

Younger PLS filter lenses: In the year 1984 Younger optics introduced a series of CR-39 lenses, called as Protective Lens Series (PLS). These lenses were design to protect the eyes by using selective filters for invisible ultraviolet and visible blue radiation. PLS lenses are neither photochromic nor tinted, rather are manufactured in a specific manner. Protective additives are added throughout the lens material uniformly so that these additives cannot be bleached or removed.

A specific wavelength is nominated to these PLS filter lenses as product code; below this wavelength these lenses literally block all of the ultraviolet and blue visible radiations.

A few specific product code lenses are summarized in Table 12.2.

Note: Using standard methods for cosmetic tint, the natural color of any of these PLS filter lenses can be changed without disturbing the lens performance.

Uses
- PLS lenses are advised to be used for protection against ultraviolet and visible blue radiations, because many researchers concluded that short wavelength radiations such as ultraviolet and blue radiations are harmful for eyes.
- These lenses are successfully used for protection in patients having ocular conditions like cataracts, corneal dystrophies, macular degeneration, and retinitis pigmentosa.

Table 12.2: Various PLS filter lenses and their properties			
Product code	Natural color of PLS filter lens	Wavelength designated	UV and blue radiation blockage (%)
PLS 400 lens	Pale yellow color	< 400 nm	Approx. 100
PLS 530 lens	Orange-amber color	530 nm	95–97
PLS 540 lens	Brown color lens	540 nm	95–97
PLS 550 lens	Red color lens	550 nm	95–97

Polaroid lenses: As discussed in Chapter 1 and as shown in Fig. 12.15 normally light beam is circularly symmetrical and unpolarized (Fig. 12.15A) but when it passes through crystals like quartz or calcite it becomes polarized (Fig. 12.15C), however, in between some light rays may also emit as partially polarized rays (Fig. 12.15B).

To manufacture polaroid filters, a thin sheet of polyvinyl alcohol is heated and then stretched so that it becomes about four times of its original length. Due to effect of stretching the molecular structure of polyvinyl alcohol get aligns in the form of long chain in the direction parallel to the stretching. The thin sheet of polyvinyl alcohol is then passed through a solution of weak iodine so that iodine molecules diffuse into layers of polyvinyl and gets attached to chains of long polyvinyl alcohol molecules. Hence, a thin sheet of polarizing filter is formed which is then laminated between two layers of coated cellulose acetate butyrate. These laminated sheets can be pressed into the desired curvature to form a lens. To create polarized glass lenses from thin sheet of polarizing material, the thin sheet is laminated between two layers of glass which then tinted and surfaced with power according to choice. In standard polarized sunglasses lenses, the tinted layer over lens has a uniform thickness, thus density of the lenses is uniform from center to periphery of lens. Sometimes, to increase the absorptive power of lens for ultraviolet radiations, special additives can be added in tint coating.

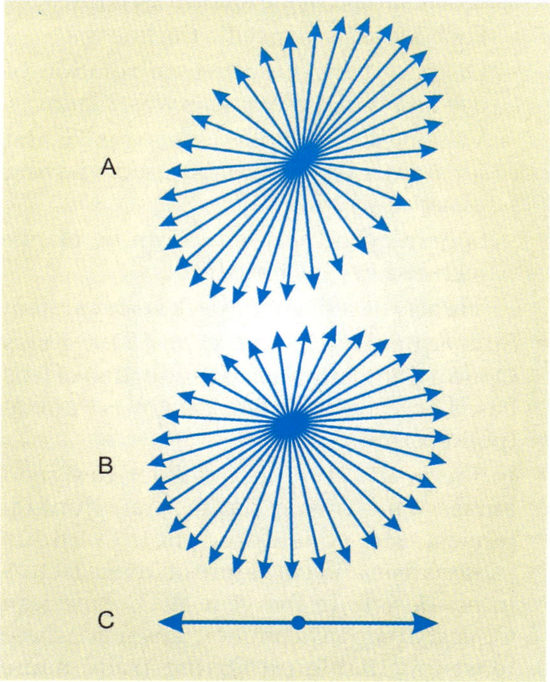

The Corlon lens: Corning manufacturers (1982) introduced a new specialized type of spectacle lens known as Corlon or bonded lenses because this lens was manufactured using both glass and plastic materials. Corlon lenses consist of following two layers (Fig. 12.16)

- Front layer of glass: Convex front layer of Corlon lens is made up of a thin glass lens, using either white crown glass or photochromic glass (photo grey extra). In case of minus power lenses, this layer has a central thickness of 1.3 mm when white crown glass material is used and 1.5 mm when photochromatic glass material is used.
- Back layer of plastic material: Concave back layer is made up of a very thin layer of special polyurethane plastic which is combined with the glass lens. Thickness of this polyurethane layer is 0.4 mm.

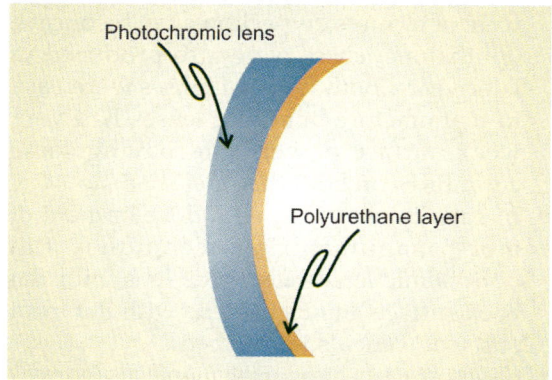

Fig. 12.15: Polarization of light. A. Unpolarized rays; B. Partially polarized rays; C. Linear polarized ray

Fig. 12.16: Corlon lens

Advantages of Corlon lens over routine spectacle lenses are

- More light in weight (up to 25%) as compared to ordinary glass lenses.
- Have thin edges (up to 25%) as compared to either ophthalmic crown glass lenses or plastic CR-39 lenses.
- Chances of scratches are less than plastic lenses because front surface is made up of glass.
- More resistant to shock caused by impacting object because of its two-layer construction. Impact of an object can break the front glass layer but polyurethane layer remains intact which protects the eyes from injuries due to glass particles.
- Its unique construction design eliminate the need for tempering because Corlon lens is more resistant from back surface infiltration as compared to both white crown glass and CR-39 plastic lenses.
- Its photochromic layer is thinner compared to a regular photogray lens so Corlon lenses darken less than regular lens.
- Polyurethane layer of the Corlon lens can easily be tinted by technicians in desired solid colors or gradient tints by using special types of water based dyes for better cosmetic looks.

SPECTACLE LENSES

Spectacle Lens Design

Spherical Lens Design

- Most primitive ophthalmic spherical lenses were of biconvex type, however, biconcave ophthalmic lenses were also produced in later years. Both types of lenses were easy to manufacture but these lenses had very weak surface powers and having same curvatures on both the sides.
- In subsequent years, with development of more manufacturing techniques flat ophthalmic lenses (flat plus lens with flat back surface, minus flat lens with flat front surface) were also produced.
- Later on, in the year 1804, meniscus (convex –concave or moon-shaped) form of lens was introduced by William Wollaston, and named them 'periscopic lenses' because of their property to provide a wider field of vision.

- Nietzsche and Gunther (German company) in 1867 developed uniform surface lenses of 1.25 D and termed them 'periscopic lens'. The plus lenses were having –1.25 D back surface and minus lenses were having a +1.25 D front surface. They also introduced 6.00 D base curve lens where plus spherical lenses had the back surface power of –6 D and a minus spherical lens had front surface power of +6.00 D.

- Tscherning (1904–1908) first identified the importance of center of rotation of the eye as a reference point in the lens design. He proposed that an oblique astigmatism might be eliminated by using two forms of bent lenses, i.e. deeper and shallower form.

- Moritz von Rohr (1908) worked on spectacle lenses with the aim to eliminate the oblique astigmatism and made following conclusions
  - Each lens has a specific thickness.
  - Distance between center of rotation of eye and back pole of lens was 25 mm.
  - Viewing angle for plus lenses was 35° and for minus lenses was 30° and viewing distance was infinity.
  - Sphero-cylindrical lenses can be manufactured in plus toric form.
  - He also described the back vertex system

- Subsequently, in the year 1913, Zeiss Optical Company started production of lens based on von Rohr's lens design as Punktal (point-forming) lens.

- In the year 1919, Edgar Tillyer designed lenses which were flatter than Punktal lenses. He considered both oblique astigmatism and curvature of image factors in his design. In the year 1923, American Optical Company commercially made these lenses available under the trade name Tillyer.

- In the year 1920, Kurova corrected curve lenses were developed by Continental

Optical Company which were later on redesigned by FE Duckwall in 1925. These lenses were having 39 base curves ranging from +2.5 to +12.5 D powers.

- Wilbur Rayton designed Orthogon lenses with the aim to correct oblique astigmatism like Punktal lens. However, correction of curvature of image was not included in this design. These lenses were slightly steeper as compared to Tillyer lenses. In the year 1928, Bausch and Lomb Optical Company initiated production of Orthogon lenses.
- On the basis of 14 base curves, Shuron Optical Company designed Widesite lenses which all were made in a positive toric form.
- In the year 1950, famous Normalsite corrected curve lens series (designed by Foster Klingaman) was developed by Titmus Optical Company. These Normalsite lenses were flatter as compared to other lenses.
- In early 1964, Univis Lens Company introduced the Best-form lenses which were negative toric lenses designed by EW Bechtold.
- In the year 1966, Shuron-Continental Company developed a negative toric lens series called Kurova Shursite. The bending curvatures of the Shursite negative toric lenses were similar to those of Shuron Continental Kurova positive toric lenses.

Spherocylindrical Lens Design

Astigmatic lenses designed for correction of astigmatism consist of a spherical surface on one side and a toric surface on the other side with two principal meridians. One meridian of lens has minimum power and other meridian has maximum power. The total sum of powers of two surfaces in each principal meridian remains fixed so that an image of the lens/eye system is aligned with axial vision. As these lens design have two powers so when light ray from a point object situated on the optical axis of the eye falls on a spherocylindrical lens, it results in formation of an astigmatic pencil after refraction, which in succession pass through two focal lines.

Negative and positive toric lenses: Previously, all corrected- curve spherocylindrical lenses were developed as positive toric lenses but many researchers have redesigned them as negative toric lenses also. Advantages of negative toric lenses are that

- Most of the multifocal lenses are negative toric lenses where bifocal addition is given on the front surface.
- Negative toric lenses play an important role in the spectacle magnification factors. In positive toric lenses two front surface powers and two back surface powers are present, whereas in negative toric lenses front surface power is the same for both meridians. Hence, front surface powers contribute in a spectacle magnification difference between two surfaces in positive toric lenses and not in negative toric lenses.

Design of High Plus Lenses

It has been seen that by using ophthalmic lenses with spherical surfaces an oblique astigmatism in the range of –23 D to +7 D can be eliminated, however, beyond this range it was impossible to remove oblique astigmatism. In regular clinical practice, patients having refractive error more than –23 D are rarely seen, however, aphakic patients usually require more than +10 D power of optical correction. Though, contact lenses are good alternative to spectacles but many of these patients being old are not comfortable with contact lens. These persons who required more than +4D to + 6D correction of oblique astigmatism in lens can be prescribed aspherical surface lens design instead of a routine spherical surface. Aspheric surfaces are the one where power of lens gradually decreases toward its periphery. In other words, an aspheric surface is the one which is axially symmetrical and is formed by the rotation of a portion of an ellipse, a parabola, or a hyperbola. David Volk (1958) developed aspheric spectacle glass lenses known as Conoid lenses. Production cost of aspheric lenses has decreased greatly due to wide acceptance of CR-39 plastic lens material because these lenses could easily be manufactured by a molding process instead of routinely used grinding process.

Terminologies in Spectacle Lenses

To understand the details of above type of lenses we need to know these terminologies related to lenses.

Blanks

Zero powered roughly finished slabs of glass are called blanks. Commonly, these glass slabs are available in different diameter sizes of 50 mm, 55 mm, 60 mm and 65 mm, however, very large size blank, say 70 mm or 75 mm are also available for specific indications. Thickness of these blanks range from 4 to 14 mm at 2 mm steps.

All ophthalmic blanks have following two refractive surfaces with a resultant zero power

- Base curve
- Combining surface

Base Curve

It is a standard fixed power curve of a blank. Available base curves are with a standard power of zero D, 1.25 D, 2 D, 4 D and 6 D, however, best form lenses have a base curve of either 1.25 D or 6 D power.

Combining Surface

This is the other surface of blank on which desired power is grounded. Net power of the lens is produced by grinding the respective combining surface of a blank provided by manufactures. To get a net plus power lens, a blank having minus base curve is used and to get a minus power lens, a plus base curve blank is used.

For example, in Fig. 12.17A, to get a lens of + 2 D, –6 D base curve blank is used and a +8 D power is grinded on combining surface of the blank to produce a net +2 D power lens. Similarly, as shown in Fig. 12.17B, to produce a –2 D lens, a +6 D base curve blank is used

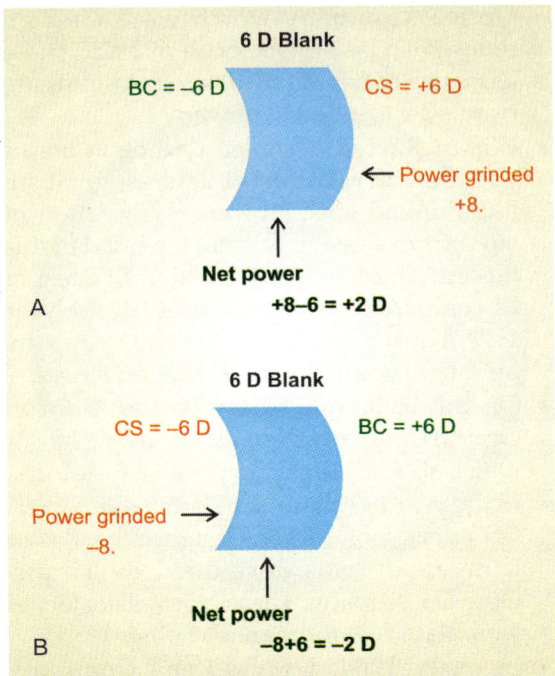

Fig. 12.17: 6 D Blanks. BC: Base curve having fixed 6 D power CS: combination surface, used to grind power. A. Minus 6 D blank; B. Plus 6 D blank

and a –8 D power is grinded on combining surface of the blank to produce a final –2 D power lens.

Lens Power

Refracting power of an ophthalmic lens can be expressed in several ways like

- Approximate power which is also called nominal power when the power of an ophthalmic lens is expressed in terms of its front and back surface powers irrespective of lens thickness.
- Back vertex power and front vertex power when ophthalmic lens power is considered in terms of refracting power for emergent rays from its back surface or front surface.
- Equivalent power when power of a thick ophthalmic lens or optical system is equated as power of a single thin lens.
- Effective power: Here the power of an ophthalmic lens is dependent upon its distance from the wearer's eye.

Note: Among all these expressions of power specification, practically only back vertex power is used by optical laboratories and practitioners to specify an ophthalmic lens power.

Approximate Power

Approximate power of an ophthalmic lens is calculated by

$$P = Fa + Fb$$

Here Fa and Fb represents the powers of front and back surface, respectively (Fig. 12.18) and can be measured by lens measure or lens clock.

In this formula for power calculation, thickness of lens is not considered as it is presumed that a lens has zero thickness. However, in reality most of the ophthalmic lenses cannot be considered to be markedly thin, thus we need a more accurate expression for calculation of lens power which includes back vertex power, front vertex power, and equivalent power.

Back Vertex Power

This is expressed as the reciprocal of the back focal length [i.e. distance from the back pole (vertex) of lens (L2) to the second focal point (F')]. The second focal point is the actual distance divided by the refractive index of ophthalmic lens media. In this Fig. 12.19 back vertex power of lens (F'v) in air is expressed as the reciprocal of the distance L2 to F'.

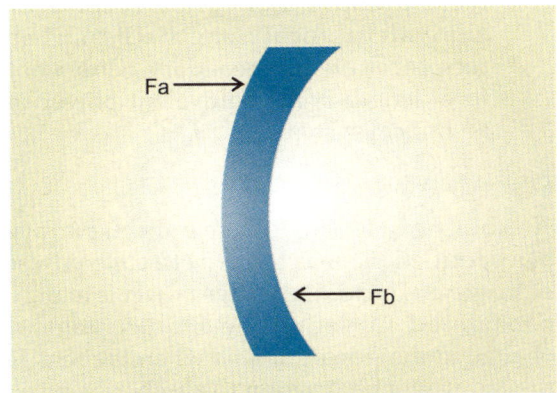

Fig. 12.18: Front (Fa) and back (Fb) powers of lens

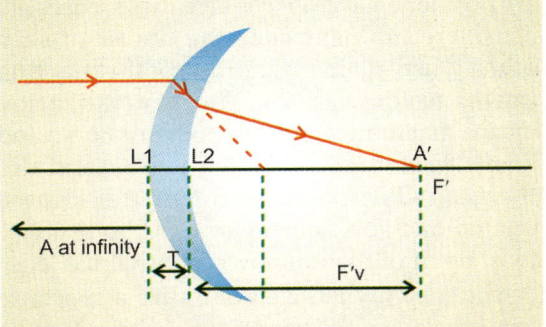

Fig. 12.19: Back vertex power of lens in air. L1, L2: Front and back refractive surfaces of ophthalmic lens respectively. F': Secondary focal point. T: Thickness of lens

Back vertex power is considered important parameter to indicate the power of an ophthalmic lens because

- As discussed above to measure back vertex power, two points, i.e. back vertex of lens and second focal point are considered. If we select such a power of lens at which the second focal point of the lens is placed at far point of the eye then lens can easily be placed at any position in front of the eye. Hence, an ophthalmic lens if placed either in a spectacle plane or on the cornea (contact lens) we can still be able to specify its back vertex power to get the expected optical effect.

- Back vertex power permits an indefinite utilization in terms of lens form like bend or cross section shape of ophthalmic lenses. We can use any form of ophthalmic lens either for examination purpose or fitting process in clinical practice. What we have to do is just to ensure that secondary focal point of our ophthalmic lens coincide with the far point of eye.

Note: Back vertex power can be measured by an instrument lensometer or vertometer.

Front vertex power or neutralizing power:

The power of an unknown ophthalmic lens can be measured by neutralizing it with trial lens of known power. When these two lenses are positioned in close contact, these lenses are considered to neutralize the power of each other when their measured total refracting power becomes zero. The neutralization means that focal lengths of both unknown and known lens are equivalent in amount and also the secondary focal point of the known ophthalmic lens coincides with the primary focal point of the unknown ophthalmic lens.

Routinely, when we neutralize a spectacle lens by placing the back pole of a trial lens on the front pole of the spectacle lens then we are measuring the front vertex power of spectacle lens. Hence, front vertex power is defined as the negative reciprocal of the reduced distance from the front pole (L1) of the lens to its primary focal point (F).

An expression for front vertex power (Fv) can be derived in a similar way as that for back vertex power (F'v). As per above definition neutralizing power is the negative reciprocal of the distance L1F in Fig. 12.20.

Equivalent Power

Many of the optical devices act as a complex optical system as they contain a series of lenses which remain separated either by air or by media of different refractive indices. Sometimes, it is suitable to consider this complex system of lens as an imaginary single thin lens

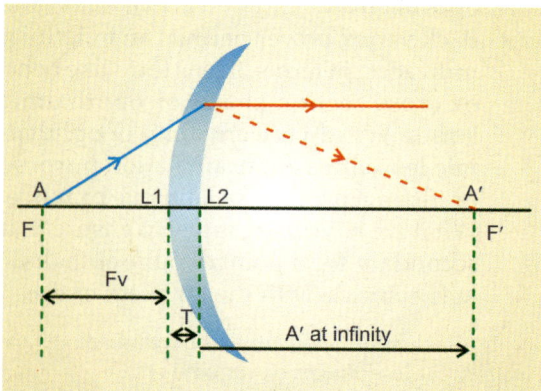

Fig. 12.20: Front vertex power of lens in air. L1, L2: Front and back refractive surfaces of ophthalmic lens respectively. F: Primary focal point. T: Thickness of lens

(equivalent lens) so that it becomes easy to find out object–image relationship of equivalent lens. It is assumed that this imaginary single lens will produce the image of a distant object of same size and at same position as produced by series of lenses of optical system. The focal length of this imaginary single lens (equivalent lens) at which image of same size and at the same position produced similar to those by optical system is known as equivalent focal length. The reciprocal of this equivalent focal length (meters) is called the equivalent power.

Position of this thin equivalent lens with respect to the system is determined by locating the principal planes of the optical system. In symmetrical optical systems only a single pair of planes is present; which poses the property of positive unity (+1) magnification (means the object and its image are of same size and image is erect). These pairs of planes are called principal planes and the points of intersection of optical axis with these planes are principal points of optical system.

- Principal plane associated with the object space is termed primary principal plane and plane with the image space is secondary principal plane.
- The distance from the primary principal point (P1) to primary focal point (F) is called primary equivalent focal length (Fe) as shown in Fig. 12.21.
- Similarly, the distance from secondary principal point (P2) to the secondary focal point (F') is called secondary equivalent focal length (Fe'). The reciprocal of the secondary equivalent focal length is the equivalent power of an optical system.

Effective Power

An ability of a lens to focus parallel light rays at a specified plane is termed effective power of that lens. The term effective power is mainly considered to define the requirement of change in the power of lens when the lens is moved from one position to another position in front of the eye.

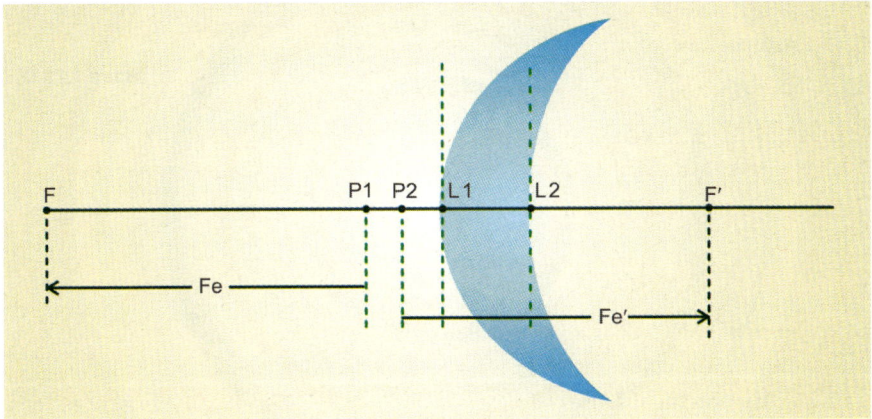

Fig. 12.21: Primary and secondary equivalent focal length. L1, L2: Front and back refractive surfaces of ophthalmic lens respectively. F: Primary focal point; F': Secondary focal point, P1: Primary principle plane, P2: Secondary principle plane, Fe: Primary equivalent focal length, Fe': Secondary equivalent focal length

Practically we consider that plus lenses are more effective because when these lenses are moved farther away from the eyes they produce more change in vergence than required. While minus lenses are considered as less effective because when these lenses are moved farther away from the eyes, they produce less change in vergence than required.

Classification of Spectacle Lenses

Spectacle lens classification is summarized in Table 12.3. The specific features of each type of lens in relation to spectacle fitting purposes have also been explained.

Various Lens Forms

Symmetrical lenses: When curvatures of both the surfaces of lenses are same, they are called symmetrical lenses as shown in Fig. 12.22.

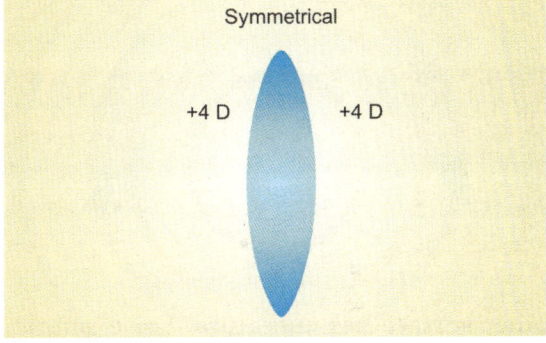

Fig. 12.22: Symmetrical lens

Asymmetrical lenses: Ophthalmic lenses having different curvatures of both the surfaces are called asymmetrical lenses as shown in Fig. 12.23.

Plano lenses: In these types of lenses one surface has zero power or plane, whereas

Table 12.3: Classification of spectacle lenses	
Based on lens form	*Based on corrective power*
Symmetrical	Monofocal lenses
Asymmetrical	Plano focal lenses
Plano	Multiple focal lenses
Periscopic	• Bifocal lenses
Deep meniscus	• Trifocal lenses
Lenticular	• Varifocal or progressive lenses
Aspheric	

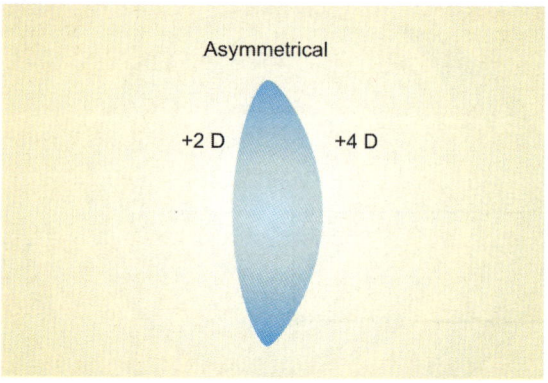

Fig. 12.23: Asymmetrical lenses

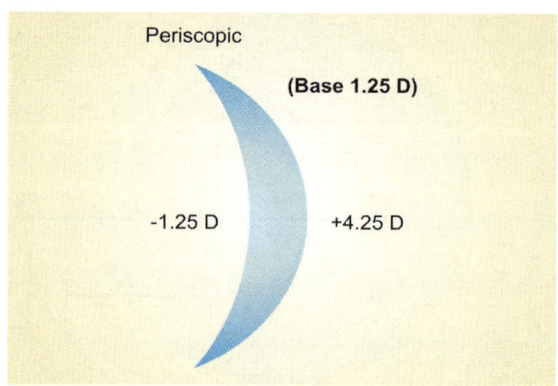

Fig. 12.25: Periscopic lens

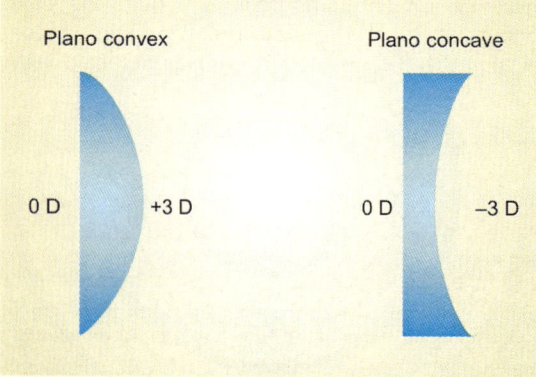

Fig. 12.24: Plano lenses

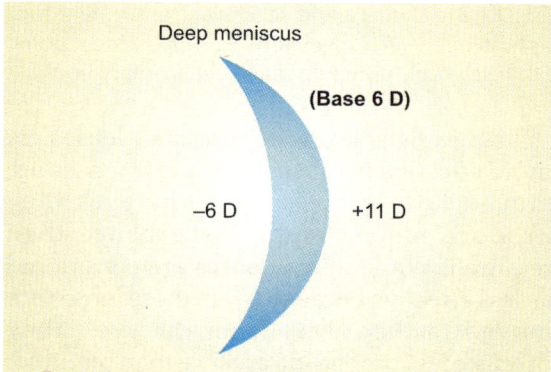

Fig. 12.26: Deep meniscus lens

other surface has curvature. For example, Plano convex or plano concave as shown in Fig. 12.24.

Periscopic lenses: These lenses are considered as best form lens having a base curve of 1.25 as shown in Fig. 12.25 and on combined surface (+4.25 D in our example) power for final lens is grinded.

Deep meniscus lenses: These lenses are also a type of best form lens where base curve is of 6 D as shown in Fig. 12.26 and on its combined surface (+11 D in our example) power for final lens is grinded.

Lenticular lenses: These lenticular lenses were designed by Obrig (1933) for correction of high degree myopia and named them Myo-disc. A small concave disc was grinded on the back surface of a Plano lens for formation of this thin and light weight Myo-disc lens as shown

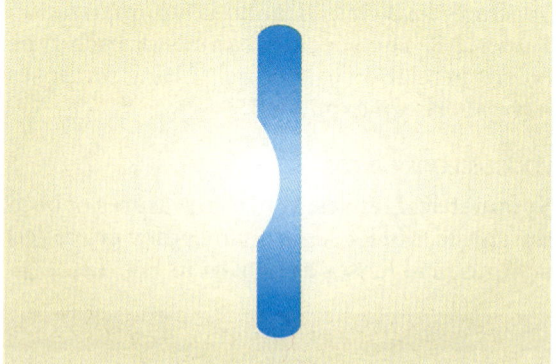

Fig. 12.27: Original Myo-disc lens designs

in Fig. 12.27. Most of the lenticular lenses which were manufactured later on were almost similar to this original Myo-disc lens in their designing.

Most of the lenticular lenses contain a powered central portion (optical zone) called as aperture which is about 30–40 mm in diameter. This aperture is surrounded by a carrier lens, having Plano or low plus power. Initially, these lenses were prepared with the aim to reduce the thickness of lens, hence in past for many years majority of the glass aphakic lenses were made in lenticular form with some minor percentage of plastic lenses.

Various types of lenticular lenses are

- **Solid state lenticular lenses:** Here the carrier is cut in a convex shape from the base lens as shown in Fig. 12.28 and this design is mainly used for plastic lenses.
- **Fused lenticular lenses:** Here aperture is fused on back surface of plus power lens under high temperatures and then desired power is grounded on the front surface (Fig. 12.29). These types of lenses are mainly used for glass lenses.

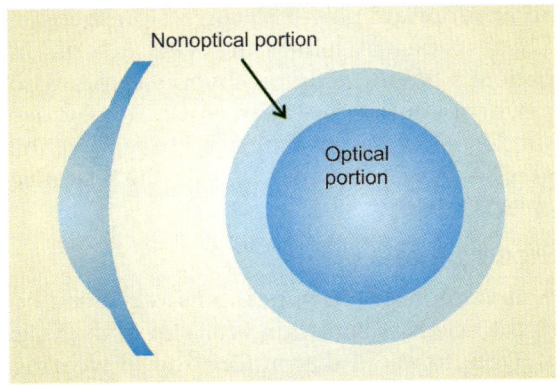

Fig. 12.28: Solid state one piece lenticular lenses

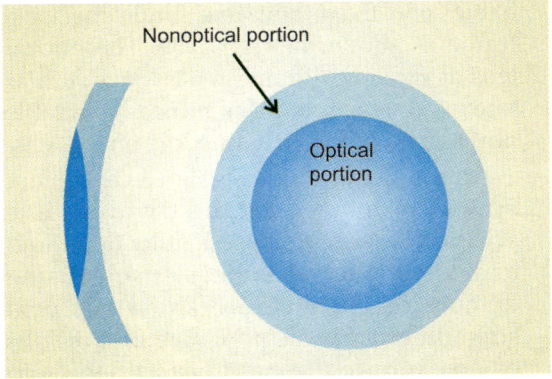

Fig. 12.29: Fused lenticular lenses

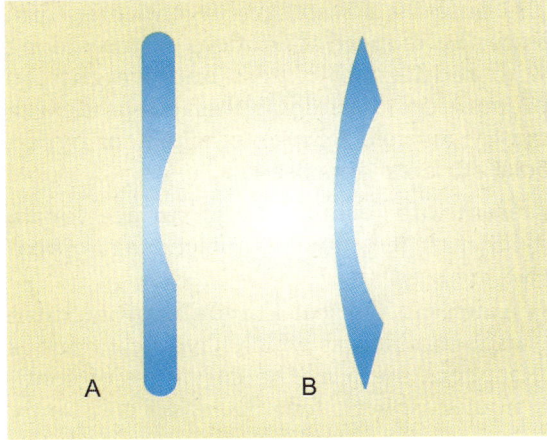

Fig. 12.30: Plano lenticular lenses. A. Concave aperture; B. Convex aperture

- **Plano lenticular lenses:** These lenses have either a convex or concave surface aperture and a plane surface carrier as shown in Fig. 12.30A and B. Initial Myo-discs are an example of minus lenticular lenses of these types.
- **Cemented lenticular lenses:** These lenticular lenses are made up of a spherical aperture cemented with a cylindrical carrier by glue. These lenses are used mainly in patients having high astigmatic refractive errors.

Advantages of lenticular lenses
  - Light weight
  - Thin lenses
  - Less optical aberrations
  - Less spectacle magnification
  - Correct high refractive errors

Disadvantages of lenticular lenses
  - Bull's eye or fried egg appearance
  - Difficult spectacle fitting

Aspheric lenses: The problem encountered during the use of lenticular design lenses for correction of high degree refractive anomalies lead to the development of new design plastic lenses known as aspheric lens. These lenses have an aspheric surface (ellipsoid) which progressively gets flat on the periphery so that power of lens also reduced gradually towards the periphery, thus especially useful in aphakic patients. In addition, aspheric lenses also pose the advantages of lenticular form lenses, i.e. reduced aberrations of lenses along with reduced thickness and weight. To prepare ophthalmic aspheric lens design mostly conicoid (ellipse, parabola, or hyperbola) surfaces were used.

Presently to form aspheric surface for an ophthalmic lens, two manufacturing approaches are used

- American Optical Fulvue manufactures aspherical lenses which have a continuous aspheric surface. The curvature of continuous aspheric lens decreases constantly from its central portion toward the periphery as shown in Fig. 12.31. Hence, there is a continuous reduction in refractive power towards the edge or periphery due to reduction in curvature of the lens.

- Annular pattern arrangement aspheric lens designs: The lens surface consists of series of different zones (spherical in shape) around the center. The surface power of each zone progressively decreases towards periphery, means the farthest zone from the center has least power and the nearest zone has maximum power. The tangents to curves of adjacent zones are arranged in such a manner that they coincide with the boundary between the two adjacent zones; thus eliminating the prominent dividing lines on aspheric surface. The junctions present between two adjacent zones are made smooth by polishing the surface with flexible pads. Armorlite multi-drop lens formerly called Welsh four drop lens is one of the examples of aspheric design lens.

Monofocal Lenses

These are the lenses used to correct either distance vision or near vision problems, hence are also called single vision glasses. These lenses are either spherical or spherocylindrical in nature. Entire surface of these lenses has the same corrective power, hence are used to correct refractive anomalies such as myopia, hypermetropia, and astigmatism with presbyopia. Various designs of these types of lenses had already been discussed above.

Plano focal lenses: These lenses are similar to bifocal lenses in the shapes and designs but the upper portion of the lens is used for distance vision correction, has no optical power or plane, whereas the near segment has an appropriate power to correct presbyopia. These types of lenses are very useful in patient's having only presbyopic errors who perform continuous near work, if they use single vision glasses they need to remove the glasses very frequently to see the distance objects clearly.

Bifocal Lenses

- Invention of the bifocal lens was done by the scientist Benjamin Franklin in the year 1785, to avoid discomfort due to wearing of two separate spectacles for distance and near vision; he cuts both the glasses into halves and fixed them in a single spectacle frame as shown in Fig. 12.32. The bifocal lens designed by Franklin has looks similar to executive single piece bifocal (available nowadays) with a dividing line on the lens.

  Although these bifocals showed excellent optical property, but the dividing line across the lens produced reflections and had a tendency to collect dust, causing discomfort to wearer. The structural strength of lens was poor as both portions of lens were kept in positions with the help of eye wire of the frame.

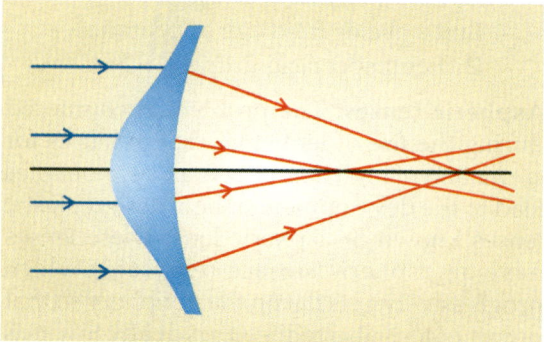

Fig. 12.31: Continuous aspheric lens design showing reduced surface focusing light rays nearer.

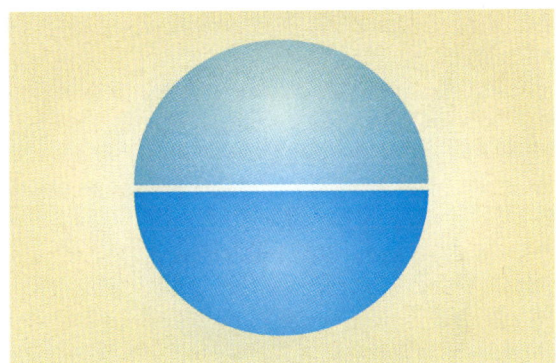

Fig. 12.32: Original Benjamin Franklin lens design

- In the year 1838, Isaac Schnaitmann developed a type of bifocal lens called solid up-curve bifocal and it was first one-piece bifocal lens which gained popularity. This lens was having good structural strength, invisible dividing line, less chances of chromatic aberration and provided wide field of view for reading than Franklin lens. However, in the distance portion of lens significant amount of aberrations were noticed, hence restricted the field of vision for distance. Moreover, a strong base down prismatic effect was seen in the distance part of lens.
- August Morck (1888) developed modified form of Franklin bifocal and named it perfection bifocal lenses. Perfection bifocal contained a curved dividing line. Each glass piece of lens had beveled edge which led to more stabilization of lens in the spectacle frame as shown in Fig. 12.33. Morck also invented cemented bifocal design in the year 1888.

- John Borsch (1889) took another step in bifocal invention and developed cemented Kryptok bifocal lenses.
- In the year 1915, Henry Courmettes further improved the design of fused bifocals; by fusing a button (segment) into the major lens, which was made up of two types of glasses.
- Subsequently, in the year 1931, Watson and Culver designed and also patented the bifocal "B" or bar segment bifocal lens (straight top) as shown in Fig. 12.34.

Almost during the same period four inventors filed identical patent applications for the "D" style segment (looks like a letter D, lying on its back) as shown in Fig. 12.35. Finally, in the year 1933, NH Stanley got the patent, for this D style segment.

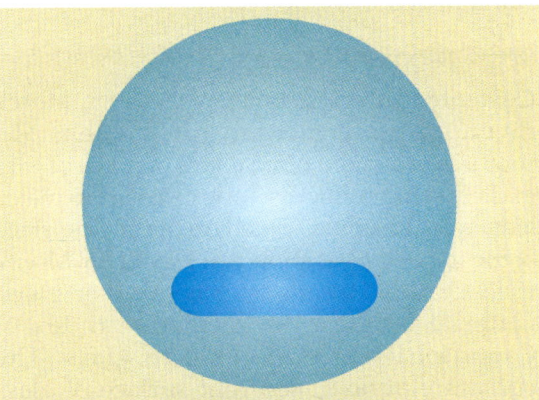

Fig. 12.34: Bifocal 'B' or bar segment lens design

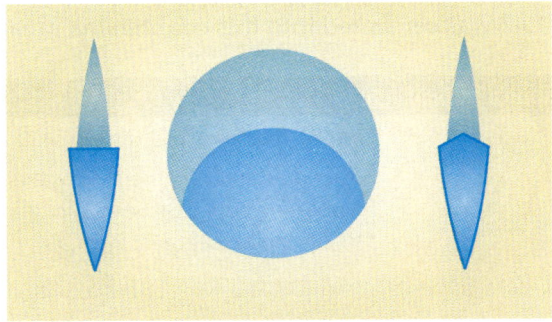

Fig. 12.33: Perfection bifocal lens design

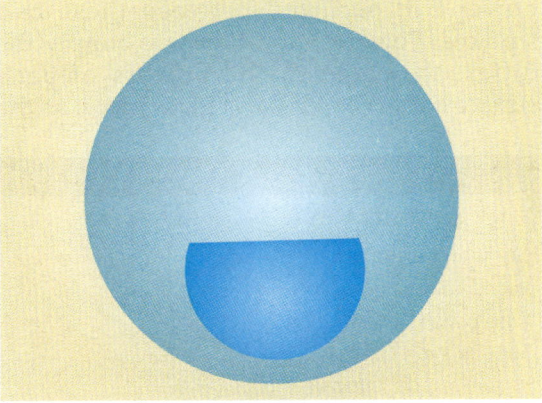

Fig. 12.35: Bifocal 'D' segment lens design

- Silverman (1932) developed the "R" or ribbon segment and patented R-compensated series of lenses; which contain 7 segments (R4 to R10) designed to compensate for vertical prismatic effects in the near vision.
- Hammon and Price modified the 'D' style design called as Panoptik (having rounded corners) and Widesite (having curved-top version).
- Charles Conner (in 1910) produced a bifocal lens which was grounded from a single piece of glass, having a uniform refraction index. He called this lens Ultex bifocal.
- American Optical Company (in 1954) took the next step for the development and manufacturing of one-piece bifocal known as executive bifocal.

Bifocal lenses are broadly classified as summarized in Table 12.4.

Single Segment Bifocals

Cemented bifocals: In the year 1888, Morck invented the cemented bifocal lens. To produce cemented bifocal lens, a piece of thin glass (having refractive index similar to major lens) was cemented/glued on the back surface of the major lens as shown in Fig. 12.36. Morck used Canada balsam as cementing or glued material because the refractive index of Canada balsam was equal to glass. The curvature of both, i.e. front surface of glass piece and the back surface of the major lens were equal hence no change in refractive power had occurred between these two surfaces. Power of addition was simply the difference between the powers of back surfaces of major lens and glass piece; as the

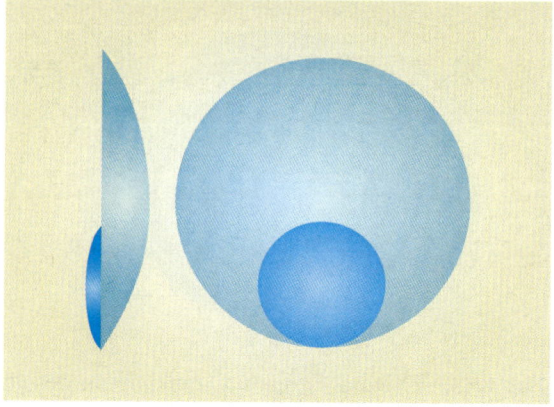

Fig. 12.36: Cemented bifocal lens design

back surface of glass piece was kept less concave as compared to the back surface of major lens.

Advantages
- Optically acceptable.
- Cosmetically widely accepted, hence was used nearly for a century.

Disadvantages
- Chances of dust collection on shoulder around the dividing line.
- Temperature changes were affecting the adherence property of the glass piece.
- Glass piece had a propensity to fall off easily with long usage.
- Cement was getting darken with use and time.

In the year 1889, Borsch developed Kryptok (means hidden) cemented bifocal lens. He created a countersink curve, like a depression on the front surface of major lens. Then a wafer or glass piece (flint glass) of refractive index 1.67 was cemented into this countersink area.

Table 12.4: Classification of bifocal lenses	
Single segment bifocals	*Double segment bifocals*
Cemented bifocals	Fused double D segment bifocals
Fused bifocals	Double segment executive bifocals
One piece bifocals	Mixed double segment bifocals
Special type bifocals	
• Minus add bifocals	
• Golfers' bifocals	

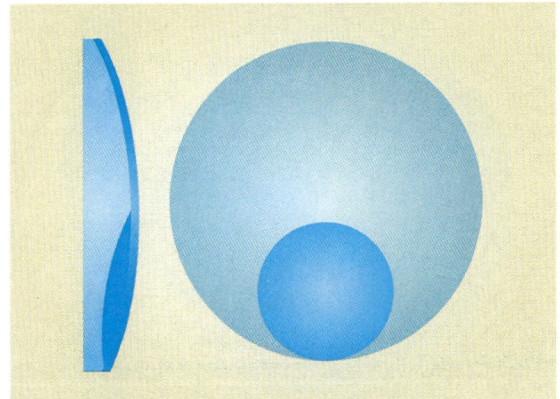

Fig. 12.37: Kryptok lens design popularly called KT

Finally, the surface of entire lens was covered with a thin meniscus of glass cemented in place (Fig. 12.37).

These were the first bifocal lens where refractive index of reading addition (near segment) material was higher (1.67) than the major lens.

Disadvantages
- Difficult to manufacture because six surfaces needed to be grounded and polished.
- Lens covering of thin meniscus glass was very fragile.
- Darkening of cementing material.
- Chances of dislocation or separation of lens

Note: Occasionally, in some special conditions like low vision aid, temporary bifocals or for experimental purposes these cemented bifocals are still used and an Epoxy resin (Araldite) is used in place of Canada balsam as cementing material for better stability.

Fused Bifocal Lenses: Most widely used bifocal lenses are fused types of bifocals and hence available in several segment styles like
- Round segments
- Straight top segments
- Modified straight top segments

Round segments bifocal lenses: Original Kryptok bifocal lenses were low in cost but made of flint glass (small nu value) segment so a large degree of chromatic aberration was present. Initially, Kryptok lenses were available in different segment sizes, but now only 22 mm segment size is available in the market.

Gradually, every lens manufacturer developed a round segment bifocal lens having a specific designed company's corrected curves. They all used barium crown glass for the segment instead of flint glass because barium crown glass has high nu value, hence chances of chromatic aberrations decreased significantly. Kryptok lenses are manufactured by fusing a round segment inside the groove of major lens as shown in Fig. 12.38.

Normally the segment size in the round fused bifocal lenses is of 22 mm in diameter, with the segment optical center located at 11 mm below the segment top in an uncut lens form (Fig. 12.39).

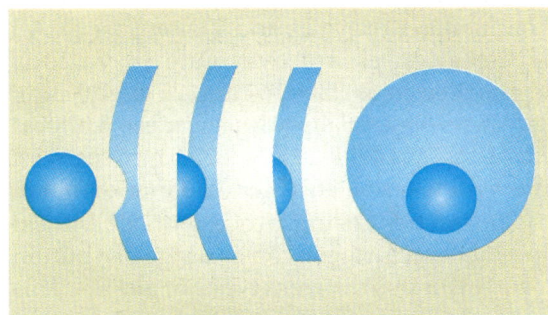

Fig. 12.38: Manufacturing process for round segment bifocal (Kryptok) lens

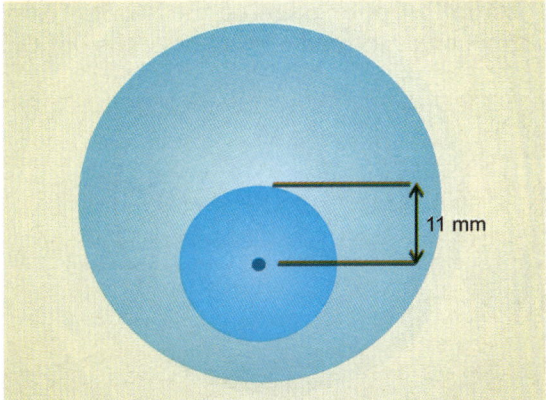

Fig. 12.39: Locations of segment and optical center in round segment bifocal lens

Several lenses belong to this category are American Optical Tillyer, Univis Unachrome, Shuron Continental Kurova and Vision Ease CRF. Round segment size in Univis R and Vision Ease R bifocal lenses is 22 × 14 mm segments and in Kurova B is 28 × 14 mm.

Straight top segments bifocal lenses: Most commonly used types of bifocal are straight top fused bifocal which was first developed by the Univis Lens Company of Dayton. Originally, Univis Sentinel D lens was made first by fusing a truncated round high index segment with small crown glass segment and then fusing this entire segment into a countersink area of major lens as shown in Fig. 12.40.

Once the patent of Univis got expired, straight top bifocal lenses were produced by many other lens manufacturers like American Optical Tillyer D, Masterpiece S, Shuron Continental Kurova D, and Vision Ease D. All of these lenses are available in various segment sizes as 22 × 16 mm, 25 × 17.5 mm, and 28 × 19 mm. Tillyer Masterpiece S bifocal lens is also available in a 20 × 15.5 mm segment and Vision Ease D in a 35 × 22.5 mm segment.

Courmettes fusing process of 'D' bifocal lens manufacturing involves usage of a button made up of two different types of glasses. This button is fused in a countersink area present in the major lens and a finally finished lens is manufactured as shown in Fig. 12.41.

Initially upper edge of the straight top segment was located 6 mm above the optical

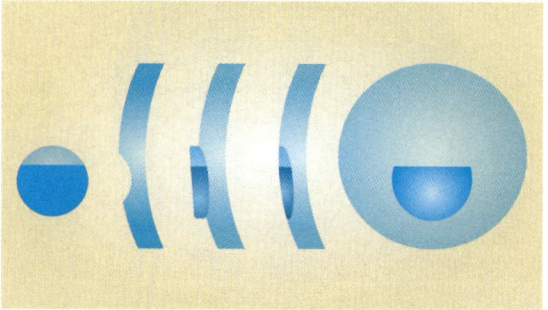

Fig. 12.40: Straight top bifocal lens manufacturing process

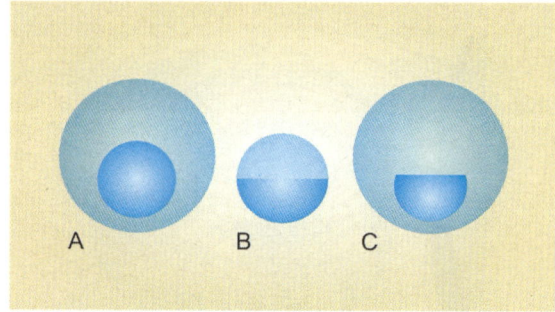

Fig. 12.41: Showing Courmettes fusing process. A. Major lens with counter sink area; B. Button made up of two glasses; C. Finally fused bifocal 'D' lens

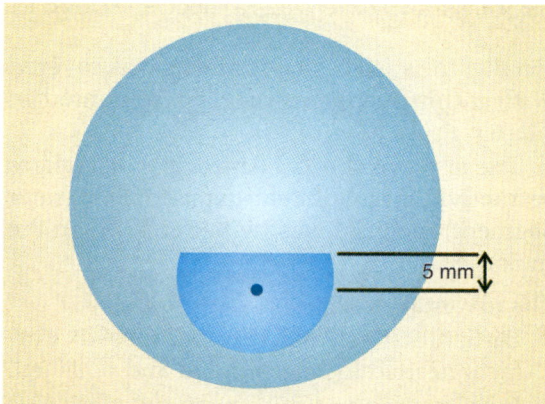

Fig. 12.42: Final 'D' bifocal lens showing 5 mm mark below top edge of segment

centre but finally after fusing the resultant segment optical center came 5 mm below the segment top margin (against 11 mm below top margin in round segment lenses) as shown in Fig. 12.42.

Modified straight top segment bifocal lenses: Enormous success of Univis straight top bifocal lenses encouraged other manufactures to develop modified forms of straight top bifocal. Panoptic design by Bausch and Lomb and Widesite lenses by Shuron were the earliest modified straight top segment bifocal lenses (Fig. 12.43).

Panoptic bifocal has a 23 × 15 mm segment with slightly rounded corners, whereas Widesite has a slightly curved top. Recently, Univis F and Vision Ease C bifocals were introduced having a similar shape as that of

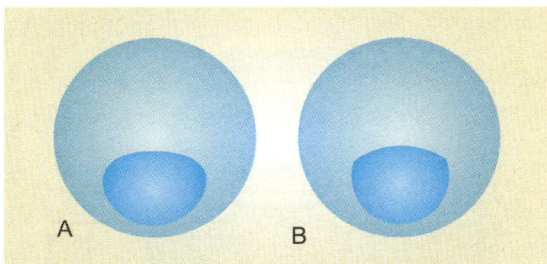

Fig. 12.43: Modified bifocal 'D' segment lens designs. A. Panoptic design with rounded edges; B. Widesite design with curved top

Panoptic while American Optical Tillyer Sovereign and Shuron Continental Kurova CT as that of Widesite.

Ribbon Segments bifocal lenses are essentially a modified type of straight top segment; here the lower part is cut off so that wearer can have distance vision from both below and above the segment as shown in Fig. 12.44.

In all designs of fused bifocal lenses, say round, straight top, modified straight top, or ribbon segments, the bifocal segment is located on the front surface of the major lens. As segment side of major lens should have a spherical surface for fusion process, in these fused bifocal lenses if a cylindrical correction is needed, then major lens must be made in a negative toric form.

One piece bifocal lenses: These lenses are available in both round and straight top segment styles. As compared to fused bifocals in most of the round one piece bifocals the near segment is located on the back surface of the major lens. Hence, if a cylindrical correction is needed, then major lens must be grounded on its front surface or in a plus toric form. However, very few types of one piece bifocals are made in a negative toric form, similar to the fused bifocals.

One piece round segments bifocal lenses: Original Ultex A and AL type lenses have large round segments. The lower parts of the segment have been cut off, hence are also called hemispherical segments. Both Ultex A and AL lenses have segments having 38 mm diameter where in A type lens the segment is 19 mm high and in AL type lens it is 32 mm high in uncut lens form. Both forms of Ultex lenses have near segment on the back surface of the major lens as shown in Fig. 12.45.

These Ultex design lenses are manufactured by chipping technique as shown in Fig. 12.46.

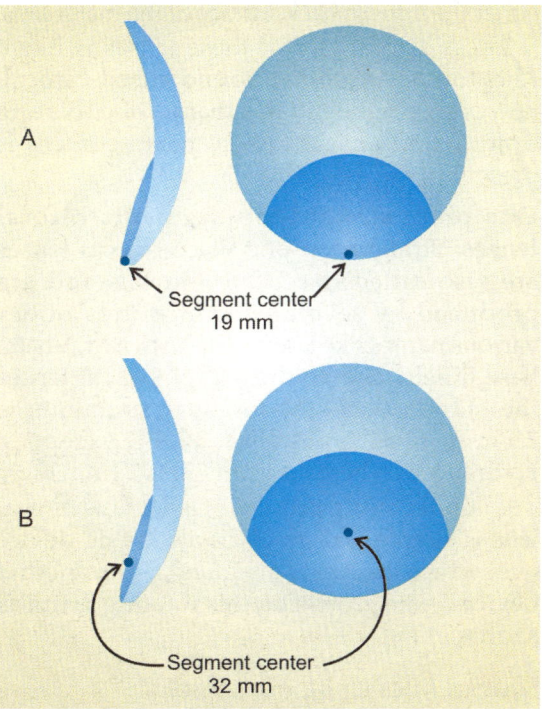

Fig. 12.45: One piece round segment bifocal lenses. A. Ultex A type having 19 mm segment; B. Ultex AL type having 33 mm segment

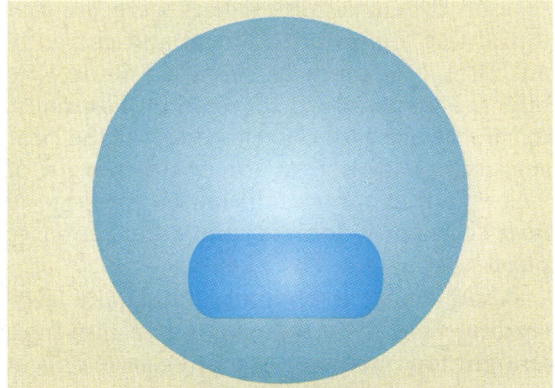

Fig. 12.44: Ribbon segment lens design

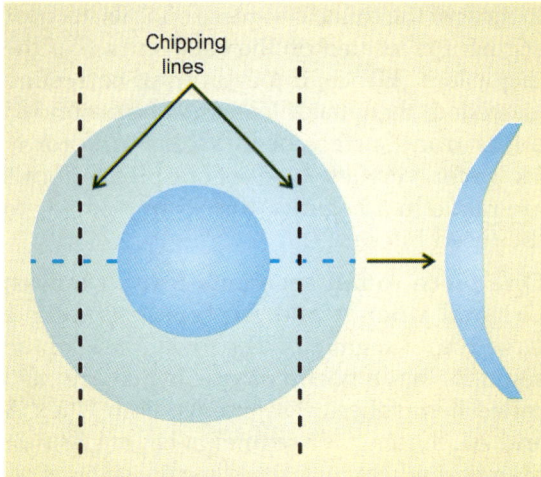

Fig. 12.46: Chipping technique for manufacturing of Ultex lenses

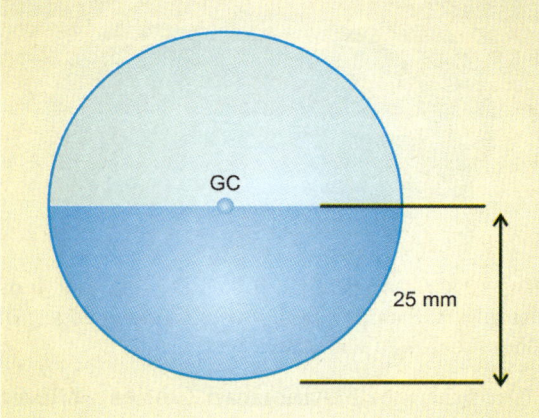

Fig. 12.47: Executive bifocal lens design

Another type of additional hemispherical one piece bifocal was developed by Robinson Houchin as Hydray having segment sizes of either a 40 × 20 mm or a 38 × 33 mm situated on either the front or back surface of the major lens.

Gross appearance of these lenses is like a Kryptok or any other round fused bifocal, however, a feeling in the change of curvature from major lens surface to near segment is present in one piece bifocals.

One piece straight-top segments bifocal lenses: Straight top one piece bifocal lenses are also called Executive bifocals and are produced by several manufactures under various names like Univis E, Kurova M, Vision Ease Bifield, and Hydray EX. In uncut lenses the standard height for near segments is 25 mm in all types (Fig. 12.47) except in Hydray lens where the segment is 29 mm high.

Manufacturing process of executive bifocal lens is simple and involves a rotating device over which the lenses are glued. Then another device create groove on this rotating drum as shown in Fig. 12.48.

Special Types of Bifocal Lenses

Minus add bifocal: These minus add bifocal lenses were especially designed to perform near work having only a small distance

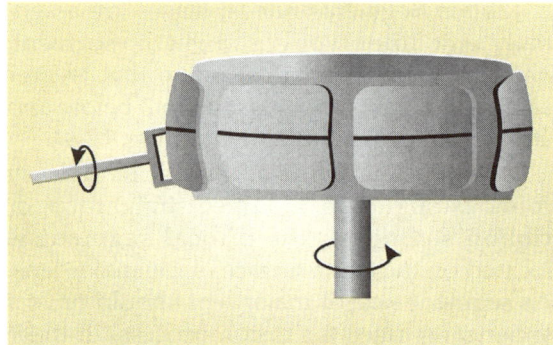

Fig. 12.48: Showing manufacturing of executive bifocal lenses

window at top of the lens. These lenses are rarely used and are prescribed only for presbyopes in profession like barber or postal clerk, who need a larger near field to work.

Solid up curve bifocal lens were the first introduced minus add bifocal and currently an Ultex one piece form called Rede Rite bifocal is available in the market. Normally, in bifocal lenses the upper edge of the near segment is located at lower lid margin of wearer but in minus add lenses the edge of near segment is located above the center of pupil as shown in Fig. 12.49A.

Another way to obtain an unusually large reading field is by the use of a 28 mm high straight top one-piece executive style bifocal as shown in Fig. 12.49B. Even the standard executive style bifocal lens can be fitted as

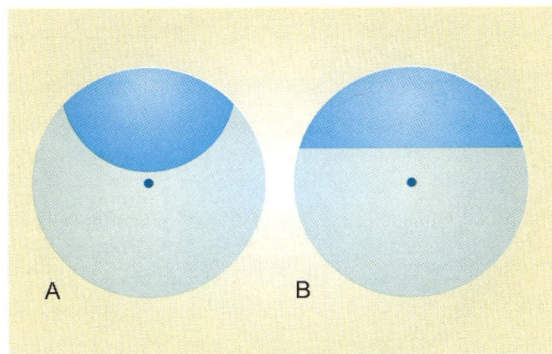

Fig. 12.49: Minus add bifocal lens designs. A. Solid up curve bifocal design; B. Straight top one piece design

high as 25 mm, this will also bring add segment top, well above the center of wearer's pupil.

Golfers' bifocal lenses: A common multifocal lens can be changed into a special design lens on demand of specific occupation simply by changing its fitting position in the spectacle frame.

For example, a 50-year-old golfer regularly complain about the near segment of his/her multifocal lenses (even progressive lenses) that near segment obstruct the view of golf ball or when he/she tries to line up a hole. To solve this problem a special type of bifocal lens was developed called golfer's bifocal lens. Here the near segment usually of round shape is placed in the outer lower corner of just one lens of spectacle as shown in Fig. 12.50.

For a right hander Golfer this near segment is placed only on right side of the spectacle and for a left hander golfer in the left side of the spectacle frame. This peculiar position of the near segment remains completely out of the way, when person is playing however, enough near vision is present to read score card or menu card.

Double Segment Bifocals

Bifocal lenses having two addition segments, i.e. one below the level of pupillary margin and another above the level are called double segment bifocals. These are mainly used by electricians, painters, and by other professionals, who do close work above the level of the eye. Majority of these lenses are of straight top variety which are available in both fused and one-piece forms. Distance between upper and lower addition segments is 13 mm in almost all varieties of these types of lenses.

The first double segment bifocal lenses were introduced by Univis as fused double D (Fig. 12.51A) and is available in either 22 or 25 mm add segments widths. Tiyler double executive lens designs are also popular as shown in Fig. 12.51B.

Several companies like Vision Ease, American Optical, Robinson Houchin and Shuron Continental make mixed double segment bifocals in various segment combinations as shown in Fig. 12.52.

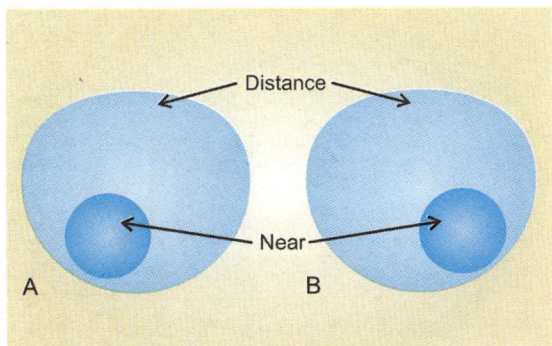

Fig. 12.50: Golfer's bifocal lens designs. A. For right eye; B. For left eye

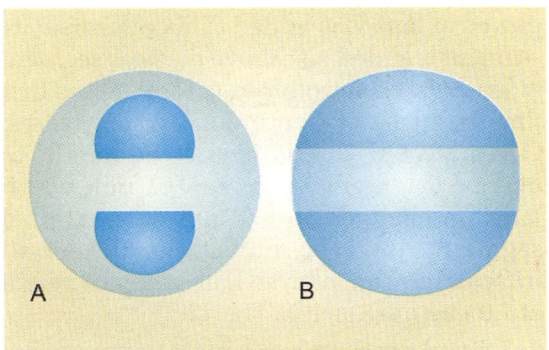

Fig. 12.51: Double segment lens designs. A. Round segments; B. Straight top segments

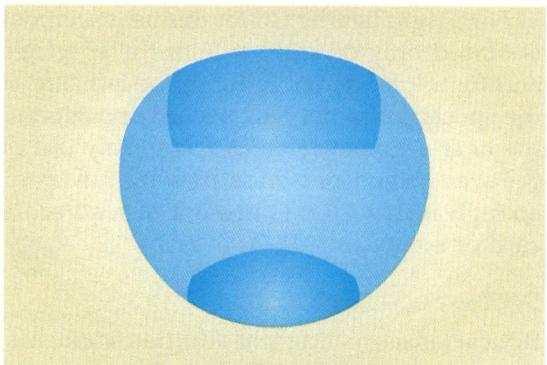

Fig. 12.52: Mixed double segment bifocal lens showing various types of segments

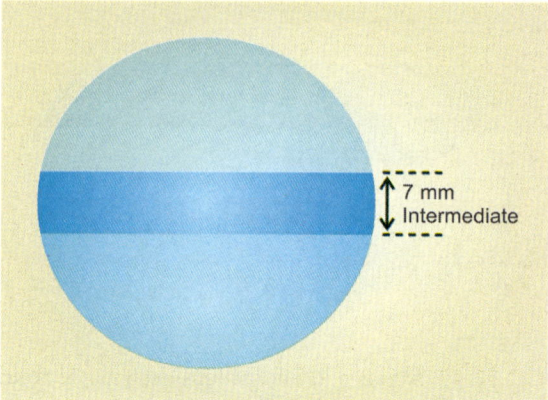

Fig. 12.53: Trifocal lens design

Note: Double segment bifocal lenses are not trifocal lenses.

Trifocal Lenses

With bifocal lens many presbyopes, wearing +2 D or more optical correction feel difficulty to see an object situated at an intermediate distance (say 1–1.5 meters) either via distance or near segment of that bifocal lens. It happens because when the presbyope see the object at this distance through the distance portion of bifocal lens, his near point of accommodation lies beyond the object of interest, while when the object is seen by person through the near portion of bifocal lens, then the far point of accommodation lies too close for the object of interest. To eliminate this problem trifocal lens were introduced in which another intermediate segment having an additional intermediate power in lens was added. This intermediate segment is added just above the near segment of lens. Univis introduced trifocal lenses first time by name of Continuous Vision lenses. Originally, in Univis lenses the height of intermediate segment was kept 6.0 mm, which later on changed to 8.0 mm occupational segment, however, nowadays almost all trifocals have an intermediate segment height of 7.0 mm as shown in Fig. 12.53.

Trifocal lenses are available in various styles and combinations in both fused and one-piece forms. Univis, American Optical, Vision- Ease, and Shuron-Continental all these companies manufacture a straight top trifocal lens, whereas American Optical, Vision-Ease, and Robinson Houchin manufacture an Executive style one piece trifocal.

For occupations like computer operator, a special design of CRT trifocal lenses has been introduced having a 14 mm high intermediate segment as shown in Fig. 12.54. CRT lens is suitable for professions where high percentage of near work is needed at an intermediate distance.

Plastic multifocal lenses: Presently, demand of plastic multifocal lenses has increased. Almost all plastic multifocal lenses are one piece design where near segment is located on the front surface of lens. These lenses are produced in finished or semi-finished form.

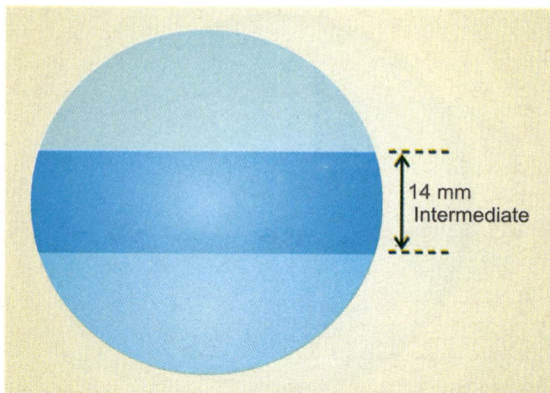

Fig. 12.54: CRT lens design having 14 mm segment

Varifocal or Progressive Lenses

These lenses have corrective power for distance and near vision along with a progressive power zone or corridor which extend across the entire width of lens and connect distance and near portions of the lens.

Central portion of the progressive lens is the functional area of progressive power zone and is known as progressive corridor or zone (Fig. 12.55). Refractive power of varifocal lens increases progressively from the distance to the near portion along this progressive corridor. All powers lying in between the distance and near powers are present in this progressive corridor. No visible reading segment and/or no dividing lines are present in this corridor, hence practically there is no image jump.

The most important factors of a progressive lens are interconnected and include

- Size of distance and reading areas
- Types and intensity of aberrations
- Depth and functional width of corridor

Various types of progressive lens designs available differ in high image performance and the severity of aberrations. An inherent astigmatism may be produced either right or left of the umbilical line (A line at center of progressive corridor as shown in Fig. 12.56) during creation of an aspherical surface with variable radius of curvatures; this astigmatism is proportional to the rate of change in the curvature.

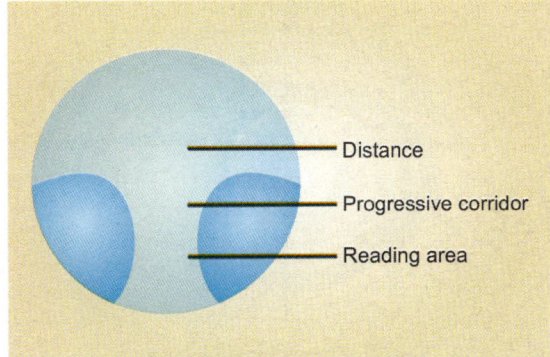

Fig. 12.55: Varifocal or progressive lens

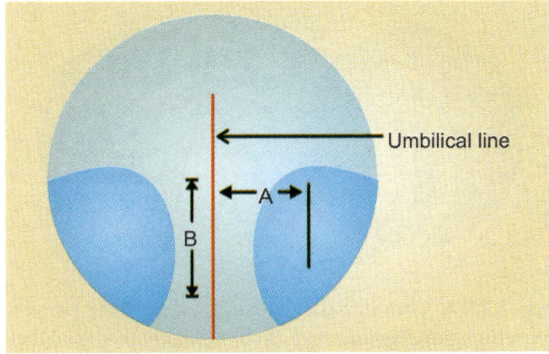

Fig. 12.56: Umbilical line and astigmatism in proportion to displacement. For same amount of astigmatism, vertical displacement B is twice the lateral displacement A

This designing principle of progressive lens developed two approaches of production of progressive lenses

- **Hard design:** Progressive lenses designed on this basis give a relatively larger area of high quality images in all areas of lens, i.e. distance portion, progressive corridor, and near portion. However, there is an associated high degree of astigmatism in lateral portions of progressive corridor.
- **Soft design:** Progressive lenses designed on this basis give a smaller area of high quality images in all areas, i.e. distance portion, progressive corridor, and near portion; but has a low degree of astigmatism in lateral portions of progressive corridor.

Several types of progressive lenses were produced till date and some important types of progressive lenses are

Omnifocal Lens: In the year 1961, David Volk and Joseph Weinberg introduced first successful progressive lens known as Omnifocal, which was manufactured by Robinson Houchin.

These lenses were made of glass and having aspherical or progressive front surface. Radius of curvature of aspheric surface of lens (front surface) progressively reduced in vertical meridian from top to the bottom, whereas in the horizontal meridian radius of curvature remained same.

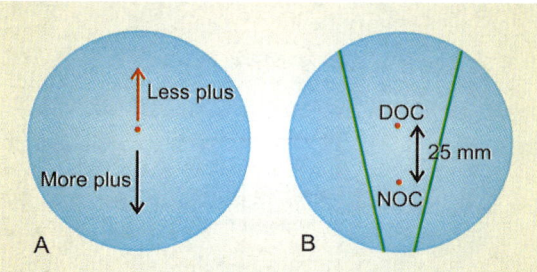

Fig. 12.57: Omnifocal lens designs. A. Plus power increases downwards from distance optical center and decreases upwards; B. Functional area of lens decreases gradually from top to bottom showing distance optical center (DOC) and near optical center (NOC)

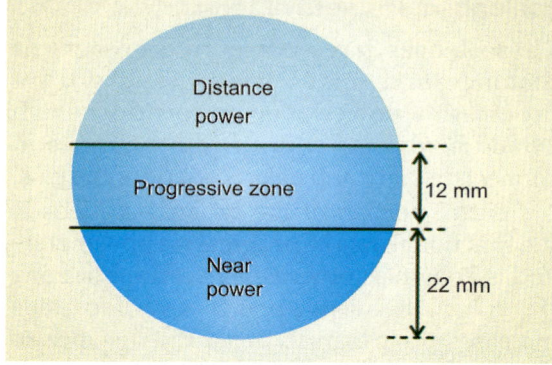

Fig. 12.58: Varilux lens design with central 12 mm progressive zone and constant power in distance and near zone.

The distance optical center of lens lies at a vertical distance of 25 mm from near optical center of lens. Total amount of plus power decreases upwards from distance optical center and increases downwards from distance optical center as shown in Fig. 12.57.

Omnifocal lens was an example of soft design because the progression of power is from top to bottom in entire front surface of lens. These lenses are now obsolete but mentioned due to its historical importance.

Varilux lens: In the year 1959, Bernard Maitenaz developed original Varilux lens and Essel Optical of France introduced them in the market. Later on in the year 1967, Titmus Optical Co introduced this lens in the United States, popularly called Varilux 1.

Varilux 1 was different in design from Omnifocal lens. The upper half of Varilux 1 had no progression in power and only 12 mm deep zone situated in the center of lens had a progressively increasing refractive power. A zone of maximum addition with a constant power having a width of about 22 mm was situated below progressive corridor of lens as shown in Fig. 12.58. In original Varilux design lens, astigmatism free progressive corridor of 5 mm width was also present but on increasing the power of near addition, the functional width of the progressive corridor decreased.

Varilux lens is considered as a hard design lens because progressive front surface is limited to a 12 mm deep zone, rather than extending from top to bottom as in soft design lenses. Varilux lenses are manufactured differentially for the right and left eyes, because the line of symmetry is inclined nasally toward the bottom of lens as shown in Fig. 12.59. Original Varilux lens were available only in glass material.

Later on after expire of patent of Varilux 1 progressive lens, the Varilux 2 lens was introduced by Essel. In this lens not only the progressive zone but also entire front surface of lens was of aspherical design. Hence, this lens was considered as soft design progressive lens. Lateral astigmatism was greatly reduced in Varilux 2 with improvised vision qualities.

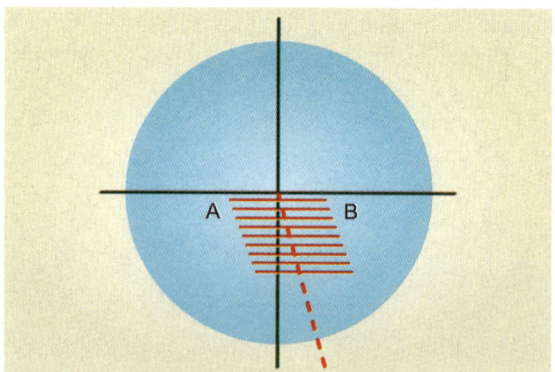

Fig. 12.59: Nasal inclination of progressive zone in right-sided Varilux lens

Once the patent on original Varilux expired several manufactures introduced their own version of progressive lenses. For example,

- In the year 1973, American Optical introduced Ultravue CR-39 plastic lens. A 25 mm wide segment corridor was present in this lens, hence was renamed as Ultravue 25. In the year 1978, another lens with same design called Ultravue 28 was introduced with a 28 mm wide segment. Ultravue lens has an advantage of a well-defined distance portion, astigmatism-free surface and wide segment area, but at the cost of higher rate of progression. This lens was of hard design category.

- In the year 1978, Younger optics introduced Younger 10/30 CR-39 plastic lens. This lens has a 10 mm deep progressive corridor with 30 mm wide functional segment area, hence the name 10/30. This lens was in hard progressive lens design category.

- In the year 1980, Silor Optical started marketing Super NoLine lens. This improvised version of original NoLine progressive lens has a progressive corridor 12 mm deep. This lens has wide distance and segment area of about 25 mm width, hence designated in hard design category. NoLine lenses are available in CR-39 plastic, ophthalmic crown glass, and photochromic glass materials.

Many more companies came up with several types of progressive lenses, although list is exhaustive but a few examples are

- Cosmetic Parabolic Sphere (CPS) progressive lens by Younger Optics
- In the year 1982, American Optical introduced Truvision lens.
- Titmus Optical in the year 1983 started marketing NuVue 75 lens.
- In the year 1984, Coburn Optical Industries started marketing of Progressive R lens.
- Sola Optical in 1984 introduced a lens called VIP lens.

- In the year 1986, Seiko Optical Products introduced two progressive lenses called P-2 and P-3.
- Polarite in the year 1986 developed a plastic polarized progressive lens by the name of Progressive M. Most recently Varilux infinity(1988) and Varilux comfort (1993) progressive lens designs were developed to increase the comfort of wearer in advancing presbyopic age.

SPECTACLE LENS FITTING

Spectacle lens fitting method: For an ideal fitting of a lens in the spectacle frame knowledge of these following components is essential

- Interpupillary distance
- Frame dimensions
- Frame specification
- Spectacle frame selection

Interpupillary Distance

Optical center or major reference point of the lens, these are two interchangeable terms which indicate a point on the lens, where maximum effect of a prescribed prism will be seen. Distance between these two points on two lenses of a spectacle lens is called interpupillary distance (IPD).

Measuring interpupillary distance: First step for accurate lens fitting in a spectacle frame is the measurement of interpupillary distance, commonly called IPD or PD and both the distance PD and near PD has to be measured. These measurements are defined as distance between two visual axes for distance and near vision, respectively at the level of spectacle plane.

As shown in Fig. 12.60 lines of sight are parallel for distance vision, hence interpupillary distance will be the same, whether measured at the level of center of rotation plane, corneal plane or spectacle plane. However, in convergence condition for near fixation, eyes rotate about their center of rotation with simultaneous convergence of lines of sight, hence distance between them decrease from center of rotation plane to

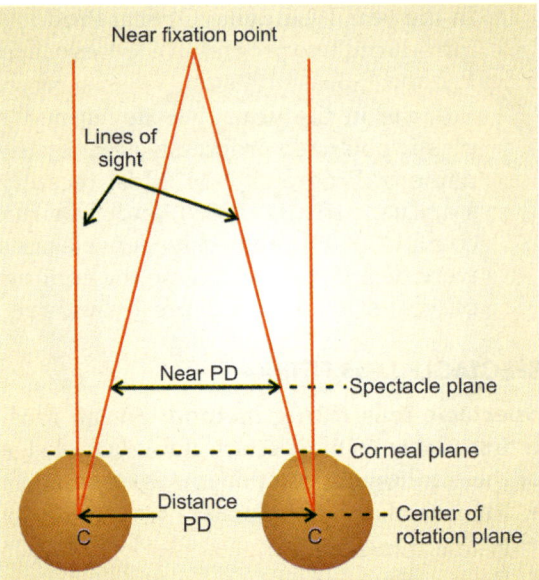

Fig. 12.60: Measuring interpupillary distance at various planes

corneal plane and further at spectacle plane level as shown in Fig. 12.61.

Visual axes distance can be measured by using:

- Millimeter ruler
- Elissor Pupilometer
- AO Grolman device
- Cal Coast PD ruler
- Bausch and Lomb PD gauge
- Topcon digital PD gauge
- Rodenstock interpupillary gauge

Similarly, pupil center and size can be measured by

- Antique Pulzone hardy rule
- Bishop Harman rule
- Fairbanks facial gauge
- Basic Pupilometer

Simplest and most widely accepted method to measure both distance and near PD is by millimeter ruler method.

Test procedure for distance PD measurement (Fig. 12.61A)

- Examiner sits in front of the patient at a distance of about one and a half feet (16 inches), holding a millimeter ruler in one hand at the level of patient's spectacle plane.
- Then examiner instructs the patient to look in his/her left eye, simultaneously aligning the temporal edge of patient's right pupil with the zero mark on millimeter ruler.
- Then the patient is asked to look at examiner's right eye, so that examiner can record the reading on millimeter ruler which is aligned with nasal edge of patient's left pupil.

Note: Sometimes it is difficult to see the pupillary border especially in patients having very dark iris, then the alignment of millimeter ruler is done with the temporal limbus of right eye and nasal limbus of left eye.

Test procedure for near PD measurement (Fig. 12.61B)

- Examiner sits in front of the patient at a distance of about one and a half feet (16 inches), holding a millimeter ruler in one hand at the level of patient's spectacle plane.
- Then examiner instructs the patient to fixate either his/her right or left eye,

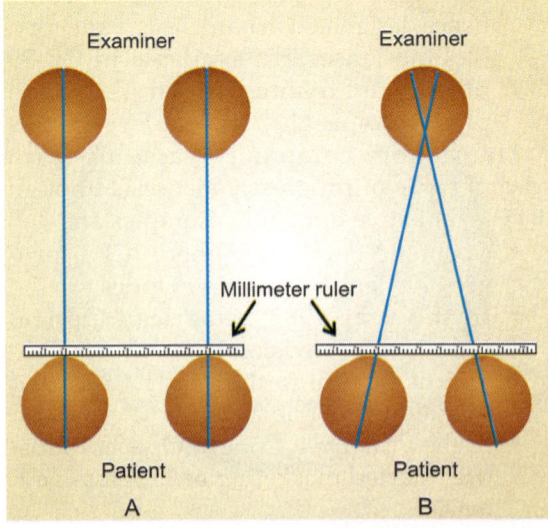

Fig. 12.61: Measurement of PD. A. Distance PD measurement; B. Near PD measurement

which is accordingly positioned on the patient's midline area by the examiner.

- Then examiner aligns the temporal edge of patients right eye pupil with zero mark on the millimeter scale, while note down reading corresponding to nasal edge of patient's left eye pupil.

Note: Normally at this measuring distance (16 inches) near PD is usually about 4–5 mm less than the distance PD.

Due to practical difficulties, it is probably advisable to measure the distance PD with accuracy and then find out the near PD by calculation with this formula.

For each eye, difference between distance PD and near PD (say d) is calculated by

$d/27 = $ ½ distance PD/427 or simply $d = 27$ (½ distance PD)/427

For example, suppose distance PD is 64 mm, then difference d for each eye, will be

$$d = 27 (32)/427$$
$$= 2.02$$

Hence near PD is 64–2 (2.02) = 59.96 mm

Following conditions can create problems while measuring the PD by using a millimeter rule

- Difference in patient's and examiner's PD can introduce a parallax.
- Anisocoria or pupil size difference in both eyes can alter dimensions.
- Asymmetry of the face
- Invisible pupil margins
- Vertical differences of the two eyes.
- Lateral head or ruler movement while measuring a PD.

To align the visual axis of eye and optical axis of spectacle lens sometimes we have to decenter the lens horizontally depending upon the frame dimensions and PD. To get the best possible visual results, it is necessary to align visual axis and optical center of spectacle lens. However, to get desired prismatic effect various types of lenses (spherical, planocylindrical or spherocylindrical lenses) can be decentered.

The lens decentration is done to control prismatic effects, means either to produce a prismatic effect or to avoid a prismatic effect.

Frame Dimensions

For measuring lenses, a system of reference points was established for spectacle frames and spectacle lenses which assist in accurate fitting of corresponding optical center and bifocal segments inside the spectacle frame. Two systems were developed to ease the lens fittings are Datum system and Boxing system.

Datum System

In the year 1935, Cole and Blackburn introduced Datum system (Fig. 12.62) for accurate fitting of lenses in spectacle frames. Various terminologies used in this system are

Datum line (AA): Placing the lens in a position as it should be fitted in a frame, the two horizontal tangents corresponding to highest (UU') and lowest (LL') edges of lens are drawn. A parallel line drawn midway between these two horizontal tangents is called datum line of reference.

Datum length (MN): The peripheral portion of the lens which bound the datum line in horizontal plane is called datum length and it represents the horizontal dimensions of a lens.

Mid-datum depth (a): Vertical line joining upper and lower horizontal tangents from lens edges is called as mid-datum depth and it represents the vertical dimension of the lens.

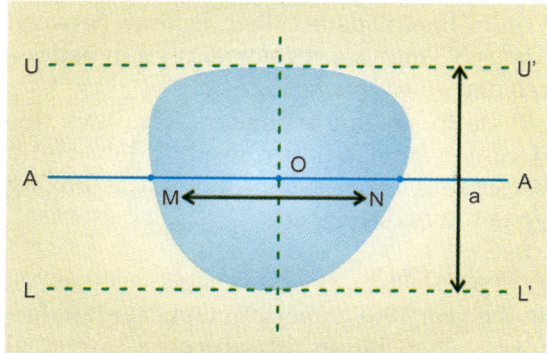

Fig. 12.62: Datum system

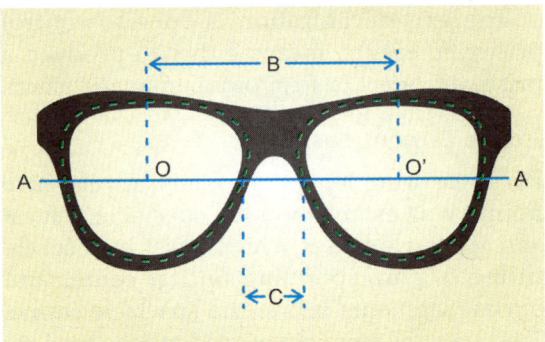

Fig. 12.63: Application of datum system on spectacle frame

Datum center (O): A cross section point present midway between the datum length and a vertical line from upper and lower lens edges is called datum center.

Application of datum system to the frame (Fig. 12.63) gives the frame dimensions and various additional terminologies are as follows

Frame difference: When there is a difference between vertical dimension and horizontal dimension of a frame, it is called frame difference. Usually it is a few millimeters, as both dimensions are also in millimeter.

Datum line of frame: It a continuous line joining Datum's line of both the spectacle lenses, i.e. AA.

Datum center distance (B): After fitting the two lenses inside the frame, a distance between datum centers (OO') of these two lenses is called datum center distance.

Distance between lenses (DBL): Distance between the nasal edges of lens measured at Datum line plane is called distance between lenses (C) and is a parameter used in various calculation of lens fitting.

Due to several technical difficulties this datum system was not used widely and a better measuring system known as boxing system was developed.

Boxing System

In the year 1961, American Optical Manufacturers Association introduced a universal system for measurement of lens and frames called boxing system. In this system the lens boxing was done by both horizontal (used in Datum system) and vertical lines (not used in Datum system). Hence, boxing system is considered as an improved version of datum system. Boxing system uses bevel apex of the edged lens as a constant reference point for all measurements in millimeters, hence the chances error in prescription interpretation were reduced.

Boxed lens: Consider the front and cross section view of a lens as shown in Fig. 12.64. Suppose a square made by the horizontal and vertical tangent lines touching the lens edges is drawn, which completely surrounds the lens is called boxed lens. Various terminologies used (Fig. 12.65) in boxing system are:

Eye size (Lens size): Horizontal measurement (A) of this box is called eye size for frames and lens size for lenses.

Frame depth: Vertical measurement (B) of this box represents the frame depth.

Box center: It is the point where two diagonals of box are intersecting with each other. It is also called the geometric center (GC) of the frame opening or aperture. It also represents the geometric center of a lens edges for a given frame.

Suppose both the right and left lenses have been boxed, as if they were inserted into the spectacle frame as shown in Fig. 12.65, then

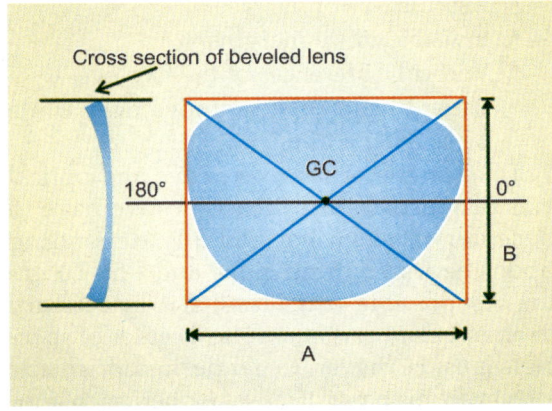

Fig. 12.64: Boxing of a spectacle lens, GC: Geometrical center.

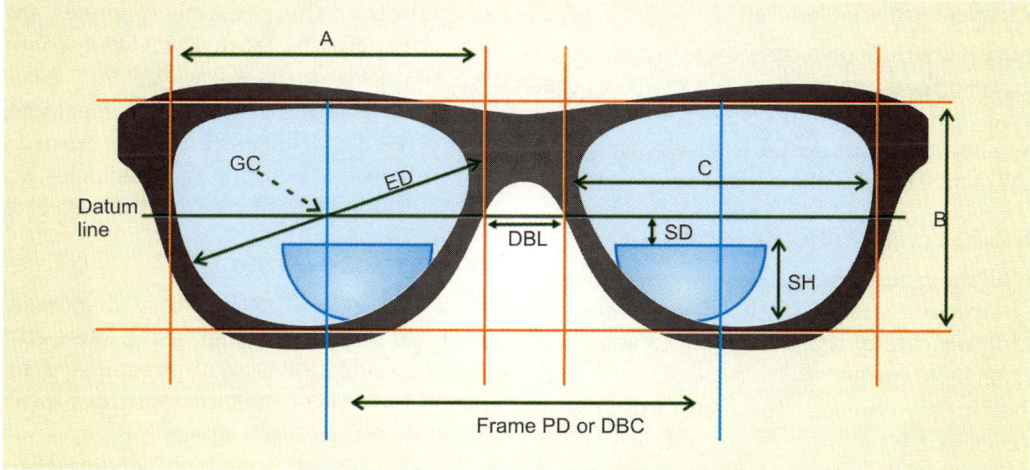

Fig. 12.65: Application of boxing system on spectacle frame

following parameters are also added in existing terminologies as

DBL: It is the minimum horizontal distance between two lenses mounted in a spectacle frame. The measuring points are the bevels of nasal side of two lenses; DBL also represents the bridge size of the frame.

Distance between centers (DBC): It is the distance between two geometrical centers of the frame (or lens) and is commonly called frame PD. This can be represented by the following formula

DBC = Eye size or lens size + DBL

Segment height (SH): Vertical distance between top edge of bifocal or trifocal segment and bottom edge of box is called segment height.

Segment drop (SD): Vertical distance between top edge of bifocal or trifocal segment and datum line is called segment drop.

Frame Specification

Size: Spectacle frames are typically marked for size, which help in calculating other dimensions of the frame. For example, marked as 50–22, where 50 represents the eye size or lens size and 22 represents the distance between lenses (DBL) or bridge size.

Effective diameter: Another important specification provided by manufacturer is effective

diameter (ED) as shown in Fig. 12.66. It is defined as twice the distance from geometrical center of lens to the peak of beveled edge of lens situated farthest from geometrical center. Effective diameter is used to determine the minimum size of blank. This blank size is calculated by doubling the amount of decentration in millimeter and adding the resultant value with effective diameter of lens.

Minimum blank size = ED + 2 × Amount of decentration in millimeter

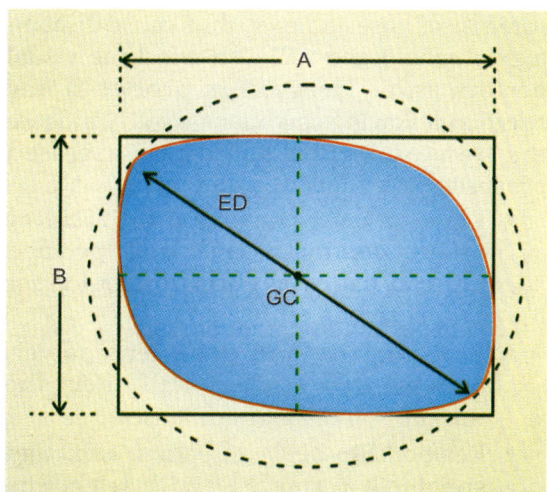

Fig. 12.66: Effective diameter (ED) and geometrical center (GC) of a lens

Spectacle Frame Selection

Primary function of a spectacle frame is to keep prescribed lenses in such a position that give an optimum visual efficiency. Also the frame should be comfortable in wearing and look attractive to fulfill the patient's expectations.

For Bifocals and Multifocal Lenses

To fulfill the requirement of optical performance and comfort expert ophthalmic personnel should take care of these facts about selection of a spectacle frame

- Thoroughly consider the factors related to prescribed lens such as refractive power, lens material, lens centration, base curve specification, multifocal type and glass tint.
- Appropriate selection of bridge design that remains stable, provide the proper weight distribution of spectacle frame and also help in maintaining the lenses in a preferred position.
- Appropriate selection of temple style and temple length, which adjusts well with the contour of wearer's ear and to shape of his/her mastoid process.
- Facilitates the lens fitting very near to face with an appropriate pantoscopic tilt along with corresponding vertical centration of lens.

Improper frame selection may cause soreness of nose and ears, thus cause discomfort to patient and will also affect the visual performance. Hence, for proper frame selection following conditions which influence the frame selection should be assessed properly

- Type of lens, because multifocal or progressive lenses will need specified minimum vertical frame dimension for proper fitting.
- Probable size and exact lens power, because these factors will affect the thickness and weight of lenses
- Relationship between patient's PD and spectacle frame PD will affect the resultant appearance of centrality of patient's eyes and also decides that

whether the prescribed lenses can be chipped out from the standard uncut blanks or not.

- To avoid the rejection of spectacles by patient always enquire about the purpose of wearing the spectacles, so that suitable type of frame can be selected.

For Progressive Lenses

For a proper and satisfactory dispensing of spectacle in case of progressive lenses fitting, the frame selection is an important step. Frame should have these specific features for proper fitting of progressive lenses.

- As shown in Fig. 12.67, for fitting of progressive lenses selected frame must have a total vertical measurement of minimum of 40 mm.
- Frame must offer a minimum vertical distance of 22 mm between the pupillary center of patient and the horizontal line tangent to bottom edge of spectacle lens, means in a Varifocal lens (having 12 mm progressive zone) this type of fitting will give reading area of 8 mm width, considering that progressive zone begins 2 mm below the pupillary center.

If the distance below pupillary center is less than 22 mm, then the remaining depth of maximum near power prescribed for reading will be very small.

- The selected frame should fit on patient's face very near (maximum 11–12 mm) to

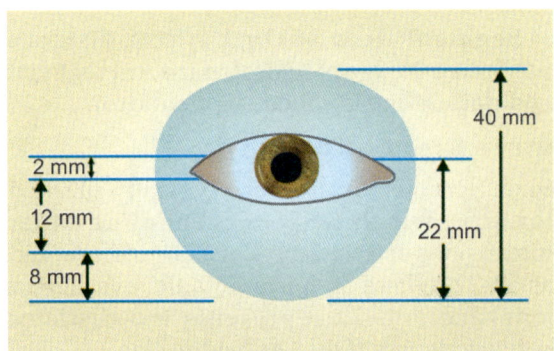

Fig. 12.67: Spectacle box vertical dimension, minimum of 40 mm

the back vertex distance, so that a wide lateral field of view and stable near vision area can be provided to the patient.

- Pantoscopic tilt of nearly 12–15° with slight amount of face forming will help in stabilization of near area and provide wider view of lateral visual field.
- Frames with an adjustable nose pads will permit flexibility in positioning the frame, while dispensing and also in follow-up.

Principles of Fitting

Once the accurate spectacle frame has been selected, the fitting of the lenses into this selected frame is an important step. For practical purposes proper alignment of spectacle frame is done by the manufacturer. The dispenser should confirm precise fitting of frame or lens on patients according to the following guidelines

- Pantoscopic tilt
- Temple angle
- Fitting triangle

Pantoscopic Tilt

Pantoscopic tilt or angle of a spectacle frame means that the bottom edge of the spectacle lens is tilted away from the vertical axis (5–8 degrees) in the inward direction (i.e. towards the cheeks of wearer) (Fig. 12.68). In other words, the upper edge of spectacle lens

is more forward than bottom edge. The inward tilting of frame improves the cosmetic looks of the spectacles, provides a better protection from flying objects, increases the field of view of wearer and decreases effect of oblique astigmatism.

Change in pantoscopic angle or tilt helps in adjustment of spectacle frame. For example, if right-sided lens appears higher on patient's face as compared to the left-sided lens, then by increasing the pantoscopic angle for the left lens will make both the lenses in level or one can decrease the pantoscopic angle for the lens which is higher (right lens in our example).

Sometimes, to achieve a satisfactory fit on wearer's face we may need to tilt the frame, so that lower part of the lens tilted away from the wearers' face, this is called retroscopic tilt, used rarely when absolute indications are there.

Temple Angle

Temple angle is an angle formed between front and temple of the spectacle frame in the horizontal plane. Degree of temple angle is dependent on elements like front width of spectacle frame and patient's head width, but in majority of the cases, frame temples are bent outwards up to a few degrees (Fig. 12.69).

Note: Recently, very large size spectacle frames are also used and these frames generated a need to bend the temples slightly inwards.

Temple angle helps us to check the distance of two lenses from the patient's eyebrow (which should be equal on both sides) and this can be observed when patient bends his/her head in downward direction. If the temple angle on one side is too small, then the patient will feel an excessive pressure on that side of head, because the lens on that side extends outward as compared to fellow lens. The problem can be solved by increasing the temple angle on this side, however; in some cases reduction in temple angle on other side can also give good results.

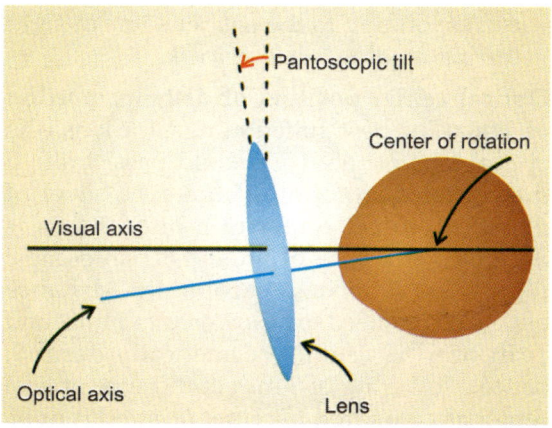

Fig. 12.68: Pantoscopic tilt

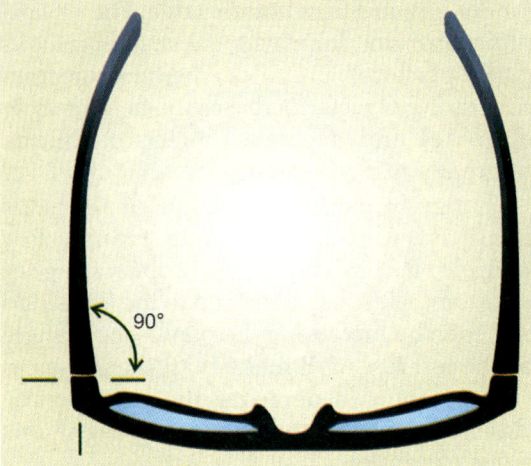

Fig. 12.69: Temple angle

Fitting Triangle

Spectacle frame or mounting may be compared with a triangle having three points of contact; one at the crest of the nose (A) and two on the apex of each ear (B, C) as shown in Fig. 12.70. Normally when head is kept in erect position, about 65% of total spectacle weight is taken up by the nose, whereas remaining (about 35%) of total weight is shared by the ears. However, on bending the head in downward direction, the majority of the spectacle weight gets transfer to the ears.

During routine work, mainly the weight of spectacles remains on the nose of individual, hence it becomes necessary to provide cushioning effect to the nose to tolerate the spectacle weight and to prevent pressure effects. It is done by prescribing spectacle frames having adjustable nose pads and the whole surface of these pads should make contact with the nose. Sometimes frames with large size nose pads (jumbo pads) can be used in those having sensitive nose skin. In case of plastic frames, as there is no adjustable pads so such a frame should be selected which provides a large area of contact with nose. Frame style having a saddle bridge is appropriate for patients who have a relatively wide, protruding, high nose crest. However, for patients having narrow and flat crest, a keyhole bridge is a better choice.

Fitting of bifocal lenses: Fitting of a bifocal lenses require knowledge of not only of the corrective powers of distance and near vision, but also the positions of optical center of the segment. This placement of optical center of segments is done in vertical and lateral positions of the bifocal lenses.

Vertical position of the segment: In bifocal lenses the vertical positioning of segment is decided by the following factors

- Optical center position of distance portion of lens.
- Optical center position of the near segment.
- Reading center which is a point in lens corresponding to the wearer's line of sight during reading or close work.

Optical center position of distance portion of lens: For best functioning of a lens, the optical axis of the lens should pass through the center of rotation of the eye. Level of distance optical center of a bifocal lens is decided on the basis of amount of pantoscopic tilt. To get 2° of pantoscopic tilt, distance optical center need to be lowered to 1 mm, and a tilt of 6° is usually cosmetically desired, hence a lowering of 3 mm of distance optical center as compared to center of pupil is done in a bifocal lens as shown in Fig. 12.71.

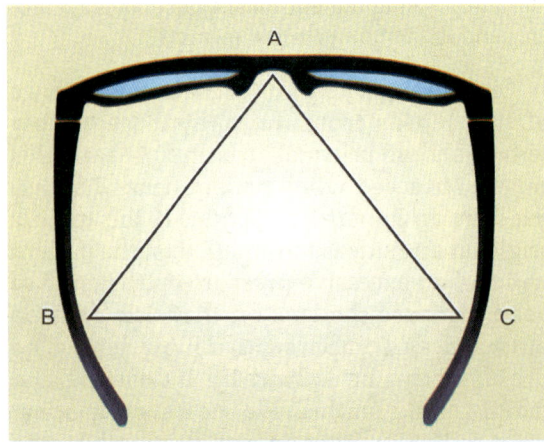

Fig. 12.70: Fitting triangle

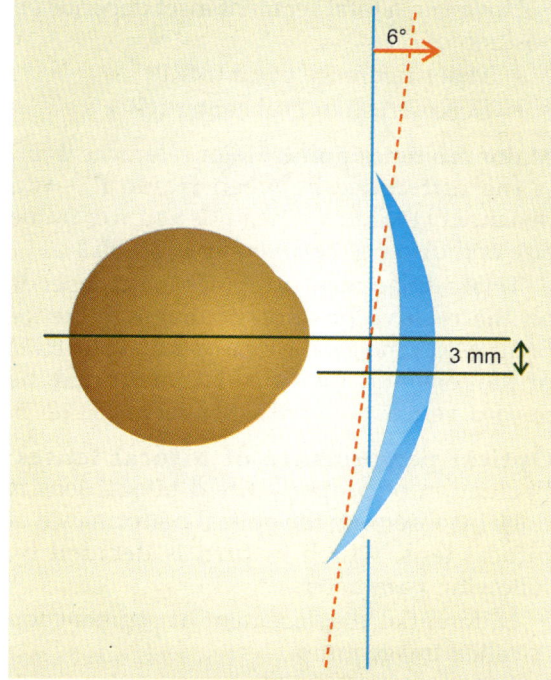

Fig. 12.71: Lowering (3mm) of distance optical center to get a 6° pantoscopic tilt.

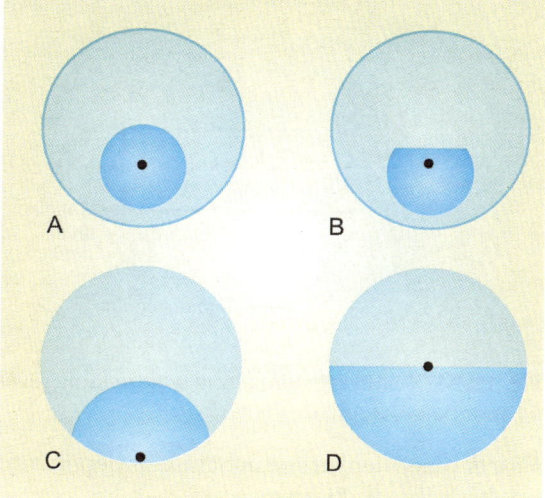

Fig. 12.72: Optical center for various bifocal lens designs from segment top. A. Fused round segment bifocal (11mm below); B. Fused straight top bifocal (5 mm below); C. One piece bifocal (19 mm below); D. Executive bifocal (at segment top)

Optical center position of near segment: Similarly, position of optical center of various types of bifocal lens segments is shown in Fig. 12.72. This clearly gives us an idea about the fitting of various types of bifocal lenses in spectacle frames, so that the reading line of wearer should be in alignment with these optical centers of near segments.

Reading center: It is considered as a point on the spectacle lens through which the foveal line of sight passes during reading. It is situated about 11 mm below the center of pupil (Fig. 12.73). As discussed above to get a pantoscopic tilt of 6° the bifocal distance optical center lies at 3 mm below the pupillary center, hence the reading center of segment is located 11–3 = 8 mm below. On this principle bifocal lenses are fitted as shown in Fig. 12.74, i.e. segment top is kept in alignment with the lower eyelid margin of wearer.

Lateral position of the segment: Normally segment optical centers are fitted in an inward

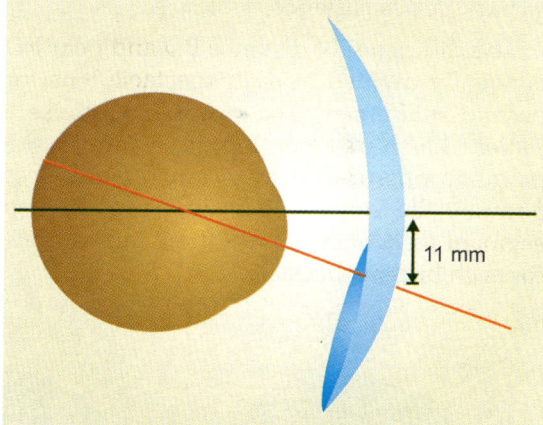

Fig. 12.73: Reading center in bifocal lens is usually 11 mm below pupillary center

position as compared to the distance optical points of bifocal lenses; this is known as segment inset. Purposes of segment inset are

- To make sure that when patient looks with both the eyes, then the field of view of two segments of bifocal glass should coincide.
- To avoid the horizontal prismatic effects at the reading center.

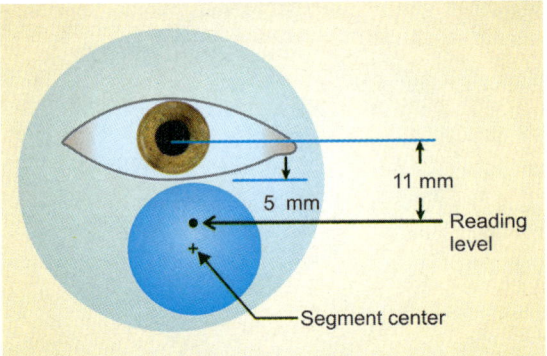

Fig. 12.74: Round segment fitting with reading level 11 mm below pupillary center

Proper placement of segment inset is dependent on the following factors

- Power of distance correction in horizontal meridian.
- Interpupillary distance usually called distance PD.
- Fixation distance of bifocal lens.
- Back vertex distance.

The difference of distance PD and near PD is equally divided in each spectacle lens for nasal displacement. For example, suppose a patient has a distance PD of 66 mm in the primary position of eyes and near PD of 62 mm in the converging position of eyes, then segment inset of 66–62 = 4/2 = 2 mm is done for each bifocal spectacle lens.

However, a total segment inset depends on position of

- Major reference point (MRP)
- Geometrical optical center (GC)

Major reference point: Major reference point is the difference between frame PD and distance PD where frame PD is a sum of frame size and distance between lenses (DBL).

Total displacement of segment inset depends on the relative position of major reference point (MRP) and geometrical optical center (GC) of the lens and total displacement may be inward, zero or outward as shown in Fig. 12.75.

Optical performance of bifocal lenses: Evaluation of properly fitted bifocal lens is done by observing the optical performance of bifocal lens, which in turn is decided by following parameters

- Differential displacement at segment top called image jump.
- Differential displacement at reading level
- Total displacement at reading level
- Chromatic aberration

Differential displacement at segment top (Image Jump): The bifocal lens consists of three optical centers, i.e.

- Distance optical center
- Segment optical center
- Resultant optical center

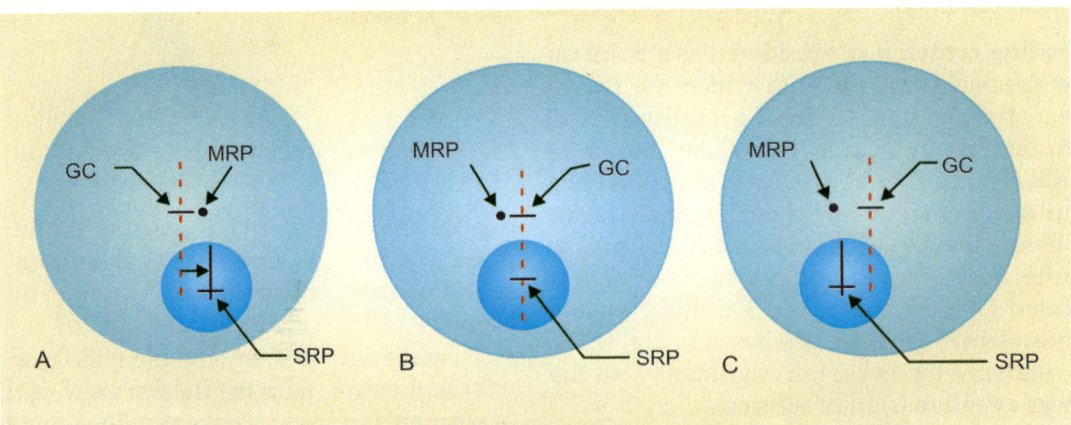

Fig. 12.75: Total displacement of segment reference point (SRP) in relation to geometrical center (GC) and major reference point (MRP). A. Inward, most common; B. Zero; C. Outward, least common

The prismatic effect in bifocal lens also exists in the segment and this prismatic effect at any given point in the segment will be equal to the sum of prismatic effects caused by both the distance lens and segment. However, the image jump occurs only due to segment and thus the prismatic power of the segment will decide the amount of image jump. Although the image jump can occur at any point on the margin of segment but it is annoying when occur from top edge of segment which is considered as zone of confusion. When an attempt is made by a bifocal wearer to look at an object through the top edge of segment, he/she sees two images because a part of bundle of rays entering the bifocal wearers' pupil is passing through the distance lens and remaining part is passing through the segment. Images formed by these two bundles of rays will differ from each other in

- Direction, i.e. differential displacement.
- Focus, because of differences in refractive power of distance and near portion of bifocal lens.
- Size, because of differences in magnification of images formed by distance and near portion of bifocal lens.

Differential displacement at reading level: Relative position of reading level in different types of bifocal lenses is represented in Fig. 12.76. These relative positions of reading level and position of segment center (solid red line) of a bifocal lens determines the differential displacement at reading level in terms of prismatic effect. Various types of prismatic effects produced are as follows

- Reading level and segment center on the same line, then no prismatic effect produced. For example, straight top D bifocal lens as shown in Fig. 12.76A.
- Reading level is above the segment center, hence a base down prismatic effect is produced. For example, Ultex AL lens as shown in Fig. 12.76B.
- Reading level is below segment center produces a base up prismatic effect. For example, executive bifocal lens as shown in Fig. 12.76C.

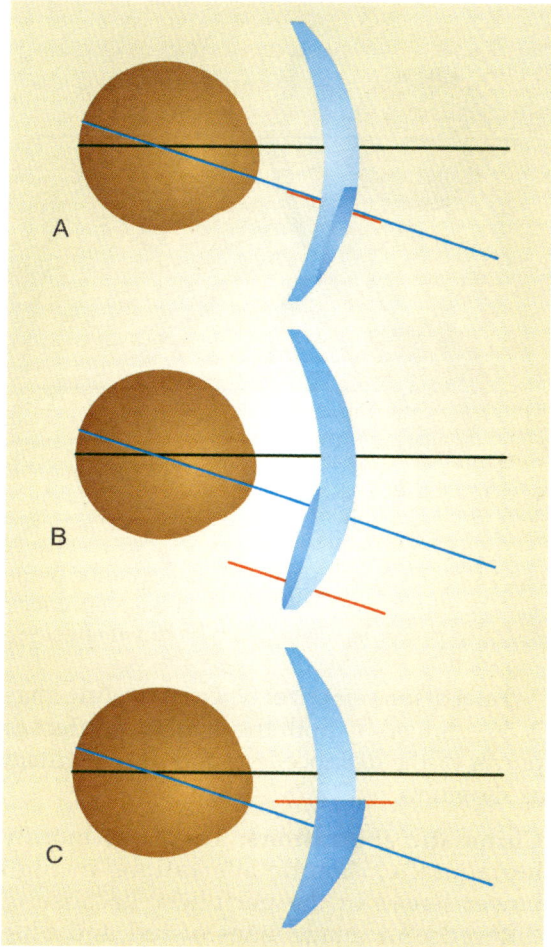

Fig. 12.76: Prismatic effects of various segment designs on reading level. A. No prismatic effect; B. Base down prismatic effect; C. Base up prismatic effect

Total displacement at reading level: Both the factors, i.e. image jump and the differential displacement at reading level, have no relation with the refractive power of the bifocal lens. However, the total displacement at reading level depends on the refractive power of the distance portion and addition power in the near segment of a bifocal lens.

In case where power of distance portion of the lens is plus, a base-up prismatic effect is added with near segment. However, in case where power of distance portion of the lens is minus, a base-down prismatic effect is added with near segment as shown in Fig. 12.77A and B.

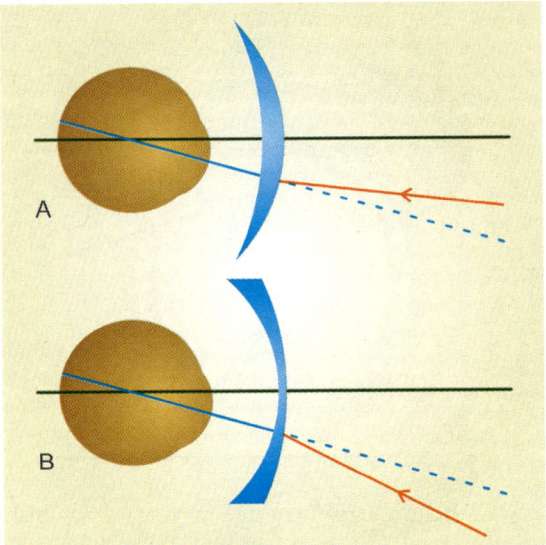

Fig. 12.77: Effect of power of distance portion of the lens. A. Plus power lens will add base up effect; B. Minus power lens will add base down effect

Total displacement of object at reading level is determined by both the combined effect of power of the distance lens and near segment as shown in Fig. 12.78.

Chromatic aberrations: There are mainly horizontal chromatic aberrations in high power lenses in the periphery because of difference in image sizes of red and blue images.

Selection of an ideal bifocal lens: An ideal bifocal segment selection criteria include following features

- *Elimination of image jump:* Bifocal segment should not have jump phenomenon. It can be achieved by selecting 'no jump' bifocals (e.g. executive style straight-top bifocal).
- *Elimination of differential displacement at reading level:* Straight top fused bifocal lenses fulfill this criterion, because these lenses have the segment pole at reading level.
- *Total displacement at reading level:* It should be zero or nearly zero and it can be achieved in bifocals where segment gives an opposite prismatic effect than that of distance lens.

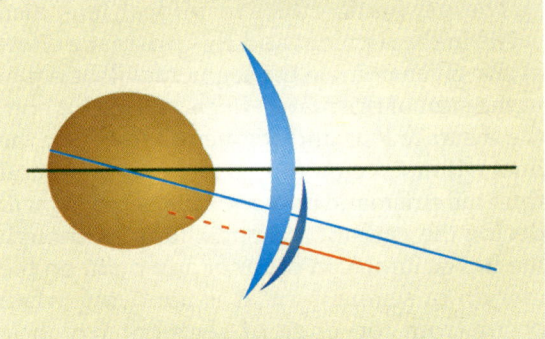

Fig. 12.78: Total displacement of reading level both by distance and near segment.

For example, a bifocal with minus distance power (means base down prismatic effect at reading) can be opposed by executive style segment having base-up prismatic effect; or a plus distance power bifocal needs base-down effect as in an Ultrex A segment, to oppose base-up prismatic effect by distance portion.

Factors required for selection of an ideal bifocal lens include: Segment size, segment height and segment shape.

Segment size or width: The size of segment of bifocal lenses has progressively increased in size as the size of spectacle frames has increased. Earlier available fused round segment bifocals had segment size of 17 mm, which has gradually increased up to 22 mm in recent years, however, segments of as wide as 35 mm are also available in special cases. Decision of segment width is made on the basis of patient requirement for near work; if more near work is requireds then a wider segment is needed.

Segment height: Initially, many practitioners thought that near segment should be placed as low as possible to avoid the interference in distance visions however, low placement of segment led to stiff neck problem in many patients. An ideal reference point for segment height is then decided as the lower lid margin. The top edge of segment is kept at level of lower lid margin or ciliary line in round top

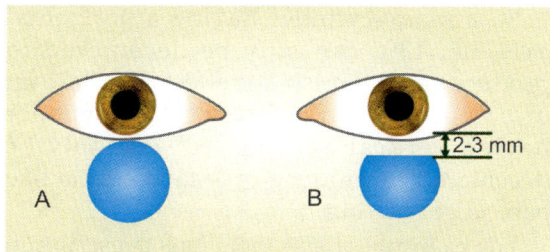

Fig. 12.79: Fitting of segment height. A. Round top segment at ciliary margin; B. Straight top segment 2–3 mm below ciliary margin

bifocals and 2–3 mm below ciliary line in straight top bifocals as shown in Fig. 12.79A and B.

Segment shape: Segment shapes are an important factor in deciding about the type of bifocal needed for various professions. Advantage of a round fused segment is that it is less visible than a straight top fused segment, hence for cosmetic reasons it is better preferred by the patients. Least visible segment is present in Nochrome round segment lens having a flesh color tint. For example, Softlite A or Cruxite A.

A very small fused round segment of about 12 mm diameter is called spot or button segment and was preferred by patients involved in profession related to distance vision. Similarly, in case of construction worker, the ribbon or bar segment bifocal lens designs with height of 9 mm was recommended because they do an occasional near work.

Lens Decentration

Lens decentration means displacement of the lens pole from its geometrical center, i.e. lens pole did not coincide with the geometric center of the rectangle of boxing system. For proper centration of the lens the geometrical center of the spectacle lens and the geometrical center of the rectangle surrounding the lens (boxing system) should correspond with each other. However, sometimes decentration is required to regulate the prismatic effects.

The prismatic effect can be added in the lens prescription by either ground the prismatic power on the lens surface or by decentering the spectacle lens. However, in a fully finished uncut lens whether prism has been grounded on the lens surface or a decentration is done to get the prism effect, the resultant prismatic effect will be the the the same. In a fully finished uncut spectacle lens decentring is generally more cost-effective as compared to grinding prism by surface procedure. Decentration is done when a small amount of prismatic effect is needed, or in high power lenses where small degree of decentration will produce desired prismatic effects. However, if prismatic effect is needed in great amount, then prism must be produced by grinding the lens surface.

Decentration of spherical lenses: Relationship between prismatic power and refractive power of the lens is represented by Prentice's rule. This rule states that on a spherical lens at any given point the prismatic effect is equal to the product of refractive power of lens and the distance of that given point from pole of the lens.

$$Ap = dP$$

Here,

Ap = Prismatic power (prism dioptre)

d = Distance from lens pole (centimeters)

P = Refracting power of lens (dioptres)

By mathematical calculation, the above formula can also be represented as

$$d = Ap/P \text{ or}$$

Decentration (d) = Prismatic power/Refracting power

The methods of decentration can be understood by this example

Consider that the spectacle lens prescription as, OD –5 DS/OS –5 DS distance PD = 66 mm, frame size = 50 mm, DBL = 22 mm.

Suppose, a base in 1Δ effect is desired in final spectacle glasses, then two steps calculations are needed for proper fitting of this minus power lens in the spectacle frame to produce this desired prismatic effect.

First step: Placement of major reference point (MRP) in alignment with pupillary center

Second step: Decentration of lens in the frame to produce prismatic effect.

First step: As discussed before, the frame PD is sum of frame size and DBL, i.e. 50 + 22 = 72 mm (in our example).

Therefore, MRP = Frame PD – IPD, i.e. 72–66 = 6 mm

Hence, in this case the pole of each lens should be moved 6 /2 = 3 mm inward (nasally) to the center of pupil when no prismatic effect is required.

Second step: According to Prentice's rule, the pole of a –5 D lens must be displaced 1Δ/5 D = 0.2 cm or 2 mm to produce 1Δ effect.

Direction of lens displacement must be outward (minus lens) to achieve a base in effect for each eye.

So, in a nutshell in first step we need to move the lens pole 3 mm inward (nasally) from geometrical center and in the second step we need to move the lens pole 2 mm outward (temporally) from pupillary center of the each eye. Hence, the total decentration of this prescription lens is 1 mm inward (nasally) from geometrical center of each lens to produce a prismatic effect of base in 1Δ.

Rule of thumb in determining the direction of decentration to produce a desired prismatic effect is that when a lens or meridian of a lens has

- A plus power then the lens decentration is done in the same direction of the base of prism.
- A minus power then the lens decentration is done in the opposite direction of the base of prism.

In the above example we needed a base in 1Δ effect for a minus 5 D lens, hence we displaced lens 2 mm in outward direction, i.e. opposite to the base of prism.

Decentration of plano-cylindrical lenses: Prismatic effect of a cylindrical lens is always perpendicular to its axis, hence a cylindrical lens can be decentered to produce a desired prismatic effect only in cases where the desired base direction is coinciding with the direction of power meridian.

So a plano-cylinder having a horizontal axis, i.e. 180° can only be decentered to produce vertical prismatic effects like base up or base down. On contrary, plano-cylinder having vertical axis, i.e. 90° can only be decentered to produce prismatic effects like base in or base out.

For example, a spectacle lens prescription has OD +2.5 DC × 90°.

Suppose we need 1Δ base in or 2Δ base out prismatic effects, then decentration of lens to be fitted in spectacle frame can be find as follows

To produce 1Δ base in effect, the spectacle lens must be decentered (using Prentice's rule) as follows

$$d = 1Δ/2.5 D$$
$$= 0.4 \text{ cm inward, because plus power in the meridian.}$$

Similarly, to produce 2Δ base out effect, the spectacle lens must be decentered (using Prentice's rule) as follows

$$d = 2Δ/2.5 D$$
$$= 0.8 \text{ cm outward, because plus power in the meridian.}$$

Decentration of spherocylindrical lenses having principal meridians as horizontal and vertical axis.

For example, a spectacle lens prescription has OD + 2 DS × –4 DC × 90°

Calculate the direction and amount of decentration to produce 1Δ base down and 1Δ base out prismatic effect.

The first step is to determine the power in each of the two principal meridians, so that we may apply Prentice's rule to each meridian, using the rule-of-thumb for the direction of decentration.

As shown in Fig. 12.80, power in the vertical meridian is +2 D and in the horizontal meridian is –2 D.

Hence, on applying Prentice rule

Base down is 1Δ/ 2 D, i.e. 0.5 cm downward displacement

Base out is 1Δ/2 D, i.e. 0.5 cm inward displacement

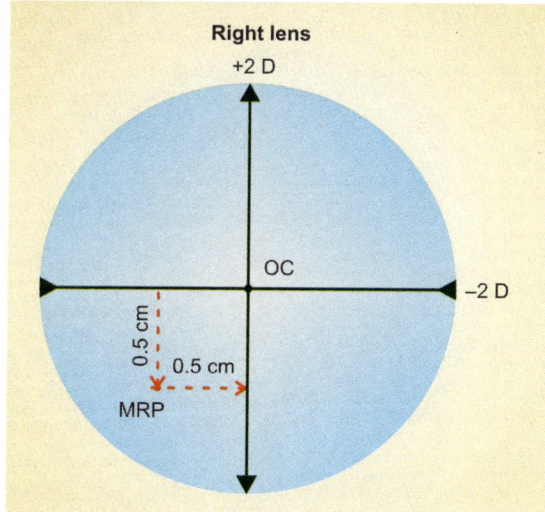

Fig. 12.80: Application of Prentice rule. MRP: Major reference point; OC: Optical center

Hence, the spectacle lens decentration will be 0.5 cm downward and 0.5 cm inward in the above prescription to produce a 1Δ base down and 1Δ base out prismatic effect.

Fitting of double segment bifocals: In most types of double segment bifocals separation distance between upper and lower segment is 13 mm, whereas normally cornea is vertically 11–12 mm in size. Hence, an ideal way of fitting a double segment bifocal lens is as shown in Fig. 12.81A and B.

Fitting of trifocal lenses: Although, trifocal lenses are not so commonly used nowadays but a proper fitting should be known to every practitioner. Upper edge of the trifocal near

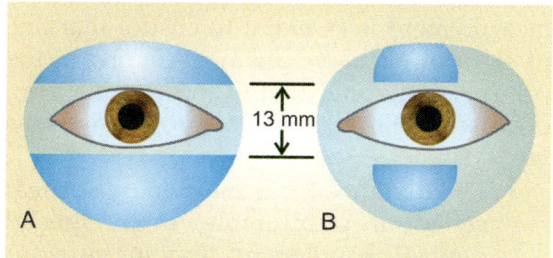

Fig. 12.81: Fitting of various double segment lens designs. A. Double executive design; B. Double straight top design

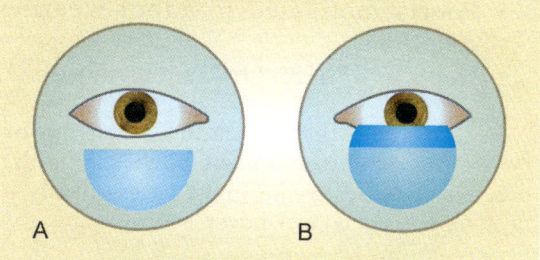

Fig. 12.82: Fitting of trifocal lens and comparing with D bifocal

segment is kept 2–3 mm below the lower lid margins same as that in a straight top segment bifocal lens as shown in Fig. 12.82A and B.

Fitting of a progressive lens: Various factors are considered in proper fitting of a progressive lens, because it is not as simple as that of regular monofocal or bifocal lenses.

Patient selection: For better results a proper patient selection is an important concern for progressive lens fitting. The main purpose of progressive lenses is to provide a continuous vision for all distances, however, many patients and optician consider it just as an invisible bifocals. Hence, it is not a good choice for those patients who want only in invisibility in lens; however, round fused bifocal lens is a good choice for these patients but intermediate vision remains blur through these bifocal lenses. Hence, if a patient wants no visibility and his requirement is for intermediate vision, then the best choice is progressive lenses.

Normally, progressive lenses should not be prescribed for the patients who are

- Having large interpupillary distance or very wide nasal bridge.
- Satisfied with their existing bifocals or trifocals spectacles.
- Comfortable with their present reading glasses and are satisfied with it.
- Need vertical prism for correction of refractive error, because progressive lenses are not available with vertical prisms.

- Poorly motivated to adopt wearing conditions.
- Nervous or of highly anxious nature.

Note: To avoid the sensation of blurring or swimming of objects in lateral visual fields, progressive lenses wearer must be essentially a head mover, not an eye mover.

In a motivated and emotionally stable patient willing to wear progressive lenses, practitioner needs to evaluate the patient's visual requirements and various factors in relation to his/her work and relaxation. Points to be considered are

- Pupil size
- Habitual eye and head movements
- Distance correction power
- Near addition power
- Relative usage of near and intermediate distance
- Previous experience with progressive lenses

Essential fitting measurements for progressive lenses: The measurements require to fit progressive lenses differ from conventional bifocal lens fittings in the following ways

- Interpupillary distance measurement should be taken monocularly by pupilometer so that each pupil aligns with progressive corridor correctly, however, single measurement is taken by a ruler binocularly for bifocal fittings.
- In progressive lens the reference point in vertical meridian (similar to segment in bifocal lenses) is the center of pupil, not the lower lid margins or ciliary line as in conventional bifocal fittings.

The progressive addition lenses consist of two types of markings

Temporary markings as shown in Fig. 12.83A consist of a fitting cross, which corresponds to center of the pupil. A distance reference point (DRP) and a near reference point (NRP) are used to check the distance and near powers of refractive correction, respectively. The

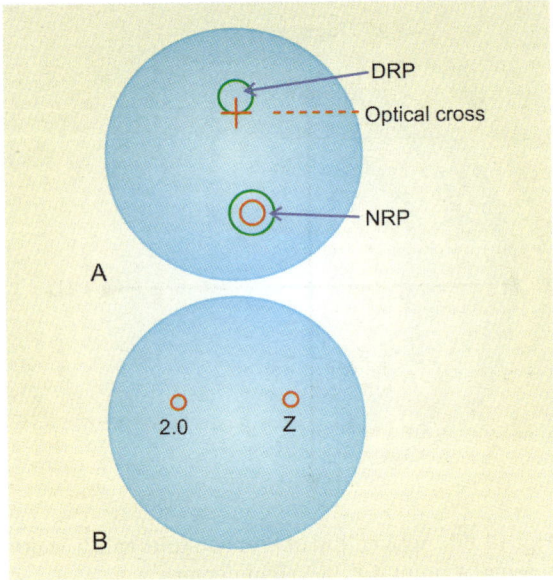

Fig. 12.83: Temporary and permanent markings on progressive lens. A. Temporary markings (DRP—distance reference point, NRP—near reference point); B. Permanent markings

height and PD of fitting cross can be confirmed from manufacturer's centering or verification chart.

Permanent markings as shown in Fig. 12.83B are partially visible; consist of two carved circles which represent the beginning of progressive zone or corridor in the form of horizontal line. Some manufacturers also put their identification mark and addition power on temporal side of lens.

A precise fitting of progress lens is mandatory, because width of progressive zone or corridor is limited. Monocular distance PD measurement is essential to ensure that line of sight of each eye always remains in the progressive zone, while eyes are moving downward. Fitting steps of progressive lens are

- The distance PD is marked by corneal reflection pupilometer or by special device provided by lens manufacturer.
- Then measure the vertical distance (D) from the center of pupil to a horizontal

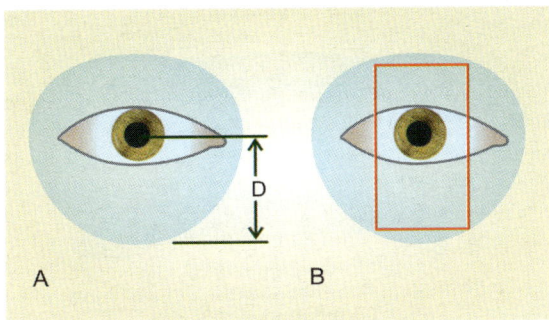

Fig. 12.84: Measurement for fitting of progressive lens. A. Vertical distance (D); B.Optical fitting box

line tangent situated at the lowest point on bottom edge of progressive lens as shown in Fig. 12.84A.

- Now place the temporary marking commonly called fitting cross on the finished lens corresponding to the center of pupil as shown in Fig. 12.84B.
- This center marking should be done on the same frame in which the patient's lenses will be mounted.
- Once the target spots are centered before each pupil, remove the frame and transfer target spot location on plastic lens using fine point pen.

There are two systems which are especially designed for progressive lens measurements are

- Grolman fitting system developed by American Optical: This system gets directly attach with patient's spectacle frame and has horizontal and vertical scales for marking of various measurements.
- Magna/Mark system: This is a magnetic based system consists of translucent targets to mark the various measurements.

In majority types of progressive lenses, the progressive corridor begins about 2 mm below the fitting cross; hence fitting techniques are modified according to the need of patient. Patients who like to use intermediate distance vision too much, fitting cross needs to be placed 1–2 mm above the pupillary center.

Glazing of Lens

Glazing of lens is the fitting process of an uncut ophthalmic lens inside the selected frame. The process of glazing has the following steps

- Lens shaping
- Lens cutting
- Lens edging and fitting

Lens Shaping

First of all the shape of lens is measured optically or mechanically, so that either manually or by a computer controlled lens grinding machine we can get an exact image of the desired lens before cutting begins.

Lens formers as shown in Fig. 12.85 also called patterns are usually supplied by lens manufacturers. These formers have similar shapes as that of desired spectacle lens, and are used to outline the shape of spectacle lens.

Lens former has a central hole which corresponds to the geometrical center and a line representing 0–180° plane. The geometrical center of former should be made coincide with the optical center of lens and by marking the side holes an axis can be marked accordingly on uncut lens.

Manual shaping of desired lens can be drawn by using Indian ink keeping the pattern on a sheet or hard board paper. Cylindrical axis, if present, is marked over the uncut lens by lensometer as three dots using greased pencil or Indian ink.

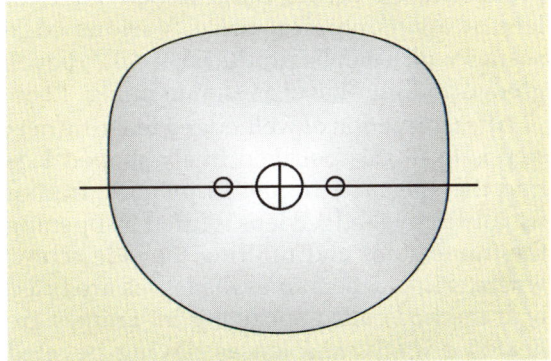

Fig. 12.85: Lens former showing 0 to 180° line for marking.

Once we had marked the uncut lens with axis of cylinder and outlined the shape of lens, the center mark and nasal side of lens is marked by using specially designed protectors in relation to cylindrical axis of lens.

Lens Cutting

After proper marking of uncut lens the extra part of lens is cut, usually a little extra than the shape marked because some margins are needed to form the edge of lens for proper fitting. After cutting the formed rough lens shape should be matched with size and shape of the frame.

The lens cutting can be done manually by using a chipper (before using chipper groove the outline of lens shape with a diamond pencil) or alternately a diamond cutter wheel or fully automated cutting machine can be used.

Lens Edging and Fitting

The partial finished lens formed after cutting also need proper edges so that it can fit properly inside the frame. Therefore, edging of lens is done either manually on a rotating diamond wheel or by fully automatic machines, although edging by manual way is more economically viable than automatic machines. For manual edging various types of grit wheels are available to grind the lens edges and to make it smooth and shiny. Nowadays diamond wheels are also present which produce faster, accurate and smooth edges of lens at an economical price. Various edge shapes which can be produced are flat, bevel, groove and mid-bevel as shown in Fig. 12.86.

After formation of well-edged lens, the next step is to fit this polished finely shaped lens into the spectacle frame. In metallic frames usually a bevel-edged lens is fitted by opening the frame sides and refitting the side screw, whereas in plastic frames the lenses are fitted by a method called springing in. Frames are heated slightly and lenses having beveled edges are just pressed inside the frames like a spring and it get fit into the frame groove.

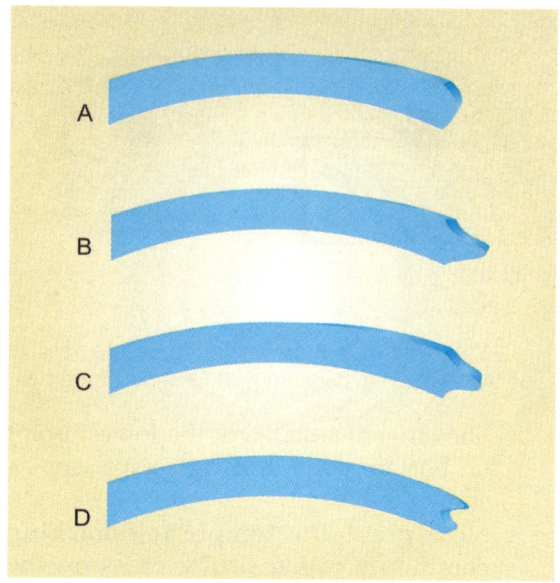

Fig. 12.86: Various types of lens edges. A. Flat; B. Bevel; C. Mid-bevel; D. Groove

Rimless fitting is a little different, it needs to make the holes in the lenses and sometimes grooves are also cut near holes on the sides of rim. Then the nasal and end pieces are fixed with lens with the help of screws and/or suction plugs.

Finally, prescription and lens power are matched, quality of lens fit is checked before cleaning and packing for dispensing of spectacle. With an expert fitter whole glazing process may take 10–15 minutes.

Verifications of Spectacles

Sometimes, the patient may complain that the lenses prescribed to him/her are not proper and there was an error in evaluating the degree of refractive error. However, on careful examination, it may be found that the problem was due to an error of either dispensing or fitting of lenses. Hence, it is mandatory to verify the spectacles before dispensing.

Spectacle verification means to verify the lens powers, cylindrical axis, optical center and prismatic effect of spectacle lenses along with any surface defects, if present. It is also essential to check the fitting of lens in the frame along with the frame alignment. Before dispensing the spectacle we should check

- Surface defects
- Lens power measurement
- Frame alignment

Surface Defects

Sometimes there may be defect in the surface which may occur during manufacturing (waves in lens) or during glazing and fitting (aberrations, chipping or dents) and can be missed many a times by dispenser.

Note: Surface defects are the most common reason for rejection of spectacles.

Lens Power Measurement

Lens power and cylindrical axis of a spectacle lens can easily be measured by lensometer; however, in the absence of instrument manual neutralization can be done to assess the parameters of spectacle lens.

Hand neutralization techniques for spectacle lenses

For spherical lenses

For neutralization of an unknown spherical spectacle lens the following method is used

- Hold the spectacle lens at about 1 meter distance while keeping its back surface towards examiner and then observe an object at 20 feet distance.
- The object should have both vertical and horizontal shapes. For example, a large cross or square or 6/60 size letter A.
- Focus on the image at central zone of the lens and slowly move the spectacle lens, both in vertical and horizontal meridians.
- Observe whether the transverse movement of object appears to be in the same direction or in the opposite direction in comparison to the movement of the spectacle lens.
- Same direction movement or 'with motion' indicates that it is a minus lens as shown in Fig. 12.87. An opposite direction movement or 'against motion' indicates that it is a plus lens.

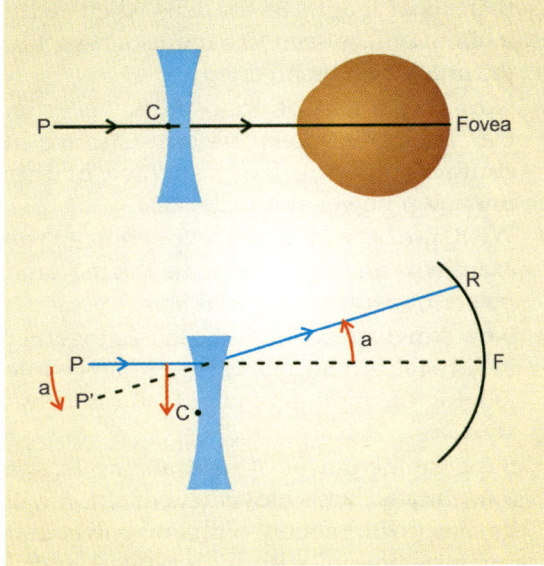

Fig. 12.87: Downward movement of minus lens, showing downward movement (same direction) of object from P to P' position.

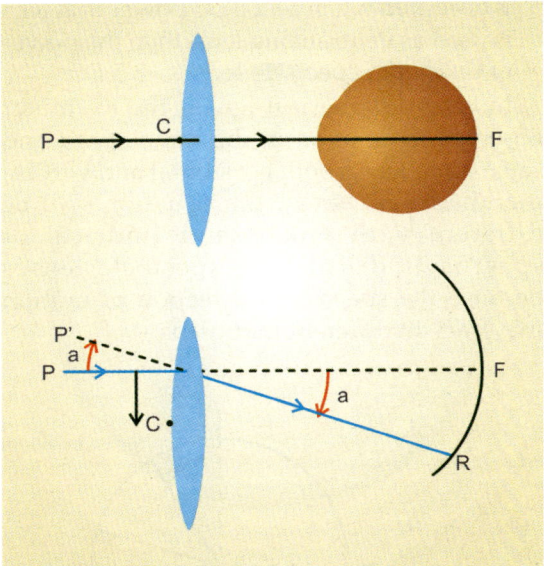

Fig. 12.88: Downward movement of plus lens, showing upward movement (opposite direction) of object from P to P' position.

- In plus lenses, 'against motion' is seen until the distance between the plus lens and observer's eye is less than focal length of plus lens (Fig. 12.88). If this distance is more than focal length of the lens, then 'with motion' will be seen like minus lenses, but the image will be inverted.

- Now take a lens of opposite power from trial lenses and keep its back surface in contact with the front surface of this unknown power spectacle lens.
- With more and more experience, the examiner can closely estimate the required power of neutralizing trial lens.
- Now slowly move both the lenses together in vertical and horizontal meridians while judging the motion of object simultaneously.
- Suppose the power of neutralizing lens is inadequate, then a movement of object will be seen ('with motion' with low power and 'against motion' with high power) and if power of neutralizing lens is sufficient or equal, then no movement of object image will be noticed. For example, if no motion is observed when a +2.5 DS power trial lens is used as neutralizing lens, then the power of unknown spectacle lens is –2.5 DS.

In case of spherical lenses the examiner observes the motion in the same speed and same direction in both horizontal and vertical meridians. However, the situation will be different with unknown cylindrical or spherocylindrical type spectacle lenses because the speed and direction of motion may vary in different meridians.

For cylindrical and sphero-cylindrical lenses: Neutralization of cylindrical or sphero-cylindrical spectacle lens is done by the following method

- Similar to a spherical lens, examiner holds the spectacle lens at one meter distance keeping its back surface towards him/her and observes an object, e.g. a plus (+) mark at 20 feet distance.
- Then examiner rotates the spectacle lens either clockwise or anticlockwise and observes a scissors like motion of the object.
- When a cross target is observed through spectacle lens, the displacement of its vertical and horizontal lines will be seen as compared to their original positions present outside the spectacle lens as shown in Fig. 12.89A.
- During rotation when spectacle lens gets oriented in a way that two limbs of target cross become parallel and continuous with principal meridians of spectacle lens, then the displacement of vertical and horizontal limbs of cross target disappears as shown in Fig. 12.89B.
- Once examiner reaches to an orientation where both limbs of target cross are parallel and continuous both inside and outside the spectacle lens, then a further rotation of spectacle lens will show a scissors motion either with or against the rotation of spectacle lens.

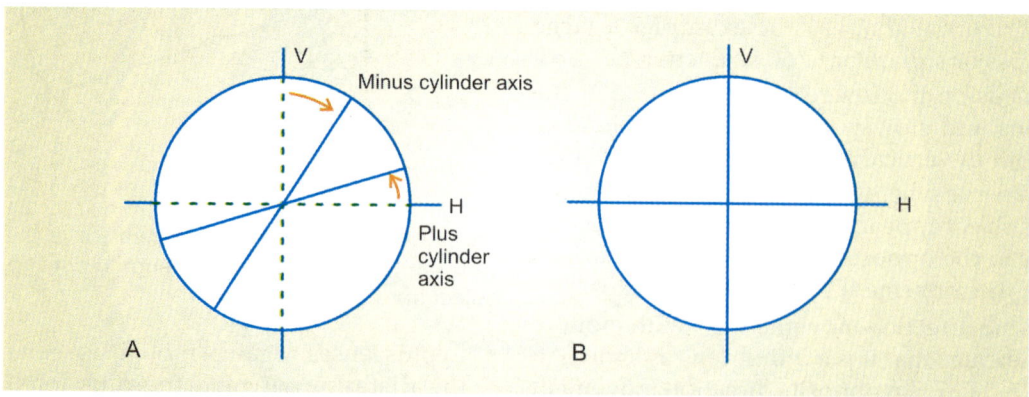

Fig. 12.89: Hand neutralization of spectacle lens containing cylindrical power. A. Off-axis cylinder showing scissor movement; B. On-axis cylinder

Hand neutralization method to determine the cylindrical power and axis.

- Observer holds the spectacle lens firmly in position where the spectacle lines are parallel and continuous with cross target limbs both inside and outside the spectacle lens.
- Then examiner draws line ABOCD in vertical axis as shown in Fig. 12.90A over limbs seen inside the spectacle lens using grease pencil on the back surface of the spectacle lens.
- Examiner then rotates the spectacle lens and observes the movement of this vertical line ABOCD.
- Suppose line seen inside the spectacle lens rotates as 'with motion' in the direction of the rotation of spectacle lens, means that line ABOCD of cross target is parallel to the minus cylinder axis as shown in Fig. 12.90B.
- When line inside the spectacle lens rotates against the direction of rotation of spectacle lens, means that line ABOCD of cross target is parallel to plus cylinder as shown in Fig. 12.90C.
- Once two principal meridians of spectacle lens of unknown power are localized, then neutralize each meridian separately using spherical lenses.
- Examiner firmly holds the spectacle lens against the line of cross on trial lens representing the axis of neutralization inside and outside the spectacle lens. Then examiner marks the axis on unknown cylindrical spectacle lens with grease pencil. This axis can be measured with the help of a lens protractor, however, an approximate ±5° will occur in manual assessment of axis.

- After neutralizing each principal meridian, power and axis are noted and a prescription of spectacle lens is written in a minus cylinder form. For example, if spectacle lens gets neutralized in horizontal meridian with –5 DS trial lens and in vertical meridian with –3 DS trial lens, it means power of unknown spectacle lens is +5 DS in the horizontal meridian and +3 DS in the vertical meridian. Prescription for unknown lens would be written as + 5 DS/ –2 DC × 180°.

Another difficult task in hand neutralization method is to mark the optical center or pole of spectacle lens.

- To mark the optical center of spectacle lens, examiner identifies the point where the two lines of target cross meet inside and outside the spectacle lens. Then mark a small dot on the lens while holding the spectacle lens in a position where the lines inside and outside are parallel and continuous as described above.

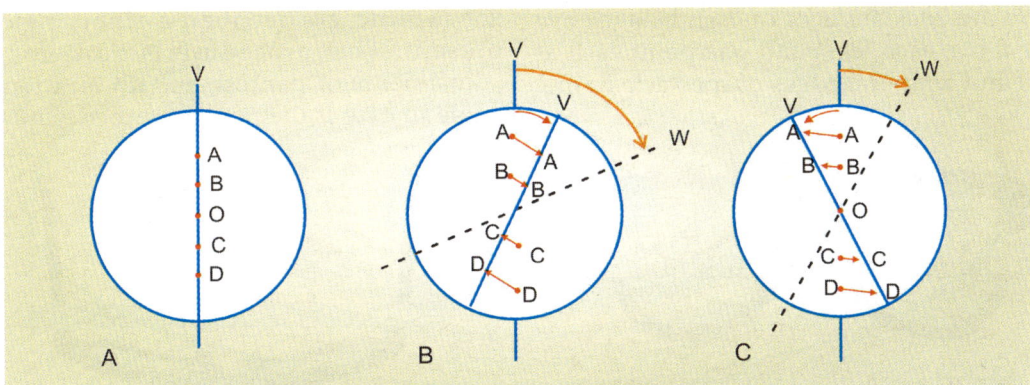

Fig. 12.90: Determination of cylindrical axis. A. Marking of axis line ABOCD over spectacle lens; B. With movement in case of minus cylinder; C. Against movement in case of plus cylinder

Frame Alignments

As we normally consider that the standard alignment of frame has been already done by the manufacturers, so we prefer to fit the lens directly. However, this is not always true and often it becomes necessary for dispenser to check the frame alignment before dispensing.

A proper frame alignment is done by the following methodology

- Front alignment
- Temple alignment

Front alignment: Front alignment is done in two steps with the help of device having straight border, e.g. a millimeter ruler.

First step: examiner places the millimeter ruler against the back of spectacle frame below the end pieces as shown in Fig. 12.91, while spectacle frame is held horizontally. Then examiner observes whether right and left end pieces are at equal distances above the ruler or not. If they are at equal distance, then no adjustment is needed, however, if they are at unequal distance, then the frame bridge is either raised or lowered so that they become equal.

Second step: Examiner then verifies the vertical alignment of spectacle frame by placing the ruler along the back surface of frame underneath or above the nose pads with temples extending upwards while spectacle frame is held vertically as shown in Fig. 12.92. In proper alignment situation the ruler should touch four points on spectacle frame. Two points are back surfaces of each lens (or eye wire above each lens) and one point each at nasal and temporal edges of spectacle frame.

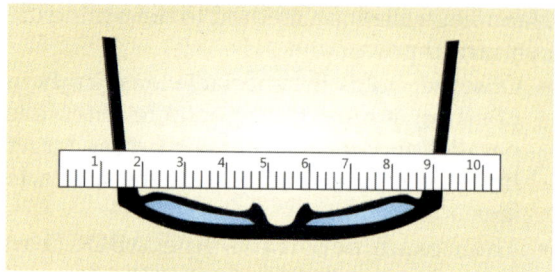

Fig. 12.92: Examination for vertical alignment of spectacle frame front

In some specific spectacle frame design the front of frame is arched in outward direction, which is commonly called face form. In these design frames the nasal edges of frame will not touch the millimeter ruler as shown in Fig. 12.93. Mostly aviation types of sunglasses are made in this design. Suppose preferred degree of face form or four point touch is absent, then it can be rectified by adjusting the frame bridge position.

Sometimes during verification of vertical alignment, examiner notices that two lenses of spectacle frame are in different vertical planes (X-ing of frame), means one side lens is tilted either outward or inward in comparison to other as shown in Fig. 12.94. Similar to face form correction X-ing can also be corrected by adjustment of frame bridge rotation.

Temple alignment: Normally in a properly aligned spectacle frame a pantoscopic tilt (generally 6°–10°) and temple angle of 92°–95° (a little greater than a right angle) is present. This procedure is done for the adjustments of pantoscopic tilt and temple angle in case if they are disturbed. Equality

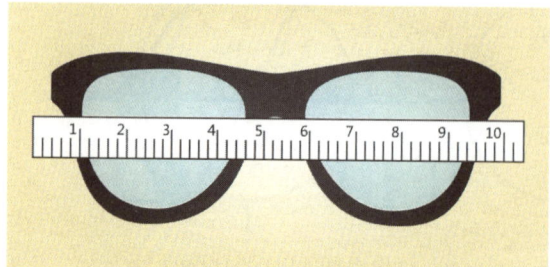

Fig. 12.91: Examination for front alignment of spectacle frame

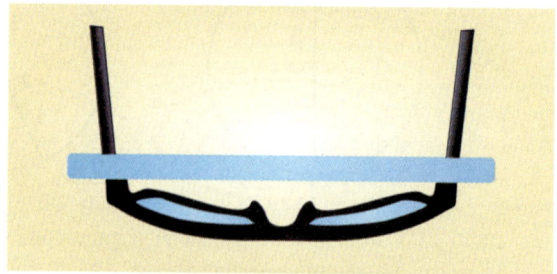

Fig. 12.93: Face form in spectacle frame

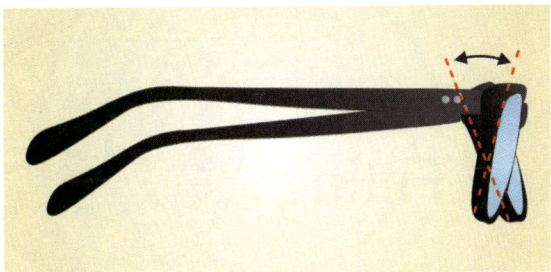

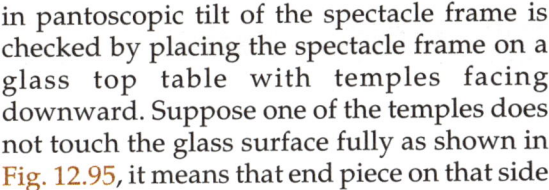

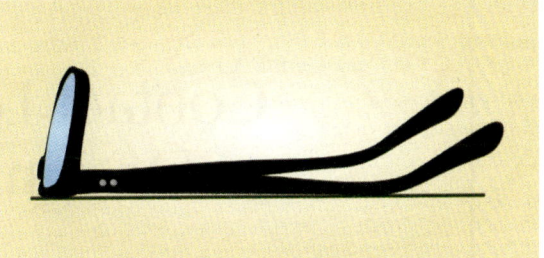

Fig. 12.94: X-ing of spectacle frame

Fig. 12.95: Unequal pantoscopic angles

in pantoscopic tilt of the spectacle frame is checked by placing the spectacle frame on a glass top table with temples facing downward. Suppose one of the temples does not touch the glass surface fully as shown in Fig. 12.95, it means that end piece on that side of frame has a larger degree of pantoscopic tilt compared to the end piece of the other side. Similarly, both sides of spectacle frame should have the same degree of temple angle. This can be easily assessed by examination of frame.

Contact Lens Optics, Design and Fitting

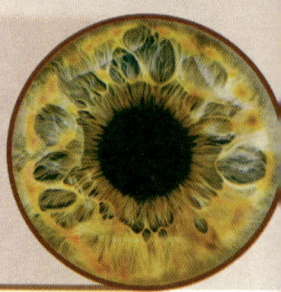

Chapter Outline

- Contact Lens Optics
  - History and events of progress
  - Concept of contact lens forms
  - Optical properties of contact lens
    - Thick lens
    - Effective power
    - Change in retinal image magnification
    - Effect on refractive status
    - Effect on accommodative demand
    - Effect on accommodative convergence
    - Prismatic effects as compared to spectacles
    - Aberrations and field of view
- Contact Lens Materials
  - Introduction
  - Terminologies in contact lens material
    - Water properties related to lens
    - Oxygen related contact lens properties
  - Rigid contact lens materials
  - Soft contact lens materials
- Manufacturing and Types of Contact Lens
  - Lathe cutting
  - Melt pressing
  - Spin casting
  - Cast moulding
  - Classification of contact lens
- Contact Lens Design
  - Regular lens design
  - Special lens design
  - Terminologies in contact lens
    - Contact lens dimensions
    - Contact lens curves and radius
  - Indications of contact lens wear
  - Contraindications of contact lens use
- Contact Lens Fitting
  - Patient work up for contact lens fitting
  - Soft contact lens fitting
  - Soft contact lens ordering
  - Insertion and removal of soft contact lens
  - Rigid contact lens fitting
  - Rigid contact lens ordering
  - Insertion and removal of rigid contact lens
  - Rigid contact lens related complications and management

CONTACT LENS OPTICS

Contact lens is a small piece of plastic which is designed to rest on the cornea and/or sclera in such a way that they are in direct contact of cornea and correct the refractive errors of eye. Along with optical uses, a contact lens can be used for various other purposes also including therapeutic, cosmetic and diagnostic.

History and Events of Progress

Basis aim of several researchers was to neutralize the front surface of cornea with the help of various devices.

- In the year 1508, Leonardo da Vinci came up with an idea that a vision of a person can be altered by immersing head up to ears with face down in half water filled specially designed bowl.
- In the year 1636, Descartes suggested that corneal surface can be neutralized by placing a tube filled with water on the cornea having a watch glass on the other end.
- In the year 1801, Thomas Young on the basis of principle of Descartes tried to neutralize his refractive power by designing long tube filled with water, having a lens of 20 mm focal length on the other end.
- In the year 1827, John Herschel done experiment with application of animal jelly in the form of glass capsule on the eyes in order to eliminate the astigmatic errors.
- In the year 1886, first proposal of hydrophilic contact appliance came from Galezowsky, who suggested the use of a gelatin disc soaked in cocaine and sublimate of mercury for post-cataract extraction cases.
- In the year 1887, FA Muller used a glass blown lens to cover the eye of a patient whose eyelids had been removed.
- In the year 1888, Fick was the first to coin the term contact lens and used a non-optical corneal contact lens for treatment of keratoconus. He also suggested the use of contact lens for aphakia and cosmetic purposes.

- Nearly for 40 years period (1895–1930) all contact lenses were made up of glass. Basically of two types
  - Blown glass from Muller
  - Ground glass from Carl Zeiss
- For another decade methods were developed to take eye cast by using material like Negocolle, a seaweed extract mainly used for dental purposes.
- In the year 1938, Obrig diagnosed that contact lens intolerance was due to limbal pressure. He also discovered that fluorescein solution with blue light can be used to check the contact lens fit.
- In the year 1937 Feinbloom first time used the plastic material for contact lens. Lenses made by him had a glass optic with a plastic scleral zone.
  - Subsequently, in the year 1943 the true corneal lenses having diameter of 11–12 mm were introduced, popularly called Tuohy lens.
- During 1950–1960 Gyorrfy revolutionalized the contact lens manufacturing world by introduction of Polymethyl methacrylate (PMMA) contact lenses for production of soft contact lenses, which shortly followed by use of hydroxyl methyl methacrylate (HEMA) in the year 1963.
- In the year 1970, rigid contact lenses (made up of PMMA) were introduced. Later on in the year 1978, rigid gas permeable (RGP) lenses were also manufactured by using Cellulose Acetate Butyrate material (CAB).
- Silicon acrylate material was introduced in the year 1975–78. Around the same period, CIBA Vision Company introduced tinted and bifocal contact lenses.
- Later on, in the year 1986, it was Johnson and Johnson Company who manufactured the weekly disposable contact lenses.

Contact lenses differ from spectacle lenses in many aspects. Important difference is that the spectacle lenses are worn about 12–15 mm away from the corneal surface, hence only vergence of incident rays hitting the corneal surface is altered. However, in case of contact lens, as it remains in contact with corneal surface, the vergence of the incident rays not altered, rather vergence of eye itself is altered. Hence in case of spectacle lens the refractive power of eye gets an accessory effort and there is no real change in refractive status of eye, on contrary, in case of a contact lens, the real refractive status of eye is changed. This change in refractive status of eye is contributed by the fact that when contact lens is in place, the anterior surface of cornea becomes optically absent, as it becomes the posterior surface of a liquid or glass lens. Furthermore, there is a chance of independent viewing movement of eyes behind the spectacles which is not seen with contact lens. The prismatic effects are observed more with the use of spectacle lens than contact lens.

Concept of Contact Lens Forms

To understand the function of a contact lens, it is essential to know the concept of glass lens and liquid lens. As we know that tear film play a significant part in corneal integrity to perform the refractive role, we should know the dynamics of tear film and contact lens together for functioning of a contact lens as corrective device.

Depending upon the curvatures of contact lens and corneal surface various lens forms are seen as

- Afocal segment
- Liquid lens
- Glass lens or focal segment
- Combined lens system

Afocal segment: When curvatures of both the surfaces of contact lens are the same, then they form an afocal contact lens. For example, contact lens having anterior surface of +6 D and posterior surface of –6 D.

As we can see in Fig. 13.1 that when three curvatures (two surfaces of contact lens and one surface of cornea) are same, the contact lens serves as afocal segment, where anterior surface of contact lens becomes anterior surface of refractive system.

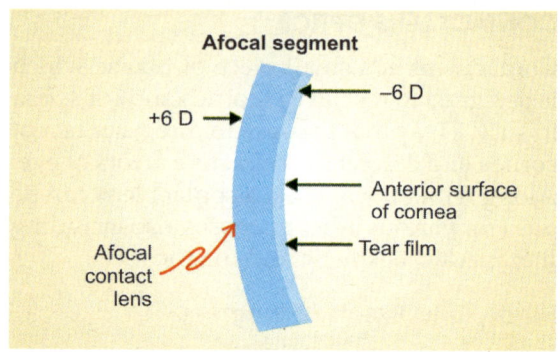

Fig. 13.1: Afocal segment

Liquid lens: When two curvatures of contact lens surfaces (both anterior and posterior) are same like afocal segment but they are different from the anterior surface of cornea, then it forms a liquid lens. The elements of refraction in this kind of system are contact lens, tear film lens (liquid lens) and anterior surface of cornea, which are separated by an invisibly thin air film. Hence in this system the effective refractive power will be exerted by back vertex power of liquid lens in the air.

As we can see in Fig. 13.2, the posterior surface of contact lens and anterior surface of the cornea forms a lens filled with liquid (tear film), called liquid lens or tear lens or fluid lens. The correction of ametropia will be due to the refractive power of this lens, which is equal to a sum of anterior and posterior surfaces of tear lens.

Glass lens: When curvature of posterior surface of contact lens is the same as that of

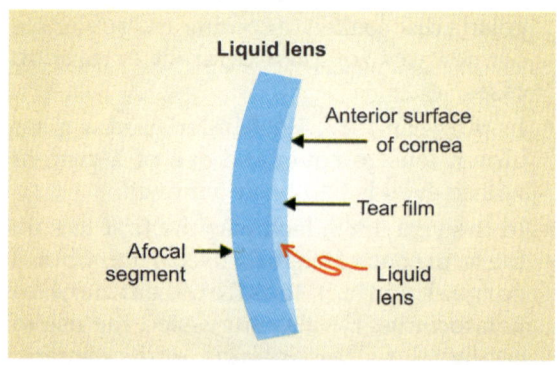

Fig. 13.2: Liquid lens

cornea, but curvature of anterior surface of contact lens is different, then they form a glass lens or focal segment or powered lens.

As shown in Fig. 13.3, a focal segment is formed due to difference in curvatures of anterior and posterior surfaces of contact lens. To understand the refractive power of this type of system, if we know the power of posterior surface of contact lens (which is usually kept fixed), then only task remains is to know the power of anterior surface of contact lens (which usually has a relationship with anterior corneal surface and decided empirically).

Suppose the posterior contact lens surface is parallel to anterior corneal surface, then back vertex power of contact lens will be equal to ocular refractive status.

Combined lens: When the curvatures of three elements, i.e. anterior and posterior surfaces of contact lens and anterior surface of cornea, are different to each other, then the effective power of system is determined by power of both the liquid lens and glass lens.

As we can see in Fig. 13.4, that two lenses are formed: Anteriorly a glass lens and posteriorly a liquid lens. Refractive status of this system is a combined power of these two lenses. Although ametropia can be corrected by tear lens alone, but in routine practice both the liquid lens and glass lens in combination are used to neutralize the refractive error.

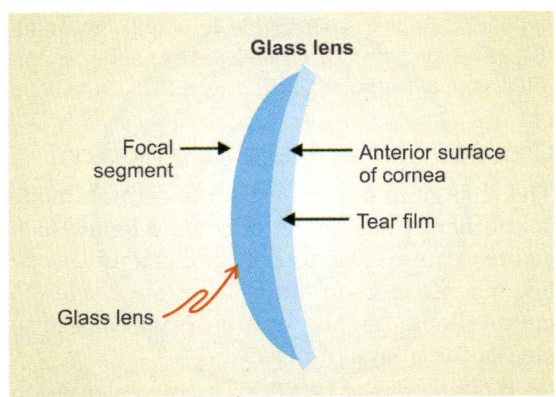

Fig. 13.3: Glass lens

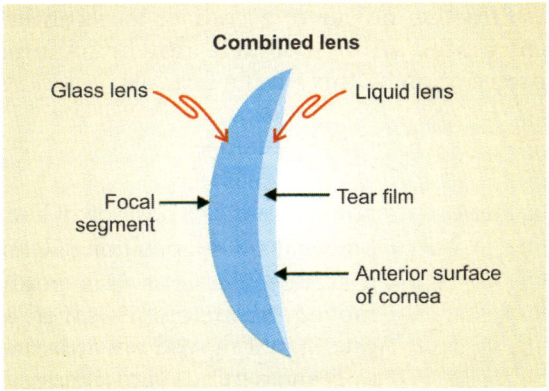

Fig. 13.4: Combined lens

Optical Properties of Contact Lens

Thick Lens

Although a contact lens physically appears thin as compared to spectacle lens but for optical reasons spectacle lens is considered as a thin lens and a contact lens is considered as a thick lens. Because the contact lens is so steeply curved, that application of an approximate power formula, as in case of a spectacle lens, will lead to serious refractive errors.

Effective Power of Contact Lens

The effective power of a correcting lens (contact lens or glasses) changes as we bring it nearer to eye. In case of a contact lens the correcting lens is brought very near to eye, i.e. it touches the eyes. Effective lens power is determined by the relative position of correcting lens with that of vertex plane. While in case of spectacles, the lens is placed at 14–15 mm in front of vertex plane, whereas in case of a contact lens, the lens is placed on vertex plane. For example, a minus lens becomes more effective when moves towards the eye, whereas a plus lens becomes more effective when moves farther away from the eye. This means that for a myope a contact lens must be weaker than a spectacle lens, whereas for a hypermetrope a contact lens power should be stronger than a spectacle lens for correction of the same amount of refractive error.

Effective power of a contact lens can be calculated from spectacle power or lens prescription by this simple formula:

$$P_A = \frac{P_O}{1 - d\,P_O}$$

Here P_O = power at original position of lens
   P_A = power at altered position of lens
   d = distance the lens has been moved (in meters), is given a plus sign if moved towards the eyes and a minus sign if moved away from the eyes.

To understand this, let us consider a myope of –8 D spectacle lens power at vertex distance of 12 mm (12/1000 meters), calculate the contact lens power (Fig. 13.5).

As per formula

$$P_A = \frac{-8}{1 - 0.012(-8)}$$

$$= \frac{-8}{1 + 0.096}$$

$$= \frac{-8}{1.096}$$

$$= -7.29 \text{ D}$$

Similarly, suppose an aphakic patient needs +12 D spectacle power at vertex distance of 12 mm, then the contact lens power will be calculated as shown in Fig. 13.6.

As per formula

$$P_A = \frac{+12}{1 - 0.012\,(+12)}$$

$$= \frac{+12}{1 - 0.144}$$

$$= \frac{+12}{0.856}$$

$$= +14.01 \text{ D}$$

The abovementioned examples clearly indicate that for myopia the power of contact lens will be less than power of a spectacle lens, whereas for hypermetropic eyes it will be more than a spectacle lens.

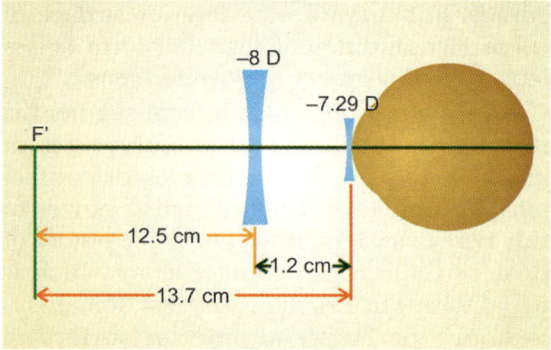

Fig. 13.5: Effective power of a contact lens for a 8 D myope; when refracted at vertex distance of 12 mm

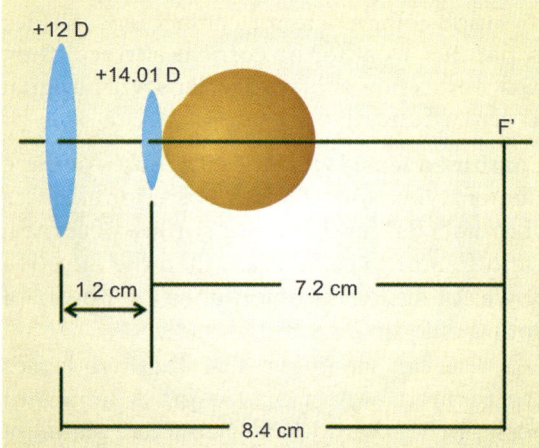

Fig. 13.6: Effective power of a contact lens for an aphakic having +12 D power; when refracted at vertex distance of 12 mm

Note: When refractive errors in eyes are of less than ±3 D, then the power difference between contact lens and a spectacle lens will be about 0.12 D, which can be considered as negligible for all practical purposes.

Change in Retinal Image Magnification

The change in magnification of retinal image is another optical effect of contact lens which is due to more closeness of contact lens to eyes. So, when a person shifts from spectacles to contact lens, he/she will observe change in size of the image of objects.

It is due to the fact that during calculation of magnification by spectacles, the distance between back of lens and entrance to pupil of eye is also included. It means if a correcting lens is brought near to eyes, the retinal image magnification will change which is seen with contact lens. Therefore, in a myopic person, the contact lens will produce a retinal image bigger in size than a spectacle lens, hence a myopic patient who starts wearing a contact lenses will usually feel happy by the fact that everything looks larger than before. On contrary, in hypermetropic patient the contact lens will produce retinal image smaller in size than spectacle lens, hence a hypermetrope especially an aphakic will be pleased by the fact that now the objects are looking nearly to their normal sizes.

Note: Usually, aphakics wearing spectacles lens have an image magnification of about 22% which is difficult to adjust binocularly, however, with contact lens the same person will have an image magnification of only 7% which is easier to adjust binocularly.

Effect on Refractive Status

As contact lenses are in direct contact of eyes, the refractive status of eye may change especially with the use of hard contact lens. On contrary, eyes are also capable to change the refractive power of contact lens especially of a soft contact lens. These changes in refractive power are of important in cases of astigmatism. A spherical hard contact lens usually hide or eliminate the corneal astigmatism, whereas a spherical soft contact lens remain confine with the toricity of cornea and produce very little or no effect on corneal astigmatism. Hence, to correct astigmatism by means of soft contact lenses, toric contact lenses should be used.

Effect on Accommodative Demand

Shift of spectacle glasses to contact lens in both myopes and hypermetropes also cause change in accommodative demand. Myopes using minus glasses has an advantage over an emmetropic person in terms of accommodative demand because the use of minus spectacle glasses decreases the accommodative demand in myopes. Suppose a myope switch over to contact lens from spectacles, then he/she has to exert more accommodative power. On contrary, in hypermetropes use of plus spectacle glasses causes increase in the accommodative demand and when they switch over to contact lens the need of accommodative demand is decreased.

The change in demand of accommodation in contact lens wearer myopes and hypermetropes as compared to spectacles lens wearer has important role at presbyopic age. In contact lens wearer myopics, the addition power for near work will be required at earlier age, whereas contact lens wearer hypermetrope will need additional power for near work at a later age as compared to spectacle worn counterpart.

An average amount of accommodation needed while wearing contact lenses is about 2.5 D irrespective to the amount or type of refractive error. Consider this fact in example, a +10 D hypermetrope wearing spectacles require 3.29 D of accommodation for a 40 cm reading distance, whereas a –10 D myope counterpart needs only 1.8 D for the same reading distance. So in this example hypermetrope has to accommodate about 0.75 D less (i.e. 2.5 – 3.29), while myope needs to accommodate 0.75 D more (i.e. 2.5 – 1.8), when these hypermetrope and myope patients wear contact lenses instead of spectacles.

Note: Persons having very high degree myopia (≥14 D) will face problems in wearing contact lenses, due to a significant increase in demand of accommodation.

Effect on Accommodative Convergence

An increase demand of accommodation in myopes due to wearing of contact lenses will lead to use of more accommodative convergence. On the other hand, hypermetrope wearing contact lens will use less accommodative convergence. As a result, contact lens wearer myope having esophoria will have to apply more negative fusional vergence than glasses wearer myope, resulting in increased eye strain. While in an exophoric contact wearer myope, increase in the accommodative convergence will decrease the use of positive fusional vergence, and thus results in reduced exophoria. Similarly, an exophoric hypermetrope contact lens wearer will require more positive fusional vergence than glasses.

The change in accommodative demand and fusional vergence due to contact lens are practically insignificant for refractive errors of small degree, however, the changes may have significant effects in cases of large refractive errors, especially if there is an associated high AC/A ratio.

As in the above example, a –10 D myope and + 10 D hypermetrope both needs more or less 0.75 D of accommodation respectively, if they wear a contact lens in place of spectacles. However, a change in accommodative demand of almost 0.75 D will be accompanied by a change in accommodative convergence. Now if they have an AC/A ratio of 6, then the change in accommodative convergence at 40 cm distance will be of 6 × 0.75 which is equal to 4.5 prism dioptres (Δ). Hence, in an exophoric myope, exophoria will be reduced by 4.5 Δ, while in esophoric myope esophoria will be increased by 4.5 Δ at 40 cm distance. It means an exophoric myope having a refractive error of –10 D will use 4.5 Δ less positive fusional vergence, when uses contact lens in place of spectacles. On the other hand, an esophoric myope in the same situation will use more negative fusional vergence of 4.5 Δ.

Similarly, a +10 D hypermetrope when switch from spectacles to contact lenses, then an exophoria at 40 cm will be increased by 4.5 Δ and an esophoria will be decreased by 4.5 Δ at the same distance.

Routinely, majority of contact lens wearers has a refractive error in the range of ±1 D to ±5 D, hence the change in accommodative convergence, needed with use of contact lenses instead of spectacles; do not present a significant clinical problem.

Note: In an aphakic patient due to absence of crystalline lens, the accommodative convergence does not exist because of lack of accommodation, hence when they switch from spectacle to contact lenses, there is no change in the demand of fusional convergence for near vision.

Prismatic Effects as Compared to Spectacles

Spectacles lens induces prismatic effect which occurs because line of sight moves away from major reference point of lenses as spectacle lens remain fixed and do not move with movement of eyes, while contact lens moves with the movement of eyes, hence no significant prismatic effects are produced with contact lenses.

For example, in case of myopes "base in" effect is produced by minus lenses, while "base out" prismatic effect is produced by plus lenses for near vision. Hence, when an exophoric myope switches from spectacles to contact lenses, he/she will be at disadvantage due to lack of base in prismatic effect for near work, whereas an esophoric hypermetrope when switches from spectacle to contact lenses, similarly will have disadvantage because of lack of base out prismatic effect for near work. A vertical prismatic effect during up and down gaze and change in demand of vergence during right and left gaze in anisometropia is seen with spectacles lenses, but wearing of contact lenses eliminate this prismatic effect.

Note: Although use of contact lens eliminates many unwanted prismatic effects of spectacles lens but due to contact lens some beneficial prismatic effects are also eliminated. For example, spectacle lens can correct a lateral prismatic deviation which is lost with contact lens.

Aberrations and Field of View

Most important types of aberrations which can be experienced with spectacle lens are oblique astigmatism, curvature of image, and distortion. All of these aberrations are minimized by the use of contact lenses which move with the movement of eyes.

Oblique astigmatism and curvature of image aberration happens when spectacle wearer rotates his/her eyes to look through the periphery of spectacle lenses, however, contact lens wearers has no such issue to look through the periphery.

Distortion of image occurs due to distance between aperture of spectacle lens and aperture (pupil) of eye. However, in case of contact lens, this distance is negligible, hence very minimum distortion of image.

Field of view is larger in majority of the contact lens wearers as compared to spectacle glasses. In a moving eye, contact lens wearer has an additional advantage of unlimited macular field of view which is absent in a spectacle worn person because due to presence of rim of spectacle's frame the macular field gets restricted as a field of fixation.

CONTACT LENS MATERIALS

Introduction

History about contact lenses tells us that initially for manufacturing of contact lens the glass material were used, mainly blown glass of Muller and ground glass of Carl Zeiss. However, a constant hunt for an ideal contact lens material was on, because contact lens of glass material were brittle, heavy and were difficult to manufacture in mass.

A revolution in contact lens material took place in the year 1943 when Kevin Tuohy introduced plastic material for manufacturing of contact lens. Although a few years back Obrig had already started the use of methyl methacrylate to produce contact lenses.

Subsequently, Gyorrfy introduced PMMA for lens, and then Wichterle changed the picture of contact lens world by introducing the hydroxyl methyl methacrylate in the year 1963. Gradually, acrylic, silicon and cellulose acetate butyrate were also introduced as contact lens materials for mass manufacturing.

Properties required in an ideal contact lens material are

- *Optical property:* Lens material should have a good percentage, i.e. 95–98% of light transmission and have a refractive index compatible with tears and cornea.
- *Ocular compatibility:* Material should be safe to wear and has no harmful effects on ocular surface especially cornea.
- *Gas permeability:* In absence of contact lens the cornea receives oxygen through tears, thus lens material should have good oxygen transmission through it so that cornea does not suffocate. Hence gas permeability through material is a major factor to decide tolerance and duration of wearing of lens.
- *Physical properties:* Specific gravity and density of the material are important properties to keep the contact lens in position because a high density material will not stay for a long period on the corneal surface.
- *Chemical properties:* Lens material should be easily wettable and water should not spread over its surface (hydrophilic), so that tear film can serve better when contact lens is in position.
- *Material strength:* This property decides that whether lens will maintain its shape and curvatures after fitting. This is important to maintain the optical property of contact lens.
- *Resistant nature:* Contact lens material should be highly resistant to chemical agents and microbial contamination, so that it will remain sterile during wearing. It should have a property to easily get sterilized by chemicals or radiations.
- *Moulding:* An easy mouldability of lens material is a prerequisite to give proper shape and curvatures to manufacture lens in large scale.

Terminologies in Contact Lens Material

For better understanding of properties of contact lens material, we should be well versed with the following related terminologies.

Water Properties Related to Lens

A hydrated contact lens has the following water elements

- Water content
- Water absorption
- Wettability

Water content: Water content means the quantity of water present in a lens. We can measure it in terms of volume or weight. It can be expressed as:

Water content = wet weight – dry weight/wet weight × 100

Water content of a contact lens is usually equilibrated in presence of 0.9% saline and change in conditions like pH and tonicity of solution and temperature can alter the water properties of lens.

Water absorption: It means the quantity of water that a contact lens can absorb, means it measures the water uptake capacity of lens and can be expressed as

Water absorption = wet weight – dry weight/dry weight × 100

Wettability: This is important to maintain the corneal tear film. Wettability indicates the adherent property of a liquid to a solid surface, despite that the liquid is held by cohesive forces. This can be assessed by contact angle which is inversely proportional to wettability. Thus a lower value of contact angle indicates better wettability than a higher contact angle. On the basis of contact angle various contact lens materials can be grouped as

- Hydrophilic = 0° contact angle
- Hydrogel = 20° contact angle
- Hydrophobic = > 150° contact angle

Oxygen Related Contact Lens Properties

Oxygen related properties of contact lenses play an important role in its usage for longer

Clinical Importance

- Increased in water content of lens improves the wearing comfort by increasing the transfer of oxygen through lens. Oxygen permeability of a contact lens doubles with an approximate increase in 20% water content, which is more significant with high absorption property of lens.
- Increased in water content also enhances the mechanical strength of contact lens by increasing its thickness.
- Low wettability increase the wearing duration and comfort of contact lens by maintaining tear film stability.

duration and to keep the cornea healthy. This includes various elements such as

- Oxygen permeability
- Oxygen transmissibility
- Equivalent oxygen percentage
- Oxygen tension

Oxygen permeability (*Dk*): It is the property of a contact lens material, which indicates the ability of oxygen to pass through contact lens material without any effort. This is called as *Dk* value of that material, where *D* means the diffusion co-efficient of oxygen and *k* indicates the solubility of oxygen in that contact lens material. The value of *Dk* of a lens material can be calculated by using oxygen electrodes in a gas chamber device. Units of *Dk* are expressed as Fatt units or Barrer

$$Dk = \frac{10^{-11}(cm^2 \times ml\, O_2)}{sec \times ml \times mmHg}$$

Note: Oxygen permeability (*Dk*) is a feature of contact lens material, not of contact lens.

Oxygen transmissibility: It is the property of a contact lens which indicates the ability of oxygen to pass through contact lens of known thickness. It means it tells about the rate of oxygen transfer across the different contact lenses of varying thickness. This is represented as *Dk/L*, where *Dk* is oxygen permeability and *L* is the central thickness of contact lens in centimeters (cm).

The oxygen transmissibility across a contact lens can be known by formula:

$$J = \frac{Dk\,(P_l - P_o)}{L}$$

Here P_l = oxygen pressure in front of contact lens

P_o = oxygen pressure behind the contact lens

L = thickness of center of contact lens (cm)

Units of oxygen transmissibility is 10^{-9} (cm × ml O_2)/(sec × ml × mmHg).

Note: Oxygen transmissibility is a characteristic of contact lens, not of its material and is inversely proportional to thickness of lens. It means thinner is the lens, greater will be its oxygen transmissibility.

Equivalent oxygen percentage (EOP): Cornea being avascular in nature, receive oxygen mainly from the atmosphere. Presence of contact lens on the cornea will hamper the supply of atmospheric oxygen to cornea. Thus EOP indicate the amount (%) of atmospheric oxygen (in volume) reaching at cornea in presence of contact lens, for a known thickness of contact lens. For example, as we all know that normally about 21% oxygen is present in the atmosphere, however, if it is stated that EOP is 4%; means that cornea is receiving 4% atmospheric oxygen, instead of 21%.

Oxygen tension: It is expressed as partial pressure applied by oxygen in a specified atmospheric condition. This is an interchangeable term with EOP and helps in deciding the health status of cornea during usage of contact lens for a long period.

Broadly, contact lens materials are divided as
- Focons
- Filcons

Focons: These are hydrophobic material, primarily used to manufacture rigid contact lenses.

Filcons: These are hydrophilic material, primarily used to manufacture non rigid contact lenses. However, elastomers of silicon rubber are highly hydrophobic, but due to its other properties these are also grouped as Filcons. On the basis of different types of substances focons and filcons are grouped as summarized in Table 13.1.

Rigid Contact Lens Materials

Initially all contact lenses were manufactured using rigid materials such as glass and thermosetting plastics like PMMA. Because of several clinical drawbacks associated with these materials subsequently better rigid lens materials such as cellulose acetate butyrate (CAB), silicon and polymers of silicon, etc. for manufacturing of contact lens were developed.

Broadly, these rigid contact lens materials can be grouped as
- Rigid non-gas permeable materials
- Rigid gas permeable materials

Rigid non-gas permeable material: Mostly the hard contact lenses were made up of thermosetting plastic like spectacle lenses. PMMA was the first commercially available plastic in this category for mass manufacturing of contact lenses. PMMA material is not permeable for water or oxygen, hence wearers have to depend on a tear pump action of eye for hydration and oxygen supply to cornea.

Advantages
- It is inert and free of toxic chemicals, because PMMA is prepared by a process of annealing (successive heating and cooling), so does not cause hypersensitivity reactions.
- Can be moulded or lathed with high degree of precision.
- Excellent visual properties and safe to wear.
- Requires minimum use of cleaning, soaking or wetting solutions.
- Can be tinted easily to reduce excessive light sensitivity.
- Durable and can be repolished to remove minor scratches, hence lasts for nearly 5–6 years.
- Economical as compared to any other type of contact lens.

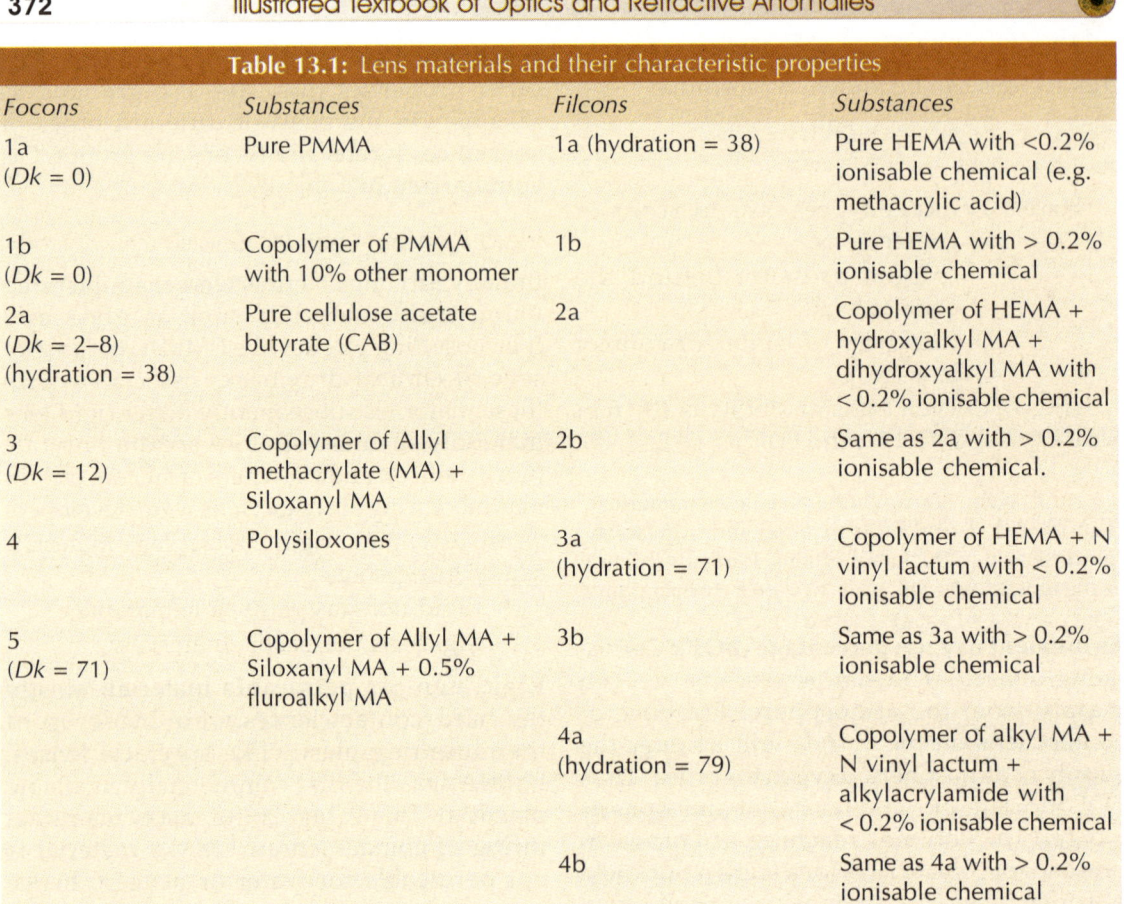

Table 13.1: Lens materials and their characteristic properties

Focons	Substances	Filcons	Substances
1a ($Dk = 0$)	Pure PMMA	1a (hydration = 38)	Pure HEMA with <0.2% ionisable chemical (e.g. methacrylic acid)
1b ($Dk = 0$)	Copolymer of PMMA with 10% other monomer	1b	Pure HEMA with > 0.2% ionisable chemical
2a ($Dk = 2–8$) (hydration = 38)	Pure cellulose acetate butyrate (CAB)	2a	Copolymer of HEMA + hydroxyalkyl MA + dihydroxyalkyl MA with < 0.2% ionisable chemical
3 ($Dk = 12$)	Copolymer of Allyl methacrylate (MA) + Siloxanyl MA	2b	Same as 2a with > 0.2% ionisable chemical.
4	Polysiloxones	3a (hydration = 71)	Copolymer of HEMA + N vinyl lactum with < 0.2% ionisable chemical
5 ($Dk = 71$)	Copolymer of Allyl MA + Siloxanyl MA + 0.5% fluroalkyl MA	3b	Same as 3a with > 0.2% ionisable chemical
		4a (hydration = 79)	Copolymer of alkyl MA + N vinyl lactum + alkylacrylamide with < 0.2% ionisable chemical
		4b	Same as 4a with > 0.2% ionisable chemical
		5 ($Dk = 200$)	Polysiloxanes

Disadvantages

- Oxygen permeability of PMMA lens is negligible, hence cannot be worn for long duration, otherwise person will develop dryness, swelling and ocular discomfort.
- PMMA material is very hard in nature so can cause corneal abrasions.
- Because of hydrophobic nature of PMMA, it has poor wettability. In PMMA lens the oxygen transmissibility is very poor so oxygenation of tears depends on renewal of tears due to blinking. As the contact lens wearer blink, there is slight movement of contact lens over the cornea so that interchange of tears occurs underneath the lens and as a result oxygen is exchanged and provides necessary oxygen to cornea.

In subsequent years many researchers tried to improve the permeability of contact lens by drilling small holes or fenestration in the lens. Hydrogel (polymers that imbibe water and swell) were also added with PMMA to improve its permeability, but still gas impermeability of material remained a major issue in its wide usage. Because of impermeability property these lenses are kept light, thin and of small size so that they do not cover a large portion of cornea. In addition, these lenses cannot be used for correction of high degree of corneal astigmatism because of their light and thin nature.

Rigid gas permeable lens material: Materials which are used for production of RGP lenses maintain the property of PMMA in terms of rigidity, but unlike PMMA these materials have good oxygen permeability, hence became popular for a long-term usage. Primarily, cellulose acetate butyrate (CAB) and silicon were used to manufacture these rigid gas permeable lenses, however, several polymers of silicon and allyl methacrylate later introduced in the market for manufacturing of better tolerable contact lens.

Contact lenses formed from these materials are also called semisoft contact lenses because of their good oxygen permeability and better Dk value.

Cellulose acetate butyrate (CAB): It was first widely used material to manufacture rigid gas permeable contact lenses. This biodegradable thermoplastic polymer was derived from yellow poplar wood fiber (YPWF) having good wettability. Advantages of this material over PMMA were good oxygen permeability, relative wettability and reduced hardness; however disadvantages as compared to PMMA were poor scratch resistance and tensile strength. Due to these reasons a constant search for better material was on, which leads to development of silicon acrylate material.

Styrene: A highly gas permeable, surface wettable, and relatively hard contact lens material used for manufacturing of RGP contact lenses is styrene (T-butyl dimethyl siloxy). This contact lens material is a copolymerization product of a reaction mixture consisting styrene, esters of vinyl alcohol and polyethylene glycol, polysiloxane along with a cross-linking agent like divinyl benzene. Initially this material looks promising, however, due to brittle nature of this material mass manufacturing became a problem.

Silicon: Silicon is highly permeable to oxygen than water. Contact lenses with more silicon will be more permeable than less silicon lens. However, silicon has its own problems like hydrophobic nature (less wettability) and relative stiffness and because of these properties it is a less friendly material for large production of contact lenses.

Silicon acrylate: In the year 1974, Norman Gaylord produced first siloxane (oxygen and silicon are combined together) based rigid lens material by cross-linking silicon acrylate with MMA, resulted in formation of trimethylsiloxy (Tris) silane. The presence of silicon provides good oxygen permeability to material while MMA provides good wetting and physical property to material. Many rigid materials now are used for production of contact lens are on the basis of these properties.

Silicon can be added in various proportions with varying Dk value in the range of 15–60 and oxygen permeability. As silicon increased, the oxygen permeability of lens increases but it also alters the surface characteristic of lens.

Fluoropolymers: Fluoropolymers were discovered during 1930 and are considered as most desirable material for mass manufacturing of RGP contact lenses because of their high oxygen permeability, wettability and resistibility to surface deposits. Fluoropolymers can also withstand high temperature and chemical attack. Free radical polymerization is basic industrial synthesis method for fluoropolymers. The polymerization process is mainly water-based method, which uses either aqueous suspension or aqueous emulsion polymerization in presence of fluorinated emulsifiers. For manufacturing of contact lenses fluoropolymers can be used either in pure form or in co-polymer forms. Flurofocon A is a polymer having high fluorine content which is commercially developed by 3M Company for mass production of extended wear contact lenses. As compared to earlier available fluoropolymers, an excellent wettability and flexibility is present in Flurofocon A. This material has very high levels of oxygen transmissibility and remarkable resistance against deposit formation. Hence, combination of physical properties and optical stability of Flurofocon A makes it the most desirable new lens material for manufacturing of contact lenses.

Soft Contact Lens Materials

First monomer material for soft lens, i.e. hydroxyethyl methacrylate (HEMA) was introduced by Otto Wichterle in the year 1950. As the name suggests that this material has a hydroxyl group, in contrast to PMMA where only methyl group was present. These soft lens materials are also termed hydrogel because they are cross-linked polymer and being hydrophilic absorbs water, get swell and make lens soft and elastic. The cross-linking provides physical stability to lens material.

During production of soft gel materials, monomers such as HEMA with the aid of a catalyst undergo polymerization which results in formation of sequence of repeating units termed Poly hydroxyethyl methacrylate or P-HEMA. This polymer is made by polymerizing two molecules of hydroxyethyl methacrylate (HEMA) monomer and using a cross-linking agent like ethylene glycol dimethacrylate (EGDMA) or polyvinylpyrrolidone (PVP). The hydrophilic nature of P-HEMA is due to the presence of hydroxyl group (OH) which creates small pores in the polymers through which fluid can enter.

When more than one type of monomer is used in production of the material, then this type of material is termed copolymers. A polymerized HEMA EGDMA lens has water content of about 38–50% and used as daily wear lens while HEMA-PVP has high water content (>50%) and used as extended wear lens. However, by using various different types of monomers different materials can be produced varying in terms of water contents, refractive indices, hardness, and strength and oxygen permeability.

Advantages

- Good hydration equilibrium of material provides better comfort of wearing. These soft lenses can be either low hydration lenses having water content of 38–50% or of high hydration lenses having water content of > 50%.
- Refractive indices of these lenses is comparable with cornea, hence quality of vision is better.
- High oxygen permeability is a major advantage and permeability increases proportionally with an increase in the water content, whereas decreases with an increase in the thickness of lens.
- Soft in nature and hence a larger portion of cornea can be covered for better field of vision and correction of refractive error.

Disadvantages

- Due to high water content and soft material nature these lenses are very fragile and get damaged easily.
- Swells up due to high water content, hence clarity of vision is less as compared to rigid contact lenses.
- Higher incidence of microbial keratitis as compared to RGP lenses.

Soft contact lenses can be produced by using several materials either as monomers, polymers or co-polymers. Broadly, we can group these soft hydrogel materials into

- Conventional hydrophilic hydrogel materials
- Silicon hydrogel materials

Conventional Hydrophilic Hydrogel Material

Conventionally, hydroxyethyl methacrylate (HEMA) is most commonly used hydrophilic monomer material for manufacturing of hydrogel lens. Although nowadays, cross-linking polymers are more used because of their better stability.

HEMA: HEMA is most widely used, original, water insoluble soft contact lens material which is used as monomer for mass manufacturing of soft contact lenses in our country. Pure HEMA lens has water content of about 38–40%. It is mostly copolymerised to form various hydrogel which are used for manufacturing of soft hydrogel contact lenses. For example, materials such as dimethyl acrylamide (DMA), glycerol methacrylate (GMA), methacrylic acid (MA), methyl methacrylate (MMA) and vinylpyrrolidone

(VP) are used for polymerization in currently available contact lens materials.

HEMA has important properties like it is not easily damaged by biodegradation, chemical or thermal sterilization and by enzymes present in tears, hence makes this material most suitable for making contact lenses used for a long period.

HEMA-NVP: Subsequently, HEMA copolymers were developed to improve water content or hydration of lens material. Copolymerization of HEMA with N-vinyl-pyrrolidone (NVP) was first commercially successful contact lens material having equivalent water content of up to 90%. These types of copolymers have rubbery feel as compared to slippery feel of P-HEMA. In addition, the amide group present in these material bind weakly with water molecule as compared to hydroxyl group, therefore, evaporation rates of water through these lens is relatively high leading to chances of instability of lens and discomfort.

Disadvantages:
- Sensitive to change in temperature: Parameters of copolymers of HEMA-NVP can change with change in the temperature, hence caution is required during lens fitting because lens parameters may change after its contact with eye.
- Corneal staining: Use of NVP containing lenses with solutions which contain polyhexanide in high amount may cause staining of cornea and increase level of discomfort. Hence, it is essential to keep in mind that if staining occurs, then solution must be changed which contains negligible amount of polyhexanide.

MMA-VP: MMA (methyl methacrylate) and VP (vinylpyrrolidone) monomers were combined to produce MMA/VP copolymer. MMA/VP copolymer showed different characteristics than HEMA/VP copolymer. MMA/VP copolymers based contact lenses may have water content from 60–85% depending upon the composition.

MAA-HEMA: To increase the equivalent water content (EWC) of material, a different hydrophilic monomer methacrylic acid (MAA) was used to manufacture hydrogels. Addition of MAA during formation of soft lens material results in formation of ionized groups within the matrix of polymer which increases water absorption property of lens. Addition of MAA with HEMA usually increases the water content up to range of 50–60%, which in turn results in significant increases in the oxygen permeability through lens.

The use of MAA in lens material is also associated with some disadvantages such as

- The lens containing MAA are very sensitive for changes in the tonicity. For example, in solutions having less tonicity (hypotonic like water) the effective water content (EWC) of lens increased, while opposite occurs in hypertonic solutions.
- EWC of this type of lens material also change with change in the pH of solution. The EWC of lens decreases in low pH conditions.
- Significant amount of protein depositions can occur on surface of lens and within its matrix. However, recently it has been found that these proteins are in non-denatured form.
- During heat-disinfection process the lens may loss its dimensional stability.

MMA-PVD: These are copolymer of polyvinyl pyrrolidone (hydrophilic), monomer VP and methyl methacrylate (hydrophobic).

Glyceryl methacrylate: Glyceryl methacrylate (GMA) monomer consists of two hydroxyl groups as compared to HEMA and thus more water soluble than HEMA. GMA in combination with other monomers or hydrogels is used for manufacturing of contact lens materials. Combination of GMA with MMA (Crofilcon A) produces a material which is more stiff and strong than P-HEMA as well as contains water contents in range of 30–42%. In addition, it can be combined with HEMA, which results in formation of non-ionic material having high water content (up to 70%). Moreover, the water balance ratio of these types of lens material is excellent because their rate of rehydration is fast, while dehydration occurs at slow rate. The chances of deposition are very less and the property of material remains unaltered with the change in pH in the range of 6–10.

Silicon hydrogel material: In the year 1999, silicon hydrogel material was successfully introduced in manufacturing of contact lens which within a decade became main type soft contact lens material representing almost 70% of total lens materials. Similar to conventional hydrogels, in silicon hydrogel materials the main chain consists of siloxane derivates like polydimethylsiloxane (PDMS), Bis (trimethylsiloxy) methylsilane, tris-propyl vinyl carbamate (TPVC) and polydimethylsiloxy bisvinyl carbamate (PBVC).

Initially two silicon hydrogel materials, Lotrafilcon A and Balafilcon A were available which were having high oxygen permeability but having low water content (25 and 38%, respectively). Hence these materials were stiffer and hydrophobic than poly-HEMA based (water soluble) materials. However, silicon containing materials are highly oxygen permeable. Later on better silicon hydrogel materials were produced and currently more than 12 different types of materials are available having desired relationship between water content and oxygen permeability. The increase in the silicon content increases permeability of material. The silicon hydrogen materials developed later on have high Dk values as well as maintain medium to high water content (> 45%).

Following surface properties of silicon hydrogels material are desirable for manufacturing of contact lenses.

- Topography and roughness
- Friction (less)
- Wettability (improved by surface treatment)
- Surface charge/ionicity (mostly non-ionic)

Several following bulk properties of this material are also contributing for manufacturing of extended wear contact lens.

- Equilibrium water content and water activity; has high percentage of free water, bound water and intermediate water.
- Oxygen permeability and transmissibility.
- Hydraulic and ionic permeability

Advantages of silicon hydrogels are

- Less chances of microbial contamination.
- Less mechanical interactions to corneal surface.
- Less protein depositions over lenses.
- Release of moisture agents like polyvinyl alcohol.
- Can also be used as drug delivery system.

A few disadvantages like sensitivity to lipid deposition, hydrophobic surface and non-ionic nature are also present in silicon hydrogel materials.

Note: Silicon hydrogels are most desirable material for manufacturing of extended wear contact lenses throughout world.

MANUFACTURING AND TYPES OF CONTACT LENS

Various processes used to manufacture contact lenses are

- Lathe cutting
- Melt pressing
- Spin casting
- Cast moulding

Lathe Cutting

Earlier this process was used for manufacturing of corneal PMMA and rigid lenses. Later on, it was also used in the manufacturing of soft hydrogel lenses. This process is used for production of both soft and rigid types contact lenses by using various types of lens materials.

Various steps in the process of lathe cutting are

- Manufacturing of buttons from material
- Back surface cutting of a lens blank
- Front surface cutting of a lens
- Wet processing of the lenses

Manufacturing of buttons from material: Firstly, the monomer material is polymerized to prepare button-shaped moulds or alternatively can be cast in the form of rods from which button can be cut later on. These buttons act as lens blanks. Polymerization process takes time, hence these button or rods are kept in a water bath at a definite temperature (depending on the type of material used) for several hours. It is followed by annealing process of buttons where the material or buttons are heated at high temperature followed by cooling at room temperature. Annealing makes the material soft so that stress is relieved inside buttons. In addition, it also prevents grooving of edges or rolling up (like cigarette) of finished lens when in hydrated state.

A soft contact lens is lathed in dry state means a smaller, steeper lens of greater power is prepared by lathe so that when it absorbs water it swells and attains required dimensions and powers.

Cutting of back surface of lens blanks: The buttons are processed on lathe to cut the back surface of lens from the buttons. Nowadays, computer-based lathe are available which can be programmed accordingly to cut buttons into numerous design and of variable parameters. Diamond cutting tools are used to cut back surface from buttons which is a two-step process. Firstly, a rough cut is given on buttons to remove excess material. Then a final cut is given to slice secondary curves and slanted edges of lens. Following the cutting, the polishing of back surfaces is done on a polishing machine. Polished materials usually contain a lanolin base and coarse diamond dust. During lathing and polishing the excessive heating of lens material must be avoided to prevent warpage and errors of curvature. Prepared semi-finished lenses are then kept in a solvent to get rid of excessive polish.

Cutting of front surface lens: The semi-finished lens blank (buttons with cut back surface) is fixed on to a mount or chuck, this process is called blocking. The mount is a cylindrical-shaped tool made of metal or plastic, having one end dome-shaped which match with the curve of posterior surface of lens blank. At this dome end, hot melted wax is applied and the posterior or back surface of lens blank is mounted with the help of this wax at dome end and centered carefully. This assembly is now loaded on the lathe machine for front surface cutting and then centration of lens blank is confirmed followed by cutting of surface by diamond tool. The front lens surface is then polished and deblocked by immersing into a deblocking solvent.

Wet processing of the lenses: The processed dry lenses go through hydration and wet processing steps which will vary according to the type of lens material. For example, non-ionic lenses are usually first washed with deionized water and then with saline. Ultrasonic baths are also used to increase the speed of hydration process. For lenses containing MAA, washing is done in tanks containing sodium bicarbonate to facilitate ionization of the lenses.

Advantages
- Can be used to manufacture both rigid and soft type contact lenses.
- Lenses usually have high quality surface finishing due to diamond cutting edges on an automated lathe machine.
- Variety of lens design, surface curvature to fit for an individual requirement and different size diameter lenses can be produced.
- High quality polishing reduces surface defects and improves the optical property of lens having a stable visual acuity which does not fluctuate.
- Lathing in dry state of soft lens gives a high dimensional accuracy so even toric lens can be designed.
- Also necessary for production of low volume and high prescription custom lenses.

Disadvantages:

- Require intense labor, hence it is both expensive and susceptible to significant human errors.
- It is a slow process.

Manufacturing errors may occur during lathe process like

- Hydrogel or soft lenses are lathed in dry state, hence they undergo final step of hydration which can be a potential manufacturing error.
- Core fractures
- Inclusions, e.g. rust
- Watermarks, bubbles or holes on lens
- Debris, e.g. fibres
- Lathe rings
- Distortion, discoloration and edge defects of lens

Melt Pressing

This method was used to manufacture PMMA and silicon contact lenses, however, now this is not widely used and is an obsolete procedure. Various steps involved in the process of melt pressing are summarized as

- The monomer is polymerized to produce a polymer (polymerization).
- This polymer is then converted into sheets, beads, granules or power.
- Moulds of desired size shape and types are taken from this polymer material.
- Compression or injection moulding is done.
- Semi-finished lens is then removed from mould.
- Lens is edged and polished for packing purposes.

Spin Casting

In the year 1961, Wichterle described a new method for manufacturing of soft lens and patented it, which is known as spin casting. Subsequently, in the year 1971 this method was further refined by Bausch & Lomb (B&L). Nowadays, manufacturing of contact lens by spin casting process is based on the same principle as developed by B&L.

Principle: The cast or mould containing mixture of desired monomers (monomer solution + cross-linking agent + initiator) is spinned at a controlled speed. During spinning the generated centrifugal forces cause ascending of the monomer mixture to the walls of cast and take the required lens shape, while simultaneously polymerization also occurs.

This process has the following steps of manufacturing the contact lens as shown in Fig. 13.7.

Manufacturing of inserts: First step is to produce inserts of excellent quality which are then used as mould to produce the casts because the quality of anterior surface and edges of each lens depend on quality of the inserts prepared.

Manufacturing of cast: Casts are usually prepared by using materials like poly propylene or polyvinyl chloride. Occasionally,

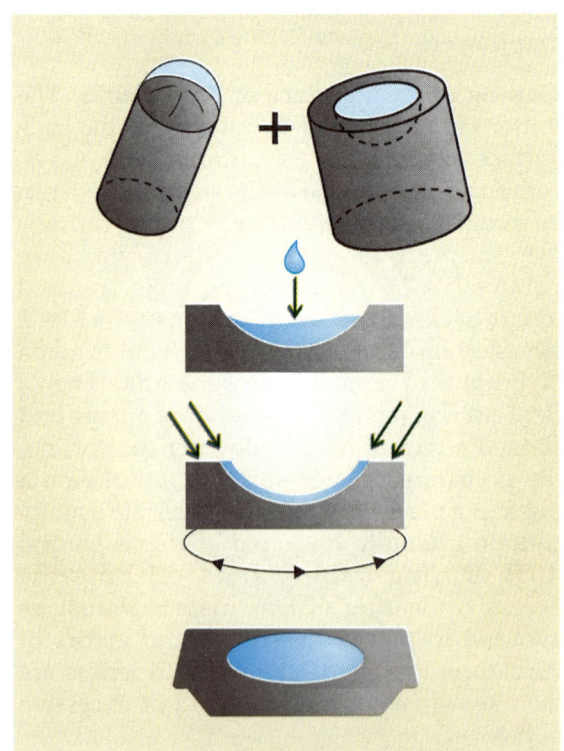

Fig. 13.7: Contact lens manufacturing by spin casting method

the surface treatment of resulting casts is done to ensure the wetting of cast material, but this treatment also increases the cost of production of lens.

Spinning process: Most important step of entire process is spinning of the cast which determines the final power and shape of the produced contact lens. Various other factors, such as combined effect of gravity, surface tension, centrifugal force during spinning, quantity of liquid monomer and the rate of spin determine the final outcome. If the radius of the produced cast is predetermined, then a contact lens of desired central thickness and back vertex power can be made by controlling the speed and dose of monomers. The rate of spin speed will decide the back vertex power while dose will decide the central thickness of lens.

- The anterior surface of lens is spheric and curvature of front or anterior surface of desired lens is provided by the inner surface of cast or mould.
- Back or posterior surface of contact lens is aspheric and the curvature of this surface depends on factors like shape and amount of speed of mould, physical properties and amount of liquid monomers in the cast.
- It is considered an ideal method for production of minus power contact lenses because the manufactured lens by this process has power of approximately equal to –3 D lens.
- However, for manufacturing of positive powered contact lens, casts with more complicated designs are required. Another method which has been adopted by manufacturers to produce the lens of desired power and curvatures is that after the spinning, lathe is also done on spin cast lens.
- The final lenses are demoulded, either manually or by an automated production line.
- These finished lenses are wet processed in a similar way to lathed lenses as explained above.

Advantages
- Generates a homogenous, consistent and properly cross-linked polymer, because a thin film of monomer is polymerized.
- Produces best quality optical surfaces.
- Accurate spin speed and precise dosing produces perfect parameters contact lenses.
- Minimum surface defects and edging errors, because surfaces formed are free and independent to cutting.
- Less expensive and easily reproducible.

Disadvantages
- Unpredictable fitting.
- Fitting of lens is not dependent on keratometer reading of patient.

Cast Moulding

Primarily this process was used as cost effective method to manufacture plastic goods but later on it was also used for production of contact lenses.

Principle: During the cast moulding procedure to prepare a contact lens the liquid monomer undergo polymerization process between two casts. The formed semi-finished lens before packaging again processed to produce desired lens.

Cast moulding: Cast moulding and its modified methods are now commonly used for production of high volume soft lenses because the unit production cost is potentially low by this method. Various steps of this process as shown in Fig. 13.8 are as follows

Manufacturing of inserts: During cast moulding process both male and female type inserts along with auxiliary insert housings are manufactured. Front or anterior surface of final contact lens is formed by using female cast which is created by the female insert, whereas back or posterior surface of the final contact lens was created by male cast which is formed by the male insert.

During this process the male inserts are manufactured in less number than female inserts, because contact lens of different

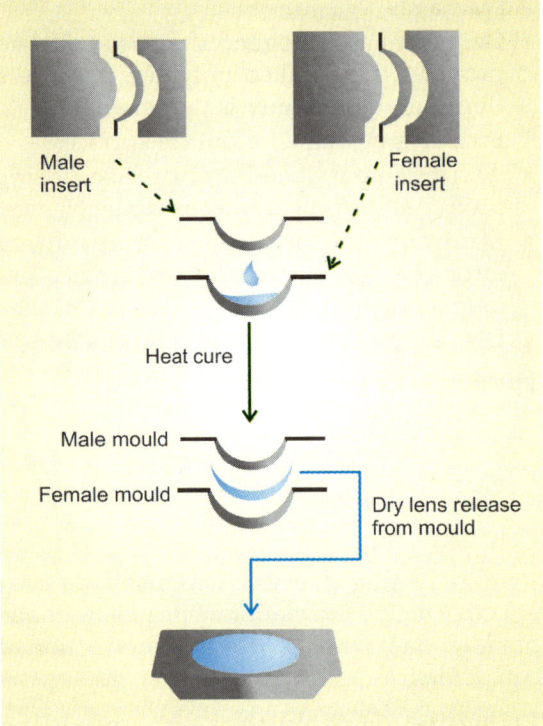

Fig. 13.8: Contact lens manufacturing by cast moulding method

powers can be produced by altering the female insert, as the radii of anterior surface and altogether thickness profile of lens get change by changing the female cast.

Manufacturing of cast: During manufacturing by cast moulding both the material used for cast and design of the casts play a vital role. The material that is used for development of cast play an important role in deciding the dimensional stability. Hence, a careful selection of chemical structure of the polymer used to produce contact lens is a vital step during cast moulding. Previously, the manufacturers faced some problems related to stability of casts which lead to low yield of lenses with correct specification for a specific manufactured batch.

The design of the cast during manufacturing of lens will decide the optical property, curvatures of surface, pattern of edge and diameter of final lens, hence resultant lens is also significantly dependent on the design of the casts.

Classification of Contact Lenses

Contact lenses can be classified on the basis of various parameters as summarized in Table 13.2.

Surface curves

- Monocurve lens has single curve on both the anterior and posterior surfaces, rarely used nowadays.
- Bicurve lens has single anterior curve, but two back curves (a central curve and

Surface curves	Anatomical position	Physical properties	Chemical nature of lens material	Hydration status	Duration of lens wear	Clinical uses
Monocurve CL	Scleral lens	Soft CL	Rigid non-gas permeable CL	Low hydration CL	Long-term or yearly wear	Optical CL
Bicurve CL	Corneo-limbal lens	Semisoft CL	Rigid gas permeable CL	Medium hydration CL	Monthly wear	Therapeutic CL
Tricurve CL	Corneal CL	Hard CL	Soft CL	High hydration CL	Weekly wear	Cosmetic CL
Multicurve CL					Daily wear	Diagnostic CL
Toric lens					Extended wear	Occupational CL
Bitoric lens						

Table 13.2: Classification of contact lens (CL) on basis of various parameters

flatter peripheral curve), most commonly used.

- Tricurve lenses are similar to bicurve except that an intermediate curve is present on back surface.
- Multicurve lenses are also similar to bicurve lenses but have more than one intermediate curve.
- Toric lens has a toric back surface, mainly used for highly toric cornea (astigmatic) cases.
- Bitoric lens has a cylindrical power on anterior surface of lens along with the toric posterior surface, mainly used in high degree of astigmatism with low corneal toricity like in cases of lenticular astigmatism.

Anatomical position in the eye

- Scleral lenses are also known as haptic or corneo-scleral contact lenses. These lenses cover the cornea, conjunctiva and sclera and are mainly used for therapeutic purposes, rarely used for optical, cosmetic or diagnostic purposes.
- Corneo-limbal contact lenses cover the entire cornea and limbus to lay over conjunctiva. Mainly used for optical and cosmetic purposes.
- Corneal contact lenses are entirely confined to cornea and are mainly used as optical and diagnostic contact lenses.

Physical properties

- Soft contact lens
- Semisoft contact lens
- Hard contact lens

Chemical nature of lens material

- Rigid non-gas permeable lenses, usually hydrophobic in nature made up of PMMA. These lenses are also called Focons.
- Rigid gas permeable lenses, made up of cellulose acetate butyrate and silicon, most commonly used as long-term wear contact lenses.
- Soft contact lenses, usually hydrophilic in nature made up of acrylic and HEMA. These lenses are also called Filcons.

Hydration status of lens material

- Low hydration lenses: Having water content in a range of 0–38%.
- Medium hydration lenses: Having water content in a range of 40–60%.
- High hydration lenses: Having water content more than 60%.

Duration of lens wear

- Long-term or yearly wear
- Monthly wear
- Weekly wear
- Daily wear
- Extended wear

Clinical uses

- Optical contact lens
- Therapeutic contact lens
- Cosmetic contact lens
- Diagnostic contact lens
- Occupational contact lens

CONTACT LENS DESIGN

Contact lens can be designed in various ways to achieve the requirement of an optimized contact lens so that it is fit for different clinical conditions.

- Regular lens designs
- Special lens designs

Regular Lens Design

These types of lens are used most commonly and usually designed for correction of simple refractive errors, because refractive status of eye in simple errors is not affected due to rotation of contact lens on the cornea. These lenses are designed as

- Single cut design
- Lenticular cut design

Single cut designed lenses may be monocurve, bicurve or tricurve containing a single continuously curved front surface as shown in Fig. 13.9. Desired base curve and peripheral curves are cut from the back surface of contact lens.

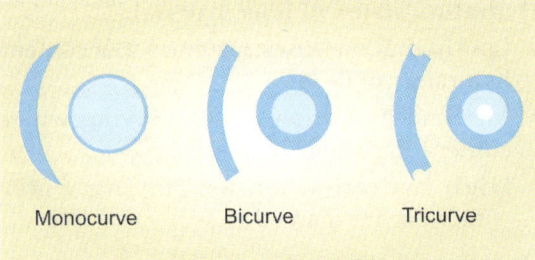

| Monocurve | Bicurve | Tricurve |

Fig. 13.9: Single cut contact lens designs

Special Lens Design

Several special types of design features are done in lens to optimize the fitting of contact lens and to prevent rotation of lens in the eye. These modifications are

- Lenticular edge modification
- Prism ballast lenses
- Truncated design lenses
- Fenestrations design
- Blending design

Lenticular edge modification: These lenses have a central optical portion which is surrounded in periphery by a carrier edge (either minus or plus powers) as shown in Fig. 13.10. This carrier edge is supported by eyelids and prevents the decentring of lens. These types of modified contact lens are designed for those persons where the optical power of gas permeable contact lens becomes more than –6.00 D or + 4.00 D. The lenticular edge modification of anterior surface of contact lens helps to improve the edge profile as well as also decreases weight

and thickness of contact lens which further improve the tolerance and centration of lens. The curve of posterior surface of lens is kept same.

Prism ballast lenses: These lenses are heavier at bottom and are indicated for correction of problems related to binocular vision related problems as in vertical phoria. As the name indicates, a prism is given in contact lens for proper orientation and to prevent rotation as shown in Fig. 13.11. The vertical base-down type of prism is prescribed in contact lens. Usually prisms are prescribed in toric (front surface) and bifocal contact lens, in both gas permeable and hydrogel material to maintain orientation.

Truncated design lenses: In these design lenses a circumferential zone in contact lens is present, which is made flat by removing lens material from a circular contact lens as shown in Fig. 13.12, the process is called truncation of lens. Like prism ballast lens, the truncation

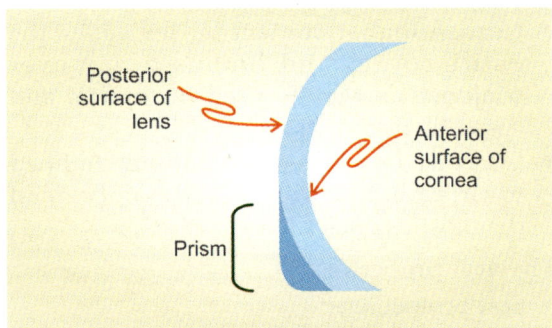

Fig. 13.11: Prism ballast contact lens design

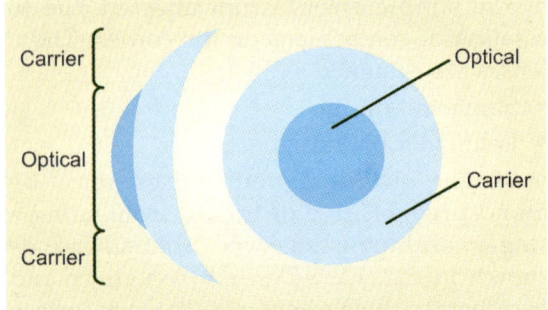

Fig. 13.10: Lenticular contact lens design

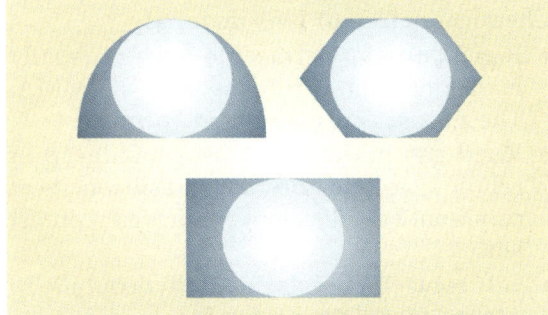

Fig. 13.12: Truncated contact lens designs

of a lens also helps in decreasing the rotation of contact lens especially with bifocal or toric (front surface) contact lens.

Fenestrations: In these design contact lenses small holes are present, which are drilled through the surface of a contact lens as shown in Fig. 13.13. This design is mainly used in contact lenses of rigid type, either PMMA or gas permeable types. The insufficient oxygen permeability through these lens material may cause corneal edema. The holes help to facilitate the oxygenation of cornea, either directly or by enhancing tear exchange.

Blending: Chances of corneal abrasion or trauma can be decreased by smoothing or blending the junctions between multiple curvatures present on posterior surface of contact lenses. Thus, blending increases the tolerance and comfort of wearing. Blending is generally conducted on gas permeable contact lenses. This can be classified as

- Light blending: When transformation or blending is clearly visible between two posterior curves of a contact lens.
- Medium blending: When transformation is minimally visible between two posterior curves of a contact lens.
- Heavy blending: When transformation is invisible between two posterior curves of a contact lens.

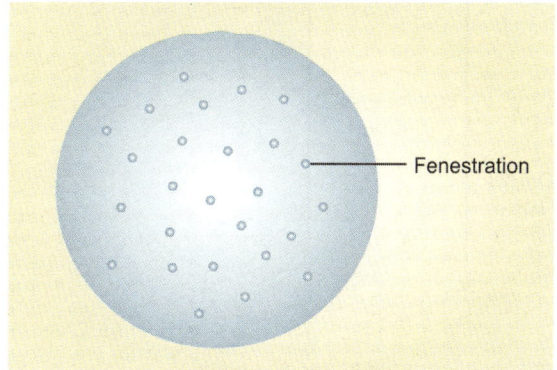

Fig. 13.13: Fenestrated rigid contact lens design

Note: Heavy blending helps in multicurve contact lenses, to improve the quality of vision.

Terminologies in Contact Lens

Most important purpose of knowing the details of contact lens design is that the posterior surface of lens must fit optimally on surface of the cornea because any discrepancy in fitting will lead to positional instability of contact lens on the cornea.

Contact Lens Dimensions

To know specifications of contact lens and to improve the fitting of lens on the cornea, it is important to know some basic information about lens dimensions which are as follows (Fig. 13.14):

Total diameter (TD): It is the linearly measured longest distance between the two boundaries of contact lens and is measured in millimeter. This is also called overall size, chord diameter or overall diameter and should not be confused with a double of radius of curvature of lens. Lenses of various types have different total diameters as follows

- Rigid non-gas permeable lenses or PMMA lenses have a TD of 7.5–8.5 mm.
- Rigid gas permeable lenses have a TD in the range of 9–9.6 mm.
- Soft contact lenses have a large TD in the range of 13–14 mm.

Back optic zone diameter (BOZD): It is a linear distance of central optical zone of contact lens which focuses rays on the retina. It is the distance between the two junctions or blend of lens and measured in millimeter. This is also called posterior optical zone diameter, back central optic diameter or optic zone diameter. Normally it should be more than 7 mm for good vision.

Peripheral curve width: It is the width of peripheral curve of lens which is flatter than the base curve and it decides the fitting of lens on the cornea. This is also called peripheral curve diameter. There may be an intermediate

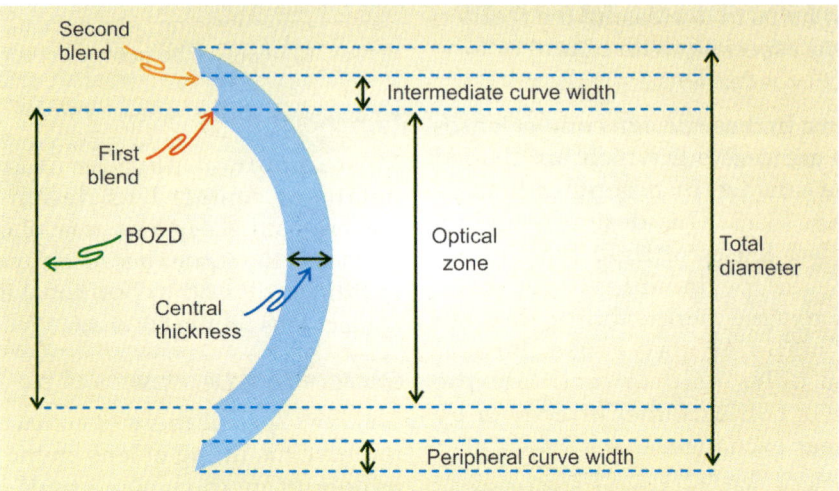

Fig. 13.14: Dimensions of contact lens

curve width, if an intermediate curve is present as in cases of trifocal or multifocal contact lenses.

Central thickness: It is the thickness of lens measured at optical or geometrical center of a contact lens. This is also called as geometrical central thickness (GCT). It is an important factor to decide the hydration and oxygenation of lens and is measured in millimeter. The value of central thickness of a lens depends on its posterior vertex power.

Contact Lens Curves and Radius

Various contact lens curves and their related radius as shown in **Figs 13.15** and **13.16** are as follows

Base curve: It is the curve of back surface of contact lens which rests on the cornea and is responsible for good fit. This is also called central posterior curve or back central optic portion. In a given lens design, back curve radii may be present in a range from 7.5 to 9.0 mm, at 0.5 mm intervals.

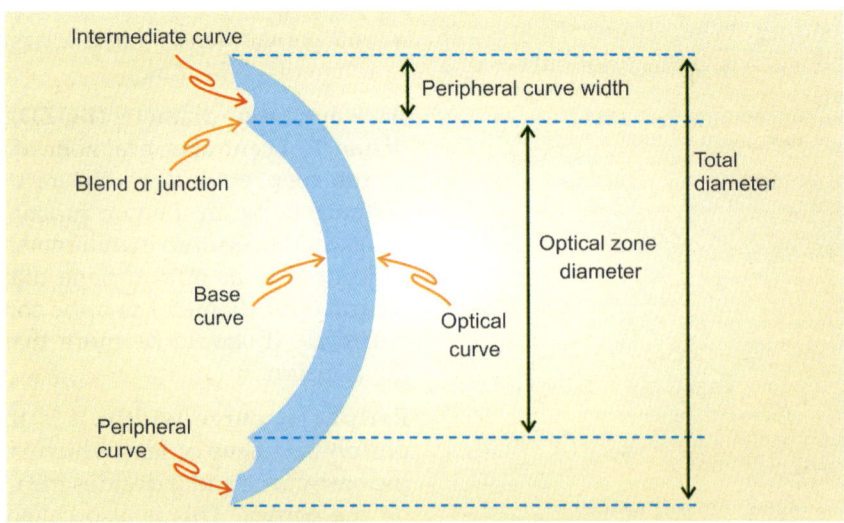

Fig. 13.15: Various terms and structures of contact lens

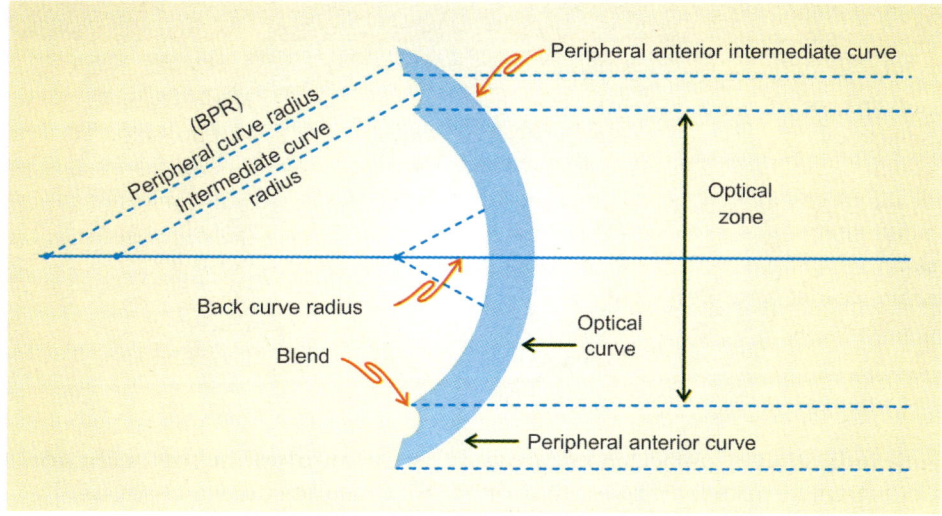

Fig. 13.16: Curves in contact lens

Note: "Longer is the radius of curvature, flatter will be the base curve".

Optical curve: It is the curve of anterior surface of contact lens, in optical zone. Optical power of a contact lens is determined by the amount of curvature of optical curve. This is also called front curve.

Peripheral curves: These curves are present on the posterior surface of lens and include intermediate curve and peripheral curve. These curves are concentric to base curve and act as reservoir of tears to facilitate a smooth lens movement over the cornea. This is also called back peripheral optic portion. Simple bicurve lens has a single peripheral curve which is larger than optical zone in radius, although two or more peripheral curves are present in tricurve or multicurve contact lenses.

Back peripheral radius (BPR): This is also known as back peripheral optic radius or peripheral curve radius. Similarly, in specific cases of high refractive errors, a contact lens with an intermediate curve and its radius are used.

Peripheral anterior curves: The slope on the anterior surface of contact lens which starts from boundary of optical curve and goes up to the edge of lens is called peripheral anterior curve, however, in specific cases there may be a peripheral anterior intermediate curve in between the optical curve and peripheral anterior curve. In high hypermetropes or high myopes the intermediate anterior peripheral curve is designed in lens for better visual quality.

Indications of Contact Lens Wear

Contact lens wear can be prescribed for various indications which can be grouped as

Optical indications: Contact lenses are used as an alternative to spectacles for correction of various refractive errors like myopia, hypermetropia and astigmatism. Several other ophthalmic conditions like aphakia, anisometropia, aniseikonia, presbyopia, keratoconus, field restrictions as seen in retinitis pigmentosa are other important indications where contact lens are advised as a better optical correction device than spectacles.

Contact lens versus spectacles: Comparison of various characteristics of contact lenses with spectacles summarized in Table 13.3.

Table 13.3: Comparison of characteristics of contact lenses with spectacles		
Characteristics	Contact lenses	Spectacles
Irregular astigmatism	Corrected (hard CL)	Not corrected
High anisometropic	Binocular vision possible	Not possible
Field of vision	Larger field obtained	Smaller field
Peripheral aberrations	Eliminated	Not eliminated
Prismatic distortion	Eliminated	Not eliminated
Wearer skill	Reasonable skill	No skill
Precautionary wearing measures	More	Less
Cosmetic acceptability	Higher	Lower
Cost	Expensive	Economical

Long duration wearing of contact lens may cause damage of ocular surface

Therapeutic indications: Contact lenses can be used as curative, supportive, palliative or preventive devices in various ocular conditions.

a. **As curative device:** As curative therapy can be used in pathology of cornea, conjunctiva, etc.
- *Corneal pathologies:* Contact lens can be used in various disease of cornea including non-healing corneal ulcers, corneal abrasions, recurrent epithelial defects, bullous keratopathy, traumatic epithelial defects, filamentary keratitis, small corneal perforations, corneal trauma, exposure keratitis and descemetocele. The extended wear type contact lenses are mainly prescribed which are also called bandage contact lens (BCL), because they serve like a bandage over a wound. Use of these lenses in corneal pathologies help in decreasing the ocular pain and discomfort by preventing mechanical trauma due to lids, also improves hydration and drug penetration which help in enhancement of the epithelial healing.
- *Conjunctival melanosis:* Lenses are used to deliver high doses of continuous radiation to conjunctiva.
- *In glaucoma:* Contact lenses are used as drug delivery device.

b. **As palliative device**
- *Iris pathologies:* Coloboma, aniridia and albinism to avoid excessive entry of light rays.

- In amblyopia for occlusion therapy (opaque contact lenses used).
- Post-surgical procedures: Pterygium excision, lamellar keratoplasty, photorefractive keratotomy, laser sub-epithelial keratomileusis, C3R for keratoconus.
- X-chrome lenses for red green color deficiency.
- In lagophthalmos to support the globe.
- Leaking conjunctival filtration bleb.

c. **As preventive device**
- Lid conditions like trichiasis, entropion and ptosis to prevent corneal abrasions.
- Giant papillary conjunctivitis to protect cornea.
- In chemical injuries to prevent symblepharon and to restore anatomy of fornix.
- Neuroparalytic keratitis to prevent corneal ulcerations.
- Glare producing iridectomies.

Note: Orthokeratology in high myopia and /or astigmatism rigid contact lens with progressive flat fit, believed to mould cornea (technique is now obsolete).

Cosmetic indications
- Corneal scars
- Microcornea
- Microphthalmos
- Heterochromia
- Deformed eyes

Occupational indications

- Actors/Actresses to change looks. Sports person involved in archery, football, etc.
- People using telescope.
- Defense people, in pilots, in shooters.

Diagnostic and operative indications

- Goldman's three mirror contact lens
- Fundus photography
- Electroretinography
- Fundus examination in irregular astigmatism
- A-scan biometry
- Gonioscopy
- For intraocular foreign body localization.
- High minus lenses for fundus examination during vitrectomy and endolaser photocoagulation.
- Goniotomy lenses during surgical goniotomy.

Research indications

- Corneal temperature measurement
- Intraocular pressure measurement

Contraindications of Contact Lens Use

a. **Diseases of Eyelids**
   - Stye
   - Chalazion
   - Blepharitis
   - Meibomitis

b. **Diseases of conjunctiva**
   - Conjunctivitis (bacterial, viral, fungal)
   - Chronic hyperemia
   - Bulbar conjunctival papillae

c. **Diseases of lacrimal apparatus**
   - Acute or chronic dacryocystitis

d. **Diseases of cornea**
   - Corneal dystrophies
   - Dry eyes
   - Tear film abnormalities
   - Corneal anesthesia as in fifth nerve palsy
   - Pannus

e. **Other ocular pathologies**
   - Episcleritis
   - Scleritis
   - Iritis
   - Choroiditis

f. **Systemic conditions**
   - *Diabetes mellitus:* There are frequent fluctuations in refractive status and corneal erosions heal very slowly.
   - Perimenopausal period.
   - Oral contraceptive usage: Lens poorly tolerated.
   - Pregnancy: Corneal shape can change due to oedamatous swelling.

g. **Allergies**
   - Contact dermatitis
   - Asthma
   - Atrophic rhinitis

h. **Occupational hazards**
   - Smoky, dusty and hot job environment
   - High altitude flyers
   - Construction workers
   - Automobile mechanics

i. **Poor general and mental health**

j. **Low hygienic patients**

k. **Old age patient with poor motivation**

l. **Arthritis or parkinsonism patient unable to use hands properly**

CONTACT LENS FITTING

Contact lens fitting require a protocol to achieve the desired results. We need to do a good work up in desired patients. Patient work up and examination remains constant in all types of contact lenses fitting whether it is soft hydrogel contact lens, rigid contact lens, cosmetic or therapeutic contact lenses.

Patient Work up for Contact Lens Fitting

Patient requiring either soft or RGP, and /or any other types of contact lenses, thorough examination is required to produce a satisfactory result which can be achieved by following examination

History: Proper history plays a major role in the outcome of a contact lens wearing results, whether a patient is new or an old patient already wearing a contact lens. Patient should be evaluated considering these facts

- Whether patient is enough motivated to wear a contact lens or not, and is mentally prepared to take all necessary precautions regarding contact lens wear.
- Understanding of patient about the advantages and disadvantages about contact lens and with this knowledge emotionally he/she is prepared to wear a contact lens.
- History of any chronic systemic illness or systemic allergy is present or not, i.e. to rule out presence of any contraindication of contact lens wear.
- Previous experience with wearing of contact lens, if present. Details of types and methods of wearing schedule of previous contact lenses.
- Occupational history (dust exposure, chemical exposure, etc.) of patient is also important.

Ocular examination: Cycloplegic refraction with a detailed anterior segment examination using slit lamp biomicroscopy should be done to rule any ocular pathology. Detailed examination includes

- General examination
- Refraction
- Keratometry
- Corneal topography

General examination:

- Eyelids should be examined to check force of lid closure, and also for any infective pathology like blepharitis, meibomitis, etc.
- Conjunctiva is examined using slit lamp to rule out any infiltrates, concretions, surface defects, limbal injection, papillae, follicles and any other infective pathology.
- Cornea transparency is noticed and detail examination is done to rule out any opacity, infiltrate and vascularization abnormality of surface.
- Tear film status is checked by Schirmer's' test and tear break up time by using fluorescein dye.

- Blink rate is calculated by a time clock. Blink rate < 15 and/ or > 30 blinks per minute are considered as defective blink mechanism and cause should be established. Blink characteristics like partial or full blink should be noticed because a partial blink is unable to wet the contact lens and chances of improper tear exchange underneath the contact lens increases.
- Corneal diameter, pupil diameter and interpalpebral width are recorded by using a plane transparent ruler. Horizontal visible iris diameter (HVID) is an important parameter to assess the best contact lens fit. It is measured from temporal end of limbus to nasal end of limbus by PD ruler. This diameter will guide clinicians to select total diameter of desired lens.

Refraction:

- Refraction under cycloplegia should be done to know the exact amount of refractive error. The recorded refraction value is expressed in minus cylinder form for those cases where we desire to prescribe only spherical contact lens.
- Vertex distance should be measured for accurate calculation of power of desired contact lens. Refractive errors with more than ± 5 D require a zero vertex distance correction at cornea because with this much refractive error effective power of contact lens will be significantly different. However, an error of ±2 D or less seldom needed any vertex distance correction at cornea.
- Spherocylindrical power should be converted to spherical equivalent power in cases of rigid lenses and in case of soft lenses where either toric lenses are contraindicated or practitioner decides to give only spherical powers. Simply half of the cylindrical power becomes spherical equivalent power, which is added with spherical power mathematically.

Keratometry:

- Corneal curvatures are measured at least in its two principal meridians (vertical or

90° and horizontal or 180°) by using keratometer either manual or automated.

- Keratometry reading is important data which is required to select the base curve radius in both rigid and soft type contact lenses.
- Any major difference in keratometry values indicates high degree of corneal astigmatism and contact lens wearing should be avoided in these cases.

Corneal topography:

- Corneal topography is performed to locate the apex of cornea because centration of lens is done according to the central corneal apex not according to geometric center of cornea which is the central point of pupil. Displacement of corneal apex will lead to the decentration of contact lens. Hence, locating of the apex will help in determining the best optical outcome with contact lens.
- Orbscan can be used to study the curvatures and surface characteristics of cornea which helps in a proper fit and avoid a flat or steep fitting of contact lens.

Various types of contact lenses will be considered as follows in detail to understand their uses and fitting methods in a better way

- Soft contact lenses
- Rigid contact lenses
- Extended wear contact lenses
- Disposable contact lenses
- Scleral RGP contact lenses
- Therapeutic contact lenses
- Colored contact lenses
- Contact lenses in special conditions such as high myopia, aphakia, presbyopia, and high astigmatism

Soft Contact Lens Fitting

- Soft contact lenses can be manufactured by using different types of polymers but mostly hydroxyethyl methacrylate (HEMA) is used because of its properties like more stability, transparent, non-hazardous and non-allergic nature.

- Soft lenses are usually bigger in size than cornea which provides a fit, where the lens edges fall under the upper and lower eyelids.
- These lenses are much more comfortable as compared to the rigid contact lens, due to its softness and an ability to bend with blinking of eyes.
- Most commonly used lenses in routine practice are soft contact lenses because of their comfort, flexibility, oxygen permeability, less glare and minimal over wear reaction.

Fitting procedures: Recommendations for fitting of soft contact lenses are provided by many lens manufactures in their brochures supplied with contact lenses. These brochures give the details of that particular lens series along with desired data and fitting parameters, however, a practitioner should be well-versed with various parameters and related nomenclature in the brochure provided with soft contact lenses.

Usually majority of lens manufactures give three choices for selection of the base curve and the overall diameter (TD) of contact lens. Practitioners need to decide the parameters for selection of contact lens on the following grounds to get the best fit of lenses.

Fitting steps include
- Trial lens selection
- Trial lens fit evaluation
- Trial lens ideal fit
- Ocular factor influencing lens fitting
- Contact lens factors affecting lens fit

Trial lens selection: Trial lens selection is done on the basis of these following criteria

- *Total diameter or overall diameter:* It must be larger (by approximately 2.5 mm) than the HVID of cornea to permit full coverage of cornea. However, this value may be more depending upon the limbal sulcus in particular eyes.
- *Lens power:* To decide the power of contact lens to be prescribed, the refraction for

spectacle should be corrected for vertex distance which is distance between the posterior surface of spectacle glass/contact lens and cornea. Suppose on refraction the cylindrical power of spectacles is more than ±1.5 D, then toric contact lenses can be used or otherwise a spherical equivalent power can be used as described above.

- *Back vertex power:* To get the benefits from contact lens, the back vertex power of contact lens should be kept as close as possible to the patients' spectacle prescription. It also helps to facilitate adaptation. If it is not possible to get same power, then it is preferred to choose a contact lens of less power to avoid accommodative spasms. For monovision, trial lens should be chosen of power as close to correct power.
- *Back optic zone radius:* Suppose choice of base curve is available with lens, then manufacturer's guidelines must be followed regarding the selection of trial lens to be tried first. This trial is done without taking the Keratometry readings in consideration. When no choice is available, then a lens with base curve flatter than keratometry reading is chosen. Amount of flattening is decided by the TD and water content of that contact lens which is taken for trial.

Following guidelines can be used to decide about selection of the trial lens parameters

- *Depending on TD:* Principle is that if larger the TD of lens, then prefer the flatter lens. For example, in a lens with TD of 13.0 mm, a lens having base curve 0.3 mm flatter than the flattest keratometry reading should be selected. Similarly for a further increase in 0.5 mm diameter, increase the flattening of base curve by 0.3 mm, means for a 13.5 mm diameter lens a flattening of 0.6 mm is needed from the flattest keratometry reading.
- *Depending on water content:* Principle is that lens of high water content usually require more steep fitting as compared to low water content lens. For example, if a high water content lens with TD of 14.5 mm needs a flattening of base curve by 1 mm than the flattest keratometry reading, then a low water content contact lens of the same diameter will require flattening by 1.2 mm.

Trial lens fit evaluation: Once the trial lens with correct parameters for fitting is selected, a sterile selected trial lens is inserted into the patient's eye. A proper fit of trial contact lens is evaluated by these parameters

- **Adaptation and patient's response**
  - *Adaptation period:* After placing the soft contact lens in the eye of patient, it is always necessary to wait for some time before (settling or adaption time) assessment of the fitting of lens because soft lenses have tendency to lose water once they are inserted in the eye. This loss of water may alter the parameters as well as fitting characteristics of a soft lens. Hence, it is recommended that the lens fit should be assessed only when the contact lens becomes in equilibrium with the tear film and established in the environment of eye. Traditionally, it is advised that about 25–30 minutes should be given for settling of a lens, however, some recent studies suggest that initial evaluation of fitting can be carry out after 5–10 minutes of insertion.
  - Although it is difficult to judge the physiological response as well as patients comfort for lens in five minutes period but its assessment should be based on lens sensation and eye movements.
  - Patients comfort is evaluated by the fact that lens should feel imperceptible on the eye by patient, especially on insertion. Lens sensation should be steady, having no appreciable difference in lateral eye movements or blinking.
- **Over refraction**
  - Normally to check the correct fitting of contact lenses, examiner should perform an "over refraction", means refraction is done while patient is wearing a pair of trial contact lenses. Advantage of an over refraction is that, rather than depending

on the predictions, whether the given contact lenses are able to correct ametropia or not, examiner can determine the actual refractive status.

- An over refraction is done with binocular balancing. There must be a clear endpoint and stable visual acuity. Any disparity in these factors show poor fit of lens and repeat retinoscopy should be carry out to confirm it.

- **Biomicroscopy examination:** Subsequent to over refraction, examination by slit lamp using a diffuse, direct illumination under medium to high magnification (which enable us to visualize the contact lens on eye) should be done to check lens fit.

Trial lens ideal fit: *"Fluorescein dye is not used to assess the lens fit in case of a soft contact lens".* The fitting is assessed by observing following parameters

- **Coverage of cornea:** Contact lens should cover full cornea before, after and during the blink in the primary position of eye. Minimum 1–1.5 mm conjunctival overlap should be seen in all movements of eyes.

- **Centration:** Lens should remain in center of cornea in primary position of gaze and should retain full coverage of cornea even during extreme lateral gaze (lens lag) and up gaze (lens sag) as shown in 13.17A and B respectively.

- **Post-blink movement:** Amount of post-blink lens movement should be judged in primary gaze, ideally recorded using a reticule marking on slit lamp. Lens movements are observed at the bottom part

(inferior edge) of contact lens during the blink. Alternatively, if lower eyelid is obstructing inferior edge of lens, then we can observe lens at 4 or 8 o'clock position for movement. Sometimes, we can displace the lower eyelid using index finger, before assessing the movement. An ideal post-blink lens movement should be of 0.5–0.7 mm. If with each blink movement of lens is more than 1 mm, then it indicates too flat fitting of lens, if it is less than 0.5 mm, then lens fitting is steeper.

Note: Recent available contact lenses has more water content and are thin with less elasticity as compared to older lenses, which were usually thicker and lower in water content; hence they show less post-blink movement.

- **Push up test:** Many a times it is difficult to assess lens movement by blink alone, hence a better assessment of lens movement can be done by Push up test. It is considered most useful way to judge dynamic fit of a contact lens in relation to eye.

Test procedure: To do this test, the examiner applies pressure on the lower eyelid by finger to move the contact lens vertically upwards and then remove the finger to release pressure on the eye so that lens returns to its original position as shown in Fig. 13.18A and B. During this test aim is to observe how easily the lens displacement occurs on pressure and then how rapidly it returns to its original position on releasing pressure.

Results: These are represented in a percentage grading system where 100% means that lens

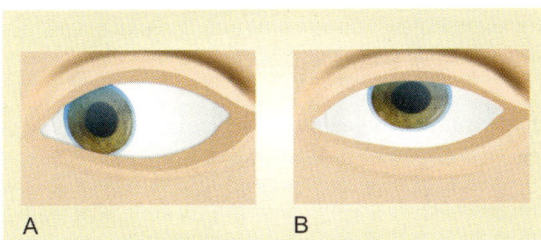

Fig. 13.17: Centration of contact lens. A. Lens lag; B. Lens sag

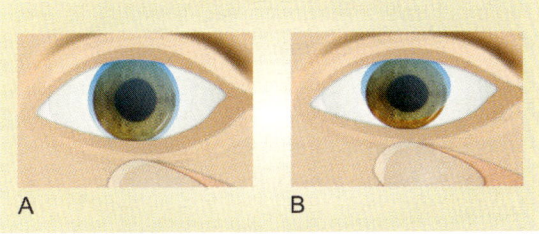

Fig. 13.18: Push test. A. Finger in position; B. Lens moved up

movement is not possible and 0% means that lens will fall away from the cornea without support of eyelids. A correct and optimum fit is considered when lens movement recorded is 50%. In addition, tightness of lens as measured by the push-up test shows a linear relationship with squeeze pressure (it is the force which exist between posterior surface of lens and front surface of the eye) and so it can also be considered in judging lens fit.

Effect of blinking is noticed not only on lens movement but also on visual acuity, retinoscopy reflex and keratometer mires.

- **Post-blink visual acuity:** Change in clarity of vision due to blinking should be checked. In case of an ideal lens fit, no change in visual acuity will be noticed by the patient. However, in a flat fit the patient complaints of blur vision while in steep fit, the vision improves immediately after blinking.
- **Post-blink retinoscopy reflex:** The changes in retinal reflex are in correlation with clarity of vision means in an ideal lens fit the reflexes are sharp, whereas in flat fit reflex becomes blur and in steep fit, it becomes clear instantly after blinking.
- **Post-blink keratometer mires:** Even the distortion of keratometer mires are in correlation with vision clarity, means in an ideal lens fit the mires appear crisp and sharp, whereas in flat fit they are blur and

in steep fit they become clear immediately after blinking.

- **Conjunctival congestion:** On slit lamp the status of conjunctival vessels and scleral indentation should be observed. In case of a steep fit limbal vessel nipping, conjunctival congestion and scleral indentation (on long duration usage) is present.

To summarize these observations and evaluations of a trial lens fit following points to be remembered as shown in Table 13.4.

Ocular factors influencing lens fitting

- *Ocular sag:* This is determined by corneal diameter, radius and shape factor and also by scleral shape and radius and any factor among these if altered will affect the lens sag, which can only be assessed by a trial lens fit.
- *Corneal apex:* Position of corneal apex will affect the centration of lens. Displacement of corneal apex will cause the lens decentration, which can be corrected by increasing the total diameter (TD). An increase in TD will increase the corneal coverage, if exposed, while changes in base curve will not affect centration.
- *Pressure of lids:* Too much pressure caused by tensed lids may lead to high riding of lens and also an excessive movement of lens. To overcome it a thin lens design and/or lens with more diameter can be used. Loose lids usually have less effect on lens fits than tight lids.

Table 13.4: Various indicators of loose fit and tight fit of contact lens	
Indicators of loose fit of contact lens	*Indicators of tight fit of contact lens*
Too much movement of contact lens	No movement of contact lens
Poor centration in primary gaze, usually in inferior lag	Constriction of limbal vessel or 'nipping'
Buckling of lens edge after wearing	Indentation of conjunctiva at lens margins
Presence of lens awareness sensation	Conjunctival congestion with redness
Change in vision, especially immediately after blinking	Ocular inflammation of low degree
Blurring of retinoscope reflex and keratometer mires, immediately after blinking	Visual improvement, immediately after blinking

- *Tear characteristics:* The change in pH and osmotic pressure of tear has important part to alter the parameters of lens, finally affecting the lens fit. Decrease in the pH of tear film causes steepening of ionic contact lens. Change in osmotic pressure like decrease in tonicity of tear will cause tight fit of both ionic and non-ionic lenses. Hence it is important to remember that if an acceptable fit is not obtained with contact lens material, then it is necessary to change the ionicity or water content of another lens material.

Contact lens factors affecting lens fit

- *Total diameter (TD):* Variation in the total diameter of lens will affect the fitting of lens. For example, increase in the TD of lens will enhance sag of lens, resulting in tight fit, while reduction in TD of lens will produce opposite effect. In case of lens with displaced apex, the TD can be increased to improve the corneal coverage by this lens. Lens fit is usually more affected by change in lens diameter as compared to change in BOZR.
- *Back optic zone radius (BOZR):* Change in the base curve of lens cause change in the movement of lens. However, studies indicate that change in the BOZR does not cause much effect on lens fit.
- *Peripheral design of lens:* The peripheral lens design may also influence the lens fit. The peripheral design indicates correlation between front and back peripheral curves of lens. It should be kept in mind that it is not necessary that lenses with different peripheral design having same TD and BOZR will show fitting characteristic in similar fashion.

Soft Contact Lens Ordering

After a detailed evaluation of the lens parameters and checking a proper trial lens fit with these parameters, soft contact lenses are ordered from a known manufacturers' series, by specifying the desired power. Usually we can specify the total diameter and power of lens, to get a proper fit soft contact lens from various manufacturers' guide.

Examination of delivered contact lens: Contact lens delivery received from the lens manufacture should be examined thoroughly before inserting it into the eye of patient as shown in Fig. 13.19. Following parameters are checked for received contact lens:

- Lens total diameter: This is checked by using a diameter gauge.
- Contact lens power: Power of the lens is determined by using lensometer, specially designed to measure the contact lens power.
- Lens edges and curves are inspected by keeping the lens on the tip of finger and observing it in bright light for any defect or abnormality.
- Lens quality and clarity is also observed while checking for its edges.

Evaluation of ordered lens fit: Once all the parameters of delivered lens are checked thoroughly, this lens is ready to use in the patient's eye. Following instructions related to lens fit along with explanation of methods of lens insertion and removal are taught to the patient.

Contact lens handling instruction to the patient: Although most of the patients are enthusiastic about wearing of a contact lens, but many of them are first time wearers. Hence, a detailed

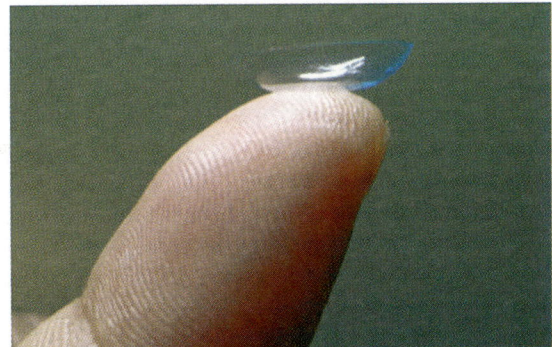

Fig. 13.19: Examination of soft contact lens before insertion

instruction about handling and caring of contact lens along with the insertion and removal techniques should be taught to majority of patients.

General instructions: Patients should be instructed that contacts should not be considered as fashion accessories or cosmetics; rather it is a type of medical devices that need proper cleanliness as explained and is vital to prevent infections of eyes. These infections are potentially hazardous for eyes; hence patients are advised to take care of lenses as per direction. Cleaning is done both before insertion and after removal of contact lens from the eye before putting the lens back in lens case.

Following instructions are important to be remembered by patients

- Strictly follow the schedule for insertion and removal of lens.
- Daily wear lenses should not be worn at time of sleeping.
- To protect from water contact lenses should be removed before bath, swimming, or doing anything, where water can go inside the eyes.
- Never touch contact lens with dirty hands. Hands should be washed with soap and water before touching lens.
- Never use tap or sterile water and saline solution prepared at home for rinsing or storage of contact lens. Use sterile contact lens solution (not tap water) for washing of case of lens followed by its drying in air.
- For disinfection of lens proper disinfectant solution should be used. Saline solution or artificial tear drops should not be used for disinfection.
- Always use a "rub and rinse" cleaning method, before insertion, after removal or before placing lens in the lens case. The contact lenses should be rubbed with clean fingers followed by rinsing with solution and then soaking. This process must be done every time for cleaning and disinfection of contact lens.

- Soft contact lenses are always stored in normal saline solution because if exposed to air, may get dehydrated and breaks due to brittleness. Rehydrate the lenses by placing them in saline solution, and wait until they become soft and regain their original shape.
- Old contact lens care solution should not be reused for cleaning and rinsing purpose and also contact lens solution should not be transferred into different container as solution may loss its sterility and infection may occur.
- Tip of lens solution container should not contact any surface. The solution bottle should be kept tightly closed after use.
- Contact lens case must be clean and ideally it should be replaced at least once in 3 months. Damaged and cracked cases should be replaced immediately.
- Over a period of time, contact lenses get damage and also its shape can alter due to cornea. Hence, check at intervals that that lenses fit is proper and the visual acuity is perfect, if not report immediately to practitioner.

Insertion and Removal of Soft Contact Lens

Before insertion of contact lenses in the eyes, we should ensure that the lens have not turned inside out, while removing from their blister packs or lens case. There are two methods to check this

- Keep the contact lens on the tip of index finger and examine its shape and edges as shown in Fig. 13.20A. In correct lens an even cup shape is seen, whereas if lens is not correct, then lens appears shallower with more pointed at its edges as shown in Fig. 13.20B.
- *Taco test:* It is another method to check whether lens is proper or in an inside out position. To do this gently folds the soft contact lens in between the index finger and thumb. Suppose the lens is in correct position, lens edges should fold inward like a Mexican Taco and touches each other

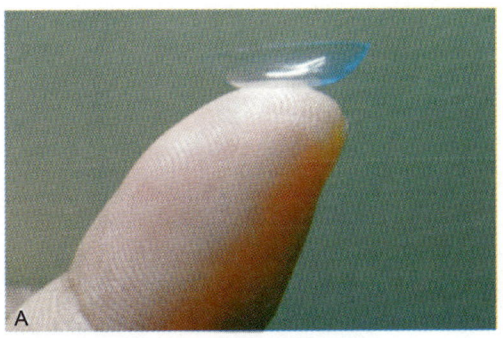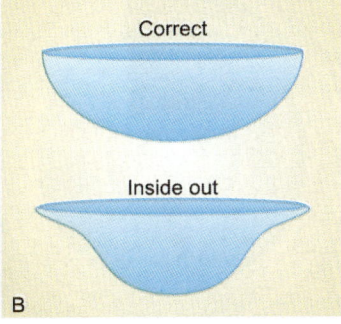

Fig. 13.20: Contact lens checking. A. CL position on fingertip; B. Check position

edges as shown in Fig. 13.21A, whereas if lens is inside out, then the lens edges will curls outward and flips out onto fingertip as shown in Fig. 13.21B.

Note: Important point to be remembered while testing the position of lens is that the lens should be held from its center not from its edges.

Lens insertion technique: Insertion of a soft contact lens is done as follows

- Wash the hands thoroughly using soap, for a few minutes and then air dry.
- Remove the lens from its case and clean as we already discussed above.
- Rinse the contact lens with cleaning solution.

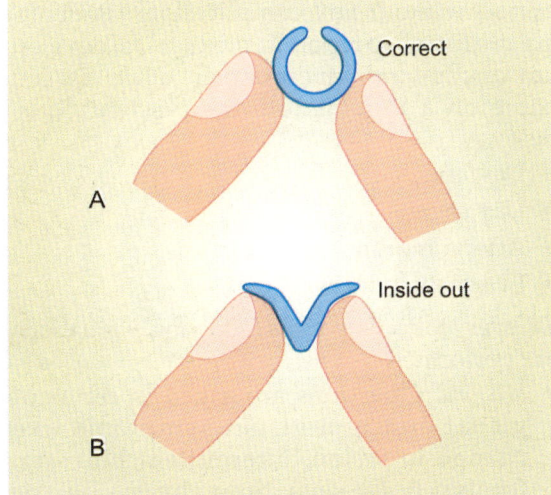

Fig. 13.21: Taco test for checking correct position of contact lens. A. Inward rolling of lens margins; B. Outward rolling of lens margins

- Place the lens on the tip of the index finger of hand as shown.
- Look up while the lower lid is retracted with the middle finger of same hand as shown in Fig. 13.22A. This is called as one hand technique.
- Alternately, the eye can be spread wide open with the index and middle finger of left hand and contact lens is placed on the tip of index finger of right hand, while the middle finger of right hand is placed over cheek bone to avoid any jerky movement of right hand. This is called as two hand technique as shown in Fig. 13.22B.
- While looking upward, gently touch the contact lens to the lower part of eye. Then slowly remove the finger, when contact lens is placed on the eye.
- Then very gently and slowly first release the lower and then upper lids.
- Close the eye and give a gentle massage over lids, to remove any air bubble in case if present underneath of contact lens.
- Open the eye and move it gently in all gazes, to center the lens. Then observe the correct centration of lens while the other eye is covered with hand.
- Similar instructions are repeated in other eye for lens insertion.

Lens removal technique
- Wash the hands thoroughly using soap, for a few minutes and then air dry.
- First turn the eyes upwards and with middle finger retract the lower lid while

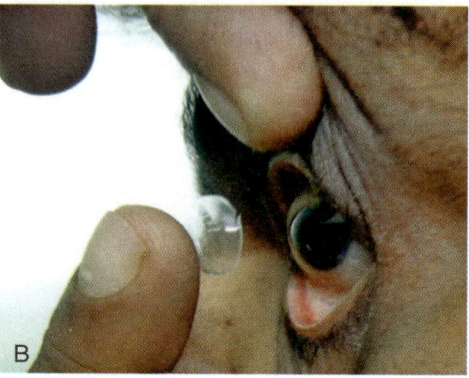

Fig. 13.22: Insertion technique of soft contact lens. A. One hand method; B. Two hands method

keeping the tip of index finger on the lower edge of the lens.

- Disengage the lens slowly by sliding the lens downwards, over to the white portion of the eye.
- Once lens slides downwards, pinch out the lens between thumb and the index finger, so that suction created under lens is broken by air as shown in Fig. 13.23.
- Slowly remove the lens from eye and do the cleaning with lens solution and place it in the lens case containing solution.

Wearing schedule for soft contact lenses: Normally soft contact lenses are well accepted and comfortable to wear from day one; hence there is tendency in patients that they may over wear it from day one. Patients should be informed about the disastrous results of over wearing of contact lenses and should be advised to follow a strict wearing schedule for best visual outcomes.

Generally the wearing schedule is totally dependent on the individual patient's profile, however, on an average patients' are instructed to wear a soft contact lens for continuous 2–3 hours and then remove the lens for a minimum period of one hour. They are advised to follow this schedule for initial 10–15 days, or till they become comfortable for longer duration wear.

Follow up: Regular follow up is must to achieve a comfortable contact lens wearing period without any complications. Patients' are instructed to report immediately if develop any discomfort, redness or pain, otherwise can come on a regular follow-up schedule as below

- Day one
- Day seven
- After a month
- Every six months

On every follow-up visits following evaluations are performed

- *History:* Questions are asked in terms of visual and non-visual symptoms like change in vision, intermittent blurring, foreign body sensations, heavy lids or ocular movements, excessive watering, discharge or decreased visual fields, etc. Examiner should be able to differentiate

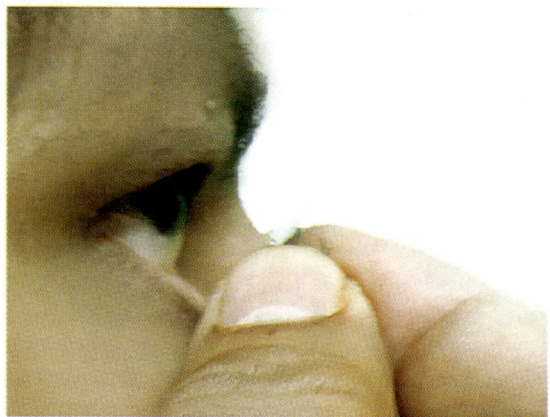

Fig. 13.23: Removal technique of soft contact lens

between physiological/psychological symptoms arising due to adaptation and actual clinical abnormalities. Usually adaptation symptoms are not present with soft lenses, however, even if present will subside on its own within 10–12 days, however, symptoms due to clinical abnormalities will start after 2–3 days and persist constantly even after 15 days.

- *Vision:* Check the visual acuity with lens in position, if visual acuity is less, then do an over refraction and recheck vision with a pin hole.
- *Ocular examination:* Detailed ocular examination is done to record head posture, lid position, periorbital edema, blinking rate and conjunctival congestion.
- *Slit lamp examination:* It is done with contact lens in the eye, and then after removal of contact lens. Position of contact lens, cornea and conjunctiva are examined in detail.

Rigid Contact Lens Fitting

Rigid contact lenses are broadly classified as

Rigid non-gas permeable lenses: Mainly manufactured from PMMA (Plexiglas) and are rarely used nowadays due to their disadvantages overweighing the advantages.

Rigid gas permeable contact lenses: These are most widely used contact lenses and are also called semisoft contact lenses. These lenses are made up of a unique plastic material which has an ability to permit oxygen to diffuse inside and carbon dioxide to diffuse outside the lens. Various polymers materials are used to make these lenses such as CAB (cellulose acetyl butyrate), silicon acrylate, butyl styrene, polystyrene, fluorine copolymers and polysulfone copolymers.

Fitting procedures: Since PMMA lenses are obsolete nowadays, hence we will discuss fitting of rigid gas permeable (RGP) contact lenses in detail.

Fitting of rigid contact lens is usually considered as more difficult than fitting of soft contact lens, but actually many fitting steps are essentially the same when practitioner needs to judge the fitting of either lens. Modern RGP lens designs are available in a wide range of lenses; which can be fitted easily in majority of normal ametropic population.

Nowadays to receive a rigid contact lens, practitioners just need to specify the total diameter (TD), back vertex power (BVP) and back optic zone radius (BOZR) of a particular lens design to manufacturer.

Fitting steps include
- Trial lens selection
- Trial lens fit evaluation
- Trial lens fit interpretation
- Corneal factor influencing lens fitting
- Contact lens factors affecting lens fit

Trial lens selection: The initial trial lens should be selected using the following parameters:

- *Total diameter:* Selection of total diameter (TD) of lens is decided by the horizontal visible iris diameter (HVID) and position of lid (size of palpebral aperture). Generally, a lens having TD 1.4 mm smaller than the HVID should be chosen. In addition, on the basis of size of palpebral aperture, the lens with smaller TD should be selected if aperture is small and vice versa.
  - Choice of TD according to HVID can be made as shown in Fig. 13.24. For small palpebral aperture, rigid lens of approximately 9.2 mm size, for an average size aperture lens of 9.6 mm diameter can be chosen, however, for very large apertures 10 mm TD size rigid lens may be required.
  - Choice of lens is also in inverse relationship with corneal curvature as summarized in Table 13.5. It means flatter the cornea, larger diameter of RGP lens will be required for a proper fit.
- *Center thickness of lens:* To enhance the oxygen transmissibility contact lenses are made as thin as possible. In majority of rigid lens materials (available nowadays), the center thickness is kept about 0.14 mm.

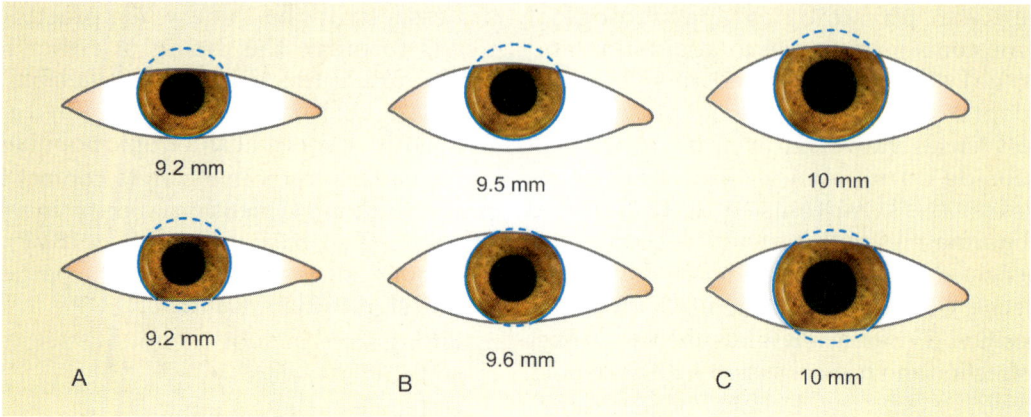

Fig. 13.24: Total diameter selection according to HVID and lid positions. A. Small palpebral aperture; B. Average size palpebral aperture; C. Very large palpebral aperture

Table 13.5: Relationship between corneal curvature and contact lens diameter

Corneal curve	Diameter of contact lens
40–43 D	9.5 mm
43.25–45 D	9.2 mm
> 45.25 D	9.0 mm

- *Calculation of power of trial lens:* Refraction should be done to determine spectacle power and then power of trial rigid contact lens is calculated. First convert the spectacle lens power into a minus cylinder form, if present. Now correct this spectacle power for a zero vertex distance by applying appropriate formula or from a ready reference chart provided by the contact lens manufacturer.

     For example, suppose spectacle power is: $8.5 \times +1.5 \times 90°$, at 15 mm vertex distance.

     First convert it in minus cylinder form as: $-7 \times -1.5 \times 180°$

     Then correct it to a zero vertex distance as: $-5.75 \times -1.0 \times 180°$.

Note: Spherical powers can similarly be corrected to a zero vertex distance and contact lens of corrected power is used directly.

- *Back vertex power:* To provide normal vision and to decrease probable changes in lens fit due to difference in lens power, the back vertex power must be approximate to patient's final prescription. The fit may vary with minus powered lens and plus power lens due to difference in their edge design and center of gravity. Hence, myopes should be assessed with negatively powered lenses and vice versa with hypermetropes.
- *Back optic zone diameter (BOZD):* BOZD is usually kept larger (≥ 1.0 mm) than average pupil size to avoid flare due to lens. To maintain corneal alignment also it is necessary to adjust BOZD because as the flattening of cornea increases, lens of larger BOZD will be required to maintain proper alignment over the cornea.
- *Back optic zone radius (BOZR):* Design of back surface of rigid lenses could be aspherical, spherical or their combination. Spherical RGP lenses can be bicurve, tri-curve or multi-curve in nature where every lens has different BOZR with different peripheral curve design. In case of spherical RGP contact lenses, initial trial lens is selected on the basis of keratometer readings using recommendations provided by the manufacturer or using the values as shown in Table 13.6. In case of an elliptical type of aspherical contact lenses usually more flat fitting is required than spherical lenses so that an alignment across the corneal surface is adequately achieved.

BOZR is chosen on the basis of keratometer readings; usually on flattest K- reading (called as fit 'On-K'), especially for spherical RGP lenses or an astigmatism <0.5 D. But for astigmatism of > 0.5 D, guidelines as shown in Table 13.6 are used to decide about the BOZR of RGP lenses.

For understanding Table 13.6 values, we can take an example, suppose keratometer readings are 45 D/46 D, means having astigmatism of 1 D; then the base curve selected will be 45.25 D. Similarly if readings are 46 D/47.5 D, then a base curve of 46.5 D will be selected, however in case where readings are 46 D/50 D, then it is better to choose a toric back optic zone contact lens.

Trial lens fit evaluation: Once the trial lens is chosen, then a sterile trial lens is inserted in the eye under all aseptic precautions. Just before lens insertion, patient is instructed that there may be feeling of foreign body sensation after insertion of lens. To reduce feeling of foreign body sensation patient is advised to look downwards after insertion of lens. *"Fluorescein dye is used to assess the lens fit in case of a rigid contact lens"*.

- **Adaptation and patients' response**
  - *Adaptation period:* After insertion of lens, as reflex tearing get stop (usually within 5 minutes), lens fit by bare eye and under white light should be examined to check the stability and centration of lens during trial period. Once an adequate lens fit is

Table 13.6: Guidelines for selection of BOZR of RGP lenses in astigmatism > 0.5 D

Astigmatism	BOZR
Spherical to 0.5 D	Fit 'On-K', means flattest keratometer reading
0.5–1.0 D	Fit on 0.05 steeper than the flattest keratometer reading
1.0–2.5 D	Fit on 0.05–0.10 steeper than the flattest keratometer reading
Over 2.5 D	A toric back optic zone is suggested

achieved, patients are advised for a longer trial period (minimum 30 minutes) which allows them to judge the comfort and problems of rigid contact lens. After trial period the subjective response of the patient is assessed. Patient must be comfortable and there must be no reflex tearing. Vision must be stable in all positions of gaze with the used power of trial lens.

- **Over refraction and visual acuity**
  - Initially to check the spherical power of contact lens, an over refraction with binocular balancing is done. The purpose of binocular balancing is to relax the accommodation, which might have been induced due to foreign body sensation of contact lens.
  - Visual acuity achieved with contact lenses should be crisp and stable in all gazes. An unstable or improper acuity indicates that a cylindrical refraction is also needed to correct the refractive status.
  - Both by subjective and objective response should be evaluated during refraction by retinoscope. The results are used to calculate the tear lens power and to adjust the central fit of contact lens, if needed.

- **Biomicroscopy examination**
  - Dynamic fit of a rigid contact lens can be evaluated and measured by using either a slit lamp or Burton lamp in the same way as for the soft contact lenses.
  - Lens-corneal alignment is assessed by help of either white light or a cobalt blue light as follows

  White light
  - Using diffuse white light and with an optic section examiner should make a judgment about centration of contact lens in the primary gaze as well as during lateral movements of eyes.
  - Along with centration, the movement of lens with blink is also judged.

Ideally, RGP lens should move downward with each blink, under the influence of upper eyelid, however, it returns to cover the pupil immediately.

Cobalt-blue light

- Alignment of posterior surface of lens with front surface of the eye can be assessed by means of fluorescein because it causes staining of the tear film, which creates a tear lens. On illuminating by appropriate wavelength of blue light (cobalt-blue filter) the fluorescein emits a fluorescent green color. The intensity of this green color is related to the thickness of the fluorescein tear film; means thicker the tear lens, more yellow will be the appearance.

- As fluorescein dye occupies the tear space present between posterior surface of lens and front surface of the cornea. The distance between these two surfaces (known as fluorescein pattern) can be assessed by looking change in the intensity of fluorescent light which occurs due to excitation by cobalt blue filter. More is the intensity (brighter) of color; more will be the distance between two surfaces.

Burton lamp

- Burton lamp is used to visualize various fluorescein patterns. It acts as a source of UV light which is used to excite the fluorescein dye. However, as compared to slit lamp the magnification achieved with Burton's lamp is less. In addition, it cannot assess pattern when polymer materials used in manufacturing of contact lens also contain a UV inhibitor where cobalt blue light with slit lamp is the choice.

- **Fluorescein assessment**
  - In RGP lenses, a fluorescein assessment of the contact lens fit is done. Fluorescein dye in small amount is introduced into the conjunctival sac while patient is instructed to blink gently 2–3 times, which spreads the dye all over the eye.
  - Lens fit should be evaluated using slit lamp or Burton lamp with a diffuse, direct illumination under medium to high magnification.
  - The brightness of fluorescein dye is assessed systematically mainly in three regions of contact lens, i.e. peripheral, mid peripheral and central. Guillon proposed a simple grading scale for the assessment of contact lens fit. According to grading if fluorescein dye is seen under the contact lens during assessment of fit, then it can range from
    - Little amount (0), means in alignment or minimal apical clearance
    - Moderate amount (+1)
    - Too much or excessive amount (+2)

Trial lens fit interpretation: Now it is important to interpret the lens fit to know whether it is correct or not, which can be done by

- **Patient's subjective response**
  - RGP lenses usually cause more discomfort after insertion as compared to soft contact lenses, however, after adaptation period of 30 minutes, patient should not feel discomfort. If after adaptation period also the patient complaints of pain and excessive reflex tearing, then it indicates that the contact lens is not correct and require modification in parameters.
  - By means of correct spherical correction the patient must have stable and crisp visual acuity. However, if vision is not stable with use of spherical lenses then a cylindrical overcorrection might be needed.
  - If residual astigmatism is suspected for the poor vision, then before prescribing a toric correction, it is essential to confirm the site of residual astigmatism because

bending or curving of lens may be also one of the causes of poor vision. If no site of residual astigmatism detected on examination, then it is most probably the lens bending causing poor vision and lens-eye fitting relationship require modification to correct the vision.

- **Over refraction**
  - Over refraction is done to calculate the tear lens values, i.e. difference in refractive power between the ocular refraction and final contact lens power required to correct ametropia.
  - In case of steeper fitting of lens than cornea, a positive tear lens will form as shown in Fig. 13.25C and final contact lens power will be either less plus or more minus as compared to the ocular refraction.
  - In opposite situation, i.e. flatter fitting of contact lens, a negative tear lens will form as shown in Fig. 13.25A and final power of the contact lens required will be either more plus or less minus than the ocular refraction.
  - In case of an ideal fit as shown in Fig. 13.25B, a slight central touch is seen.

Note: Simple guidelines in calculating tear lens powers are that if there is 0.5 DS difference in over refraction, it means a 0.1 mm difference is present between corneal radius and contact lens radius.

- **Lens centration and movement:** During lateral gaze and in between blinking, the position of lens must be centered over the

visual axis. Various positions of lens may be seen due to these factors.

- Corneal opacities, against the rule astigmatism and oblique astigmatism may decenter the contact lens either temporally or nasally. Smaller lens with a steeper fit will correct this horizontal decentring.
- Vertically lens movement is about 1–1.5 mm, but sometimes lens may ride high, means the upper edge of lens crosses the upper limbal margin or lens hook on to upper lid.
- Similarly, lens may ride too low or rapidly drop after blink, means lower edges of contact lens crosses the lower limbal margin.
- Some degree of decentration is acceptable in case of rigid contact lens fitting.

Various contributing factors and the management of lens decentration are summarized in Table 13.7, along with the available options to improve the centration of contact lens.

- **Fluorescein patterns**
  - Analysis of fluorescein patterns helps to find out the tear lens shapes in relation to lens fit. Thus help to confirm the relationship of contact lens and the eye. For example, steep looking fit will show positive tear lens pattern while a flat looking fit will show a minus tear lens pattern.
  - Sometimes, even when using the contact lens with BOZR which was matched with keratometer readings of cornea, then also a steep or flat fit looking fluorescein patterns may occur. It may be due to either BOZR of trial lens is inaccurate or due to difference in the eccentricity of cornea.

Corneal factors influencing lens fit: Eccentricity (e) of cornea decides rate of flattening of the cornea toward the periphery. Normal cornea has average eccentricity value of 0.2 to 0.5. If cornea has e value lower (i.e. e <0.5) than

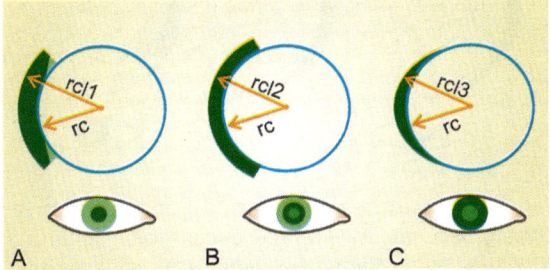

Fig. 13.25: Various tear lenses and over refraction. A. Flatter fit; B. Ideal fit; C. Steep fit

Table 13.7: Various possible causes and management of lens decentration

Lens location	Possible causes	Management
Lens riding high or not dropping after blink (superior decentration)	Flat and wide peripheral zone High minus lens Large diameter lens and tight lid Too thick edge lens With the rule astigmatism Displacement of optic cap in upward direction	Steepen the base curve Use plus carrier lenticular design Reduce diameter and use prism ballast lens Reduce Tc and Te of lens Use toric peripheral design
Lens riding low or dropping rapidly after blink (inferior decentration)	Lens too small in diameter Lens too thick No lid attachment Displacement of optic cap in downward direction	Use large lens (increase TD) Reduce Tc Add peripheral negative carrier
Continue to be on one side (lateral decentration)	Corneal apex decentered Too small lens Flat contact lens Against the rule corneal astigmatism	Increase the diameter of lens and use soft lens Steepen the base curve of lens Use back surface with toric design or toric periphery design
Stationary Lens	Too steep lens	Flatten the fit
Excessive decentration of lens (beyond limbus)	Excess lacrimation Lens too flat Excess corneal astigmatism	Correct symptoms Steepen the design Use back surface in toric design

average, means it indicates that cornea has steepen central cornea (more flat peripheral cornea), while high e value (i.e. e >0.5) indicates flatter central cornea than peripheral cornea. Relationship of corneal eccentricity with contact lens fit is shown in Fig. 13.26.

- *Cornea with average eccentricity:* Spherical contact lens will show an ideal lens fit, as apical appearance, mid-peripheral touch and peripheral clearance pattern as indicated by a bright green periphery with faintly appearing central portion as shown in Fig. 13.26A.
- *Cornea with lower eccentricity than an average eccentricity:* Means cornea steepens out faster towards periphery at faster rate, hence spherical contact lens of the same central radius prescribed for this type of cornea will show peripheral pooling as shown in Fig. 13.26B. This lens fit will need a modification, as if dealing with a flat fitting lens.

- *Cornea with more eccentricity than an average eccentricity:* Means cornea flattens out faster towards periphery at faster rate, hence spherical contact lens of the same central radius will show central pooling as shown in Fig. 13.26C. This lens fit needs a modification, as if dealing with a steep fitting lens.

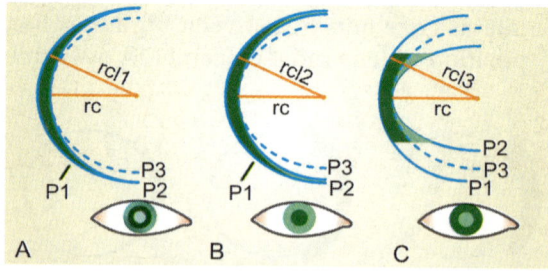

Fig. 13.26: Corneal eccentricity and respective contact lens fit. A. Average eccentricity, ideal fit; B. Lower eccentricity, flat lens fit with peripheral pooling; C. Higher eccentricity steep lens fit with central pooling

Contact Lens factors affecting lens fit

- *Contact lens base curve is flatter than corneal curvature (flat fitting):* Chances of excessive movement of lens and fluorescein pattern will show a central black area with peripheral pooling. Fluorescein pattern in this case will show a central black area indicating a direct lens corneal touch (means there is no tear layer between lens and cornea) and diffuse green portion in mid-peripheral and peripheral zone due to pooling of dye in these areas as shown in Fig. 13.27.

- *Contact lens base curve is steeper than corneal curvature (steep fitting):* A lens having base curve steeper than corneal curvature will show very little or no movement with presence of air bubbles underneath the contact lens. Fluorescein pattern will show a central pooling and bright green band at periphery, with a broad dark mid-peripheral zone which indicates intense lens touch in mid-peripheral zone as shown in Fig. 13.28.

- *Contact lens base curve is equal to corneal curvature (ideal fitting):* A lens having base curve equal to corneal curvature will show desired movement of lens with rotation of eyeball. Fluorescein pattern will show an apical appearance and light green clearance at periphery, with a dark mid-peripheral zone which indicates that an adequate amount of tear lens is formed with an ideal lens fit as shown in Fig. 13.29.

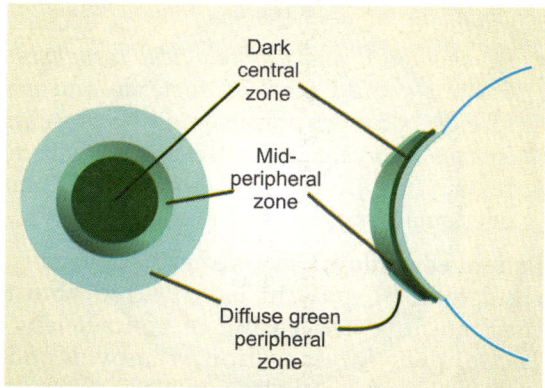

Fig. 13.27: Flat lens fit showing central dark area

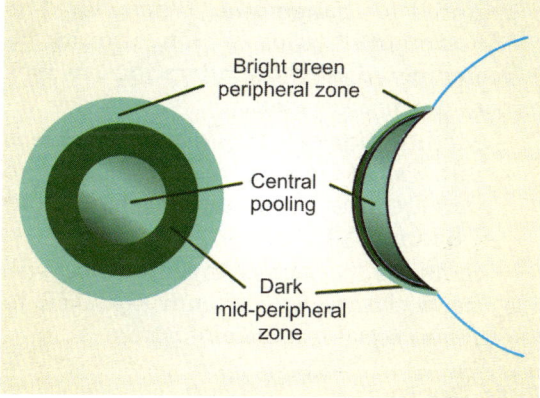

Fig. 13.28: Steep lens fit showing central pooling

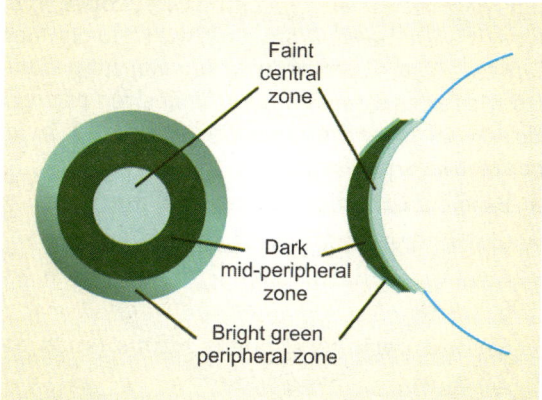

Fig. 13.29: Ideal lens fit showing apical appearance and peripheral clearance

- Base curve in RGP lenses is an important parameter to decide about the lens to be ordered. Sometimes, a selected lens of particular diameter may need change in diameter due to change in the base curve as both are directly correlated to each other. Usually, a large diameter lens should have a small base curve to produce the same effect as that of a small diameter lens with steeper base curve. On an average, a change of 1 mm in the diameter requires a change of 0.01 mm in the radius of curvature of lens.

- Various parameters used for selection of a rigid lens are dependent on each other, so to get an ideal lens fit, if one parameter is changed, then simultaneously it is also required to change other parameter. The fundamental rules which should be remembered to make alterations in lens parameters are as follows.

- Modification of 0.05 mm in BOZR of lens will cause change in power equal to 0.25 D considering radius of lens is about 7.8 mm.

- Similarly, 0.5 mm change in BOZD will need change of 0.05 mm in BOZR to retain equal fluorescein pattern.

Rigid Contact Lens Ordering

After doing a detailed evaluation about the lens parameters and checking of a proper trial lens fit with these parameters, the rigid contact lenses are ordered from a known manufacturer's series by specifying the desired power. Following parameters are specified in a contact lens prescription

- Base curve radius (such as 7.8 mm)
- Optic zone diameter (such as 7.0 mm)
- First peripheral curve radius (such as 8.0 mm)
- Second peripheral curve radius (such as 8.6 mm)
- Back peripheral zone (such as up to 8.2 mm)
- Total diameter (such as 9.0 mm)
- Contact Lens power (such as –5 DS)

Above parameters will typically be written in a perception form as

7.8: 7.0/8.2: 8.0/8.6: 9.0, power –5 DS

Examination of the received lens: Contact lens delivery received from the lens manufacture should be thoroughly examined, before inserting it into the eye of patient. Following parameters are checked for received contact lens

- Lens total diameter is checked by using a diameter gauge.
- Contact lens power is determined by using lensometer, specifically designed to measure the contact lens power.
- Base curve is measured by using a specially designed instrument called Radiuscope.

- Contact lens central thickness should be measured by a thickness gauge.
- Lens edges and curves are inspected by keeping the lens on the tip of finger and observing it in bright light for any defect or abnormality.
- Lens quality and clarity is also observed while checking for its edges.

Evaluation of ordered lens fit: Once we had examined the received lens as per specification, this sterile rigid contact lens is inserted in patient's eye under all aseptic precautions. After an extended adaptation period of about 25–30 minutes, evaluation of ordered lens is done to check the lens fit on the same guidelines as described for trial lens fit evaluations. However, some important points of lens fit for evaluation are as follows

- *Position of the lens:* Well-centered lens indicates an ideal fit. High ride or low ride lens indicates an abnormal fit.
- *Movements of lens:* 1–1.5 mm vertical movement or lateral excursion in horizontal gaze indicates an ideal fit. Excessive lens movement in all gazes shows a flat fit and less or no movement indicates a steep fit.
- *Fluorescein pattern:* As described above the distinctive fluorescein patterns will be seen in an ideal, flat and steep fit lenses.
- *Visual acuity:* Should be crisp and clear which remain stable before, during and after the blinks. Over refraction can be done to rule out any under or over correction of power.
- *Psychological and physiological responses:* Patient should feel comfortable and no foreign body sensation should be present. In case of an ideal fit corneal metabolism remain healthy, hence no corneal erosions or edema is noticed after adaptation period.

Patient education: Once we get a satisfactory rigid lens fit, patient is educated about the handling and caring of contact lens. Techniques for insertion, removal and recentration of contact lens are also explained to patient.

Handling and caring of contact lens: To prevent infection, it is essential to educate the patient about proper handling and caring of the contact lens. Following instructions are given to the patient at the time of dispensing of a rigid contact lens

- Thoroughly clean the hands with soap and water and air dry them before inserting, rinsing, cleaning or removing the contact lens.
- Never apply excessive pressure while cleaning the lens, because they are very thin and can easily get fractured.
- Clean the lenses after removal and before placing them in lens case, keeping the concave side upwards.
- Always use antiseptic solution or a commercially available multipurpose contact lens cleaning solution, to rinse, clean, soak or disinfect a RGP lens, never heat or use running tap water.
- These lenses should be disinfected by chemical treatment at regular intervals for maintaining the sterility.
- Patients are advised not to sleep or do underwater swimming, while wearing these lenses.

Insertion and Removal of Rigid Contact Lens

Patient is taught to insert the contact lens in his/her eyes very comfortably.

Insertion Technique

- Insertion steps of a rigid contact lens are similar to that of a soft contact lens as instructed above.
- Lens is kept on the tip of index finger as shown in Fig. 13.30A and is inserted in eye as described for soft contact lens (Fig. 13.30B). Important point in rigid lenses is identification of right and left eye lens, especially in cases where there is a vast difference in refractive powers of two eyes.

Note: Letter 'R' is engraved on the lens periphery for right eye lens, hence when patient keeps the lens on the tip of finger, he/she should search for this mark for right eye.

Removal Technique

Removal procedure for a rigid lens is different from soft contact lens removal technique. Here lens can be removed by two methods as per convenience.

Method 1 (Fig. 13.31)

- Head is bended down to make it parallel to the floor, then patient places the thumb/middle finger of right hand on right lower lid margin and index finger of the same hand over right upper lid margin.
- Cup the left hand under the right eye to grasp the falling RGP lens.
- Then patient draw both the eyelids away from the lens, while pressing them tightly together and keeping the straight gaze.

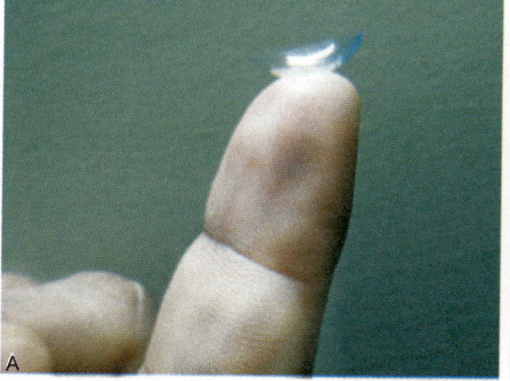
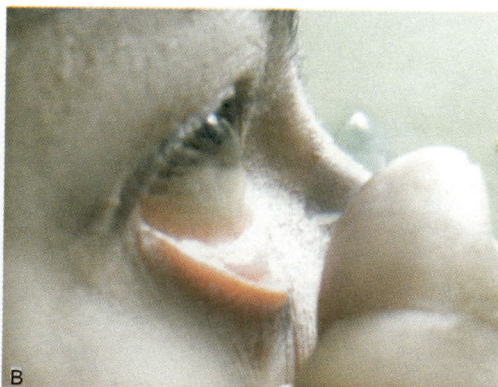

Fig. 13.30: Technique of RGP lens insertion. A. Lens placed on index finger; B. Lens insertion

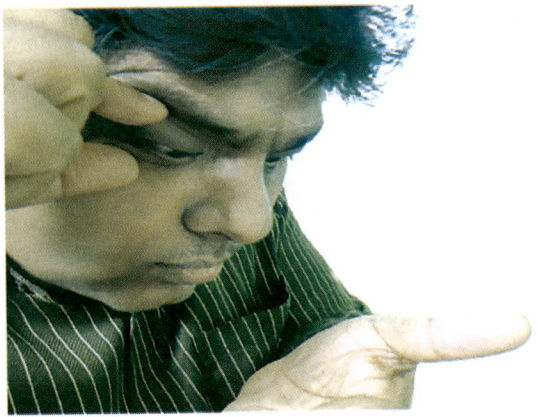

Fig. 13.31: Method 1 for RGP lens removal

- Suppose lens did not fall by this manoeuvre, then alternatively both the hands can be used to pull the upper and lower eyelids using right and left hands.

Method 2 (Fig. 13.32)

- Similarly bend the head down, now place index finger of right hand over the upper lid margin.
- Cup the left hand under the right eye to grab the falling lens.
- Look downwards keeping both the eyes wide open, now pull the index finger upward and outward.
- Suppose lens did not come out, then patient is instructed to blink simultaneously while pulling the upper eyelid.
- Left hand is used to remove the lens from the left eye.

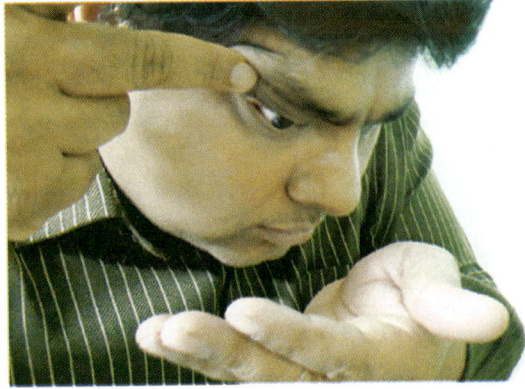

Fig. 13.32: Method 2 for RGP lens removal

Recentration Technique

- *Suppose if lens is beneath the upper lid:* Pull the upper eyelid in upward direction and look downwards, while firmly holding the upper lid upwards. Now make rapid horizontal eye movements, slowly look straight, and then downwards, now gently leave the eyelid.
- *Suppose if lens in beneath the lower lid:* First widely open both the eyelids by right hand fingers and locate the contact lens. Slowly slide the lens upwards by placing the upper eyelid margin at lower edge of lens. Once centered, look straight and then downwards, while slowly leaving the eyelids, first leave lower lid then upper lid.
- *Suppose if lens is in the corners of eye:* Wide open the eyelids as above, now locate the lens by lateral eye movements. Once lens gets centered, look straight and then downwards. Now slowly leave the eyelids one by one, first lower followed by upper lid.

Wearing schedule

- Patients are advised to practice the insertion and removal of RGP lenses for initial 2–3 days, once they feel confident and comfortable, regular wearing of lenses should be started.
- Gradually the wearing time is increased, in case of RGP lenses. First wear the lens for 1–2 hours and see the response in terms of visual acuity, comfort and ocular symptoms. If comfortable, then wear the lenses regularly for 2 hours everyday, for 3–4 days.
- When there is no symptom then gradually the wearing time is increased on daily one hour basis, at 3–4 days interval.
- Once a constant wearing of 6–8 hours is reached, say roughly in 30–45 days, then patient can wear these lenses regularly during their duty hours.
- Always remember to remove the lenses after a constant wear for 8 hours and before sleeping time.

Follow-up: Regular follow-up is must to avoid the complication of contact lens wear. Following follow-up visits are mandatory for a comfortable and successful RGP lens wearing

- Day one
- Day three
- Day seven
- After a month
- Every three months
- Every six months
- After one year

Follow-up visit evaluations are essentially similar as in case of a soft contact lens, by taking history, vision and slit lamp examination.

Rigid Contact Lens Related Complications and Management

- **Pain:** Intolerable pain can be experienced after using rigid lenses at various time intervals, which gives a clue about the cause of pain as follows
  - Immediately after wearing rigid lenses the pain may be due to improper insertion technique, foreign body behind the lens, torn lens edges or due to dry lenses.
  - Severe pain a few hours after wearing rigid lenses may be due to corneal edema or abrasions caused by steep fitting lens. Replace the lens after evaluating the lens fitting with fluorescein dye.
  - Sometimes pain may be felt 2–3 hours after removal, which indicates occurrence of over wear syndrome due to micro corneal abrasions and edema caused by tight lens fitting. Give rest period for 2–3 weeks and then advice a flatter lens, once cornea is healed.
- **Watering:** Continuous excessive watering may occur due to unfinished lens edges which cause mechanical irritation, inadequate blinking and corneal edema. Change the lens and advice to clean the lens surface properly before insertion.

- **Burning or scratchy eyes:** Irritation in eye if occurs immediately after insertion of lens, then it is most likely due to contamination of multipurpose cleaning solution or dirty lens. However, if burning or scratchy sensation is felt after 1–2 hours of insertion of lens, then it indicates lens has a steep fit. Sometimes dry eyes, poor blinking and polluted environment may also give this kind of sensation. Change the cleaning solution and sterile the lens. Use a flatter lens if steep fit is found as the cause of irritation.
- **Excessive blinking:** During adaptation period frequent blinking is common however; if it persists even after a few days of wear, then it is essential to find the cause. Small size lens or presence of small foreign body over lens are the common causes of excessive blinking, however, a mucus strand or fogging of lens because of scratches will also induce excessive blinking.
- **Excessive dryness sensation:** Patient may experience continuous dryness feeling due to poor lacrimal secretions, inadequate blinking or tight fit lenses. Treat the cause for better tolerance of lenses and prescribe artificial tears eye drops.
- **Foreign body sensation:** During adaptation period a little foreign body sensations are acceptable, however if they present for a long duration, then search for the causes of it. Mostly the torn edges or too flat lens causes these kinds of sensations, although too thick, large or scratchy lens with conjunctivitis may also give continuous foreign body sensation. Treat the causes and change the lens of appropriate fit.
- **Lens coating in morning:** Sometimes in early morning a milky fluid coating may be seen over the lens. This may be due to collection of Meibomian gland secretions, mucus, proteins or epithelial cells debris over the lens. Rarely, in low grade infections abnormal secretions will deposit over lens. Treat with antibiotics and clean the lens with anti-infective solutions.

- **Lid swelling in evening:** During adaptation period very mild swelling of lids may be seen which subsides on its own once patient is accustomed to lens. If lid swelling is present even after adaptation period, then probably edges of lens or steep fit lens is the cause. Remove the lens and change as per proper fitting guidelines.
- **Visual disturbances:** Several visual disturbances may occur while person is wearing a rigid contact lens. These symptoms can be grouped as
  - *Fluctuation in vision:* Initial fluctuation in vision may be present during adaptation period, which improves on its own. However, if it appears later then excessive watering or small size lens are the causes. Treat the cause of watering and change the lens size to achieve a stable clear vision.
  - *Visual changes with head posture:* Flatter lenses move excessively over the cornea, so patients have tendency to tilt their head upwards to keep the lens in the center position for better vision. Change the lens with smaller diameter for central fit and thus decreases the lens movement. Sometimes the visual acuity may improve by head shaking or head bending, this is due to poorly centered lens. Change the base curve and TD of lens to achieve better centration and stable vision.
  - *Blurring in distance vision:* Blurring for distance vision may be seen in early phase of lens wear. Common reasons are excessive watering, improper lens power or uncorrected astigmatism, poor quality lenses or scratched lens surfaces. Do an over refraction and examine the lens in white light, check the power of lens with lensometer. In late phase blurring of distance vision may be caused by corneal edema or warpage of contact lens. In both conditions simply change the lens with appropriate fit.
  - *Blurring in near vision:* In a pre pre-sbyopic age group, if distance vision is clear and blurring of near vision is present with contact lens, then the probable causes are improper lens power, decentred lens, and poor fluid exchange underneath lens or severe convergence insufficiency. Change the contact lens if incorrect power or decentration is present. Advice patient to blink frequently for proper tear exchange and do convergence exercises in convergence insufficiency cases.
  - *Blurring in vision after contact lens removal:* Many patients experience blurring of vision, when they remove contact lenses and start wearing spectacles commonly called 'spectacle blur'. Reason for this spectacle blurring are corneal edema or lens-induced corneal curvatural changes.

CHAPTER 14

Contact Lens Specific Conditions, Complications and Maintenance

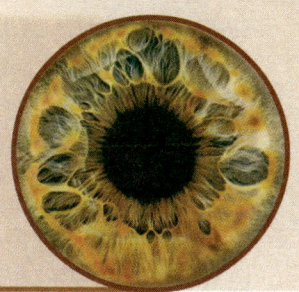

Chapter Outline

SPECIFIC CONTACT LENSES

Extended Wear Contact Lenses

Since invention of contact lenses, some patients either desired, or were selected by their clinicians to wear contact lenses during sleep also. Hence the need for type of contact lenses arose which could act for extended period. In attempt to this, extended wear and continuous wear contact lenses have been developed. Extended wear (EW) lenses are the one, which the patient can wear for six nights continuously followed by a night of no lens wear. Similarly, continuous wear (CW) lenses can be worn up to 30 nights continuously followed by a night of no lens wear.

Indications of extended wear contact lenses

Ideally every person should be prescribed daily wear contact lenses. However, in following situations extended wear contact lens can be used

- In certain persons who are engaged in night duties or irregular working shifts like in case of doctors and nurses, armed force personnels, security persons and emergency staff members, etc. the use of extended wear contact lens is more convenient.
- Young infant or elderly aphakics may also benefit from these lenses because they are incapable or frightened for contact lens insertion, thus to overcome complications related to lens handling and vision limitations, extended wear can be used.
- When patient is not keen to use daily wear contact lenses, because of convenience of extended wear lenses.
- Persons habitual of over wearing or sleeping with contact lenses, require extended wear lenses to avoid complications.

Broadly on the basis of material used and properties, we can group these EW lenses into
- Rigid extended wear contact lenses
- Silicon hydrogel extended wear contact lenses
- Soft hydrogel extended wear contact lenses

Rigid Extended Wear Contact Lenses

Almost all types of rigid contact lenses manufactured for extended wear are gas permeable lenses with medium and / or high Dk values. It is well known that insufficient oxygen supply to eye may cause edema of cornea. Extended wear contact lenses either RGP or silicon hydrogel allow sufficient supply of oxygen to the cornea and meet criteria of zero additional swelling.

Indications: RGP extended wear lenses are indicated in the following conditions in addition to abovementioned indications.
- Patients facing visual problems with toric extended wear soft contact lenses.
- Severe metabolic problems such as edema and hypoxia with soft hydrogel extended wear lenses.
- Medical problems like allergies, giant papillary conjunctivitis, or superior limbic keratoconjunctivitis associated with use of soft extended wear contact lenses.
- Patients having high refractive errors (hypermetropia or myopia) requiring thick lenses or toric bifocals lenses.

Several studies showed that rigid contact lens wear is usually associated with greater degree of hypoxia leading to decrease in corneal epithelial barrier function. Hence, recommended RGP contact lenses for extended wear purpose should have the highest oxygen transmissibility and fastest rate of tear exchange so that an adequate barrier function of corneal epithelium remains maintained.

Lens fitting and wearing schedule are essentially similar to basic RGP lenses of daily wear type. Although in some specific cases, such as papillary conjunctivitis, corneal decompensation, etc. extended wear RGP lenses are not recommended.

Initially, patient is advised to wear RGP contact lens on daily basis for a week, and then gradually extend their wear duration, preferably up to 5–6 nights continuously. For a successful, uncomplicated extended lens wear, lens should be removed for one night, then after cleaning and rinsing lens can be worn again for 6 nights.

Follow-up: Regular follow-up is must to prevent complications related to extended wear; a usual follow up schedule is after

- 24–48 hours of initial lens wear
- One week of lens insertion
- One month or at time of removal, cleaning, disinfecting and reinsertion of lens

On every follow-up visit a thorough examination for proper lens fit and clinical signs are done. Generally during slit lamp examination a special attention is given for:

- Contact lens depositions
- Lens adhesion
- 3–9 o'clock staining
- Persistent corneal striae
- Epithelial microcysts
- Contact lens bending or indentation

Complications of rigid extended wear contact lenses: Complications and lens related problems in extended wear lenses are more common and more pronounced as compared to daily wear RGP lenses.

Chances of infections are less but caution is required in case of lens adhesion because of increased risk of corneal ulceration. Low riding lenses should be avoided because there is increase risk of adhesion to cornea. Risk of adhesion further increased with use of lens material having high *Dk* value, thin lens and inadequate edge lift of lens. To avoid adhesion it is advised to use thick, flatter fitting rigid lens with medium *Dk/t* value (~100) with adequate edge lift.

3 and 9 o' clock staining usually does not cause discomfort but with continuous use of lens severe injection of conjunctiva can occur. It is more common with use of low riding, thick edge lens as well as in person who blink incompletely. Prolonged 3 and 9 o' clock staining may lead to vascularization in horizontal meridian. Sometimes, there may be contact lens induced papillary conjunctivitis due to hypersensitivity reaction or irritation.

Silicon Hydrogel Extended Wear Contact Lenses

The silicon hydrogel (Si-Hy) lenses were introduced in 1999 with the aim to increase the oxygen transmission through lens which was main limitation factor with the use of soft hydrogel lenses. As a result the wearing of lens for extended period became safer and comfortable with availability of these types of lens. The Si-Hy lenses contain both properties, i.e. increase oxygen permeability due to presence of silicon and hydrophilic nature of hydrogel lens. However, these lens material demonstrated less wettability and more chances of lipid depositions than hydrogel lens materials. As a result to improve the wettability the lenses were surface treated or added with other materials.

A wide range of Si-Hy material extended wear lenses are available, for up to 30 nights of continuous wear and/or for six nights of extended wear. These lens materials show a significant advancement in lens design, so that complications usually associated with lens induced corneal hypoxia, such as limbal redness, epithelial and stromal edema, vascularization of cornea, endothelial polymegathism and myopic shifts are rare.

Although several advantages are present with Si-Hy lenses, but a few disadvantages are

- Si-Hy materials are more stiff in nature as compared to soft hydrogel material (HEMA or Etafilcon A), hence during blinking can create more negative pressure beneath the contact lens. As a result, chances of development of mechanical arcuate lesions and local papillary conjunctivitis are more.
- Increased frequency of formation of mucin balls with overnight wearing for a long period, especially more common in eyes having steeper corneal curvature.

Various hydrogel contact lens materials and their respective properties are summarized in Table 14.1.

Table 14.1: Various hydrogel contact lens material and their respective properties

Material	Water content (%)	Max Dk/t	Min Dk/t	Surface modification	Other technology
Asmofilcon A	40	161	70	Nanoglass plasma coating	Menisilk
Balafilcon A	33	84	38	Plasma oxidation	None
Comfilcon A	48	145	64	None	Aquaform technology
Enfilcon A	46	125	55	None	Aquaform technology
Filcon II 3	58	86	–	None	Aquagen process
Galyfilcon A	47	107	37	None	Hydraclear technology
lotrafilcon B	36	101	45	Plasma polymerization	Aqua moisture system
Etafilcon A	58	26	8	None	None
Narafilcon A	46	118	47	None	Hydraclear technology
lotrafilcon A	24	203	68 to 140	Plasma polymerization	Aqua moisture system

Soft Hydrogel Extended Wear Contact Lenses

Soft hydrogel extended wear lenses were familiarized by John de Carle with Permalens and in the year 1981 soft hydrogel extended wear contact lenses got an approval from FDA for cosmetic purpose. Soft hydrogel extended wear contact lenses can be used continuously for 30 nights. After 30 days lens should be removed, cleaned, disinfected and then reinserted. However, these lenses as compared to rigid gas permeable and silicon hydrogel (Si-Hy) do not allow sufficient oxygen to the cornea, thus incapable to accomplish the criteria of zero additional swelling with overnight wear.

Lens fitting: Instrumentation required for fitting of extended wear soft contact lenses is essentially same as for all other basic contact lens fitting. History and symptoms are elicited from patient before fitting extended wear contact lenses, specifically to fully understand and to find out the reasons of patient's desire for overnight lens wear. Although, the fundamental principles of extended wear soft contact lens fitting are similar to fitting for daily wear, however, most important concern is to provide maximum oxygen supply to the eye along with enough tear exchange so that debris formed behind lens can be removed effectively.

Wearing schedule: Initially it is recommended to wear soft lenses for 24 hours and observe the symptoms and clinical condition of eyes. If patient is asymptomatic and comfortable, then these lenses wear can be extended for week period. Gradually, these lenses can be worn for longer durations, usually 25–30 days.

Follow-up: Regular follow-up is the key to avoid complications such as microbial keratitis and lens depositions. Normal follow-up visits are planned after:
- Day one
- One month
- Two–four months or during removal and reinsertion of lens

On every visit a detailed slit lamp examination for lens fit and corneal condition is done. In case of any complication lenses are removed and reinserted after resolution of problem.

Complication with soft EW lens: The EW soft lenses can cause all those complications related to daily wear soft lenses. However, use of EW soft lenses carry more risk for development of

- Ulcerative keratitis: Wearing of lens for extended period may alter morphology of corneal epithelium and predispose to infections.
- Corneal vascularization
- Deposition of protein and mucus on contact lens
- Tight lens syndrome: There is sudden development of painful red eye. On examination, lens is immobile and moderately dehydrated. Corneal edema develops due to poor oxygenation, also flare and cells are seen in anterior chamber. To treat this condition, lens should be removed for 1–2 weeks for healing and to prevent infections. Once the eye is normal, lens with looser fitting should be prescribed.

Rigid versus soft extended wear contact lenses: High *Dk/t* RGP extended wear contact lenses have several advantages and disadvantages over soft hydrogel lenses as summarized in Table 14.2.

Extended wear versus daily wear contact lenses: Extended wear contact lenses have several advantages over daily wear lenses such as

- Simple and convenient for patients to wear.

Table 14.2: Various advantages and disadvantages of rigid EW lens over soft extended wear contact lenses

Advantages	Disadvantages
Enhanced oxygen transmissibility	Adhesion phenomenon
Active tear pump mechanism	Poor initial wearing comfort
Lesser lens deposits	Difficult fitting procedure
Better reproducibility	3 and 9 o'clock staining
Superior optical quality	
Maintenance of lens parameters for a long period	
Zero additional swelling with overnight wear	

- Needs lesser handling and maintenance as compared to daily wear.
- Cost effective.

However, extended wear lenses has a few disadvantages such as

- Greater incidence of overall complications as compared to daily wear lenses.
- Increased risk of microbial keratitis, because of overnight use.

Patients should be given full information regarding associated risks and benefits with an overnight or extended wear and then asked to make the choice of contact lens type. Hence, it is important that a discussion should include risk comparison with other lens types and wearing modalities even a comparison to refractive surgery. Once patient accepts this increased risk with extended wear, then clinician decide on best course of action.

Disposable Contact Lenses

These may be grouped as

- Daily wear disposable contact lenses
- Extended wear disposable contact lenses

Daily wear disposable contact lenses: These daily wear disposable lenses are sometimes confused with simple daily wear contact lenses. The daily wear disposable lenses are the one, which are worn during awakening time, only for one day. Once removed from the eye, these lenses are thrown away and not used again, whereas daily wear lenses after removal from the eye can be worn again in the next morning after overnight treatment in cleaning solution.

Over past decade, a significant increase in the demand of daily disposable contact lenses has been noticed all over the world because these lenses provide more convenience of wearing and are associated with decreased risk of complications. Various types of 'comfort enhanced' daily disposable lenses have been developed to decrease the chances of dryness and discomfort among the wearers. Selection of daily disposable contact lens for a patient will depend on the total of convenience offered by lens to the wearer as well as on the health and compliance of patient for wearing the lens. As compliance is better and risk of complications is less in the teenage group, these lenses are more preferred in this age group.

Comfort enhancing daily wear disposable contact lenses is mainly classified into three groups depending on their mechanism of action

- *Lens made up of poly HEMA materials and co-polymers:* The copolymers have property to retain water. For example, Acuvue Moist contact lens (Etafilcon A) has an embedded copolymer called polyvinyl pyrrolidone (PVP), which works as a water holding agent, hence rate of dehydration of lens is reduced during lens wear.
- *Lens made up of poly HEMA materials with lubricating additives:* These are also made up of poly HEMA material, although in place of water retaining molecules these lens materials have lubricating additives coatings. These lubricating additives are usually present in packaging saline, used for storage of lens. For example, in case of SofLens daily disposable, a high water content material poloxamine is added in the saline solution which coats the lens surface and then slowly released into tear film when these contact lenses are inserted in the eye.
- *Lens made from polyvinyl alcohol (PVA):* PVA is a water-soluble non-toxic polymer, commonly used in lubricating eye drops and lens solutions. When these lenses are prepared using PVA, some of the PVA remains in unpolymerized (free) form in the matrix of contact lens. After wearing the lens due to blinking this free form of PVA is slowly released from the contact lens into the tear film. For example, Focus Dailies All Day Comfort (Nelfilcon A). Furthermore, addition of other substances like hydroxy propyl methylcellulose (HPMC) and polyethy-

lene glycol (PEG), which are present in packaging saline, further maintain the release of PVA for a long period. For example, Focus Dailies Aqua Comfort Plus (Nelfilcon A Plus).

For daily wear disposable lenses, maximum wearing time suggested is summarized in Table 14.3.

These types of contact lenses are indicated particularly for daily disposable wear, hence should be discarded after removal from the eye. As these lenses are disposed of after every single daily use, risk of developing giant papillary conjunctivitis is reduced significantly. Daily disposable lenses provide more comfort in patient than other contact lenses which are worn for a long period especially, in those patients who feel discomfort and itching due to allergies.

Extended wear disposable contact lenses: These lenses are also disposed off, once removed from the eye, however, these lenses can be worn continuously for either six days (weekly) or thirty days (monthly), once inserted in the eye. Because of their longer duration of continuous wear, these lenses are called extended wear contact lenses. However, they differ from simple extended wear contact lenses which can be used again after removal from the eye.

Introduction of weekly replaced disposable lenses has resolved two major issues, i.e. corneal hypoxia and corneal edema. These lenses are worn for six continuous nights and then disposed, hence are referred as disposable extended wear lenses.

Table 14.3: Wearing schedule of daily wear disposable contact lenses

Day	Hours
1	4–6
2	7–8
3	9–10
4	11–12
5	12–14
6 and afterwards	All awakening hours

Disposable contact lenses are available for various wearing and disposing schedules such as they can be worn either on the daily basis or on extended wear basis. These lenses are available for daily, weekly, fortnightly or monthly disposable schedule. Generally wearing schedule is decided by the treating consultant, however, it vary a little for daily wear or extended wear disposable contact lenses.

Patients should be given following warnings related to extended contact lens wear:

- Eye discomfort
- Excessive tearing
- Eye redness
- Visual changes or diminution of vision

Note: Several ocular problems including corneal ulcers may develop rapidly which can lead to visual loss.

Extended wear disposable hydrogel contact lenses as compared to conventional non-disposable continuous wear lenses are found beneficial only in carefully selected patients with strict follow-up schedule. However, a significant hypoxia related adverse events and marked microbial keratitis is noted in many EW lens wearers as compared to conventional non-disposable continuous wear lenses.

Examples of disposable contact lenses are

- AVAIRA contact lenses exist in various lens designs form such as spheric, aspheric, toric and multifocal. These lenses are prepared using material comprising 46% water and 54% Enfilcon A (silicon containing

hydrogel). A tint (phthalocyanine blue) has been added, so that the contact lens becomes more visible, hence can easily be handled. An additional UV absorbing monomer is also added in lens to block UV radiation.

- Various disposable lenses and their properties are summarized in Table 14.4.

Scleral RGP Lenses

RGP lenses when rest over sclera are termed scleral RGP lenses. These lenses cover the entire corneal surface and form a fluid vault for oxygenation of cornea. Majority of newer types of scleral contact lenses are made up of high oxygen permeable materials for better tolerance.

Scleral RGP lenses are grouped into following categories, depending upon overall diameter as

- Corneo-scleral (12.9 to 13.5 mm)
- Semi-scleral (13.6 to 14.9 mm)
- Mini-scleral (15.0 to 18.0 mm)
- Scleral (>18.0 mm)

Indications

Corneal conditions:

Scleral lenses are indicated in cases of irregular cornea, diseased cornea and healthy cornea. Usually corneo-scleral lenses are used in irregular cornea and healthy cornea, whereas scleral lenses are used for scarred and severely pathological cornea.

Several conditions where scleral lens can be used are

- Naturally occurring ecstatic cornea: Like in young children and adults with keratoconus,

Lens series	Lens material	Water content	Lens diameter
Precision UV	Varsurfilcon A	74 %	14.5 mm
Actifresh 400	MMA / VP	55%	14.3 mm
Proclear	Omafilcon A	62%	14.2 mm
Soflens 66	Alphafilcon A	66%	14.2 mm
Acuvue	Genfilcon	48%	14 mm
Dalies	Nelfilcon A	69%	13.8 mm

Table 14.4: Various types of disposable contact lenses and their respective properties

pellucid marginal degeneration and forme fruste keratoconus.

- Secondary corneal ectasias: Post-surgery ectasias, post-corneal transplantation, post-infarcts corneal cross-linking.

Intolerance to corneal RGP or hydrogel lenses

is seen in the following conditions like

- Refractive conditions: Lens decentration in high refractive errors
- In dry eye
    - Due to ocular disease: Alkali burn, ocular pemphigoid, Steven Johnson syndrome, neurotrophic keratitis, Sjögren syndrome, filamentary keratitis.
    - Due to reduced tear meniscus, decreased tear production, conjunctival hyperemia—as seen in early or contact lens related dry eye.

Scleral Contact Lens Fitting Technique

Insertion technique

- To check lens fitting, fill the lens completely with isotonic, non-preserved artificial tears and add one drop of fluorescein from a strip.
- Scleral lens is either supported on a large DMV scleral suction cup or a tripod made by using thumb, middle, and index finger, as shown in Fig. 14.1A.

- Retract upper and lower eyelids as shown in Fig. 14.1B with the help of thumb and index finger of other hand while keeping the face parallel to the ground.
- Slowly raise the contact lens onto the eye in one continuous motion, then slowly release the eyelids before lowering the supporting suction cup.
- Suppose a large air bubble is seen underneath lens, either the lens was not inserted in one continuous motion or the lens cup was not completely filled with solution.
- Remove the lens and reinsert as shown in Fig. 14.1B.

Lens removal technique

- Scleral lenses are generally held by the force of suction so always loosen these lenses before removal.
- Put a few drops of rewetting solution and then inferior peripheral portion of lens is gently pushed in repeated motions for some seconds.
- Keep the upper eyelid in steady position and lower eyelid is used to raise the lower portion of contact lens, away from the eye. Otherwise, a medium DMV suction cup can be placed over the lower peripheral portion of contact lens, slowly pull the cup in

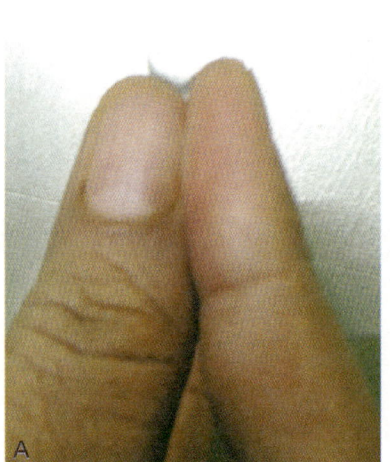
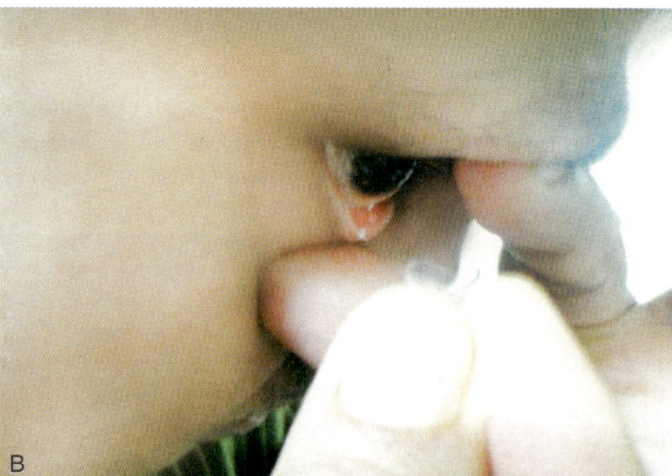

Fig. 14.1: A. Tripod of fingers; B. Insertion technique of scleral contact lens

downward and outward direction with force directed perpendicular to the lens surface.

Fitting principles: Most important principle for scleral lens fitting is that lens should vault the cornea entirely while lens is aligned to the bulbar conjunctiva. To achieve this fit following parameters need to be checked

Overall diameter

- Generally, lenses with large diameter can retain more fluid in the corneal chamber thus allow more clearance over the cornea, hence are more convenient for the user, whereas lenses smaller in diameter vault the cornea more strongly thus they require more accurate central fit.

- In case of irregular corneas, always choose a lens of larger diameter, although some lens manufacturers provide guidelines for selecting an overall diameter based on HVID.

Initial trial lens

- We can follow the lens manufacturer's fitting guide to select a trial lens, however, a simple clinical approach can be tried to assess the trial lens base curve.

- Stand on the side of the patient while examining shape and profile of the cornea. Suppose cornea appears very steep, select a steeper base curve similarly, if cornea appears flat then select a flatter base curve. For an average profile cornea, select an average base curve.

- Scleral lenses are fit on the basis of sagittal height, hence clinical assessment is an effective method when properly done.

Corneal fit examination

- On slit lamp optical section is made using white light and then in high illumination with medium magnification, examine the central corneal clearance.

- Various layers can be observed in cross section, the outermost band of dark black color is due to scleral contact lens. This dark area is surrounded by two thin reflections from the front and back surface of contact lens. Now, compare the thickness of this black layer with the green layer of tear lens.

- Suppose, if thickness of black layer (trial lens) is 300 microns and on examination the green layer is appearing approximately of half thickness than black band, then it tells that lens is vaulting the cornea by 125–150 microns which is considered an ideal clearance for a non- fenestrated lens design. Different trial lens are tried until a proper central corneal clearance value is not obtained.

- Usually all types of scleral lenses take 30–40 minutes time to settle into the conjunctiva. Scleral trial lenses showing gross excessive vaulting should be removed and replaced with a flatter base curve lens.

Correlation of corneal and peripheral fitting

- Scleral contact lens fit can be considered in two parts
  - Central fit is over the cornea and commonly called "corneal chamber"
  - Peripheral fit is over the conjunctiva.

- Entire corneal chamber should be examined with diffuse cobalt blue light in high illumination and medium magnification. Observe areas of lens-corneal touch (bearing) as in case of a corneal RGP contact lens.

- In an irregular cornea, commonly we observe a bearing in mid-peripheral or peripheral regions of cornea however, it is acceptable once central corneal clearance is present. In such a situation an additional clearance is produced in peripheral area, without increasing the central corneal clearance.

- An excessive lens movement or bubble formation underneath lens indicates that peripheral curves are too loose. To correct this condition simply tighten the peripheral curve by choosing scleral lens of an appropriate base curve.

An ideal scleral contact lens fit

An ideal scleral contact lens fit is expressed by the following factors:

- Centered lens
- Minimum 2 mm larger than limbus
- Minimum corneal vault
- No touch or bearing
- Good coverage to limbus
- Edge alignment
- No movement of lens

Over topography

- Many a times it is useful to perform a computerized topography, keeping the scleral contact lens in place, once it had settled for about 15–20 minutes. Topography will show any kind of lens flexure, if present.
- Toricity of >0.5 D may be clinically significant and may affect the vision. It can be corrected by increasing the central thickness of contact lens.

Tear exchange evaluation

- Before dispensing a scleral lens to patient, tear exchange evaluation is done.
- Insert a sterile scleral lens without adding fluorescein dye in filling media.
- Once lens is properly placed, wait for settling period of about 10–15 minutes. Now instill fluorescein dye with a dye strip over the lens surface.
- Periodic examination of tear lens is done to see the presence of dye which moves behind the contact lens into the corneal chamber.
- In ideal conditions, after 20–30 minutes a small amount of dye should be seen in the corneal chamber. Although tear exchange underneath contact lens is not so rapid, but it is significant for a proper lens fit.
- Suppose on examination after sufficient waiting period of 30–40 minutes, no fluorescein dye is observed in the corneal chamber; means it is a steep fit, hence to correct it either peripheral fit must be flattened or overall diameter should be increased.

Therapeutic Contact Lenses

Introduction

Therapeutic contact lenses (TCL) or bandage lenses have emerged as an effective alternative for the management of various eye diseases especially, in recalcitrant cases which show poor response to other treatment modalities. Although TCL is not used as first line treatment in majority of ophthalmic disorders but it can work as an effective adjunctive treatment in various ophthalmic disorders. Due to higher risk of development of microbial infections with TLC, the decision to use these types of lens should be taken with great precautions.

The most important purposes of prescribing the therapeutic contact lenses are

1. To provide relief and comfort from eye pain due to corneal disorders
2. To assist in healing of corneal wound
3. To provide mechanical support and protection to cornea
4. To maintain proper hydration of corneal epithelial surface
5. Also used as drug delivery system

Types of TCL: Therapeutic contact lenses made from both hard and soft lens materials are available, although hydrogels types TLC are more used. Silicon rubber and copolymers are also used to produce specific types of TLC, having good oxygen permeability.

TLC can be classified as

1. Soft hydrogel lens
   - Low water content (38–45%)
   - Mid-water content (45–55%)
   - High water content (67–80%)
2. Hard (PMMA) and gas permeable scleral lenses
3. Hard scleral rings
4. Silicon rubber and silicon hydrogels (38%)
5. Collagen shields having $Dk/L = 63\%$ water content soft lens.

Various commercially available therapeutic contact lenses are summarized in Table 14.5.

Table 14.5: Various types of commercially available therapeutic contact lenses and their properties

Lens type	Lens material	Water content	Total diameter (mm)
Hydrogels			
Plano	HEMA	38.6%	14
Plano	Polymacon	38.6%	13.5 /14.5
Plano ES 70	MMA / VP	70%	15
Troy		85%	15–20
Igel	Igel 67/ 77	67% / 77%	14.5
Collagen shields			
Bio-Cor type I	Porcine		
Chiron type I	Bovine		
Silicon rubber			
Silflex	Polysiloxane		11.7–13.7
Scleral lenses	Scleral sealed		~ 22

Choice of TCL from available TCLs will depend on main purpose for use (as discussed above) and on the physiological requirement of a pathological cornea, etc.

Fitting of a TCL: Fitting of a TCL is very simple if following guidelines are follows which are chiefly for soft TCL because these are most commonly used TCLs in various ocular conditions.

- Keratometry is usually of very little help because due to associated underlying corneal pathology there may be formation of irregular mires. Thus, a trial lens fitting is suggested. However, keratometry readings of other normal eye may be helpful.
- During fitting the use of topical anesthetics (except in a few conditions) should be avoided because it will mask the pain arising due to poor lens fit.
- Ideally, to check the dehydration effects on lens, the fitting must be evaluated at an interval of 20 and 60 minutes.

TCL fit should be assessed on slit lamp both in terms of central fit and peripheral fit.

- An ideal central fit TCL will provide good corneal coverage with proper mobility characteristics.
- Similarly, peripheral lens fit is also necessary to check because flared edges of

lens may give rise to discomfort to patient and adhered edges indicate tight lens fit.

- It is recommended to keep several lens designs with similar parameters available at time of insertion because if one particular lens design fails to produce desired lens fit, then another lens design may fit well.
- Generally, the excessive steep or flat lens should not be used for fitting. However, in some conditions like corneal edema or cornea epithelium defects, a TCL of flatter fitting may be preferred. On the other hand, steeper fitting TLC may be used in patients having irregular corneal topography.

Indications for use of therapeutic contact lenses: Therapeutic contact lenses are used in various diseases of cornea. In treatment of various ocular conditions which cause abnormalities in epithelium of cornea, the relief from pain is the most common and important part of treatment and these lenses can be used to relieve the pain effectively in these conditions.

Bullous Keratopathy: Use of TCL in following patients of intractable bullous keratopathy is very useful

- Patient of bullous keratopathy presenting with a painful blind eye.
- Patient is not fit for graft surgery.

- As a temporary relief measure in those patient who are waiting for penetrating keratoplasty.

These patients should be prescribed with TCL as early as possible. Use of TCL in these patients is associated with relief in pain as well as some improvement in vision. Relief in pain is probably due to protection of nerves by TCL which are exposed due to rupture of bullae. In some patients vision is also improved as irregular cornea is covered by regular surface of contact lens. In bullous keratopathy patients the movement of lens should be minimal but must be sufficient enough to allow adequate tear flow beneath the TCL. Hydrogel TCL of large diameter having high water content (Duragel 75, Plano ES70, etc.) can be used which maintain maximum oxygen permeability for constant wear. For temporary purposes, a thin high water content TCL can be used to decrease the risk of corneal vascularization.

Thygeson's superficial punctate keratitis: It is a recurrent and chronic disorder described by presence of small and oval punctate corneal opacities of grey white color on cornea. Exact cause is not known but may be viral or immunological in origin. Corneal opacities cause warpage of corneal epithelial surface and reduced visual acuity. High water content extended-wear TCL (sometimes low water content) can be used for treatment of severe cases. The lens acts as a pressure bandage and improves symptoms of pain and foreign body sensation by covering the corneal lesions and nerves.

Superior limbic keratoconjunctivitis: It is a chronic inflammatory disease involving conjunctiva (superior bulbar), limbus and upper part of cornea, characterized by foreign body sensation, photophobia, and ocular pain. Along with other therapeutic modatilities soft TCL especially of large diameter are very effective in relieving the severe pain and symptoms associated with superior limbic keratoconjunctivitis cases. TCL with relatively large TD is used till symptoms and signs are disappeared.

Filamentary keratitis: It is a disease of eye in which filaments of mucus and degenerated epithelial cells get deposit on surface of cornea, usually it is self-limiting in most of the cases. The treatment includes topical therapy with artificial tears and lubricants. Cases which do not respond to lubricants alone, low water content disposable TCLs can be used along with steroids, topical antibiotics and atropine. Filaments get resolved usually in 4–5 days and within 2–3 weeks a complete disappearance of filaments may be seen; however filaments may recur after some time.

TCL are also effectively used for corneal healing in various recalcitrant cases which are poorly responding to routine medical treatment like in the following conditions.

Recurrent corneal erosion: Disturbance of corneal epithelial basement membrane due to anterior membrane dystrophies (Map dot finger dystrophy or Cogan dystrophy) or trauma may result in recurrent breakdown of corneal epithelium causing damage of corneal surface (corneal erosions). Majority of patients usually remain asymptomatic throughout their life but nearly 10–15% may develop recurrent erosion syndrome manifesting in form of pain and photophobia and foreign body sensations. Most patients of recurrent erosions are treated with lubricants and hypertonic saline, however, a disposable bandage contact lens (usually thick, high water content extended wear type preferred) can be used as an extended wear lens for 2, 3 or even 6 months duration, as per requirement. Before placing TCL, the affected area of corneal epithelium should be debride completely and irrigate with saline. Ultra thin TCL are not indicated due to possible chances of buckling of lens. Corneal abrasion (<5 mm) due to trauma can be managed by topical eye drops and eye pad. If the size of abrasion is more than 5 mm, then it can be treated by the use of TCL, because epithelium heals more quickly with disposable TCL as compared to conventional methods of treatment.

Persistent epithelial defects of cornea: When an epithelial defect of cornea does not heal or remain persistent for more than two weeks, the cornea get highly vulnerable to infection, ulceration, perforation and scarring.

Soft disposables TCL are very useful as they protect corneal surface from mechanical trauma by eyelids and gives time to newly formed epithelial to get attach to newly secreted basement membrane. Soft contact lenses with high oxygen permeability are more preferred to reduce chances of corneal edema and neovascularization. Collagen shields hydrated with acidic fibroblast growth factor (FGF) can be also used to promote healing of epithelial defects.

Chemical injuries: Chemical injuries to eye result in breakdown of collagen leading to widespread damage to cornea, epithelial surfaces, etc. and formation of stromal ulcer. The purpose of TCL is to prevent the further progression of ulcer formation by preventing transfer of photolytic enzymes from tear fluid to corneal stroma. Due to presence of chemosis and epithelium defect, TCLs of small total diameter (~12 mm) are first choice of treatment. Hydrophilic lens with high oxygen permeability are more preferred because they help in epithelial migration and promote epithelial stromal adhesion. Scleral lens can also be prescribed if lids are also involved in injuries. In case of corneal melting due to injury cyanoacrylate tissue adhesive can be applied and then covered with TCL.

Epithelial disorders following surgical procedures: Temporary corneal epithelial defects may occur after many surgical procedures on eyes like vitrectomy, cataract extraction, post-penetrating keratoplasty, epikeratoplasty, kerato-refractive procedures (PRK, LASIK), etc. Soft and/or collagen TCL can be used to decrease the chances of epithelial trauma after surgery which promotes rapid epithelial healing.

Penetrating keratoplasty: In case of perforation of an existing corneal graft the silicon rubber TCL can be used. TCL can also be used if epithelial healing is delayed, epithelial filaments are formed or loose sutures are present after PK procedure.

TCL, in various designs and of different materials can also be used to provide mechanical protection and support like in cases of corneal thinning, perforation or corneal trauma so that the need of immediate surgery or corneal grafting is delayed or minimized. Various types of lens like hydrophilic TCL, scleral lenses or rings and silicon rubber lenses can be used to provide mechanical support to cornea.

Corneal perforation: Use of a TCL gives structural support and maintains integrity of an eye if applied in case of small corneal perforation (<2 mm) with no loss of tissue. Healing rate is faster if lesions are small and noninfected. In addition, lacerations or perforations which lie adjacent to limbus and in well vascularized area respond faster on TCL application. As compared to suturing the small corneal perforations heal better and with very less degree of resultant astigmatism. Thin, low water content soft contact lenses are usually first choice.

Corneal wound leakage: Anterior segment wound leakage may occur secondary to surgery like post-cataract surgery and penetrating keratoplasty, trabeculectomy etc. Majority of leaks are mild and self healing. In moderate wound leakage thin low water content soft TCL can be placed. The lens will help in the wound healing by decreasing flow of aqueous to wound and promotes re-epithelialization and vascularization. Sometimes, even collagen shields can be placed in the eye at the time of surgery and then hydrophilic TCL after 24 hours of surgery. Post-trabeculectomy a leaking drainage bleb may form either just after procedure or after several days or weeks. TCL of large size (TD = 20 mm) with high water content (e.g. Mega soft 76.5%) can be placed which compress over the leaking bleb to prevent excessive drainage.

Thinning of cornea: Patients with a thin cornea have very high chance of perforation and usually present with a descemetocele. In such cases, hydrophilic TCL can be prescribed which act as a corneal splint and slows down the rate of corneal thinning and ultimately prevent corneal perforation. If corneal thinning is due to dry eyes, then silicon rubber lenses are better choice.

Protection of the cornea: In various conditions of eyes like entropion, trichiasis, eye exposure due to lid deformities, cranial nerve palsies, etc. epithelium of cornea can easily damage due to trivial trauma, hence TCL are used to protect the cornea. TCLs especially scleral lenses, are very useful to provide protection to cornea and comfort in cases of trigeminal or facial nerve palsy.

Various ocular pathologies can lead to dehydration of cornea which ultimately leads to corneal blindness, hence TCL are used to maintain corneal hydration in various conditions as follows

Cicatrizing conjunctival disease: Cicatrization of conjunctiva with involvement of cornea may occur in diseases such as Stevens-Johnson syndrome, ocular pemphigoid, chemical burns, trachoma and dry eye. In Stevens-Johnson syndrome, a thick TCL of low or medium water content having large TD (15–20 mm) can be used to prevent formation of adhesions, however, scleral lenses are more useful. Alternatively, a silicon rubber lens can also be effective in selective recalcitrant cases. Chemical burns due to strong alkali lead to severe ocular damage. The TCL can be prescribed in the later phase of treatment to promote epithelial healing and to protect the fornix from mechanical forces of eyelids. TCLs like Mega soft bicurve TCLs or scleral lenses or scleral rings can be placed to prevent symblepharon reformation.

Dry eye: It is most commonly encountered clinical problem in ophthalmology. Dry eyes occurring as a result of secondary causes like keratoconjunctivits siccca, Stevens-Johnson syndrome, ocular pemphigoid, etc. can be prescribed lens specially silicon rubber lenses which provide hydration to the cornea.

TCL as drug delivery devices: TCL can be used as drug delivery devices for treatment of some ocular diseases. Hydrogel soft lens impregnated with medications when placed on the cornea usually delivers high levels of medication in eyes as compared to topical eye drops. Several drugs such as pilocarpine, corticosteroids, antibiotics, antifungal and antiviral, etc. can be delivered through contact lens for treatment of glaucoma, herpes simplex infections, fungal ulcers, etc. The thickness and water content of lens and molecular weight may affect delivery of drug through contact lens. The use of TCL for drug delivery for prolonged time may be associated with increased risks of harmful reactions due to direct contact of cornea with drugs.

General instructions to patients: Proper care as per following guidelines of therapeutic contact lenses is must to achieve the best results.
- Cleaning and disinfection of TCL are done at least once in every 15 days.
- Proper size and adequate water content are prerequisite for good outcome; hence TD and water content are kept as per the requirement in a particular ocular condition.
- Specific suitable prophylactic topical antibiotic drops are used to prevent secondary infections.
- Never use a TCL for more than 6 months duration, however, some TCL requires to be changed even at 1 or 2 months intervals.
- Never apply certain topical drops such as fluorescein, hypotonic saline, phenylephrine or gels over TCL.
- In case of severe burning, irritation, chemosis or enhancement of symptoms report immediately to ophthalmologist.
- Always consult before insertion or removal of a therapeutic contact lens.

Complications of therapeutic contact lenses: Although, complications related to TCL are similar to those seen with an extended wear contact lens. Several complications related to therapeutic contact lens wear are
- Microbial keratitis is most serious complication.

- Ulcers induced by TCL wear.
- Giant papillary conjunctivitis (GPC).
- Neovascularisation.

For prevention of complications prophylactic antibiotics with TCL can be beneficial in short term, although role of antibiotic is highly controversial.

Colored Contact Lenses

Introduction

Colored contact lenses can be used for cosmetic, therapeutic, occupational or prosthetic purposes. Although, by many practitioners, all colored contact lenses are considered as cosmetic contact lens but soft hydrogel contact lenses are colored for various clinical indications also. Generally, hard or rigid contact lenses are not colored because it is difficult to center them on the cornea and are small in size, hence they do not serve the desired purpose. Several lens manufacturers have developed colored soft hydrogel contact lenses for cosmetic or prosthetic purposes. These lenses are also available in various refractive powers and thus can be used as an alternative to the regular soft contact lenses.

Various desirable properties in an ideal colored contact lens are

- Clarity and purity
- Quality and safety
- Color stability
- Reproducibility
- Variable lens designs
- Biocompatibility
- Heat tolerance

Indications: Colored lenses can be used in various ocular and non-ocular conditions

Ocular conditions: As a prosthetic colored contact lenses either to treat or as an adjuvant treatment modality can be used in the following ocular conditions

- Corneal pathologies like disfigured cornea or scarred cornea, either due to disease or trauma. In patients having leucocoria or white opacity with no light perception, these dark colored lenses are used to produce cosmetic relief.
- Visual problems due to photophobia or diplopia need colored contact lenses as treatment modality. Conditions like albinism, aniridia, fixed pupil causes excessive light entry and macular complications; here black colored contact lenses with small clear central pupillary area are needed. Similarly, amblyopia and diplopia due to any reason need an occluder contact lens having black pupillary area.
- Heterochromia is a condition where color of iris is different in both eyes. These patients need colored contact lenses to match the color of both the eyes.
- In young children, colored lenses can be used for the treatment of strabismus and amblyopia as occlusion therapy. These lenses have black pupil and iris pattern with a clear periphery, so that light does not pass through these lenses.
- Specific type of custom colored tinted lenses are used as low visual aid where central pupillary area is tinted with a specific material to reduce the glare, hence patients having poor vision due to macular pathologies or retinopathies gets benefit by these lenses.
- X chrome colored lenses are used in color deficiency patients which support in identification of colors. ChromaGen tinted color lenses are used to assist in color identification especially, in cases of deuteranopes.
- Colored contact lenses with power can be used in young persons with refractive errors, especially during festive seasons and social gatherings to enhance the looks.

Non-ocular conditions: Colored lenses are used by many persons to enhance the look or for occupational requirements

- Sports persons use colored contact lenses to decrease the glare while driving or playing games.

- Similarly, cinema or television actors need to change the color of eyes according to the demand of role they are performing, hence several colored lens designs are used for this purpose like having black pupil with white iris or different shape large pupils with colored iris patterns.
- Many persons use colored lenses to enhance their looks by wearing various iris patterned contact lenses. These lenses have clear pupil with different iris patterns and tints with a clear periphery. Sometimes power is also incorporated in these lenses if person has associated refractive error.
- ChromaGen custom tinted contact lenses are useful in patients having learning disorders such as dyslexia.

Fitting methods: Fitting guidelines for color lenses are similar to those of a soft hydrogel contact lens.

- Initially a trial soft lens is tried to record the fitting parameters; once the lens fitting is checked as per guidelines, same type of soft lenses with same parameters, material and design are ordered to get tinted as per requirement of patient.
- Commercially several lens manufactures are providing these tinted colored lens in series of power and lens parameters in terms of thickness, total diameter and color pattern.
- In majority of cases where colored lenses are indicated as prosthetic lens to cover up the corneal deformities. The iris size, color and pattern of normal eye should be taken as standard to decide the required lens for deformed eye.
- Ideal fitting of color lens is decided not only by the type of fit, i.e. steep or flat, rather the color comparison between the two eyes is also important.

To summarize the fitting requirements of colored lenses are:

- Measure the pupil size in normal illumination
- Perform keratometry readings and obtain base curve by using a trial lens.
- Measure HVID, if not possible of diseased eye, then of normal eye.
- Get photographs of patient for color matching of lens.

Types of colored CL: Various types of colored lenses have been designed for cosmetic, prosthetic, and occupational purposes. These lenses can be grouped on the basis of colored patterns as follows

- Black pupil with clear mid-periphery and periphery (star burst, **Fig. 14.2A**): These lenses are mainly used to occlude the entry of light in cases such as amblyopia and diplopia. Sometimes, also used for cosmetic purposes in cases such as inoperable mature cataract, subluxated lens or in film industry. Generally, lenses are available with pupil size in the range of 2–5 mm and total diameter of 11–14 mm.
- Black pupil with iris pattern and clear periphery (iris pattern, **Fig. 14.2B**): These types of lens are also available in wide range of pupil size with various iris patterns to meet the requirement of different conditions. Mainly, used for cosmetic purpose in disfigured ocular conditions.
- Clear pupil with iris pattern and clear periphery (limbal rings, **Fig. 14.2C**): These types of lens are available in power (ranging from +6 D to –10 D) as these lenses are mainly used by patients (having refractive errors) during social gathering or special occasions to change the colors of eyes. Lenses are available, in various iris patterns and colors such as blue, hazel, brown, green, etc. according to different requirements. This type of lens can also be used as prosthetic lenses in conditions such as aniridia, heterochromia, albinism, polyocoria, post-iridectomy, and fixed pupil. These lenses have a clear pupil size in the range of 2.5–4.5 mm with iris pattern diameter from 9 to 11.5 mm, having a total diameter up to 15 mm with a clear peripheral zone.

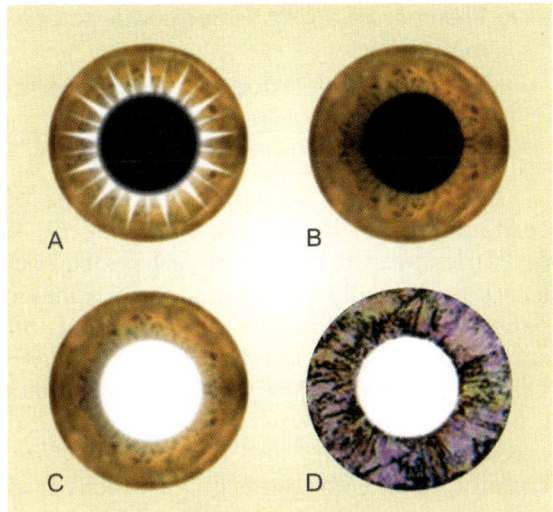

Fig. 14.2: Various types of colored contact lenses. A. Star burst; B. Iris pattern; C. Limbal ring; D. Under print

- Clear pupil with dark periphery (under print, Fig. 14.2D): These lenses are mainly used to cover up the white cornea or disfigured cornea as in cases of leucomatous corneal opacities or phthiscical conditions for cosmetic purposes.

Complications of colored CL: Several complications related to colored contact lenses are similar to those encountered with use soft contact lenses like:

Corneal edema: May be due to decreased oxygen permeability, which in turn is because of excessive thickness of colored lenses as compared to the normal soft hydrogel lenses. In colored lens, the color coating is done in between the two layers of polymer to reduce the dissociation of dye in surrounding tissue, hence the two layers of polymers lead to increase in the thickness and decrease in the oxygen permeability of colored lens. Although in a large number of patients, the ocular condition is severely compromised, hence corneal edema is not a major issue to handle, however, in selected cases these colored lenses needs to be discontinued, if corneal edema occurs.

Protein and lipid deposition: Like all other contact lenses there may be protein and lipids depositions on colored lenses also, rather chances are more of depositions because these lenses are used as prosthetic lenses for longer duration than routine lenses. Chemical treatment can be done to deproteinize these lenses as done for other soft contact lenses.

Similar to soft lenses there may be belching of vessels or discomfort due to tight fit, hence lenses should be changed with a proper fit lenses.

In addition, because of color tinting, many other complications can also occur with these cosmetic lenses such as

Toxic effects: These lenses are colored by using various types of dyes or chemicals to produce the tints and patterns, however, some of these may react with ocular or surrounding tissues to produce the toxic effect. There may be water soluble dye which is poorly hold by polymers and thus slowly dissociates into the surrounding tissues.

Discoloration of lens is another common problem encountered. In most of these colored lenses, water soluble dye is used which slowly dissociate with time and thus clear pupil and/or periphery of lens becomes discolor with time. Strict follow up and timely changing of lens is must to avoid these problems.

Care of colored CL: Care and handling of colored contact lenses are similar to those of a soft contact lens. These lenses are quite stable and heat tolerable, hence can be worn safely. Lens color withstands the chemical disinfectant and enzyme cleaning, hence can safely be cleaned like regular soft lenses. The tints of lenses are quite UV tolerant, so can be worn in hot climate without any additional problem.

Regular follow up and timely cleaning of lenses is the key to a successful wearing of colored contact lenses. Regular follow-up schedule is similar to those of a soft contact lens. In case any problem like red eye, pain, blurring of vision or intolerable foreign body sensation is felt, report immediately to an ophthalmologist.

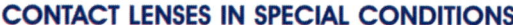

CONTACT LENSES IN SPECIAL CONDITIONS

High Myopia

Contact lens prescribed in the patients of high myopia (>–8 D) not only provide optical benefit (retinal image is larger and normal than glasses) but also helpful for cosmetic purposes. However, contact lens fitting in high myopes needs special attention due to two reasons

- Contact lenses usually ride high due to larger diameter and thick edges.
- Contact lenses base curve should be relatively flatter for proper fit.

As the degree of myopia increases, the edge thickness of contact lens will increase due to increase in the power of contact lens. As a result, thick edges create a base-up wedge effect and lens is pulled up by upper eyelid and lens tends to rise high. It can be reduced by reducing the peripheral thickness and by using lenticular or aspherical lens design. These lens design will decrease the irritation of lids and will prevent tugging of upper eyelid on lens. To minimize the flatness a smaller diameter lens can be used with better fitting, so that flatter edges will not create any problem. Hence, RGP lenses and lenticular design lenses are preferred choice of contact lenses in case of high myopes.

Aphakia

Aphakia means absence of crystalline lens, either due to surgical removal or any congenital condition. In surgical extraction placing an intra-ocular lens at the time of surgery is an ideal option, however, sometimes in very young children or with some associated conditions surgical implantation of intra-ocular lens is not possible. To have a clear vision these patients are dependent either on spectacles or contact lenses.

Contact lenses gives far better quality vision as compared to spectacle in case of aphakia because spectacles in an aphakic patient can produce the following problems

- Magnification of retinal image by 20–25%
- Reduced field of view and poor eccentric acuity
- Presence of a ring scotoma due to prismatic effect
- Pin cushion effect due to spherical aberrations
- Increased demand on convergence

These problems are eliminated by use of contact lenses, hence are very useful in pediatrics and adult patients. Aphakic contact lenses are specially used in monocular aphakic patients with good results. Both RGP and soft contact lenses are used in aphakics with variable results. Majority of aphakic contact lenses are made with a tint to prevent excessive light entry and thus reduce glare. Usually a grey color tint is given which act as a density filter and protects from UV rays.

Soft Contact Lenses in Aphakia

For correction of aphakia by contact lens, both daily wear and extended wear type soft contact lenses can be used. The aphakic contact lenses are rarely used in adult because of availability of newer intraocular lens implant techniques, however, in pediatric and elderly patients these contact lenses are still used with variable results.

- In young children, an extended wear lens is better choice than daily wear lens, because it is difficult to teach them the insertion and removal techniques of lens.
- In infants, the contact lenses should be prescribed immediately after cataract extraction because of potential risk of developing amblyopia, however, in adults it is advised to wait for at least two months after surgery, so that corneal topography and keratometry gets stabilized.
- There is an increased risk of neovascularisation and infection with use of extended wear contact lenses, hence daily wear lenses should be preferred wherever possible.
- Soft aphakic contact lenses are relatively thick and pose discomfort, hence lathe cut lenticular design lenses are used to increase the comfort and wearing time.

- For fitting these lenses in pediatric patients select the appropriate power, usually +1–1.5 D more than refraction value in children more than 2 years and +2 D more in children younger than 2 years age.
- Try for a steeper fit with good tear exchange as compared to flatter fit to minimize the lens loss.

RGP Contact Lenses in Aphakia

Rigid gas permeable contact lenses has following advantages over soft contact lenses in aphakic patients

- Oxygen transmissibility is high
- Optically better as compared to hydrogel and/or silicon lenses
- Flexibility in design
- Economical
- Easy to handle: Can be insert and remove easily
- High safety profile: Chances of bacterial infection and protein adherence are less

RGP lenses of excellent optical property are used in aphakia because in aphakic person strong plus power lenses are required and an unwanted cylindrical error may present with these high spherical powers which is not corrected by soft contact lenses. Mainly following lens designs are suitable for aphakic patients such as

- Single cut lens design
- Lenticular design

Fitting of RGP in children

- *Total diameter:* It is usually kept 1–2 mm smaller than the corneal diameter but relatively larger than adult TD to prevent loss of lens.
- *Power:* Based on the trial lens and over refraction, also correct for vertex distance. For example, suppose spectacle power is +20 D, then give +26.3 D contact lens. Similarly, if spectacle power is –15 D then give –12.75 D contact lens. In high power more than 10 D we also need to correct for tear layer, usually in the range of 2–3 D lacrimal lens.

- *Base curve:* Fit steeper than usual to prevent the loss of contact lens.
- *Material:* Usually material having high or hyper Dk is used for long-term results.

RGP lenses prescribed for aphakia usually ride low because RGP lenses have more central thickness (due to increase plus power) which creates a base down edge effect and the lens is forced down below by upper lids because of more weight and central thickness. To eliminate this problem a small lens with steeper fit is preferred. The single cut lens design RGP lenses have a diameter of 7.5–8.5 mm. However, in spite of small size the centration of these lenses are poor; hence lenticular design lenses having an anterior central optical zone with a minus power carrier (peripheral zone) can be prescribed which has better centration.

Although RGP lenses have several advantages, but a few disadvantages of these lenses are

- More adaptation time
- Poor comfort of wearing
- Needs higher skill to fit
- High chances of lens loss or dislocation
- Increased possibility of self trauma

Presbyopia

Contact lenses for presbyopia correction may be considered an effective alternative to spectacles because they offer faster visual adaptation and more freedom of movement as well as increase in the quality of vision than ophthalmic lenses. Before prescribing contact lens it is essential to know the lifestyle, working distances, etc. of patient so that proper lens design can be selected for every patient depending on the information. For correction of presbyopia, multifocal contact lenses which contain distance and near vision in the same lens are used. There are several contact lens options which can be given to presbyopes including full monovision, modified monovision and bifocal or multifocal contact lenses of gas permeable or hydrogel or silicon-hydrogel materials.

One piece back surface hard bifocal contact lenses are most commonly used to correct presbyopia. In these bifocal lenses the power of addition is equal to the difference between the back surface interface powers in two portions of contact lens as shown in Fig. 14.3.

Broadly, three classes of lens design can be used to fit in presbyopes such as

- Non-rotational design lenses
- Rotational design lenses
- Simultaneous vision design lenses

Non-rotational lens designs: Non-rotational contact lenses are similar to multifocal spectacle lenses, consist of a distance optic segment in the upper portion and a near optic segment in lower portion and are developed to move vertically on the eye. In addition, trifocal non-rotational lens design in which half of the add power is incorporated in the intermediate zone have been also designed which moves vertically on the eye. These lenses are manufactured using RGP material and are in the solid form (Fig. 14.4).

Basically, these non-rotational lenses are designed in such a manner that movement of eye is independent from the lens, i.e. depending on the direction of fixation of eyes (straight or downward gaze) of person either a distance or near zone of lens are positioned in front of the pupil.

As it can be seen in Fig. 14.5A, the distance portion of the lens lies in front of the pupil with the primary or straight ahead gaze of the eyes, whereas near portion comes in front of

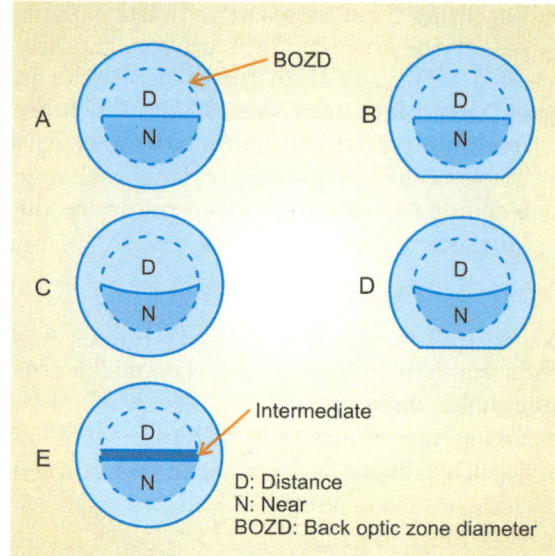

Fig 14.4 A to E: Various non-rotational multifocal contact lens design. A. Straight top non-truncated; B. Straight top truncated; C. Crescent non-truncated; D. Crescent truncated; E. Trifocal

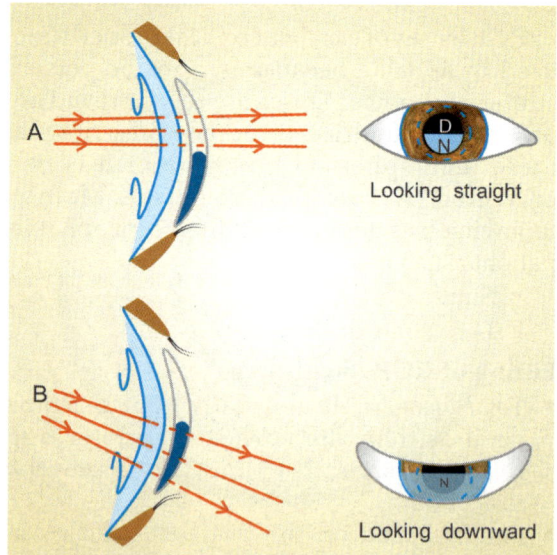

Fig. 14.5: Position of non-rotational design contact lens in various gaze. A. Straight gaze; B. Downward gaze

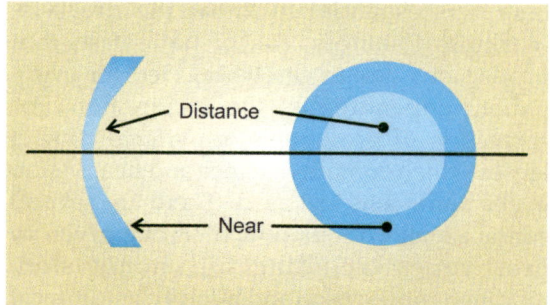

Fig. 14.3: One piece back surface bifocal contact lens.

the pupil with the downward gaze of the eyes (Fig. 14.5B). As the gaze is shifted in downward direction, the lower eyelid pushes the contact lens upwards. Due to this effect the lower portion of contact lens (having near addition) gets aligns with the pupil. Non-rotational contact lens design are similar to spectacles, i.e. allow an independent movement with simultaneous alignment with lower eyelids. Base-down prism is usually added in the lower portion of the lens so that thickness of lower portion of lens is increased as well as center of gravity of the lens is lowered. As a result, lens remains in a lower position on the eye and lens rotation also not occurs. Sometimes, base-down prism alone is insufficient to control the lens rotation and its position, hence truncating a lens design along with lower edge of prism base, enhances the effect of base-down prism by increasing the area of contact between contact lens edge and lower eyelid so that lower lid can push the lens up during downward gaze.

For example, routine non-rotational contact lens parameters are lens diameter (8.7–10.5 mm), BOZR (6.0–9.4 mm), distance power (±20 D), add power(+0.75 D to +4.5 D), stabilization prism (1 to 3Δ), stabilization height (1 mm above to 2 mm below the geometric center) and truncation (0.4–0.6 mm).

Non-rotational lens designs are more preferred in presbyopes who are having

- Lower eyelid is just at or above the lower limbus with moderate to tight lower eyelid tensions.
- Flat corneal topography.
- Pupil of small size with normal illumination.
- Persons who need larger optical zones or back toric or bitoric lenses.
- Persons having residual astigmatism, with front toric designs.
- If add requirement is higher (>+3.00 D) means in case of advanced presbyope or who do frequent close work.

Rotational lens designs: Rotational lenses for presbyopes are designed in such a manner that distance or near segments of the contact lens remain in correct position even when the lens rotates. These lenses have concentric optical zones, hence rotation of the lens over the eye has no effect. Like non-rotational lenses, mostly these are also RGP lenses, where the concentric optical zones may be spherical or aspheric as shown in Fig. 14.6.

In these lens designs, when the individual's gaze is focused straight ahead then he/she will observe the distance objects through the center of the lens, whereas when his/her gaze shifts for reading (downward gaze) then the near vision will be observed through a surrounding annulus as shown in Fig. 14.7A and B respectively.

Unlike non-rotational lens, with rotational lenses there is no need of incorporation of

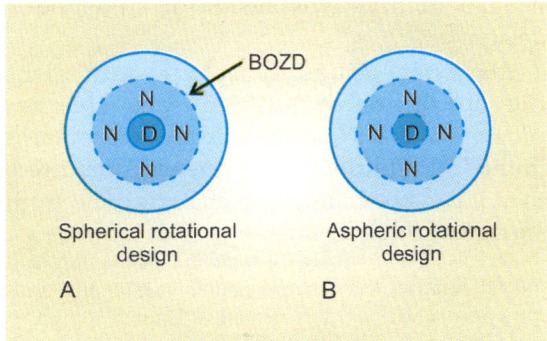

Fig 14.6: Rotational bifocal contact lens design

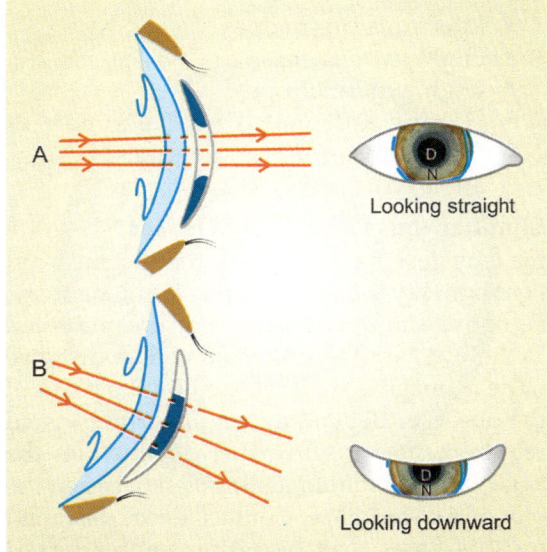

Fig 14.7: Position of rotational design contact lens in various gaze. A. Straight gaze; B. Downward gaze

prism or truncation to stabilize the lens rather these lenses can rotate due to blinking, but still gives continuous optic power for distance as well as for near vision.

Concentric optical zones in a rotational lens may have

- Spherical design in front or back surface
- Aspherical design in back surface, or on both surfaces

Spherical design: Normally in spherical design on the front surface of lens, a central distance zone is present which is surrounded by a transition zone followed by a spherical near zone. The back surface of lens has a normal tricurve lens design or an aspheric design.

Aspherical design: In aspheric design lens the curvature of back surface changes progressively so that the add power remains limited. If additional add power is required, then it can be obtained by changing the front surface of these lenses.

> **Note:** Smaller the distance zone, higher the add power; and steeper the lens must be fit.

Rotational lens designs are preferred in those who are

- Low adds presbyopes
- High myopes
- High hypermetropes
- Having steeper corneal geometries (especially aspherical rotational designs are used)

Simultaneous vision design lenses: These are the lens designs where both the distance and near light rays enter the pupil simultaneously, i.e. both distance and near vision are presented to the eyes at the same instant. The distance or near image is then selected by the brain of the observer depending on his or her visual requirements which further depends on the ability of the brain to distinguish between the blur and clear image. Contact lenses designed on this basis may be either center based (center-distance or center-near) monovision or modified monovision designs

Centration based designs: While prescribing simultaneous lens designs it is important to maintain lens centration with minimal lens movement because decentration of lens may result in visual symptoms. Simultaneously, too tight fit has to be avoided to maintain the proper corneal metabolism. Centration based design is mainly used for soft lenses. The lens designs may be

- *Center-near (CN) designs:* In center-near design, most of the plus power exists at the lens center while most negative power at the periphery as shown in Fig. 14.8A. It means the central portion of lens design focuses near objects while peripheral portion focuses distance objects. The center-near based bifocal and aspheric lens designs have been developed mainly to deal with problem of contraction of pupil occurring while working at near.
- *Center-distance designs:* In this lens design the central part is for the correction of distance vision while the peripheral part is for near vision correction as shown in Fig. 14.8B. This lens designs are mainly suggested for initial stage of presbyopia, requiring add up to +1.25 D.

Monovision: Monovision contact lenses means where in one eye (usually dominant eye) the full correction is given for distance vision, whereas the fellow eye (usually non-dominant eye) is corrected for near vision,

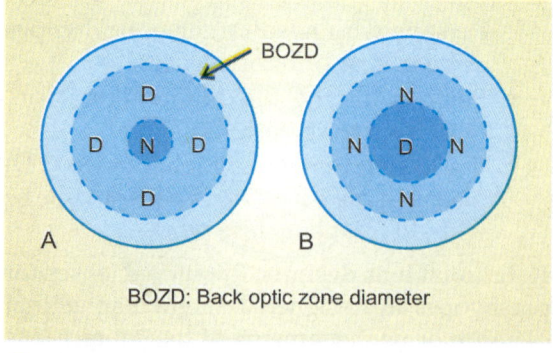

BOZD: Back optic zone diameter

Fig. 14.8: Rotational center based aspherical contact lens design. A. Center near; B. Center distance

using RGP or soft hydrogel contact lenses of bifocal or multifocal lens designs. Thus, in monovision the distance and near images are presented simultaneously to the brain or visual system. After a period of adaptation, the brain becomes versed to suppress the blurred image and thus the object of interest whether distance or near can be seen clearly. However, some patients complain of visual problems and are intolerant to monovision. In these cases, multifocal contact lenses or partial monovision can be tried. Monovision contact lenses are effective way to correct presbyopia with low reading addition. As the presbyopia increases, the adaption to monovision becomes difficult for patients. There may be loss of stereopsis as well as patient experience more difficulty to carry out distance and near tasks. Furthermore, patients having amblyopia should not be prescribed monovision contact lenses, prescribe multifocal contact lenses in such patients.

Modified monovision: Modified monovision technique can be used in advanced case of presbyopia where monovision may pose problem to patient. In this method, the center distance lens design is used for dominant eye while center near design is used for contra-lateral eye. Modified monovision provides the advantages of monovision while along with keeping some multifocal function. However, in modified monovision usually bifocals or multifocal contact lenses are used to correct both distance and near vision.

For example, modified monovision combination can be as done as shown in Table 14.6.

Table 14.6: Various modified monovision combinations

Dominant eye	Non-dominant eye
Rotational multifocal (center distance)	Simultaneous multifocal (center near)
Rotational multifocal (center distance)	Near single vision lens
Distance single vision lens	Simultaneous multifocal (center near)

Diagnostic criteria to judge regarding whether to prescribe monovision, modified monovision or multifocal lenses can be done by performing this simple test. First do an assessment to know which eye is dominant eye, now try to give over plus lenses in non-dominant eye which are just enough for good near vision. Suppose patient develops no symptoms and is comfortable in near vision, then he/she is a good candidate for prescribing monovision. On contrary, if the patient feels dizziness or an imbalance with significant difference in clarity of vision between two eyes, then avoid monovision and prefer binocular bifocals or multifocal lenses.

Contact Lens Fitting in Presbyopes

Fitting of rotational lens designs

- Examination of the patient to find out the lens related parameters
  - Lens diameter: Size of palpebral aperture (PA) and/or HVID can be used to calculate the diameter of lens. It is recommended that a lens with slightly larger diameter should be used to avoid discomfort to patient except if PA is extremely narrow in the size. The estimation of lens diameter on the basis of PA and HVID can be understood by Table 14.7.
  - Back optical zone radius (base curve): Corneal topography/keratometry readings are used, to select the suitable BOZR of the lens as per the manufacturer's instructions. Rotational lens with front surface spherical design usually has a tricurve shaped back surface and BOZR is fit to achieve an alignment fitting

Table 14.7: Estimation of lens diameter according to palpebral aperture (PA) and horizontal visible iris diameter (HVID) in rotational lens design

Lens diameter (mm)	PA (mm)	HVID (mm)
9.0–9.3	<8	10–11
9.4–9.6	8–11	11.5–12.5
9.7–10.0	>11	>12.5

relationship. However, rotational lens with back surface aspheric design, BOZR is kept steeper than flat K (about 0.15–0.80 mm) depending upon the total add power required (e.g. for high add reading it is more steeper).

- Calculation of distance power: Distance power is calculated according to change in BOZR, e.g. for every 0.05 mm change of BOZR, 0.25 D is added.
- Calculation of near power: Calculate as per requirement of patient.

• Select the diagnostic contact lens according to BOZR, calculated power, near/reading add and total diameter. Insert this contact lens and allow it to settle for 15–30 minutes.

• Evaluation of lens fit: Assess position of contact lens and assess near vision in following terms
  - Lens centration and diameter: Ensure the centration of lens.
  - Lens movement with blink: 1–2 mm of lens movement is perfect.
  - Fluorescein pattern: In spherical rotational lens, the fluorescein pattern should appear centrally with optimal edge clearance (0.5 mm). For aspheric rotational lens, slightly high riding, with some central pooling and a wide band of peripheral edge clearance should be seen.

• Accuracy of lens prescription is checked by doing a binocular over refraction for distance and then for near, with the patient holding reading material under normal illumination.

Fitting of non-rotational lens designs: Fitting of non-rotational lenses is considered more difficult than rotational lenses as more parameters are taken into consideration for optimal visual performance.

First lens related parameters are calculated

• Assessment of lens parameters
  - Diameter of lens: Palpebral aperture (PA) size and/or HVID are used to calculate the lens diameter as summarized in Table 14.8. Like rotational lenses, lens

Table 14.8: Estimation of lens diameter according to palpebral aperture (PA) and horizontal visible iris diameter (HVID) in non-rotational lens design

Lens diameter (mm)	PA (mm)	HVID (mm)
9.0–9.3	<8	10–11
9.4–9.6	8–11	11.5–12.5
9.7–10.0	>11	>12.5

with slightly larger diameter should be used to avoid discomfort to patient except if PA is extremely narrow in the size.

- Proper BOZR should be selected for fit alignment. The BOZR should be modified according to corneal astigmatism, as the corneal astigmatism increased, select steeper BOZR. If cornea is spherical, then BOZR can be taken equal to flattest keratometry reading.
- Measurement of segment height: Determine the distance between lower edge of lens (or lower eyelid) and lower margin of pupil. Otherwise, segment height is kept 1 mm lower than the geometric center of contact lens.

• Stabilization using prism: In the absence of truncation, start stabilization with prism of 1 Δ in case of minus prescription lens and start with a prism of 1.5 Δ in case of plus prescription.

• Prism axis: Initially start with prism axis at 90°. Suppose there is a nasal rotation of 5–10°, then balance the prism axis, clockwise for right eye and counter-clockwise for left eye, means to 95° or 100°, respectively. Suppose the position of inferior prism marking is rotated towards examiner's left, then add same degree of rotation to prism axis. On the other hand, if rotated to right then subtract the same degree of rotation from the prism axis (LARS principle means left add, right subtract).

• Assess distance power: Using diagnostic lens, perform binocular over refraction to calculate distance power.

• Assess near power: Keeping distance over refraction in position, add an additional power for reading. Make sure that patient's head is tilted slightly downward, with eyes set at a down gaze which ensure upward translation of contact lens.

- Truncation: If upward translation of contact lens does not happen, then truncation is necessary to avoid lower eyelid from sliding over the inferior part of lens.
- After evaluating lens parameters order of lens can be done and then check the lens fit and assessment of ordered lens
  - *Lens centration and diameter:* Lens should be well centered or slightly low
  - *Lens movement with blink:* 1–2 mm of lens movement is ideal
  - *Lens translation on down gaze:* 2 mm of lens translation is ideal; which enables the near segment of lens to translate over the pupil.
  - *Lens rotation:* Usually 5–10° generally nasally, for both distance and near gaze
  - *Near segment position:* Near segment top should be present, at or just above lower pupillary margin.
  - *Fluorescein pattern:* An aligned fluorescein pattern should be seen; which indicates perfect lens centration, lens translation and movement of lens.
  - *Distance/near vision:* Should be optimal at working distances.

Fitting of center near designs: In these designs, centration and minimal lens movement is necessity to attain a good lens fit; because objective is to offer both distance and near vision, simultaneously. The lens fitting steps are similar to other lenses, i.e. evaluate the lens parameters and select the lens according to parameters. To get an ideal fit the lens diameter can be increased and steepening of optical zone can be done, i.e. either steepen BOZR or increase BOZD and reducing the axial edge lift.

Ideal lens fit of center near lens is checked by
- Lens centration and diameter: Lens should be well centered with good corneal coverage.

- Lens movement with blink: About 1 mm of lens movement is required.
- Fluorescein pattern: Should show centered lens with an adequate edge clearance.

Follow-up: On follow-up visits, if required alteration in parameters can be done if essential for comfortable visual performance like
- If too much lens movement is there, then TD can be increased or BOZR steepening is done.
- Ensure that a balance exist between distance and near vision requirements because on adding more minus power to improve the distance vision will affect the near vision on contrary, adding of more plus to improve the near vision will affect distance vision.

High Astigmatism

Correction of astigmatism by contact lens, especially of high degree, needs proper selection of contact lens design which may vary with each case.

Elements responsible for production of astigmatism are
- Cornea (mainly)
- Crystalline lens
- Retina (rare)

Cornea is considered major refracting surface of the human eye. Even a minor change in the curvature or radius of the corneal surface can induce change in the refractive power of the eye. Different types of astigmatisms usually appear due to toricity of the anterior corneal surface. Astigmatisms can also be induced by the crystalline lens (lenticular astigmatism) and retina and is termed internal astigmatism, however, still clinically most significant astigmatism is contributed by corneal surface.

The sum of corneal and lenticular astigmatism is termed total refractive astigmatism. Hence, for correction of astigmatism by contact lenses, both types of ocular astigmatisms should be taken into consideration. As we know that most of the astigmatism is contributed due to cornea but if there is large difference between corneal and total refractive astigmatism, it indicates presence of significant amount of lenticular astigmatism in that individual. For example, if in a case having higher refractive astigmatism as compared to corneal astigmatism and when a spherical rigid gas permeable (RGP) contact lens is prescribed to this case, then a significant amount of residual astigmatism (lenticular astigmatism) will remain uncorrected which will affect visual acuity. These types of cases require fitting of a RGP contact lens having toric design or alternately a toric soft contact lens can also be used.

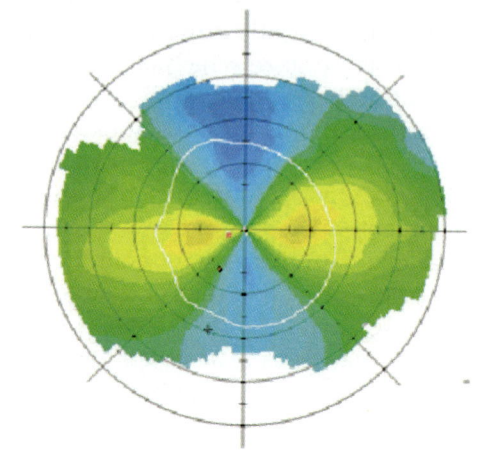

Fig. 14.9: Corneal topography showing regular astigmatism

Types of astigmatism: Depending on the angle between two principal meridians astigmatisms are classified clinically in two different types. The corneal surface can be assessed by performing keratometry and corneal topography. Keratometer is commonly used for measurements of corneal curvature. Corneal topography is an advance method for corneal assessment which does complete corneal examination.

Corneal topography is a useful method to assess and classify corneal astigmatisms. Broadly, astigmatism can be divided as

- Regular
- Irregular

Regular astigmatism: Astigmatism is said to be regular when corneal meridians representing maximum and minimum refractive powers are perpendicular to each other. Further regular astigmatisms can grouped as with the rule, against the rule or oblique astigmatism. In regular astigmatism, corneal topography appears like a tie, having two perpendicular main meridians as shown in Fig. 14.9.

Irregular astigmatism: When the principal meridians do not lie perpendicular to each other and the meridians representing maximum and minimum refractive powers are not separated by an angle of 90°, it is called

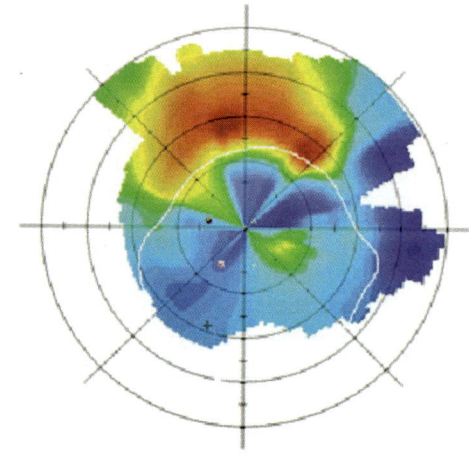

Fig. 14.10: Corneal topography showing irregular astigmatism

irregular astigmatism. Irregular astigmatism is more commonly seen with keratoconus, after surgical procedures or in scarred cornea. In irregular astigmatism, corneal topography will show that two principal meridians which are not perpendicular to each other as shown in Fig. 14.10.

Contact lens for astigmatism: Various types of contact lens designs can be used to correct astigmatism, however, to avoid rotation of lens during blinking, different systems in the form of prism ballast, truncation, or thin zones are provided.

Correction of Regular Astigmatism

General rule for selection of a contact lens is that lens choice mainly depends on the amount of refractive astigmatism as summarized in Table 14.9 and shown in Fig. 14.11.

Soft contact lens correction

- *Spherical soft contact lenses:* Spherical soft contact lens is the first choice to correct astigmatism in cases having astigmatic error up to 1 D and less than 1/3 of the spherical error. If visual acuity remains poor with spherical soft contact lenses,

then soft toric or spherical RGP contact lens should be used. Generally, improvement in the visual acuity is observed better with use of spherical RGP lenses as compared to soft contact lenses in astigmatism. For example, a patient having refractive error as –6 DS × –1.25 DC, can be corrected with an equivalent soft spherical contact lens, and patient remains comfortable with fair amount of visual acuity. Whereas, a patient having refractive error as –2.5 DS × –1.25 DC will be uncomfortable with an equivalent spherical soft contact lenses.

- *Toric soft contact lenses:* Patients having astigmatic error more than 1.25 DC need toric soft lenses. In these cases, soft spherical lenses are unable to rectify the error and RGP lenses may be intolerable, hence soft toric contact lenses having different radii are used. These lenses are fitted as per the guidelines provided by the lens manufacturer; however, fitter should make sure that

Table 14.9: Choice of type of contact lens on the basis of degree of astigmatism

Degree of astigmatism	Lens of choice
< 1.00 D	Soft or RGP spherical lens
1.00 to 4.00 D	Soft toric lens or RGP spherical lens
> 4.00 D	RGP toric lens or custom soft toric lens

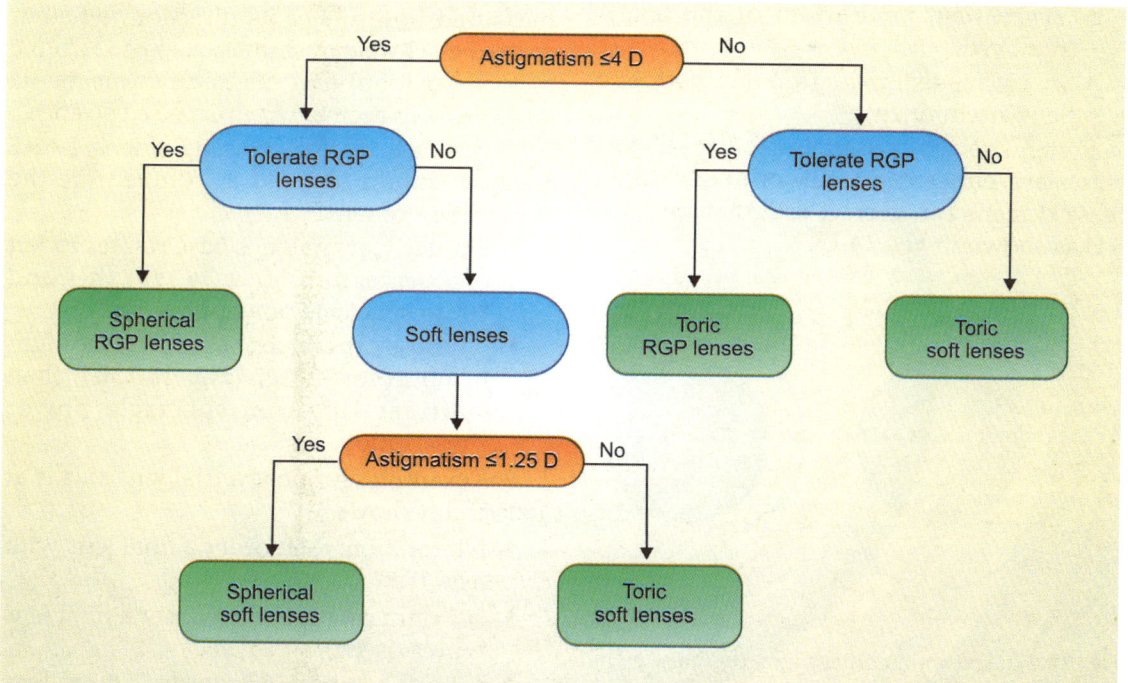

Fig. 14.11: Selection cascade for contact lenses in regular astigmatism

the patients refractive error should correctly match with contact lens parameters.

Soft toric lenses are available as

- *Standard lenses:* Consist of low cylinder amount and are available easily on order.
- *Custom lenses:* These lenses have high cylinder amount or nonstandard diameters and usually require long time duration to receive from the laboratory.

Soft toric contact lens design

- Back surface toric (most common, good for toric cornea)
- Front surface toric (better for spherical cornea)

Stabilization: The soft toric lenses need to be stabilized, so that rotation of lens does not occur during blinking. Stabilization can be done by various methods

- *By using prism ballast,* i.e. in the inferior portion of lens additional material is added, generally 0.75 – 2 Δ of ballast added.
- *Prism ballast with truncation* (usually used in custom designs).
- *Truncation,* i.e. bottom of the lens is removed.
- *By making thin zones* (top and bottom of lens are thinned).

Systems generally used to stabilize soft toric lenses are, either thin zones or prism ballast; these designs can correct astigmatism up to 8 D as shown in Fig. 14.12.

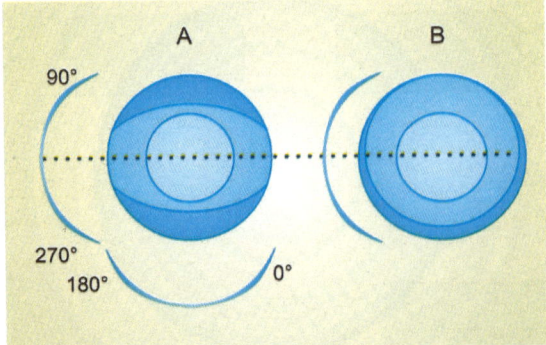

Fig. 14.12: Soft toric contact lens design. A. Thin zone toric stabilization system; B. Prismatic stabilization system

Contact lens fitting methods are

- *Empirical fitting method* requires spectacle power and K readings adjusted by using type of guaranteed fitting program provided by manufacturer, however, eyelid force and interaction between the eyelid and contact lens is not accounted.
- *Diagnostic fitting method* requires spectacle power corrected for vertex distance in both the meridians (for example, –4 DS × –2.5 DC × 180 will become –3.5 DS × –2 DC × 180, at corneal plane where vertex distance is 10 mm) along with K reading.

Assessment of lens fitting: The overall lens fit as well as rotation of the lens should be assessed in terms of coverage, centration, movement and rotation. An ideal lens fit is considered where contact lens remains in a stable position and does not rotate markedly after blink (Fig. 14.13A). Improper lens fit is considered when contact lens rotates to an off axis position which needs compensation at the time of ordering the lens. If on examination, lens rotation is found, then it should be measured in terms of its direction (whether rotated clockwise or counterclockwise from 6 o'clock position) and magnitude (means its degree of displacement from expected position).

In this case, during ordering of lens, LARS method should be used to compensate the misrotation of lens.

- Similarly, if trial lens base rotates to left of observer in 10° (Fig. 14.13B), then add 10° to spectacle power prescription.
- Suppose if trial lens base rotates to right of observer in 10° (Fig. 14.13C), then subtract 10° from spectacle power prescription.

For example, suppose a trial lens axis is at 180° and it shows

- No rotation, then order a final lens with axis 180°
- 10° right rotation, then order a final lens with axis 170°.
- 10° left rotation, then order a final lens with axis 10°.

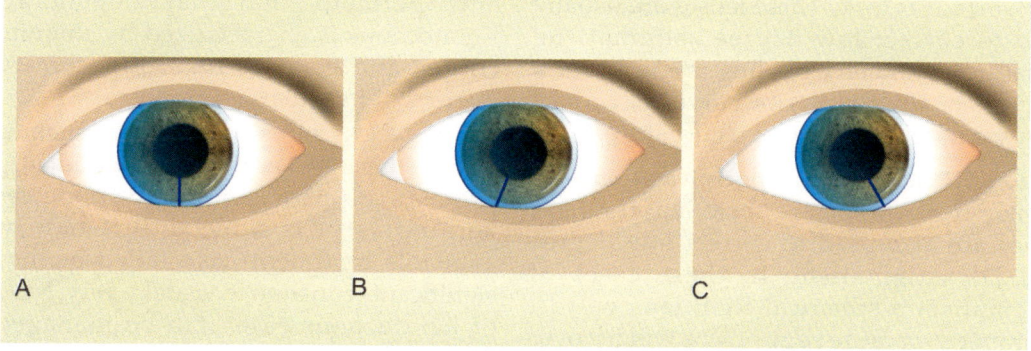

Fig. 14.13: Assessment of soft toric contact lens fit. A. No rotation, B. Left rotation, C. Right rotation

Stability of contact lens rotation is determined by
- Ask the patient to move eye in different directions of gaze and record the time of return of lens to its resting position.
- Observe the effect of fast blinks and complete blinks on rotation of lens.
- Move the contact lens by hand off axis and record time of return of lens to resting position.
- Assess the effect of convergence on rotation of lens.

Rigid gas permeable (RGP) contact lens

RGP contact lenses offer useful choices to correct regular astigmatism with high quality of visual acuity. Various RGP lens design can be used depending upon patient's astigmatism. Generally, in cases having low degree of astigmatism, spherical RGP contact lenses are recommended, however, with high degree of astigmatism, a toric RGP lens is recommended to correct astigmatism. Toric RGP contact lenses can also be required for correction of astigmatism in cases of lenticular astigmatism.
- *Spherical RGP contact lens:* Primarily used to correct low degree astigmatism, means up to ≤4 D. These lenses are not useful in correction of moderate to high degree astigmatic refractive errors. Patients having corneal astigmatism to the tune of 4 D can be corrected by spherical RGP contact lenses, although these lenses are made with diameter 0.2–0.3 mm smaller than usual diameter.

- *Toric RGP contact lenses:* To correct moderate to high degree astigmatism mainly toric RGP lenses are used. These lenses are available in various designs to fit in different types of refractive errors.

RGP toric contact lens designs are available as
- Front surface toric RGP lenses
- Back surface toric RGP lenses
- Toric RGP lenses with peripheral curves
- Bitoric RGP lenses

Note: Generally in RGP toric lenses stabilization is done by creating back toric surfaces, although RGP front toric lenses needs an additional stabilization system.

Front surface toric RGP lenses: Front surface toric RGP lenses are used to correct high degree residual astigmatism or lenticular astigmatism in patients having spherical cornea. Stabilization in these types of lenses is done by an additional system such as prism blast or truncation method. In blast method usually a base down 2 D prism is added on the front surface during manufacturing of contact lens, however, sometimes more dioptre prisms may be required to center a very high degree minus power contact lens.

In truncation method contact lens diameter is reduced in one meridian, usually by cutting (nearly 0.5–1 mm) an entire edge of contact lens.

Back surface toric RGP lenses: Usually stabilization of toric RGP lenses is done by creating back surface as toric. These lenses are usually used to correct low degree astigmatism. Usually Keratometry reading are used for a proper lens fit of posterior curves of contact lens, accurately with corneal curvature.

Toric RGP lenses with peripheral curves: Similar to back surface toric lenses, these lenses are also used to correct low degree (2–3 D) astigmatism. In these cases of astigmatism a spherical RGP lens will fit improperly, because edge of lens will lift over steepest meridian of cornea; which may cause decentration and loss of contact lens. Hence, to correct this problem additional steeper peripheral curves are made in steepest corneal meridians, whereas standard lens curves are fitted along the flatter corneal meridian.

Bitoric RGP contact lens: Bitoric RGP contact lens is used in patients who are presented with moderate degree astigmatism along with a residual astigmatism. Usually, a RGP contact lens is fitted with a posterior curve, same as that of keratometry reading however, when this toric back surface RGP lens is placed on the cornea the interface between contact lens and tear film forms a toric surface. This newly formed toric surface causes a state of an induced astigmatism and to correct this condition, an additional anterior surface toricity is created which forms a bitoric RGP contact lens.

Correction of irregular astigmatism: Correction of an irregular astigmatism using RGP contact lenses provides a considerable enhancement of visual acuity than spectacle correction. Hence, RGP contact lenses became the first choice of management, in some corneal pathology having an irregular cornea such as keratoconus, post-keratoplasty, complicated refractive surgery, corneal trauma and post-herpetic keratitis.

Contact Lens Fitting in Primary Corneal Ectasias

Keratoconus is one of the most common types of primary corneal ectasias seen in clinical practice. Others less common are keratoglobus and pellucid marginal degeneration. Keratoconus is characterized by thinning of cornea and ectasias resulting in varying degrees of irregular astigmatism.

Spectacles can be used for management of initial stages of keratoconus, while surgical procedure (most commonly penetrating keratoplasty) is done only when other available treatment have failed or there is significant reduction in visual acuity. Majority of keratoconus cases can be managed by prescribing contact lenses.

Classification of degree and type of keratoconus is important in making the decision about type of contact lens fitting method. Position and size of cone in the eye affect the selection of contact lens fitting method, hence it is advised to do computerized corneal topography to identify the type of cone. Basically there may be three types of cones as follows

1. *Nipple cones:* Mostly these cones are located below the visual axis (sometimes central), small in size with variable conicity.

2. *Oval cones:* These cones are also located below the visual axis having larger inferior conical area.

3. *Globus cones:* These cones are rarely seen, where about 75% of cornea gets affected and clinically Munson's sign is present in majority of cases.

Ideal fit in keratoconus: Keratoconic patients or other primary corneal ectasias patients require high levels of comfort, because they need to wear contact lenses for longer duration, hence appropriate lens materials should be chosen. Cases where steep high minus lenses are required, lens material having high dimensional stability should be prescribed so that chances of the contact lens distortion are less.

Contact lens of different Dk/t (moderate to high values for large or flatter lenses, low value for stability and wetting purpose) can be used.

Rigid contact lens fitting: Rigid gas permeable (RGP) contact lenses for correction of keratoconus are the most common and most successful method which provides a new anterior surface to cornea. Several contact lens designs are available and can be fitted accordingly at different stages of keratoconus and cone types. Various fitting methods of RGP lenses are summarized as

Apical clearance method: In this method the contact lens rest on the paracentral cornea and vaults the cone. Central cornea is not covered, hence chances of trauma and scarring of central cornea is reduced. These types of lens are of small diameter, having less back optic zone diameter which may result in significant flare and glare problems. In addition, there may be corneal edema, decreased tear exchange, air bubbles under contact lens (may creep into central optic zone, causing poor visual acuity).

Apical touch flat fitting method: In this method nearly entire weight of contact lens lies on the cone, with wide edge standoff. The lens remains in position due to top lid. Due to apical touch better visual acuity is obtained and improvement in visual acuity is noticed immediately probably because of corneal molding by RGP contact lens. These contact lenses can cause to development or progression of apical changes and/or abrasions and scarring of cornea. It is more successful in early keratoconus cases, but still can be used in certain cases where corneal apices are displaced.

Three-point touch method: It is most commonly used fitted design for keratoconus especially for multicurve contact lens designs. The main principle used is to distribute the weight of contact lens uniformally between the cone and peripheral cornea. Hence, a three-point touch fitted lens will show an apical contact area of about 2–3 mm and an annulus rim of mid peripheral contact zone. The area and shape of the contact zones may vary due to cone asymmetry, e.g. mid-peripheral contact zone may assume more crescent shape, if cone is vertically asymmetrical.

Contact lens designs for primary corneal ectasias: Various lens designs are used to correct and improve visual acuity in patients having keratoconus and other corneal ectasias. These lens designs are broadly grouped as

- Multicurve design contact lenses
- Aspheric/elliptical design contact lenses
- Large diameter contact lenses
- Combination or Piggy back lenses

Multicurve lenses Standard form of multi-curve lens designs may be used in persons having early keratoconus, however, for advanced stage of disease more specific lens designs are available to use like Woodward multicurve lens design. Most important advantage with these lenses is that practitioner knows all the parameters of this type of lens design which are already provided by manufacturer, hence any modifications in lens can easily be ordered by practitioner. The multicurve lenses are designed on the basis of the fact that in early or moderate keratoconus the periphery of cornea is not much changed, thus multicurve lenses have normal curves in the periphery, but steeper base optical zone radius (BOZR).

Central keratometry decides the selection of cone radius and for each cone radius a number of peripheries with different diameters are available. For example

- Shepherd NLK (Northern Lenses) also called acuity lenses
- Profile lenses (Jack Allen)
- Rose K system

Among these lenses the most widely used is Rose K system, which is mainly useful in cases having central cone, however, in cases having inferiorly displaced cones, Rose K is not very useful.

- *Rose K system:* On the basis of statistical data collected from keratoconus patient by Dr Paul Rose of New Zealand, these contact lens designs were developed having complex computer generated peripheral curves. The important characteristic of these lenses are
  1. To obtain an ideal edge lift of 0.8 mm, these contact lenses include triple

peripheral curve system, i.e. standard, flat and steep.

2. Rose K design lenses are existing in wide range of base curve (4.75–8 mm) and diameters (7.9–10.2 mm). As the steeping of base curve increases, the optic zone diameter of lens decreases.

3. Toric curves are available on all surfaces of lens, i.e. front, back and periphery. Traditionally, Rose K lenses are made from Boston ES material, however, Boston XO material was also used by some laboratories to increase oxygen permeability property.

Aspheric/elliptic lenses are the one in which lens flatten in curvature progressively from the center to the periphery. Many aspheric lenses designs like Quasar K No 7 lens, Jack Allen KD lens, and Persecon Elliptical K lens are available for early keratoconus cases. These lenses have large optic zones thus very useful in patients having large pupils and/or oval type cones. Aspheric lenses are available in wide variety of materials, and can be made in specific material on order.

Large diameter lenses: These contact lenses are large in diameter (up to 14.5 mm) having bicurve or multicurve and are available in a number of lens designs such as

- *Soper cone design:* These contact lenses are of bicurve design having two posterior curves, one curve is fitted on the central cone and the second curve is fitted on the normal peripheral cornea (like a hat on the head). Lens has small diameter and fixed back optic zone. As the base curve is decreased for a given diameter, the vaulting effect of lens get increase.

- *McGuire lenses:* It is a modification of Soper cone lens design and consists of four peripheral curves (primary, secondary, tertiary and quaternary) instead of two which are blended together. These

four peripheral curves are 3, 6, 8 and 10 D more flatter than the base curve of the lens. This lens system contains three diagnostic lens sets, i.e. nipple, oval or globus types of cones. Fitting principle is to achieve a three-point touch which in turn is dependent on the size of optic zone in relation to cone size. The optic zone sizes differ from 6 mm for the nipple cone to 6.5 mm for the oval cone, and 7 mm for the globus.

- *Dyna Intra Limbal (DIL):* These large diameter lenses are specifically designed for cases having inferiorly displaced keratoconus, pellucid marginal degeneration and post-keratoplasty where stability of lens is difficult to attain by using smaller diameter lenses. These lenses are mainly used to provide stability. These lenses are available in various diameters ranging from 10.8 mm to 12.5 mm, diameter range. Ideally, the total diameter of lens is kept 0.2 mm smaller than that of corneal diameter because it allows a lens movement of approximately 0.5–1 mm. Epithelial/stromal scarring may occur with lens due to 'settle back' tendency of these lens. Usually materials having high DK/t are recommended for manufacturing of these lenses.

- *S-Lim lenses (Jack Allen):* These semi-scleral contact lenses mainly remain on the limbus with very little movement. These lenses are mainly designed to vault the corneal grafts by changing the sag depth according to requirement. For exchange of tears, 2–4 fenestrations are present in the lens.

- *Kerasoft lenses (Ultra vision):* Normally soft lenses, e.g. hydrogels or silicon hydrogels are not preferred for correction of irregular cornea as these lenses have propensity to drape on the surface of cornea, hence soft lens, e.g. Kerasoft have been specially manufactured for treatment of keratoconus which does not drape over the cornea. Kerasoft lenses (58% water content terpolymer) has a back surface cylindrical design and are available as lens series called A, B and C with total lens diameters of 14 mm, 14.5 mm and 15 mm respectively. Among these lenses series B lenses are most commonly used and has flatter fit as compared to series A lens. Kerasoft lenses are mainly used for early keratoconus and for those patients who have difficulty in wearing RGP lens. These lenses offer more comfort and prolonged wearing time in patients who cannot tolerate RGP corneal lenses.

- *Hybrid soft perm lenses:* These lenses are manufactured by using RGP material for the center portion of lens and soft 25% water content HEMA in the periphery. The total diameter of lens is about 14.3 mm with 8.0 mm of central portion. These lens provide good centration, better visual acuity and less discomfort as compared to RGP lens, hence are preferred in RGP intolerant patients. However, these lenses have very less oxygen transmissibility (Dk/t), chances of giant papillary conjunctivitis and corneal neovascularisation are more. Research and advancement in lens manufacturing are coming up with newer versions which give higher oxygen permeability (Dk 100–105) and 40–45% water content HEMA skirt.

Combination or Piggy back lenses As we know that soft contact lenses are recommended in cases where patient is sensitive to RGP lenses or excessive lid sensation to RGP lenses are present. However, good visual acuity is difficult to attain with use of only soft contact lenses. Hence, a concept of combination or piggy back lenses means fitting a RGP lens over a soft lens (silicon hydrogels) gained popularity so that same level of visual acuity can be obtained as with a single lens. Generally, silicon hydrogel with the steepest base curve is preferred for piggy banking lens

manufacture especially in cases of early keratoconus and irregular astigmatism. As compared to conventional soft lens, silicon hydrogels have more oxygen transmissibility and rigidity. However, in severe cases of keratoconus particularly in inferiorly displaced cones, a piggyback combination is not so successful because silicon hydrogels tend to pucker and do not fit well. Fitting of RGP lens should be done first and an apical touch of slight larger area is tolerable.

Problems arising due to lens fitting in keratoconus

- *Peripheral staining:* Staining in the form of three and nine o'clock may occur. It usually develops due to dryness in the areas surrounding the contact lens. It can be managed by using lenses of large diameter, decrease lens edge lift, performing blinking exercises and instillation of ocular lubricants.
- *Vortex staining:* This type of staining is more common with flat fitting contact lenses which may damage corneal epithelium. Recommended measures are steepening of contact lens (causes reduction in pressure over the cone), and increasing Dk/t of lens material.
- *Dimpling:* Air bubbles trapped under contact lens which acts like smooth foreign bodies causes dimpling. Usually this happens when normal GP lens designs are used in early keratoconic cases or when an excessive apical clearance is present. In case of dimpling, reduction of BOZD and addition of peripheral curve by using a different multicurve design will help to correct the situation.
- *Stromal scarring:* It is usual in advanced stages of keratoconus which can affect visual acuity. In cases of significantly decreased visual acuity, graft surgery is indicated.
- *Thinning:* Corneal thinning may occur which can be managed in a similar manner to stromal scarring. In cases of severe thinning graft surgery is required.

- *Giant papillary conjunctivitis:* As kerato-conus is generally associated with atopic disease, hence GPC is commonly seen in patient with keratoconus. If develops can be managed by preservative free eye drops, mast cell stabilizers (e.g. sodium cromo-glycate) in the initial stages, however, in severe conditions steroids are used to control the situation.
- *Neovascularisation:* Most commonly associated with use of Softperms and PMMA scleral contact lenses. It is recommended that development of neovascularisation should not be allowed in any case because this will seriously affect the success rate of corneal graft surgery to be done in the future.
- *Nebulae:* Nebulae means a small raised area of scarring developed in the superficial corneal stroma due to wearing of flat fitting contact lens leading to discomfort and decreased wearing time. It can be debrided by mechanical means (using a scalpel blade) or by an excimer laser (phototherapeutic keratectomy).

Contact lens fitting in keratoconus
Before fit assessment
- Fleischer's ring and Vogt's striae are hallmark signs of keratoconus.
- In cases of keratoconus, on doing corneal topography the steepest area of cornea usually measures more than 48 D. Furthermore, if eccentricity value ≥ 0.8, then it is more likely to be because of keratoconus.
- In absence of corneal topography facility, patients having moderate to advance keratoconus can be assessed by clinical examination. When a +1.25 D trial lens is placed over patient's side of keratometer, then the range of value extends about 8 D in case of keratoconus.

Contact lens fitting
- In centrally located cone having relatively small apex, usually small diameter RGP lenses are used.

- Cases having large oval or globus cone and inferiorly decentered apex: hybrid design lenses, intra-limbal, scleral, or piggyback lenses are successful.
- However, most of the lens designs used for keratoconus needs minimal apical clearance or mild touch; because excessive apical bearing can cause corneal staining and probable corneal scarring while excessive apical clearance can cause peripheral seal off.
- Sometimes, when patient is prescribed RGP lens and there is poor centration, discomfort to patient or scarring then piggyback combination can be tried. For example, soft silicon hydrogel contact lens of very low power (0.5 D) is placed under RGP lens, however, in combination the GP material of hyper Dk (>100) should be used. Sometimes, soft contact lens of moderate plus power (+6 D) having thicker center can also be used with RGP lens if positioning of RGP lens over soft contact lens is low due to presence of low corneal apex.

Orthokeratology

Orthokeratology or ortho-K is reversible, non-invasive method used as an alternative to refractive surgery for correction of visual acuity in low to moderate degree of myopic cases. This approach was known since many years, however, its clinical applications have increased in recent years because of availability of lens materials having high oxygen transmissibility and availability of better contact lens manufacturing techno-logy.

Principle of orthokeratology is that reshaping (change in curvature) of corneal surface occurs due to constant wearing of a specially designed RGP contact lens, for longer period of time. These types of lenses are worn overnight or on alternate nights, then removed in the morning and not worn during the day. By orthokeratology there is flattening of the cornea so that overall refractive power of the eye is reduced, however, effects on the shape of cornea are temporary and cornea regains its original shape on discontinuation of lens. Sometimes, due to compromised corneal epithelium, serious complications can occur. Orthokeratology does not affect shape of posterior cornea or depth of the anterior chamber. Reverse geometry design lens have been designed to improve centration and refractive effect which consist of central optic zone more flat relative to cornea while surrounded peripheral zones are more steeper with reverse curves.

Assessment before lens fit

- Ideal candidates for this technique are
  - Myopic having refractive error less than 5 D.
  - Cylindrical error of ≤ 1.50 D, in case of with the rule astigmatism or ≤ 0.50 D in case of against the rule astigmatism.
  - Pupillary diameter less than 6 mm.
- Important screening tests to be done are refraction, slit lamp examination and corneal topography. Topography provides values of corneal eccentricity and also helps to rule out those patients which are having irregular cornea.

Lens fitting Process

- Base curve radius of RGP lens is determined by using "Jessen formula", which uses FAP (flat add plus) tear lens factor. This results in a final contact lens power of +0.75 D, which permits regression of corneal surface during daytime. For example, suppose patient has a refractive error of –3 DS × –0.75 DC × 180 with keratometry values 44.00 D at 180°/horizontal meridian and 44.75 D at 90°/vertical meridian. Base curve of contact lens should be, equal to flatter by 3.75 D (3.00 D + 0.75 D) than K (44 D), which becomes 40.25 D (44 D–3.75 D).
- Selection of initial diagnostic lens is based on achievement of bull's eye fluorescein pattern (means there is central and mid-peripheral bearing with narrow tear circulation zone and slight peripheral edge lift).

- Before evaluating lens fit it is advised to wait for 10–15 minutes. Ideally, during evaluation there must be good centration of contact lens with a minimum ≤ 1 mm lag during blinking.
- Again patient must be examined in the morning as follows
  - Check the fitting relationship of lens and cornea; remove contact lens for assessment of corneal integrity.
  - If on examination, a consolidated staining of cornea is observed, then it indicates that contact lens is too flat in central portion.
  - Do corneal topography which should show bull's eye pattern (central flattening with paracentral steepening) in ideal fit. If there is flattening in superior part with an steepening of inferior arc (smiley face pattern) then it indicates that lens is too flat in fit. If, there is presence of slight central steepening (central island pattern) then it indicates that lens is too steep. Cases where no obvious topography patterns noticed during examination, then patients are advised to wear contact lenses for another 2–3 days, then again re-evaluate the fitting.
- On an average, the favorable results are obtained in about 10 days of lens wear although, duration may vary with degree of myopia, i.e. less for lower myopic and more for moderate to severe myopic patients.
- During treatment period, daily disposable lenses of progressively decreasing power should be prescribed to patient and then re-evaluate after one week time.
- Once treatment period is over, these contact lenses are worn on a retainer basis; which is every night for severe myopic patients and once a week for low myopic patients. These patients can self-monitor their retainer wear time, whenever patients notice blurring of vision for distance they can wear contact lenses overnight.

Precautions during lens wear

- To obtain optimal lens centration and to decrease corneal staining it is recommended to use highly viscous artificial tear drops before insertion of contact lens.
- Lens should not be removed immediately after awakening. Rewetting drops should be applied before removal of contact lens.
- To break the suction (if present), lower eyelid margin can be used to gently push the lower lens edge.

CONTACT LENS RELATED COMPLICATIONS

Contact lenses can cause a wide range of changes in eye and complications related to contact lens include inflammatory, mechanical, or metabolic changes. Although risk of complications is low, but poor hygiene and improper handling of contact lenses can cause several complications. Majority of lens related problems are insignificant and without any consequences, however, sometimes serious ocular and vision threatening complications can occur. Recent advancements in contact lens materials and multipurpose cleaning solutions have reduced several risks related to extended wear but some problems still exist today.

Risk Factors Related to Complications with Contact Lens Wear

Factors related to contact lens itself

- *Materials used for contact lens:* Generally complications are more frequent in soft contact lens wearer as compared to RGP contact lens users. However, hydrogel and silicon hydrogel lenses are commonly used as daily wearer or monthly/three monthly disposable lens. As compared to other soft lenses silicon lenses have less chance to develop limbal injections, protein deposition, corneal neovascularisation and less damage to epithelium and its functions.
- *Various deposition and risk of contamination:* A large number of proteins and lipids present in the tear film can deposit on the surface of contact lenses, although on silicon hydrogel materials proteins deposition is least as compared to other materials. The deposition starts as soon as lens is placed in the eye and increases with time of wear. Deposition of proteins on surface of lens appears as thin hazy layer, and it is mostly due to deposition of denatured lysozyme, sometimes due to albumin and gamma globulin. Lipids deposition on surface appears as oily appearance on the lens surface. Sometimes excessive deposition of lipids and mucin as jelly bumps may elicit immunological reaction in conjunctiva. In daily wear lenses the quantity of deposition on lens also depends on factors like water content, chemical and ionic characteristics of hydrogel lens materials. Generally lenses with low water content show less deposition than high water content lens. Similarly, deposition of proteins is more with ionic lenses as compared to non-ionic lenses. In addition, the environmental contaminations and pollutants such as oils, dirt, lotions, make-up, powders, smoke, aerosols like perfumes and hair sprays can also deposit and contaminate the lens. There may be deposition of bacteria, such as *Pseudomonas aeruginosa* and *Staphylococcus epidermidis*, along with several fungi and protozoa on lens surface. Bacterial infection lead to formation of a bio film on lens surface and can penetrate into lens material, especially in high water content lens, leading to increase risk of development of bacterial keratitis.
- *Deformation and damage of contact lens:* Contact lens warpage may occur due to change in various parameters of lens which can be confirmed by using a spherometer. Change in parameters of lens is indicated by bad lens fit and increased or decreased lens movement on the cornea, which further lead to injury of corneal epithelium and other complications.
- *Cleaning and care solutions for contact lens:* Complication may occur due to improper

cleaning of lens. Multi-purpose solutions used to clean contact lenses, must have cleaning agents, disinfectants, preservatives and polymers or softeners to make contact lenses wearing more comfortable. Regular and proper cleaning of contact lens is must, however, improper handling of lens or solution can lead to contamination of solution itself; which gives continuous problems because patients do not change the multipurpose solution regularly.

Factors related with contact lens wearer

- *Ocular pathology:* Many eye related conditions such as vernal conjunctivitis seasonal and constant allergic conjunctivitis, atypical keratoconjunctivitis, dry eye syndrome or keratoconjunctivitis sicca, systemic diseases like thyroid diseases and dermatological conditions related to meibomian glands dysfunction act as limiting factors for contact lens wearing because the risk of complication due to contact lens wearing is increased in compromised ocular state.

- *Blinking pattern:* Chances of dryness of lens and deposition on lens are increased with less frequent blinking or incomplete blinking. There is diminution of tear exchange between contact lens and cornea which may cause retinal hypoxia. To prevent these complications it is essential to achieve full blinking by blinking exercises.

- *Intake of medicines:* Medicines like diuretics, anticholinergics, antihistamines, and antipsychotic may increase dryness of eye surface by decreasing production of tears. Constant use of steroids and other immuno-suppressant drugs is associated with alteration in body defense mechanism leading to increases risk of infections in contact lens.

- *Smoking:* Due to smoking there is change in the stability of tear film as well as sensitivity of conjunctiva and cornea is reduced because due to smoking lipid layer of precorneal tear film is damaged.

- *Wearing schedule of contact lens:* Generally, contact lens wearing is associated with some physiological changes like thinning of epithelium and decrease rate of epithelium cell exchange in the eye which is further increased with use of continuous wear or extended wear contact lenses. Silicon hydrogel lens which have high oxygen transmissibility may also produce these changes but in lesser frequency. Furthermore, wearing of contact lens during night is also associated with increased risk of complications and it is assumed that silicon hydrogel lens can be prescribed for night wear if required, because of their high oxygen transmissibility.

- *Frequency of replacement of contact lens:* With continuous wearing there is ageing of polymers material of lens and chances of deposits over lens increased which are not removed completely with regular cleaning and disinfection of lens. Nowadays, although lens with better materials are available which show less deposit formation but it is advised to prefer disposable or daily wear contact lenses causing less complications.

- *Contact lenses wearing without professional advice:* Many wearers buy contact lenses without a prescription through internet and use them irregularly with improper handling. Due to poor compliance and without professional control a large number of complications related to contact lens wear may arise.

- *Maintenance of lens in hygiene conditions:* Appropriate hygiene is very necessary for proper maintenance of contact lenses, lens cases, and cleaning solution bottles so that chances of contamination decreased. Occasionally, contact lens wearers do not follow hygiene during insertion and removal of contact lens and predisposed to infections.

Complications and Diseases Related with Contact Lens Wear

Contact lens related complications are declining gradually because of better lens material, wetting solution, awareness among wearer, and better sterility maintenance. In spite of these factors some amount of insult to ocular tissue is caused by regular wearing of contact lenses.

Problems occurring due to contact lens wear in relation to various ocular structures are summarized in Table 14.10.

Problems related to eyelids

- **Unusual blinking pattern:** Blinking abnormality may already be present in contact lens wearer however, it may precipitate due to lens wearing. Blinking abnormalities may be in the form of forced blink, partial blink, inadequate number of blinks, and dry eye. These abnormalities may lead to drying of ocular surface, lens deposits, accumulation of tears behind contact lens, corneal hypoxia or hypercapnia, epithelial erosions specifically at 3 and 9 o'clock positions, reduction in tear break up time. Blinking training or exercise will help to improve blinking and thus reduction in signs and symptoms.

- **Ptosis:** It is commonly seen in RGP lens wearers, there may be reduction of palpebral aperture due to edema of ocular tissue. Edema may occur due to injury obtained during frequent insertion and removal of contact lenses. Other factors which may predispose it are forced pressing of eyelids, extension of lateral eyelid, papillary conjunctivitis (GPC) and blepharospasm. To treat these conditions RGP lenses should not be wear for up to three months, treat GPC with proper anti-allergic and lubricants, use soft contact lenses and in very severe cases eyelid surgery shall be performed.

Table 14.10: Contact lens wear complications related to various ocular structures

Eyelid	Tear film	Conjunctiva	limbus	Cornea		
				Epithelium	Corneal stroma	Endothelium
Unusual blinking pattern	Dry eye	Conjunctival congestion	Limbal redness	Epithelial erosions	Edema of corneal stroma	CLPU (CL peripheral ulcer)	Endothelial bubbles
Ptosis	Mucin balls	Papillary conjunctivitis	Vascularized limbal keratitis	Corneal microcysts	Thinning of corneal stroma	CLARE (CL induced acute red eye)	Polymegathism/ Pleomorphism
Meibomian glands dysfunction			Superior-limbal keratoconjunctivitis	Epithelial edema	Corneal neovascularization	Infiltrative keratitis	
External hordeolum				Vacuoles	Deep stromal neovascularization	Acanthamoeba keratitis	
Internal hordeolum					Corneal stromal pannus		
Squamous blepharitis							

- **Dysfunction of Meibomian glands:** It is due to mechanical blockage of Meibomian glands ducts leading to collection of yellowish creamy secretions and drying of eye. Contact lens does not receive sufficient hydration, hence causing dry eye and intolerance to contact lens. This condition can be treated by applying warm compressions over eyelids, using lubricants eye drops, improvement of eyelid hygiene. In severe cases antibiotics therapy and eyelid scrubbing can be done.

- **External hordeolum:** Commonly known as stye. It is characterized by an inflammation of eyelash root tissue or sometimes associated with inflammation of gland of Zeis or Moll. It is an acute infection caused by Staphylococcus common in those having associated staphylococcal squamous blepharitis. It manifests as infectious swelling of external lid edge and cause discomfort and pain. Treatment includes removal of eyelash related to that gland along with hot compressions which facilitates the spontaneous drainage of abscesses outside. Topical and systemic antibiotics are also prescribed for 5–7 days period along with other symptomatic drugs. Use of contact lens should be avoided during acute phase, usually about 7–10 days.

- **Internal hordeolum:** An acute staphylococcal infection of meibomian gland is called internal hordeolum and it is also frequently associated with staphylococcal squamous blepharitis. Patient presents with lid swelling with eyelid edge inversion and discomfort, pain and intolerance to contact lenses. General treatment includes application of hot compressions and antibiotics for 5–7 days, along with other symptomatic drugs. Contact lens wearing is not recommended during this acute phase, usually about seven days.

- **Squamous blepharitis:** Infection by Staphylococcus may cause conjunctivitis, staphylococcal infection of follicles of eyelash and toxic punctal epitheliopathy. Patient will present with diffuse redness, scales at roots of eyelash, sticky eyelashes, along with feeling of warmth, intense itching, and photophobia with foreign body sensation leading to an intolerance of contact lenses. Treatment includes antibiotics, corticosteroids (as ointment), artificial tears, and improvement of eyelid hygiene. Contact lenses should not be worn during this acute phase, usually variable in duration, because of periods of remission and recurrence of this condition.

Problems related to tear film

- **Dry eye:** Dry eye in contact lens wearer may occur due to increased evaporation of tear film. In contact lens wearer the tear film remains compromised and there is limited mobility as well as exchange of lipid deposits on the surface of lens. As a result disintegration of lipids occurs at rapid rate leading to decrease in lubrication of lens. Other mechanisms proposed for dryness are decrease production of tears due to increase in osmolality, ocular surface inflammation and lack of biocompatibility of the lens surface. Treatment measures include change of contact lens thickness, material and design, along with solution used for caring of lenses. Artificial tear drops, control of tear evaporation, reduction of tear drainage and reduction in time of contact lens wear are other measures to be done to control the dry eye situations.

- **Mucins balls:** With contact lens wearing, the production of mucus may alter, leading to change in characteristics of tear film and lens surface. There may be accumulation of balls of mucin under the lens surface which appears as tiny grey points on slit lamp examination. Normal corneal defense mechanism of cornea and visual acuity may compromise due to mucin balls. Usually more common with use of silicon hydrogel contact lenses. This condition can be corrected by fitting of a flatter contact lens, contact lens must be replaced frequently along with change in lens material. Artificial tear drops along with mast cell stabilizers should be added. A drastic improvement in condition will occur soon after contact lens is taken out of eye.

Problems related to conjunctiva

- **Conjunctival congestion:** Due to presence of contact lens, toxicity of contact lens solution or change in pH may lead to irritation, immunologic reaction, hypoxia, hypercapnia and relaxation of smooth muscles, causing vasodilatation of conjunctival vessels. This condition is usually asymptomatic, however, sometimes itching, slight irritation along with feeling of hot or cold sensation may be seen. If severe redness occurs, then contact lenses should not be used until complete healing occurs.

- **Contact lens associated papillary conjunctivitis (CLAPC):** Due to immunological mechanism, deposits present on contact lens (especially proteins) act as allergen and causes thickening of conjunctiva. Patients having allergic conditions like asthma, hay fever or general allergies are more prone for development of papillary conjunctivitis. Common symptoms are itching which is more intense at time of removal of lens because of more degranulation of mast cells due to handling on eyelids, more mucus discharge (especially in the morning), discomfort to contact lens and intense photophobia and slight blurring of vision. On examination, giant papillae on upper tarsal conjunctiva (like cobble stone) along with conjunctival oedema and hyperaemia are seen. Management includes removal of contact lens (until inflammation is over), reduction in time of lens wear, change of lens material, reduction in time of lens change, change of lens care solution and improvement of eye hygiene. Mast cell stabilizers like sodium cromoglycate and steroid eye drops are used to treat these papillae for nearly a period of 4–6 weeks. However, these giant papillae may remain for weeks, months, or even years, hence contact lenses can be worn with control of acute phase with all the precautions mentioned above.

Problems related to limbus

- **Limbal redness:** It is similar to conjunctival congestion and may be partial or complete. There is vasodilatation, contributed by hypoxia, hypercapnia, mechanical irritation, immunological reaction, infection, inflammation (acute red eye). Management includes removal of cause and fitting of a silicon hydrogel contact lens.

- **Vascularized limbal keratitis:** It is a complication usually seen in rigid contact lens wearer involving cornea, limbus and conjunctiva. On examination, an elevated vascularised epithelial lesion is seen at limbus along with conjunctival oedema and corneal vascularization. Corneal infiltrates are present near the limbus, with positive fluorescein staining around limbus. Common presentation is discomfort, lacrimation and photophobia. Management includes shortening of contact lens wear time and changes in lens design, i.e reduce the overall diameter, increase edge lift and/or more flat base curve. Antibiotic, ocular lubricating and steroid eye drops are given for 5–7 days and RGP lenses should be removed during this phase; however, soft contact lenses can be fitted later on. Prognosis is usually good and condition heals within 1–2 weeks time.

- **Superior or upper limbal keratoconjunctivitis:** It is another contact lens related inflammatory condition, mainly occur due to hypersensitivity to preservatives of contact lens solution, especially thiomersol. Patients generally complain of foreign body sensation with redness, itching and photophobia. In case of extensive pannus there may be an associated diminution of visual acuity. On examination limbus, bulbar and tarsal conjunctiva, and cornea involvement seen in the form of redness on superior limbus with infiltrates, micro-pannus, and micro-erosions of cornea and/or conjunctiva are seen. Irregular superior cornea and epithelial and subepithelial infiltration of superior cornea along with hypertrophy of superior bulbar conjunctiva also found. Management includes immediate removal of lens and application of lubricating eye drops along with non-steroidal anti-inflammatory drugs until inflammation disappears. Usually redness disappears early but epithelium takes time to heal, hence treatment is continued for 3 weeks to a few months. Later on patient can be prescribed lens with different design or polymer which cause less mechanical irritation of limbus. Patients should also be instructed about change of lens care solution, reduction in time of lens wear and use of preservative free contact lens.

Problems related to cornea

Contact lens can affect epithelium, stroma and endothelium of cornea leading to various complications.

Effect on epithelium of cornea: Wearing of contact lens may cause erosion and edema of epithelium and formation of microcysts on epithelium of cornea.

- **Corneal epithelial erosions:** The surface defect of corneal epithelium or breakdown of epithelium in contact lens wearers may present as small lesions or large lesions with different shapes and locations. The lesions can be identified through fluorescein test as staining areas because fluorescein dye will enter in the inter-cellular space where epithelium is eroded. Healthy epithelium remains unstained with fluorescein. Small lesions affecting superficial layer of epithelium generally do not pose any problem to patient and can be treated by prescribing lubricating eye drops. Symptoms in the form of foreign body sensations, severe pain and rarely photophobia arise when there is involvement of large area and epithelium is affected up to deeper extent. Erosions may be seen at different areas of cornea

1. *Erosions at three and nine o'clock position:* Usually more common in persons using RGP type contact lens and appears mainly due to interruption of tear flow leading to local dehydration and death of epithelial cells. Lesions are mainly present laterally and inferiorly on the cornea, the sites where upper and lower lids are in contact during blinking. Thus, insufficient or incomplete blinking and elevations of lids (due to thick edge of lens) so that a gap is created adjacent to lens edge leading to drying of tissue. To prevent this it is advised to patient to perform blinking exercises with tears supplements. Fitting of contact lens having small diameter or reduced thickness can be considered.

2. *Superior epithelial arcuate lesion (SEAL):* More commonly seen in silicon hydrogel lens users, wearing lens of improper design and elasticity. The upper lid creates an inward pressure on the contact lens and results in excessive mechanical friction pressure on the epithelium and ultimately its disruption. The lesions involve the full thickness of epithelium and seen in that area which is covered by upper eyelid, i.e. within 2 to 3 mm of superior limbus and parallel to it. Patient usually remains asymptomatic, however, sometimes may complaint of slight discomfort in wearing contact lenses for longer duration. To manage this contact lens of either less elastic material or a hard RGP lens, should be chosen.

3. *Inferior epithelial arcuate lesions:* The arc-shaped lesion (smile stain) is present parallel to the inferior limbus, usually associated with soft contact lens with less mobility. It also results from insufficient blinking causing drying out of contact lens and consequent necrosis of epithelium. Management includes changing the contact lens with more thickness with better movability on

corneal surface. Material of soft contact lens is changed or select a hard RGP lens.

4. *Central corneal epithelium erosions:* More common in extended hydrogel lens wearer. There is complete loss of epithelium from large area of cornea, seen as circular staining with fluorescein. Exposure of epithelium to hypoxia for prolonged time results in loss of its function and ultimately epithelium get completely detached when lens is removed. It is advised to remove the lens for recovery of epithelium which may take 7–10 days. Contact lens having high oxygen transmissibility should be prescribed later on.

Sometimes, any foreign body entrapped beneath hard contact lens can also damage the corneal epithelial surface, seen as irregular lines with fluorescein stain. Management includes removal and thorough rinsing of contact lens in multi-purpose solution and then reinsertion.

- **Corneal microcysts or microbullae:** Microcysts are small (15–50 micrometer diameter) circular or oval-shaped points scattered on the cornea. Usually common with extended hydrogel contact lens wearers. The microcysts formation occurs due to chronic hypoxia, trauma or mechanical irritation caused by lens, poor movement of lens and accumulation of debris in intercellular spaces. Microcysts in small number are well tolerated and do not need treatment. If present in large numbers and causing discomfort and decreased vision, then use silicon hydrogel or hard RGP contact lenses instead of extended hydrogels. After discontinuation of contact lens, the number of microcysts are increased in the first few days due to increased metabolic activity, however, then they start to decrease and completely disappear within two months.
- **Epithelial edema:** During adaptive phase of lens wear especially of hard contact lens there is reflex tearing which results in decrease tonicity of precorneal tear fluid. Due to this hypotoncity of precorneal tear film, water get enter in the epithelial cells of cornea. Commonly this condition is asymptomatic, however, halo effects can be seen in a few cases. Management includes changing the adaptation regime for hard contact lens.

- **Vacuoles:** Like microcysts these are also small (5–30 micrometer diameter) circular scattered points filled with clear fluid. These vacuoles differ from microcysts in a manner that their shadow is formed opposite to the direction of light as compared to formation of shadow in the same direction of light in case of microcysts. Vacuoles are formed due to hypoxia and are usually asymptomatic. Usually no treatment is required for vacuoles because they disappear soon after removal of contact lenses.

Effect on stroma of cornea: Change in thickness and transparency of corneal stroma may occur due to chronic hypoxia induced by contact lens wearing. Various changes observed in stroma of cornea due to contact lens wear can be grouped as

- **Edema of corneal stroma:** Accumulation of fluid into corneal stroma leads to increase in the thickness and distortion of the cornea. The main factor responsible for stromal edema is chronic hypoxia. Due to hypoxic stress (anaerobic respiration in stroma) there is increased production of lactates in the stroma causing elevation of osmotic pressure within the stroma and ultimately tissue swelling or edema. Other factors like hypotonic characteristic of tears, hypercapnia and low temperatures also contribute in edema. Percentage increase in the thickness of cornea is correlated with amount of edema. Up to 2% increase in the thickness of cornea is not associated with significant damage and hence no treatment is needed. Thickening of cornea up to 8% due to edema is dangerous and on examination striae and folds are seen in posterior stroma. To manage this condition, contact lenses with materials having higher oxygen transmissibility, thinner design and better movement on the cornea should be fitted. In severe edema it is recommended to remove contact lenses for longer duration (3–4 months).

- **Thinning of corneal stroma:** Edema of corneal stroma for prolonged period results in decrease of stromal mass which ultimately become visible as stromal thinning (measured by Pachymetry after disappearance of the edema). It is important to treat the cause of stromal edema for prevention of stromal thinning. This tissue loss is irreversible and corneal thickness remains permanently the same which cannot be recovered to original state before onset of stromal edema. Management includes removal of contact lens permanently, if not possible, then use contact lenses having high oxygen transmissibility.

- **Corneal surface neovascularization:** Surface neovascularization may occur due to chronic hypoxia or release of inflammatory mediators from damaged epithelium. Due to hypoxia, accumulation of lactates promotes softening of stroma which further induces in growth of new vessels. Release of inflammatory mediators also promotes migration of inflammatory cells which stimulate growth of vessels in stroma of cornea by releasing vaso-proliferative agents. Usually, in mild to moderate cases the person remain asymptomatic. In severe case if central cornea is involved, then loss of vision may occur. In severe corneal neovascularisation, the use of contact lenses should be stopped permanently. However, in mild to moderate cases contact lens can be used with proper care and maintenance, contact lens with higher oxygen transmissibility, i.e. more gas permeable lens should be used and daily wearing time of lens should be reduced.

- **Deep stromal neovascularisation:** Deep neovascularisation can develop in deeper layers of stroma, but it is slow in onset. Corneal hypoxia induced by lens especially by low oxygen permeable lens and thick lens results in softening of stroma due to edema. Furthermore, neovascularisation can also be precipitated by infection and toxic reactions due to lens solutions. In mild case progression of neovascularisation can be stopped by improving the handling of contact lenses, using lens of high dK/L value, reduction in schedule of daily lens wear and careful monitoring of condition. In severe cases, wearing of lens should be completely stopped.

- **Corneal vascular pannus:** Corneal pannus means growth of fibrovascular limbal tissue and fine blood vessels on the surface of cornea. Hypoxia induced by lens wearing (causing stromal edema) and damage of epithelium of cornea due to infection are important precipitating factors for formation of pannus. Generally, it does not cause difficulty to patient, but in extreme cases it can cause reduction of visual acuity. In mild cases, replace lens material with better oxygen transmissibility, reduce schedule time of daily lens wearing and careful monitoring of pannus progression. In cases of severe pannus, contact lens wearing should be permanently stopped and pannus is treated surgically.

- **Contact lens peripheral ulcer (CLPU):** It is rare with daily wear, more commonly seen with extended contact lens wear. A small (0.5–1.0 mm), distinctive circular ulcer or infiltrate with clear defined margin appears at periphery of the cornea. It is noninfectious and usually develops due to action of toxins on hypoxic cornea released from gram-positive bacteria. There is redness of eyes, pain, foreign body sensation and mild photophobia. Management includes removal of contact lens, start appropriate antibiotics, analgesics and steroids in topical and systemic form as per severity of condition.

- **Contact lens induced acute red eye (CLARE) or tight lens syndrome:** It is an acute inflammatory reaction affecting cornea and conjunctiva, presents in early morning when patient use an extended wear contact lens for overnight and eyes remain closed for long period. There is hyperaemia of conjunctiva and periphery of cornea. It occurs due to release of endotoxins from gram-negative bacteria contaminating beneath lens or in lens care solution. Symptoms are characterized by severe pain, excessive lacrimation, severe photophobia and severe conjunctival injection. On examination, punctal and diffuse infiltrates are seen in corneal periphery along with signs of inflammation. Management includes immediate removal of contact lenses, antibiotic treatment and anti-inflammatory drugs. Once the red eye is completely settled, contact lenses with high Dk/t for daily wear use can be fitted.

- **Infectious keratitis (IK):** A unilateral inflammatory reaction in anterior corneal stroma is seen where numerous small infiltrates of irregular shape are present in peripheral area along with bulbar redness. It occurs due to infection of corneal epithelium and stroma by microbes mainly pseudomonas, leading to inflammatory reaction and necrosis of tissue. There is loss of corneal epithelium with stromal infiltration and corneal ulcer. Patient presents with extreme red eye with surrounding swollen and inflamed ocular tissue, severe pain, irritation, excessive lacrimation, photophobia, purulent discharge diminished visual acuity. The incidence of infectious keratitis is more with extended hydrogel lens than daily wear RGP lens. Other predisposing factors are warm climate, poor hygiene, non-compliance with contact lens wear and care instructions, swimming with contact lenses, hypoxia, mechanical trauma, dry eye, smoking, diabetes. Treatment includes immediate removal of contact lens, proper antibiotics and anti-inflammatory drugs.

- **Acanthamoeba keratitis:** Infection by protozoa acanthamoeba is not so common in contact lens wearer usually persons having poor immunologic response are more affected. Infection can occur with any type of lens but more common with soft type of lens. Early signs of acanthamoeba keratitis appear as dendriform keratitis, sub-epithelial infiltrates and diffuse coarse punctate epithelial keratopathy. Later on, it can invade the stroma also. Treatment includes removal of contact lenses and application of topical neomycin and propamidine isethionate with or without oral ketoconazole. After recovery the RGP lenses with high Dk/t can be fitted with the instructions regarding the wearing and handling of contact lenses.

Effect on endothelium of cornea: The endothelium of cornea has important role in preventing the excessive swelling of stroma. The various changes may occur in endothelium by all types of contact lens but these are more common with the use of low gas permeable lens.

- **Endothelial bubbles (blebs) response:** The bleb response (focal, circumscribed defects in endothelium) occurs due to edema of endothelium which is precipitated by acidic pH change caused by corneal hypoxia. It may appear within a few minutes after insertion of contact lens and is subsides rapidly after removal of lens (i.e. reversible). Endothelial blebs usually do not require any treatment but development of blebs indicates presence of hypoxia in the eye due to lens wearing. Occasionally, blebs are in large numbers, then a contact lens with higher Dk/t should be prescribed.

- **Endothelial cells polymegathism and pleomorphism:** Endothelial polymegathism (i.e. significant variation in the size of endothelial cells) and pleomorphism (i.e. variation in shape of endothelial cells) may occur due to use of lens of poor oxygen transmissibility (PMMA wearers or extended wear lens) for a long period. Chronic hypoxic stress and hypercapnia due to contact lens wearing lead to weakening of junctions between endothelial cells followed by change in their shape and size. The cornea in presence of polymegathism swells at faster rate than normal cornea. Wearers will complaint of discomfort and intolerance with lens. Management includes fitting of contact lenses with high oxygen transmissibility and reduction in duration of daily lens wear.

MAINTENANCE AND CARE OF CONTACT LENSES

Introduction

Maintenance and care of contact lenses by its wearer is most critical step to decide the success rate and satisfaction in contact lens wearer patients. Different regimen can be used for care of lens and choice of regimen will depend on many factors including type of lens and its material, specific patient needs, lifestyle or wearing schedule of contact lens. Triad of prescribed good contact lens, patient compliance for lens and monitoring by professional at periodic interval decide the outcome of safe and effective contact lens wear.

Aims of care and maintenance of contact lens are

- Provide comfortable lens wear
- Minimize and/or prevent contamination by microbes
- Decrease deposits formation on contact lens
- Maintain availability of contact lenses in ready wear status

To achieve these aims, various maintenance products are used, which serve following functions to keep the contact lens in wearable state

- Keep the lens clean
- Maintain wetting/re-wetting of lens
- Prevention of infection
- Removal of protein deposits
- Maintain physical and chemical state of contact lens

Elements of maintenance and care: The maintenance and care system of contact lenses consists of following elements to deliver an effective result

- Personal care
- Contact lens solutions
- Disinfecting agents
- Preservative agents
- Protein removal process
- Lens storage system

Personal Care

Personal hygiene of contact lens wearer remains the most important first step in maintenance and care of contact lens. Person using contact lenses should keep his/her nails properly trimmed and hands should be washed thoroughly with soap and water prior to using contact lenses. Then, dry the hands and use antimicrobial rubs, if possible before removal of lenses from lens case. Use of any oil-based solutions like cream or ointments before handling the contact lenses should be avoided because, it may cause deposition of lipids over lens surfaces. Hence, foremost important aspect of a good contact lens wear outcome starts with a proper handling and caring of contact lens during insertion or removal.

Contact Lens Solutions

Various solutions are used for care and to maintain contact lens in good condition and for comfortable wear. These solutions are routinely used by the contact lens wearer and purchased by users along with lenses. For convenience of understanding we can group these contact lens care solutions as

- Cleaning agents
- Rinsing solutions
- Wetting and lubricating drops
- Multipurpose solution

Cleaning agents or solution: Lens surface can be cleaned manually by rubbing and rinsing with saline or by using cleaning solutions on daily basis. These cleaning solutions generally consist of surfactants which act on the contact lens surface to remove most loosely attached foreign substances like lipids, residues, dirt, mucus, proteins, microbes or other deposits. Cleaning of lens is very important step to remove the cysts and trophozoites of acanthamoeba from surface of lens. The cleaners may be available in a separate bottle or may be combined with disinfecting/soaking solution in one bottle. Along with surfactants other agents can be added in cleaning agent like

- Different non-ionic or ionic chemical substances, added to decrease contact between lens and the solution
- Agents acting against microbes are also added in daily cleaner
- Agents which maintains osmolality
- Buffer system to regulate the pH
- Chelating agents for removal of contaminants from lens
- Abrasive material as adjunct to remove adherent substances or muco-proteinaceous deposits from surface of lens which cannot be removed by surfactant itself. However, use of abrasive material or excessive rubbing can lead to scratches and may induce change in power to contact lenses.
- Agents like polyvinyl alcohol or methylcellulose as viscosity enhancers
- Alcohol to remove lipids

The cleaning agents may be of two types

Surfactant cleaners: These agents have detergent like action and by reducing surface tension act as surface active agent. Surfactants have both hydrophobic and hydrophilic components and molecules of surfactant combine with different type of debris or residues and deposits on lens, as a result, a layer of surfactant molecules is formed over contaminant (micelles formation), surface tension get decrease and it causes dispersion of contaminant from contact lens surface which get suspend in surrounding liquid and finally removed by rinsing. Some common examples of surfactants are isopropyl alcohol, hexylene glycol, polyvinyl alcohol, poloxamine, poloxamer-407, octylphenoxy ethanol,

etc. Surfactants are able to remove lipid, inorganic deposits, mucus, etc. however, they are not much effective for removal of proteins.

Enzymatic cleaners: As surfactants cannot remove protein effectively, hence enzymatic cleaners can be used which contain proteolytic enzymes to break down proteins from surface of lens. However, use of these cleaners is not obligatory and not used on daily basis. Enzyme cleaners are usually used for types of lens which are not replaced frequently and are nondisposable.

Cleaning procedure: Principle is Rub and Rinse of lens. Contact lenses should be cleaned every time before insertion and after removal to get a complication free result. Following steps are done for cleaning of lenses

- Thoroughly wash hands and dry them (avoid moisturizing cream/perfumed soaps before cleaning)
- Place the contact lens in palm of hand.
- Pour 4–5 drops of cleaning agent on each surface of contact lens.
- Gently rub contact lens using pulp of forefinger, for about 15–20 seconds per side in a circular motion. Slowly roll forefinger in both directions to clean periphery of lens.
- Rinse well using rinsing solution.

Process of rubbing and rinsing is important because it significantly helps in removal of loose debris and many microbes from contact lens surface. Cleaning should be done on daily basis for all types of contact lenses including disposable lenses.

Rinsing solutions: Cleaning of lens is followed by rinsing. The purpose of rinsing is to remove surfactant cleaners, microorganisms and suspended residues from the surface of lens completely, irrespective of the type of cleaning agent. It is advised to rinse all types of contact lenses and before and after overnight soak. Various types of solutions which can be used for rinsing are

- Unpreserved saline
- Preserved saline
- Multi-purpose solutions.

Rinsing should not be done with tap water due to increase risk of infection with acanthamoeba.

Buffering agents are also added in rinsing solution and usually buffered isotonic saline is more preferred as compared to un-buffered saline.

Wetting and Lubricant drops: These drops are used, while contact lens is in the eye and before insertion of lens in eye where these agents provide lubrication and rewetting of contact lens surface. Standard wetting drops contain following components in a proportionate amount, to increase the comfort and duration of contact lens wear.

- Non-ionic surfactant in very low concentrations to promote cleaning of lens
- Polymer for lubricating the lens surface
- Buffering agents to compile pH of tears
- Viscosity agents to reduce friction
- Preservatives for maintaining the sterility of drops.

In patients, who use extended wear or continuous wear contact lenses, use of these wetting and lubricant drops are very helpful for wearers, although drops can also be used with daily wear lenses. These are especially indicated on those patients who have relative tear deficiency and use contact lens during sleeping also, who work in dry atmosphere and work for prolonged period on computers, etc. These wetting and lubricants prevent the contact lens from dryness due to wind exposure, low humidity and high temperatures. Patients facing difficulty in removing soft hydrogel lenses because of dehydration or the one who frequently damages his/her lenses on removal will also be benefited by use of lubricants.

Wetting and lubricating drops are also formulated with various viscosity enhancing agents like

- Polyvinyl alcohol
- Methylcellulose and hydroxyl methylcellulose
- Hydroxy propyl methylcellulose (HPMC)

- Polyethylene glycol
- Polysorbate 80

Presence of viscous agents in lubricants helps to increase the contact of solution with lens and also help to decrease the friction. These viscosity agents help to maintain the relative density of cleaners, soaking solution and lubricants. Usually, cleaners are kept more viscous than lubricants while lubricants kept more viscous than soaking agents.

Note: Viscosity order: Cleaners> lubricants> soaking agents.

Multi-purpose solutions: Most widely used solution for maintenance and care of contact lenses is multipurpose solution. As name suggests this single solution performs functions of several components of lens care system, hence reduces the requirement of actual number of lens care solutions.

For patient convenience and ease of utilization, this multi-purpose solution performs a combined function of cleaning, rinsing and disinfection. Moreover, in newer solutions even protein remover agents are also added to enhance efficacy of solution and reduce another maintenance step in contact lens care.

Disinfecting Agents for Care of Contact Lens

Disinfection means removal and/or killing of microorganisms (microbes, fungi and viruses) from contact lenses and is important step to be followed after daily cleaning and rinsing of lens. In contact lens wearer the natural defence mechanism of eye remains compromised, i.e. protective barrier function of corneal epithelium affected and there are more chances of infection by microorganisms. Thus, disinfecting contact lens care solutions are used to minimize or kill potentially harmful micro-organisms (bacteria, viruses, amoebas, fungi) along with maintenance of contact lens hydration. By disinfection the living or vegetative microorganisms are destroyed but not the spores of microorganisms. Sterilization is a process which kills all life form of microorganisms including their spores and it is impossible to achieve sterilization with normal lens care solutions.

The disinfection for contact lens can be done mainly by two techniques

- Disinfection based on heat (thermal disinfection)
- Disinfection based on chemical methods (chemical disinfection)

Disinfection based on heat: As the name indicates heat is used to deactivate or kills most of living contaminants from contact lens. Normally sterile thiomersol, persevered (with potassium sorbate) saline or unpreserved saline are used as medium to boil the lens. Boiling of lens can be done by keeping it in a bowl filled with saline and boiled for 10–15 min in range of 70–90°C. A saline-based solution containing thiomersol with EDTA can also be used, where EDTA helps in removal of calcium from contact lens surface. Thermal disinfection method should not be used with high water content lens.

Advantages
- Very effective method for disinfection
- No associated allergic reactions or discomfort

Disadvantages
- Decreased life span of lens due to alteration in property of lens
- Discoloration of lens with time due to heating
- Reduction in water content of lens especially high water content lens
- Change in optical and physical properties of lens due to exposure to heat
- Warpage of lens due to denaturation of proteins

Chemical-based disinfection systems: Wide varieties of chemical-based disinfection systems are present for disinfection of contact lenses that can grouped as follows

- Conventional cold chemical disinfectant-based solution

- Hydrogen peroxide-based system
- Chlorine system

Conventional cold chemical disinfectant-based solutions: Ideal characteristics required in chemical disinfectants are

- Non-toxicity
- Non-irritating
- Compatible with other ingredients
- Stable over time
- Effective against a wide range of micro-organisms

Many chemical agents such as chlorhexidine, benzalkonium chloride, thiomersol, and sorbic acid are used as disinfectant solution, although with caution because they may cause sensitivity reactions.

- *Chlorhexidine gluconate (CHG):* It is a biguanide antimicrobial agent, mainly effective against bacteria. It has no antifungal activity. It can be used as preservative and disinfectant with thiomersol for both soft and hard contact lenses. It can bind with lens materials and with protein deposits and cause allergic reactions. Its breakdown product may cause yellowish discoloration of lens.

- *Benzalkonium chloride (BAK):* It is a quaternary ammonium compound and can be used as disinfectant and preservative with ophthalmic solution for PMMA lenses. It acts as cidal agent against many bacteria and fungi. BAK is not used in solution for hydrogel lens (e.g. silicon acrylate and fluorosilicon acrylate) because it binds with lens materials, lens being gas permeable also absorb BAK which can accumulate to toxic levels and may cause eye injury. Additionally, BAK also increases hydrophobicity of lens surface, chances of deposit formation increased. Normal concentration of BAK in contact lens care solution is 0.001–0.01% and it is more active at alkaline medium (pH = 8). It shows synergistic action with EDTA and require in low dose when combined with it.

- *Thimerosal:* It is a mercurial compound having bacteriocidal activity against many bacteria and fungi. It can be used both as a preservative (0.001%) and as a disinfectant (0.0005%) and acts by inhibiting the activity of cellular enzymes leading to killing of micro-organism. Its activity is maximal at neutral or slightly alkaline pH and usually used in the concentration of 0.001–0.2% in the solution. It is comparatively nontoxic but in some patients it may cause allergic reactions especially in persons wearing hydrophilic contact lens. It should not be combined with EDTA because its activity is reduced with EDTA. When compared with BAK, it shows less activity against some gram-positive and gram-negative micro-organism than BAK. To achieve effective antimicrobial action it can be combined with other preservatives like chlorhexidine, etc.

- *Sorbic acid:* Sorbates or sorbic acid act as antibacterial and antifungal agent and is added in contact lens saline as enhancing agent. When used alone it usually does not cause any allergic reactions but in formulation with other compound it may cause burning sensations due to change in the pH of solution (as it is acidic in nature). It may cause yellow or brown discolouration of contact lenses by reacting with amino acids present in tear proteins.

Hydrogen peroxide-based system: In this system, microorganisms are exposed to oxidative atmosphere by using 3% peroxide concentration with an acidic pH of 3–4. Hydrogen peroxide is effective against majority of all microbes responsible for infection in contact lens wearer. Residual hydrogen peroxide on lens after disinfection process may cause irritation on eyes, hence it is necessary to do neutralization of peroxide by using substances like sodium pyruvate, sodium bicarbonate, sodium thiosulphite, and catalase. The hydrogen peroxide get decompose into saline and oxygen. Disinfection by hydrogen peroxide for bacteria and viruses requires its exposure for about 10–15 minutes (45 minutes for fungi, 2–3 hours for acanthoemaba) followed by neutralization for about 30 min–3 hours.

The disinfecting solutions based on hydrogen peroxide may contain preservative or may be preservative free. Depending on the method adopted to neutralize the peroxide, two types of peroxide lens care systems can be used for disinfection with hydrogen peroxide

- One-step disinfecting system
- Two-step disinfecting system

One-step system: These systems are formulated in such a manner that both disinfection and neutralization of hydrogen peroxides is done in a recommended time period (30–60 minutes). This is very simple to use and usually most of the hydrogen peroxide get neutralize in first 30–60 minutes. These systems are either tablet using systems or a disc-based system. In tablet using systems delay period is done during neutralization phase, whereas in disc-based systems no delay is done during neutralization phase. The effectiveness of this system can be improved by controlling the rate of neutralization of hydrogen peroxide.

Two-step system: System where neutralization of contact lens is done as a separate step is called two-step disinfecting system. Thus in this system the neutralizing agent in the form of tablets is added separately during disinfection process. These tablets release catalase enzyme to neutralize the hydrogen peroxide so that it reaches to safe residual level. The main advantage with this system is that the neutralization of hydrogen peroxide can be delayed according to requirement so that high peroxide concentration remains maintained for a long time which will enhance the antimicrobial effect of solution compared to one-step system. Recommended method for two-step system disinfection is that contact lenses are kept in hydrogen peroxide solution overnight, then neutralize the lenses just before their usage.

Advantages of hydrogen peroxide system

- Rapidly kill most types of micro-organisms in large numbers
- Takes very short time period, usually a soaking time of 10–20 minutes.
- High anti-microbial efficacy
- Decomposition products (oxygen and water) are non-toxic in nature.

Disadvantages of hydrogen peroxide system

- If not neutralized properly, it can cause irritation to eyes
- Once completely neutralized, has no anti-microbial activity
- Occasionally not compatible with contact lenses such as high water content, ionic contact lenses; where this system can alter (reversibly) lens parameters and water content.

Note: Multi-step hydrogen peroxide systems although available; but are very complex and can confuse patients.

Chlorine Systems: For disinfection of soft contact lenses anhydrous effervescent tablets of either stabilized halane or halazone benzoic acid are used in convenient blister pack, where both these tablets differ in amount of available chlorine (4–8 ppm).

These chlorine releasing tablets are dissolved in unpreserved saline (~10 ml), which forms a disinfecting solution having pH in range of 5.5–7.5. Recommended exposure time is usually four hours, however, concentration of undissociated hypochlorous acid decides the effectiveness of antimicrobial activity. Contact lenses should be rinsed thoroughly before insertion into eyes.

Dissociated hypochlorous acid produces hypochlorite and chlorine which also act as bleaching agents, hence contact lenses tinted with reactive dyes may change color.

Preservative Systems

Preservatives are used usually with other chemical agents. These are used to either kill or inhibit the growth of microorganisms. An ideal preservative present in contact lens solution

1. Should provide effective degree of disinfection in the existing environment
2. Should be nontoxic
3. Should be compatible with lens material and tear film, i.e. no effect on wettability and parameters of lens

Commonly used preservatives are

- Benzalkonium chloride
- Chlorhexidine
- Thiomerosal
- Chlorbutanol
- Benzyl alcohol
- EDTA
- PAPB and PHMB
- Quaternary ammonium compounds

Chlorbutanol: It is an unstable volatile preservative with a characteristic smell. Basically, it is used as chlorinated alcohol (0.5%) along with other preservatives. Although it has broad spectrum action on bacteria in acidic pH, however, it acts slowly. Initially, it was used to disinfect PMMA lenses, but now it is rarely used. It remains stable at low pH, at high pH it get break into hydrocarbons and HCl.

Benzyl Alcohol: It can be used both as a preservative and disinfectant. Pure benzyl alcohol because of its physio-chemical properties is considered as ideal preservative. It has low molecular weight and can enter easily into intermolecular spaces of lens polymers. Being bipolar molecule it has low polarity. It is more stable than chlorbutanol, water soluble and can be used to disinfect and preserve RGP and PMMA lenses. Benzyl alcohol is not suitable for hydrophilic materials because it can interact with contact lens and may cause irritation and toxicity to eye. It is converted into aldehydes, leading to hardening and discoloration of soft contact lens. It is effective against both bacteria and virus but not active against *Pseudomonas aeruginosa*.

EDTA (Ethylene diamine tetra acetic acid): EDTA *per se* is not a true preservative rather it acts as a chelating agent, preservative enhancers and potentiator. It has no antimicrobial action but it potentiates the antibacterial action of other quaternary ammonium preservatives against gram-negative microorganisms especially pseudomonas. In addition, because of chelating property it binds with divalent cations like calcium and magnesium present in solutions or on the cell walls of gram-negative organisms which is necessary to prevent cell growth of microbes. EDTA does not interact with lens material and is used in combination with BAK and other preservatives in most contact lens solution.

Poly aminopropyl biguanide (PAPB) and Poly hexamethlene biguanide (PHMB): PAPB and PHMB both are high molecular weight preservatives, specially developed to avoid the problem of ocular irritation and hypersensitivity occurring due to previous preservatives. PHMB is used in the concentration of 0.001% and show broad spectrum antimicrobial action and less toxicity.

PAPB which is also known as Dymed contains positively charged biguanide group which selectively bind to negatively charged phospholipids of membrane of micro-organisms, leading to disintegration of micro-organism. It is nonirritating, nonsensitive and has more antimicrobial effect as compared to chlorhexidine. It can be used as preservative and disinfectant in very low concentration of 0.00005–0.0005%.

Quaternary ammonium compound (Polyquad): These high molecular weight cationic polymers like poly quaternium-1, polidromium chloride, Onamer M are effective antibacterial but show less antifungal activity. Polyquad in the concentrations of 0.001–0.005% can be used as disinfectant and preservative for both rigid and soft lenses. Quaternary ammonium compound being large in mole-

Note: Opti-Free and Opti-Free Express (Alcon): contain Poly quaternium-1.

cular structure cannot adhere and enter into lens material, thus chances of ocular reactions are less.

Protein removal process or enzymatic cleaners: Enzymatic cleaners contain proteolytic enzymes like papaine, pancreatin, lipase, subtilisin, etc. and are included in lens care systems for removal of proteins from surfaces of contact lens. The enzyme cleaners can be used once a week or more frequently depending on the length of lens wear, for example: Disposable lens usually do not require treatment with enzymatic cleaners while soft and some RGP lenses require it because they are not replaced frequently. Papaine containing cleaners are not compatible with hydrogen peroxide and thermal disinfection.

For protein removal, the enzyme tablets are dissolved in saline or distilled water and lens is placed in this solution for 4–6 hrs. Lens should be cleaned and rinsed before and after process of protein removal. This mechanism of enzyme tablets only loosens the proteins hence patients are advised to clean and rub their contact lenses after completion of deproteinization process.

Lens Storage System

Storage system for soft lenses and RGP lenses is slightly different because soft lenses are stored in a hydrated state, while RGP lenses are stored in a dry state.

All soft contact lenses once removed from their sterile packing are kept in a lens case (filled with rinsing or multipurpose solution) in such a manner that entire lens is merged in solution. Normally lenses are removed from the case and cleaned with cleaners before inserting in the eye. Similarly after removal from the eyes, lenses are rinsed and kept back in the lens case containing multipurpose solution. However, these lenses need to be treated chemically at least once a week to prevent contamination and to remove debris and proteins.

RGP lenses are stored in dry state in a simple shape (usually flat), fitted inside a lens case which can be kept in purse or pocket. After removal from the case these lenses are cleaned and rinsed before inserting in the eye. Similarly, after removal from the eyes these lenses are cleaned and rinsed with multi-purpose solution before keeping them inside the lens case.

Care of Lens Cases

Improper care and maintenance of contact lens case may cause contamination of contact lenses by various microorganisms by formation of a biofilm or glycocalyx on its surface. Contamination may occur by pathogens like *Pseudomonas aeruginosa* and Serratia marcereens which in turn can produce biofilms. The glycocalyx formed on lens surface protect bacterial cells from action of chemical disinfectants or preservative and also helps in trapping of nutrient particles for micro-organism growth. To avoid chances of contamination it is necessary to rinse the lens case after every use and to discard all used solution from lens case. Thereafter, lens should be stored in fresh solution so that disinfecting efficacy of solution remains maintained which might loss due to mixing of fresh solution with used solutions. Lens cases should be scrubbed with a toothbrush preferably with oil-free soaps or detergents, usually on weekly basis. Then rinse with hot water and rub thoroughly with clean and dry tissue. Colonization of microorganisms like protozoa can be prevented by keeping lens case dry, because protozoa needs moist or wet environment for their growth.

CIBA vision has introduced a unique lens case called Pro Guard. In this lens case an anti-microbial agent is already incorporated which prevent contamination of case by micro-organisms. This type of case comprises electrically charged silver ions which help to reduce the chances of contamination up to 40%.

Note: Ideally, the lens case should be replaced at regular intervals.

Maintenance and Lens Care Methods

Newer approach for better lens care is to simplify the cleaning, storing and disinfecting systems required for maintenance and care of contact lenses which can easily be understood by patients and they can comfortably adopt them. Various lens care methods for better outcome that are recommended for RGP and soft contact lens wearers and also for allergy sufferer patients are as follows

Simplified RGP lens regimens: RGP contact lens solutions usually used are in a sequence initially for cleaning followed by disinfecting, then wetting and lastly for conditioning and cushioning purposes. Most of the commercially available solutions serve all these function in one solution, however, if patient is switching to a solution which serves purpose of cleaning, disinfection and conditioning but not of wetting and cushioning, then an additional solution should be added to the lens care regime.

Soft contact lens regimens: Most common approach adopted by majority of patients wearing soft contact lenses is to use one bottle lens care system. For example, commercially available soft lens care products like ReNu (Bausch and Lomb), Opti free and Opti one (Alcon) are very popular. These solutions have very low toxicity. Simply a digital cleaning with rinsing (use clean hands) followed by soaking of lens in a clean case is needed for maintenance and care a soft contact lens by these solutions. Although these solutions has very low toxicity and allergic reactions because they avoid use of preservatives like thimerosal, chlorhexidine and hydrogen peroxide exposure, better compliance and results are still doubtful with these solutions.

Sometimes one bottle lens care systems which contain surfactants can cause Sicca like syndrome. To prevent these patients are advised to adopt a saline rinse technique before insertion of contact lens, preferably with sterile saline which may be sorbic acid preserved or non-preserved.

Care regimes for allergy lens wearers: Patients suffering from allergies should use topical eye drops of either anti-histaminic or mast cell stabilizers or non steroidal anti-inflammatory drugs before and after lens wear to minimize the discomfort.

In a nutshell, care regimen is selected on the basis of patients wearing schedule, type of lens selected for wearing, ocular sensitivity, replacement schedule and patient's convenience. Patients are advised not to mix different types of solutions and brands and take advice from clinician before substituting any solution for lens care.

Radiuscope

Measurement of the base curve (i.e. radius of the curvature of back surface) of a contact lens is done by using an instrument called Radiuscope. In the year 1900 eminent scientist Drysdale described a principle which is used in all types of Radiuscope although they may vary from each other in design and method of displaying the readings.

Principle: When a parallel beam of light is directed on center of a concave reflecting surface, the light gets reflected along the same path as that of incident light. Now if this parallel beam of light is directed to the center of curvature of same concave reflecting surface; it will again reflect back along the same path, as that of incident light.

As both center of a concave reflecting surface and center of curvature of the same surface are reflecting incident light along its original path sometimes we call these points as self-reflecting points. It means that center of curvature and surface of the lens are two positions where the object and image coincide.

Thus the examiner needs to focus the Radiuscope upside and downwards until two clear images (one from center and second from center of curvature of contact lens) of the same

target are seen at two different positions as shown in Fig. 14.14A and B. Radius of curvature of contact lens is the distance between the two positions of Radiuscope, where target images are focused clearly.

Main parts of Radiuscope are
- Compound microscope
- Internal illuminated target
- Half-silvered mirror

Radiuscope includes a compound microscope having an internally illuminated target, such as a radial line target (Fig. 14.14) which is projected along visual axis of Radiuscope in such a manner that image of target is seen clearly through an eyepiece by an observer. Half-silvered mirror is fitted above the microscope objective, which is set at an angle of 45°. When an object is focused (through Radiuscope), either on its concave reflecting surface or at its center of curvature image of this target is seen clearly in both the situations.

Procedure: To measure the back radius of a contact lens following steps are done

- Place the contact lens (keeping its concave surface upward) on the platform of Radiuscope, while convex surface of contact lens is kept in downward direction and float on fluid or wetting solution. The fluid helps to reduce the reflections from the lower (convex) surface of the lens when the reflections from upper (concave) surface of contact lens are observed.

- Slowly move the stage of Radiuscope so that illuminated target gets aligned with mirror and a real image is formed at working plane of objective lens from the light reflected through mirror.

- Once alignment is done, now move the microscope downward, toward contact lens surface, until working plane of microscope coincides with plane of back surface of contact lens.

- At this point reflected light (passing through half-silvered mirror) form an

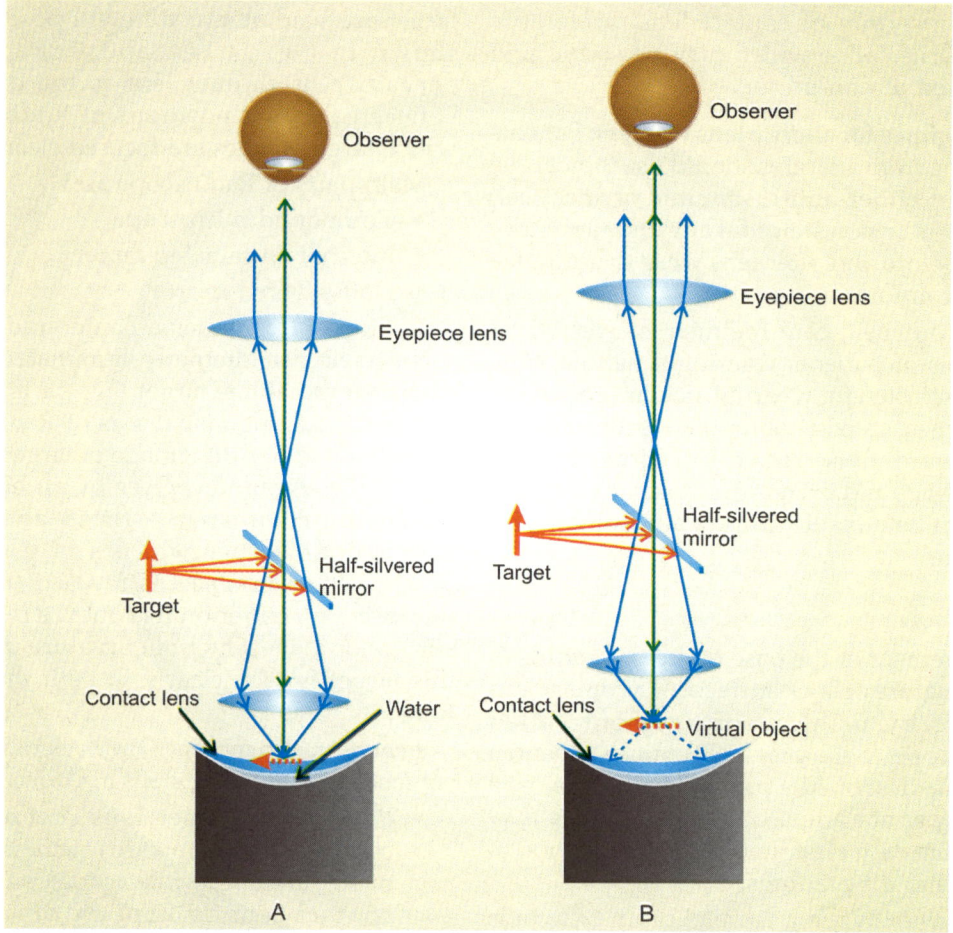

Fig. 14.14: Radiuscope; Zero position (First focus): When microscope objective focuses at back surface of contact lens. Final position (second focus): When microscope objective focuses at center of curvature, of back surface of contact lens.

image in focal plane of microscope eyepiece, where it is seen clearly by the observer, as shown in Fig. 14.14A. This point is termed zero point and observer notices the reading on the scale of Radiuscope.

- Now slowly observer raise the microscope, until a second point is found where image of target is in finest focus; which occurs when working plane of objective lens align with center of curvature of back surface of contact lens.

- At this point concave surface of contact lens is again returning the light, along its own path. This point is called second focus point (Fig. 14.14B) and observer again notices the reading on the scale of Radiuscope.

Measure the distance covered by microscope between zero point and second focus point; where images were clearly focused. This distance denotes real length of radius of curvature of concave surface (base curve radius) of contact lens under examination.

Refractive Surgery

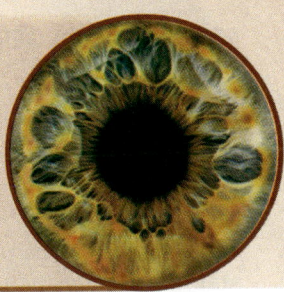

REFRACTIVE SURGERY

Introduction and Classification

Recently, the refractive procedures done for correction of refractive errors have become very popular especially in younger populations. To perform the refractive surgery it is necessary to wait until refractive errors get stabilize which usually occurs at the age of 19–20 years in the females and 20–21 years in the males. These refractive procedures took a long curve of evolution and techniques have improvised continuously. In recent decades a steep change has taken place in refractive surgery techniques which made several older techniques obsolete. We will describe only those techniques in detail which are presently in trend.

Refractive procedures are classified on the basis of type of incision, laser used or site of refractive correction. The classification of various refractive procedures is summarized in Table 15.1.

Lasers in Refractive Surgeries

Following lasers are used to perform the refractive surgery on the cornea.

- Excimer laser
- Solid state UV laser
- Femtosecond laser

Excimer Laser

Excimer literally means excited dimer, where 'exc' part is taken from excited and 'imer' part from dimer. In a molecule, where components of that molecule are bounded together in the excited state and not in the ground state, then that molecule is termed diatomic molecule. In ground state two-component molecules are not bounded, in reality they are repulsive in nature. When these component molecules are excited by electrons they attract each other and become a stable molecule. Hence, in Excimer laser when these stable excited molecules dissociate and separates into two molecules, i.e. they come to their ground state level from

Table 15.1: Classification of various refractive surgeries				
Incisional refractive procedures	Lamellar refractive surgery	Laser refractive surgery	Intraocular refractive surgery	Miscellaneous refractive techniques
Radial keratotomy (RK)	Freeze Keratomileusis of Barraquer	Photorefractive keratotomy (PRK)	Phakic refractive lenses (PRLs)	Conductive keratoplasty (CK)
Relaxing incisional procedures	Epikeratoplasty/ Epikeratophakia	Laser in situ Keratomileusis (LASIK)	Refractive lens exchange (RLE)	Orthokeratology
Astigmatic keratotomy (AK)	Non-freeze keratomileusis	Laser subepithe-lial Keratomileusis (LASEK)		Intrastromal corneal ring segments
Hexagonal keratotomy	Keratomileusis in situ (BKS technique)	Custom laser in situ Keratomi-leusis (C-LASIK)		Intracorneal hydrogel lenses
Ruiz procedure	Automated lamellar keratoplasty (ALK)	Epithelial laser in situ Keratomi-leusis (E-LASIK)		
		Femtosecond LASIK		
		Small incision lenticule extraction (SMILE)		

their excited state level they emit energy. This property makes these molecules suitable for laser because ground state is not stable and excited state molecule keep on forming by population inversion (details in Chapter 1).

Majority of these excimer molecules acts as an active laser medium (details in Chapter 1) and forms laser by an electric high voltage discharge through a gas chamber having noble gas mixture. Wavelength of laser coming out is determined by the type of gas mixture used to produce it and a few examples are summarized in Table 15.2. Usually, Krypton and Xenon are mixed along with argon, chloride and fluoride.

Excimer system to be used as a medium of laser was first defined by Houtermans in 1960s, but was extensively used for medical purposes since early 1980s. In medical field these excimer lasers are primarily used for tissue surface ablation. These excimer laser system work efficiently in relation to absorption coefficient of tissues and as cornea has high absorption coefficient, it becomes the most desirable target tissue for laser ablation.

During the year 1980s, frequency doubled organic dye lasers and frequency quadrupled Neodymium: YAG lasers were commercially available which were capable of producing a laser in the range of 280 nm (UV spectrum), however, these lasers are not used for corneal surface ablation. Instead excimer laser are used for surface ablation because of the following characteristics of laser outputs:

- Firstly, it is considered as 'cool laser' because thermal effects of excimer laser are almost negligible because of very short pulse duration (12–15 nanoseconds) which does not allow thermal energy to diffuse into corneal tissue to cause thermal damage. Thus, it is considered appropriate to carry out surgery on delicate cornea.

- Secondly, the pulse to pulse energy level of excimer laser can be reproduced and the variation remains in acceptable limits. The pulses can be repeated (pulse repetition rate) in a wide range of frequency ranging from 1 to 50 Hz.

- Thirdly, these excimer lasers have enough energy to produce large beam. Laser energy typically up to 450 mj is obtainable in order to produce large beam of laser which can ablate the corneal surface effectively. This large laser beam can remove the corneal tissue and alters the shape of the central corneal portion in 4–7 mm diameter area without any limitations on pulse energy.

Most of the continuous wave or pulsed wave lasers cause ablation of the surface by the principle of photothermal process, however, excimer lasers ablate cornea by photochemical process instead of routine photothermal mechanism. The short wavelength (193 nm) photons are capable of breaking the molecule bonds in corneal tissue without producing any thermal or acoustic damage to surrounding tissue. Damage to deeper corneal structures like descemet's membrane and endothelium is mainly prevented by an advantageous property of limited penetration of excimer laser. Corneal endothelial damage is greatest by Krypton fluoride laser (248 nm wavelength) as compared to other excimer laser wavelengths. Similarly, Xenon chloride laser can penetrate deeper tissues and damage crystalline lens or even retina in case of aphakics. Longer wavelength (>280 nm) lasers causes photo-keratitis, thermal damage, and has mutagenic properties.

In a nutshell, Argon fluoride laser with 193 nm wavelength is the most suitable excimer laser for clinical purposes. Argon

Table 15.2: Examples of gas mixture with respective output wavelengths of LASER

Gas mixture	Laser wavelength
Argon fluoride	193 nm
Krypton chloride	222 nm
Krypton fluoride	248 nm
Xenon chloride	308 nm
Xenon fluoride	351 nm

fluoride laser is capable of eliminating microscopic amount (0.1–0.4 nm) of corneal tissue without producing any thermal injury to the cornea. A well-defined exceptionally smooth corneal surface is produced by this laser, because it delivers an accurate amount of energy per pulse and also the precise numbers of pulses are applied to the specified area of the cornea. Excimer laser can produce tiny (10 μm wide) corneal incisions even up to 95% depth of corneal thickness.

Excimer laser machines: Excimer laser machine or system had been improved constantly since its advent so that various types of beam are delivered by these machines. These photoablating excimer laser machines can be grouped as summarized in Table 15.3.

Solid State UV Laser

Energy absorption coefficient of cornea is high and relatively stable in the range of 190–220 nm, hence laser pulses in the similar range (193–220 nm) can be used for corneal surface ablation. Several scientists introduced fifth node of Neodymium-YAG laser as an alternate source of laser for photoablation of cornea. These solid state UV laser radiations are generated in a laser crystal by frequency conversion of an infrared laser light. The wavelength of this solid state laser radiation is in a range of 208–213 nm. For example,

LaserSoft is a diode pumped solid state laser generating 0.2 mm flying spot short pulsed laser beam with a repetition rate of 4 kHz and ablation zone of 1–10 mm diameter.

For accurate custom ablation (C-LASIK) solid state laser is more preferred to excimer laser because of various advantageous features as summarized in Table 15.4.

Introduction of solid state laser (SSL) has improved the corneal refractive surgeries as it provides more advantages over excimer laser to the surgeons. The smaller (0.2 mm) spot size in SSL helps to obtain an accurate and defined ablation, thus resulting in reduction of corneal microirregularities (i.e. high order abberrations) and a smooth and homogeneous corneal surface is obtained. While, in excimer laser the large spot size produces more mechanical stress due to larger acoustic shock waves, hence there is more damage of collagen structure of cornea. Furthermore, high repetition rate in SSL causes significant lesser collateral damge to surrounding corneal tissue, hence chances of post-procedure corneal haze is significantly low in SSL.

Femtosecond Laser

Advancement in research to eliminate the collateral damage to surrounding tissue leads to the invention of femtosecond laser. This newer improvised medical technology

Table 15.3: Classification of excimer laser machines with properties	
Laser types	*Properties*
Broad beam laser	These first generation machines produced a wide-ranging beam of laser about 7 mm in diameter. These lasers had high energy per pulse and also beam irregularities, hence need lower number of pulses but forms the central corneal islands.
Scanning slit laser	To reduce beam irregularities a scanning slit was introduced, which provide sequential ablation. Formation of central corneal island reduced to a significant level.
Scanning spot laser	In these next generation machines a scanning spot was added to previous version. The spot passes around the proposed area of ablation.
Flying spot laser	These fourth generation machines had wavefront technology and an eye tracker. While performing the procedure these advanced features demonstrated to be very useful for patient's comfort.

Table 15.4: Excimer laser versus solid state laser (SSL)

Laser features	Excimer laser (193 nm)	Solid state UV laser (213 nm)
Beam quality	Require beam forming elements and is multimode in nature	No beam forming element needed, hence produces Gaussian bean of single mode
Flying spot size	0.8–1 mm	0.2 mm (five times smaller)
High order aberrations	Not treated	Treated
Eye tracking system	Speed 150 Hz	Speed 1 kHz
Repetition rate	50–500 Hz	1 kHz
Thermal effect	Temperature rise in corneal stroma during procedure is up to 7°C	Temperature rise in corneal stroma during procedure is 0.8°C
Corneal drying	Required during transepithelial treatment	Not required
Damage due to acoustic shock waves	Minimal	Almost nil
Post-procedure corneal haze	Present	Significantly less
Post-procedure visual recovery	Slower	Faster
Post-procedure scarring	Minimal	Almost nil
Maintenance cost	Higher because require gas storage system	Lower

initially came for the creation of accurate and precise corneal flaps, however, its use expanded slowly in field of other ocular surgeries especially cataract, lamellar kerato-plasty and penetrating keratoplasty.

Presently, Femtosecond laser systems utilize photodisruptive laser of 1053 nm wavelength in infrared spectrum. Various types of femtosecond lasers are

- Solid state bulk lasers, for example, diode pumped lasers like neodymium-doped or ytterbium-doped and Titanium-sapphire lasers.
- Fiber lasers
- Dye lasers
- Semiconductor lasers
- Free electron lasers

Femtosecond laser has several advantages and specific features as follows:

- Femtosecond (FS) laser system works on the principle of photodisruption. Target tissue absorbs the femtosecond laser energy to form plasma state. This plasma quickly expands to create cavitation bubble where, the force generated in creation of cavitation bubble separates the target tissue. Thus, laser energy is converted into mechanical energy and this process is called photodisruption.

- Femtosecond laser system literally produces no collateral damage to the surrounding tissue, hence it is used as an effective tool to create tissue planes and flaps in LASIK surgery.

- Earlier FS laser systems had repetition rate of 30 kHz (excimer has up to 500 Hz and SSL has 1 kHz) which gradually reached to the present stage of 160 kHz, thus FS laser can create corneal flaps within a few seconds duration.

- FS laser has pulse frequency in the range of 50–160 kHz, pulse duration 400–800 femtosecond (fs, where 1 femtosecond = 10^{-15} second) and energy range 1–50 in microjoules (μj, where 1 microjoule = 10^{-6} joule)

- Due to these specialized features FS laser can be focused at 2–3 μm size spot within a range of 5 µm in cornea and high speed delivery of laser abolishes the possibility of damage to the surrounding target tissue.

- Excimer laser and solid state laser can be used only for surface ablation, whereas femtosecond laser can be focused very accurately in transparent medium like cornea and due to high speed this laser can be used to cut deep within the target tissue without damaging the surrounding tissues.

In a nutshell, femtosecond laser technology produces high speed, microscopic accuracy and precise photodissection of target tissue.

The effective outcome of various refractive surgical procedures mainly depends on the following factors

- Proper selection of patient
- Proper evaluation of patient before procedures (preoperative)

Selection of an Ideal Patient

Criteria for good patient selection include the factors such as

- **Age of patient:** Patients less than 18 years of age are not considered suitable for refractive surgery because the refraction below 18 years generally remains unstable. If refractive status is corrected before this age, then any further change in refractive status later on will destroy the whole purpose of refractive procedure. Usually procedure is performed on those patients who are having stable refraction over a period of one year. These procedures preferably should be done up to 45 years because presbyopia will develop after age of 40–45 years and again the patient will need glasses for correction of presbyopia, however, this is not the rule that refractive surgery cannot be done after 45 years of age.
- **Occupation of patient:** The procedure like radial keratotomy is avoided in the persons having profession like night driving job or sportsman or security personnel. After RK, the chances of glare or eyeball perforation is increased in this kind of jobs.

- **Desire or expectation of patient towards procedures:** Enthusiasm of patient plays an an important role in effective and desirable outcome of any refractive procedure because an unmotivated patient will usually remains unhappy and unsatisfied with the outcome. Those patients who have a strong desire to have good visual acuity without spectacles or contact lenses as found in actor/actresses or in other occupations, show satisfaction after surgery. Generally the patients think that laser is a full proof and 100% accurate and precise method for correction of refractive errors. This thought will increase their expectations about refractive outcomes very high, which eventually is a major cause of dissatisfaction. Hence, counseling before procedure should be done to inform patients that a second procedure may be required in selected cases to achieve the desirable visual acuity and also there may be a few procedure related complications after surgery. It is also important to inform that the refractive procedure will not eliminate the requirement of near correction for presbyopia.
- **Associated eye diseases:** Various ocular conditions where refractive procedures are absolutely or relatively contraindicated are summarized in Table 15.5.
- **Informed consent:** It is also essential to obtain a written informed consent from patients before surgery. Patients must be aware of the type of refractive procedure and its possible complications. Detailing about the outcomes and individual variations along with risks and benefits of proposed refractive procedure is done in the language which the patient best understands.

Preprocedure Examination

In motivated patients who are selected for refractive procedure following examination is must to improvise the visual outcome.

- **Systemic examination:** Elaborative systemic examination is done to rule out any systemic debilitating illness like connective

Table 15.5: Ocular condition where refractive surgery is contraindicated

Absolute contraindications	Relative contraindications
Corneal ectasias like keratoconus	Dry eye
Herpes keratitis	Chronic blepharitis
Thin cornea	Large size pupil
Connective tissue diseases	Ocular surface disorders (OSD)
Chronic use of steroids or antimeta-bolite in autoimmune disorders	Monocular (one-eyed) individual
Blepharophimosis	Diabetes mellitus
Glaucoma	Uveitis
Corneal aberrations due to contact lens usage	Pregnancy
	Ocular infections (recent onset)

tissue disorders, juvenile diabetes, chronic asthma, etc.

- **Visual examination:** Both distance and near visual acuity are measured using standard charts, with and without glasses. Ideally a cycloplegic refraction is done to evaluate the exact amount of refractive error so that an accurate amount of correction will be done by refractive procedure.
- **Ocular examination:** Detailed ocular adnexal examination is done to rule out any squint, nasolacrimal blockage or other orbital anomalies.
- **Anterior segment examination:** Thorough anterior segment examination is done with slit lamp to rule out any ocular disorders which are contraindicated for refractive procedures.
- **Fundus examination:** Meticulous posterior segment examination is done by dilating the pupil and using an indirect ophthalmo-scope with scleral indentation technique, to exclude any condition which can create any complication pre- or post-procedure. Special

attention is given to retinal lattice degenera-tions or small retinal holes which can lead to retinal detachments during or after refrac-tive procedures in high myopes. These lesions if present must be treated before performing the refractive procedures and patient must be kept well-informed about them in detail.

- **Pupil size assessment:** Measurement of the size of pupil before refractive procedure is an important aspect to avoid many post-procedure complications especially intole-rable glare. Ideally pupil should be measure in non-accommodated state under mesopic conditions at low intensity light. Pupil size can be measured by the following methods
  - Rosenbaum card method
  - Colvard pupillometer
  - Procyon pupillometer
  - Aberrometer
  - Pupilscan
  - Neuroptic devices

  Normally, in scotopic conditions average pupillary size in a young individual is considered as 6 mm however, a larger pupil size more than 6 mm, is not necessarily an abnormality because pupil is a dynamic structure. Total ablation zone is kept larger than pupillary size to prevent any post-operative complications like glare, halos or poor visual acuity.

- **Intraocular pressure measurement:** Most important examination step in refractive surgery is to record the intraocular pressure (IOP) preferably by applanation tonometer. Glaucoma is an absolute contraindication for refractive surgery hence in case of any doubt a complete evaluation of glaucoma is done before procedure.

- **Corneal examination:** A detailed corneal examination is done by performing:
  - *Tear film status:* Schirmer's test and tear film break up time test using fluorescein dye is done to rule out any dry eye situation, which is a relative contraindi-cation for LASIK procedure. There are high chances of developing severe dry

eye post-LASIK in patients, who are at borderline dry eye state.

– *Keratometry:* This gives a gross idea about the corneal curvatures and any irregularities in corneal surface.

– *Pachymetry:* Corneal thickness is measured by Pachymetry. This is an important data to be known before performing any refractive procedure to rule out thin cornea, which is an absolute contraindication for corneal refractive surgeries. The most preferred way of corneal thickness evaluation is ultrasonic pachymetry because it is easy to perform and quite accurate method to evaluate the corneal thickness.

– *Corneal topography:* This is the method to study the shapes of corneal surfaces and is generally called keratoscopy. Different types of keratoscopy are:
- Placido-disc keratoscopy
- Photokeratoscopy
- Videokeratoscopy: This is most widely used method to evaluate the corneal surface abnormalities and is useful in detecting borderline cases of keratoconus.

Note: Commercially available topographic systems are Orbscan and Pentacam. Keratometry, Rastersterography, and Interferometry are other methods to evaluate the corneal surface irregularities.

– *Aberrometry:* Measurement of any optical deviations (aberrations) is called aberrometry. There may be low order or high order aberration in the eye. Nowadays even aberrometry is done before refractive procedures so that these optical deviations can be abolish during laser ablation of cornea. Important types of aberrometer having the same basic principle are:
- Hartmann-Shack aberrometry
- Tscherning aberroscopy
- Ray tracing aberrometry

REFRACTIVE PROCEDURES FOR MYOPIA

Refractive surgeries for myopia have developed very fast as compared to hypermetropic or astigmatic refractive surgeries. A few procedures are now obsolete but mentioned for historical values. Various refractive surgeries done for myopia are summarized in Table 15.6.

Table 15.6: Various refractive procedures for correction of myopia			
Refractive lamellar surgery	*Refractive laser surgery*	*Refractive intraocular surgery*	*Miscellaneous techniques*
Freeze Keratomileusis of Barraquer for myopia (MKM)	Photorefractive keratotomy (PRK)	Phakic refractive lenses (PRLs)	Orthokeratology
Non-freeze keratomileusis	Laser *in situ* Keratomileusis (LASIK)	Refractive lens exchange (RLE)	Intrastromal corneal ring segments
Keratomileusis *in situ* (BKS technique)	Laser sub-epithelial keratomileusis (LASEK)		Intracorneal lenses
Automated lamellar keratoplasty (ALK)	Epithelial laser *in situ* keratomileusis (E-LASIK)		Gel injection adjustable keratoplasty
	Custom laser *in situ* keratomileusis (C-LASIK)		
	Corneal lenticule extraction procedure (SMILE)		

Refractive incisional procedure (e.g. Radial keratotomy) and refractive lamellar procedures are now obsolete.

Radial Keratotomy (RK)

The idea of radial keratotomy for myopia was initiated by Japanese scientist Tsutomu Sato (1939) who performed surgery for correction of myopia by creating 40 radial incisions in Descemet's membrane (posterior layer) and 40 radial incisions in anterior surface of cornea. Subsequently, this procedure was not accepted by many because it was associated with increase chances of bullous keratopathy. During 1970s and 1980s, many Russian scientists mainly Fyodorov and his colleagues improved the technique by making incisions only on the anterior surface of cornea and thus reducing the chances of bullous keratopathy. After this many attempts have been taken to refine the method of incision for RK and availability of better microsurgical instruments and advancement in corneal topography measurements played an important role in improvement of RK-based surgeries.

Procedure: In RK, under topical anesthesia using Neumann corneal marker eight radial lines are marked on the cornea. Then eight centripetal radial corneal incisions of nearly 90% corneal depth are made by diamond knife in the peripheral part of cornea. A central optical zone of nearly 4 mm is left clear as shown in Fig. 15.1.

These incisional corneal wounds while healing, contracts the peripheral cornea and flattens the central cornea. Thus, the RK procedure provides a new shape to cornea, i.e. flat in central and steep in periphery. This flatten cornea has less refractive power and hence myopia gets corrected. Most popular hypothesis is that due to normal intraocular pressure the weak peripheral cornea (due to incisions) is pushed and thus central cornea becomes flatter as shown in Fig. 15.2. A moderate degree (2–7 D) of myopia can be corrected by this method.

Advantages

- There is rare possibility of central corneal haziness because the central 4 mm zone is not incised.
- Very economical as compared to PRK or LASIK
- Post-operative wound healing is earlier in RK as compared to PRK.

Disadvantages

- Chances of eyeball rupture following even a trivial injury are very high after RK as compared to PRK or LASIK, because cornea is weakened by multiple incisions in RK.
- Significant glare and halos especially during night time is experienced by large number of patients.
- Improper healing of corneal incisional wounds can produce high degree irregular astigmatism.
- Overcorrection or undercorrection of refractive error is not very uncommon with RK.

Note: Newer, safer, effective refractive procedures with predictive outcome, like LASIK and LASEK, have made RK procedure obsolete.

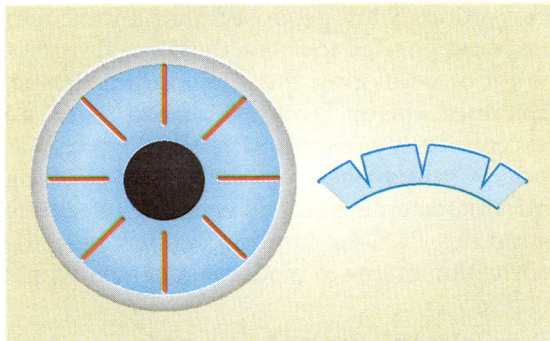

Fig. 15.1: Radial keratotomy

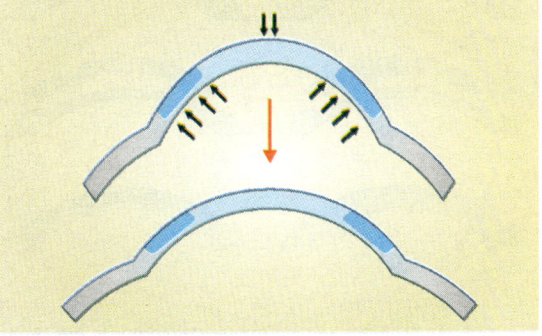

Fig. 15.2: Myopia correction by radial keratotomy

Keratomileusis

It is a lamellar corneal refractive procedure which was first described by scientist Jose Barraquer who is known as Father of all the lamellar corneal refractive surgeries. Keratomileusis term is derived from Greek words (Kerato = cornea and mileusis = carving or chiseling) which means chiseling of the cornea. In lamellar keratoplasty, the refractive power of cornea is altered by placing a lenticule on or within the cornea. This procedure became the milestone for all the recent corneal refractive procedure.

Freeze myopic Keratomileusis of Barraquer (MKM) and hyperopic Keratomileusis of Barraquer (HKM): This technique is similar for correction of both myopia and hypermetropia. A thin lamellar button or disc of corneal tissue is removed from its superficial surface with a microkeratome as shown in Fig. 15.3. This corneal button is then reshaped into a new desired shape for correction of myopia or hypermetropia after freezing it as shown in Fig. 15.3. This corneal tissue is freezed and then cryolathe reshapes it. This newly shaped corneal disc is then stitched to the patient's corneal stromal bed at appropriate place.

Epikeratomileusis or Epikeratophakia or Epikeratoplasty: In the year 1979, scientist Kaufman developed this technique of epikeratomileusis. In this procedure in place of a corneal wafer, a portion of corneal epithelium is removed. Under the edge of remaining epithelium, a pocket is created and a cryolathed donor homograft is inserted inside this pocket. Sometimes, a preserved material is used instead of homograft.

Non-freeze keratomileusis: In the year 1983, Krumiech and Swinger described this technique.

Keratomileusis *in situ* (Barraquer-Krumiech-Swinger technique): In the year 1985 a modification and combination of both techniques was developed by these three scientists popularly called BKS technique.

Automated lamellar keratoplasty: In late 1980s, Ruiz introduced the technique of automated lamellar keratoplasty. In this technique two keratectomies are done with help of automated microkeratome. This lamellar procedure revolutionalized the corneal refractive surgery and laid a ground for recent laser baser keratectomies.

Photorefractive Keratectomy (PRK)

Photoablation of corneal stroma by use of excimer laser is called photorefractive keratectomy. PRK is used to correct myopic, hypermetropic and astigmatic refractive errors, though it is very successful in myopic cases.

Excimer laser for medical purposes was available since early 1980s, however, it was Trokel and colleagues in the year 1983 who used excimer laser to perform PRK for myopic correction. They proposed that an excimer laser can be used to ablate the corneal surface without damaging the surrounding tissue. Excimer laser ablation produced an exceptionally even corneal surface, which was not possible even by the latest existing microkeratome used in lamellar refractive surgeries. PRK similar to RK is effective in the correction of low to moderate degree myopia (1.5 to 7 D).

Principle: For correction of refractive error a selected optical zone of anterior corneal

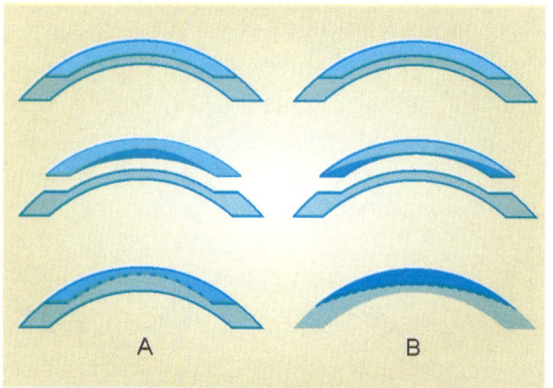

Fig. 15.3: Barraquer Keratomileusis. A. Myopic correction; B. Hypermetropic correction

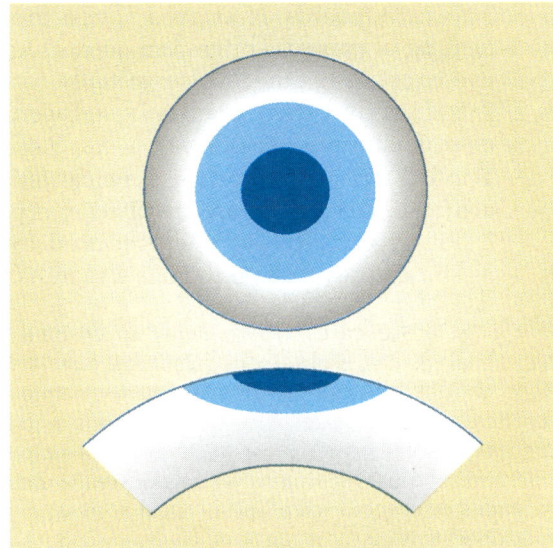

Fig. 15.4: Photorefractive keratectomy (*see* text)

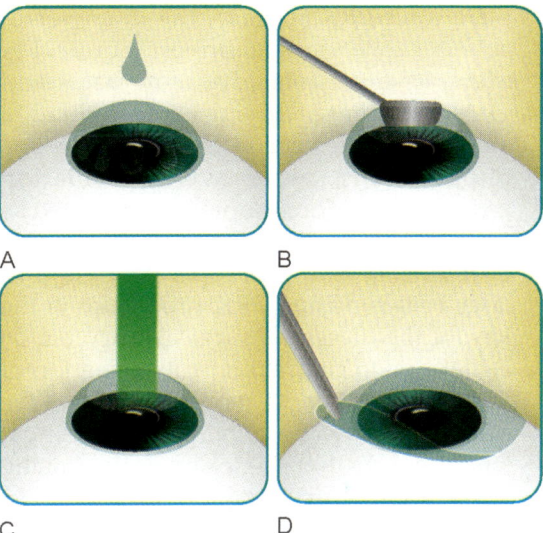

Fig. 15.5: Surgical steps of photorefractive keratectomy. A. 20% Ethyl alcohol drop for epithelial loosening; B. Mechanically removal of epithelium; C. Laser treatment; D. Bandage contact lens placement

stroma is photoablated with excimer lasers. This ablation causes the remoulding of cornea and hence leads to change in the refractive status of the cornea. For example, in case of myopia central optical zone of anterior corneal stroma is ablated as shown in Fig. 15.4, which causes flattening of the central cornea and thus decrease in the refractive power of cornea. This decrease in corneal refractive power leads to the correction of myopic error.

Surgical steps (Fig. 15.5)
- PRK is a day care surgery and can be performed comfortably under topical anesthesia, however some surgeons prefer to give additional mild sedatives.
- Corneal epithelium removal: To deliver the excimer laser at corneal stromal bed, removal of corneal epithelium is a prerequisite. This can be done by any one of the following methods
  - Mechanically: Using microsurgical blade or rotating brush.
  - Chemically: Using cocaine or 20% ethyl alcohol (for about 25–30 seconds)
  - Laser method: By use of excimer laser
- Normally, epithelium in 0.4–0.8 mm area larger than the calculated central ablation

zone is removed to avoid any procedural accidents.
- Once epithelium is removed and Bowman's membrane is visualized, the patient is instructed to focus on the target light, while surgeon adjusts the centration of microscope with the treatment area of cornea.
- Without any delay the laser treatment is started with the use of eye tracker system to safeguard against eye movements. Surgeon should try to minimize the time gap between epithelium removal and laser delivery to prevent excessive drying or wetting of corneal stromal surface.
- Once laser ablation is complete the corneal surface is irrigated and simple antibiotic ointment is applied. The eye is patched for an overnight period. Alternately, some surgeons apply bandage contact lens and start preservative free antibiotics in high frequency dosage.

Important surgical aspects of PRK
- *Ablation zone:* To prevent complications like halos around vehicle lights and intolerable

glare after PRK surgery, the diameter of ablation zone plays an important role. For example, small zone give more halos and glare during night driving because ablation area boundaries are within scotopic size pupil. Ideally, on an average, ablation zone diameter for myopia is considered as 6–6.5 mm and for hypermetropia 8.5–9.0 mm.

- *Centration of ablation:* Proper centration of laser beams during PRK procedure is the key for the successful surgical outcome. To achieve good centration proper fixation of the eyeball is perquisite. Fixation of globe can be done by operating surgeon using a hand held suction ring or by patient using self fixation during ablation. Fixation light on operating microscope should be coaxial with line of vision of patient and surgeon during ablation. Surgeon instructs the patient that during procedure this fixation light will become dim but still remain visible, so keep on trying to fixate the light. Fellow eye is patched to prevent any cross fixation during procedure. Laser beam is always centered to the pupil of patient. Decentration of ablation should never occur during treatment.

Post-surgical treatment

- Once surgery is complete, eye patching for overnight period is done after applying the topical plain antibiotics ointment and cycloplegic drops (atropine).
- Next day the eye patch is removed and complete ocular examination is done and then to prevent infection and to reduce the post-operative pain and inflammation following topical medications are prescribed
  - Topical preservative-free antibiotics are started 4–6 times a day to prevent any infection for 7–8 days and then are reduced to three times a day for 2–3 weeks duration.
  - Topical non-steroidal anti-inflammatory eye drops 4–6 times a day to reduce post operating pain and inflammation for 8–10 days and then frequency can be reduced over one and a half month duration.
  - Topical steroids is started (once the healing of corneal epithelium occurs) as eye drops 4–6 times a day initially for 7–8 days and then gradually reduced over one month period.
  - Topical preservative-free lubricants/artificial tear drops are instilled every 2 hourly initially and then reduced to 3–4 times a day for a period of 2–3 months.

Note: In those cases where delay in corneal epithelial healing is observed, a Bandage contact lens should be applied to promote the rapid corneal healing. Use of topical steroids and frequent use of preservative-free lubricants help in better corneal healing as well as decrease the chances of corneal haze and corneal regression postoperatively.

Complications: Various complications can occur during photorefractive keratectomy which can be grouped as follows.

- **Intraoperative complications**
  - *Photoablation zone decentration:* It can occur due to improper alignment of the laser beam in relation to the central fixation or may occur because of the sudden accidental ocular movements by the patient during delivery of laser. Decentration of photoablation will produce symptoms like glare, diplopia, halos and also the residual astigmatism associated with poor visual acuity. In majority of cases, over a period of time gradual corneal remoulding will decrease the effect of decentration, however, in remaining cases where symptoms are significant and no improvement is noticed with time then a computer assisted analysis of the center of pupil and center of ablation zone is performed. Suppose an ablation zone of irregular orientation in relation to the pupillary center is found, then to neutralize the effect of decentration a second ablation at 180° to first ablation is done. The center of this second ablation zone is decenterd from the pupillary center by the same

amount as the first ablation is decentered from pupillary center, but at 180 degree. This process will make the average center of two ablations in a line which passes through the pupillary center.

– *Sub-retinal hemorrhage:* It can occur during surgery due to rupture of fragile retinal vessels. In PRK a shock wave of high amplitude disrupts the tissue of stromal bed and this shock wave can cause the retinal hemorrhages.

- **Postoperative complications**
  - *Overcorrection:* Usually, a slight amount of overcorrection is desired in PRK because in majority of the cases regression (about 0.5–1.0 D) will occur after a few months of procedure. Suppose a patient presents with greater degree of hypermetropia even after more than a month postoperatively, then it is advised to taper the corticosteroid rapidly so that the process of wound healing is increased. Due to tapering of corticosteroids there are chances of additional remodeling of stroma and as a result the amount of hypermetropia will decrease. However, this rapid tapering of steroids may cause increase amount of corneal haze, which require close monitoring of the patient. Generally, improper healing of wound during postoperative period is common cause of overcorrection of the refractive error, hence it is suggested to do scraping of epithelium and stroma after procedure to enhance the process of wound healing.
  - *Undercorrection:* Residual myopia due to undercorrection can occur commonly because of increased rate of wound healing or in some cases due to thickened hyperplastic epithelial layer. Topical steroids can be started in mild to moderate degree residual myopia to delay the wound healing, however, long term usage of steroids can cause potential complications like glaucoma or cataract in otherwise normal eyes. Residual myopia can be managed by using spectacles or contact lenses, however, it is advisable to wait at least for six months before prescribing contact lenses because use of contact lens can further cause regression.

  - *Central islands:* Postoperatively, small central elevations may be seen on the corneal surface during analysis with corneal topography (usually cornea shows a central area having high refractive power than its adjacent paracentral area). Several hypotheses have been postulated to explain this phenomenon of island formation. Some considered that corneal tissue hydration may vary in different corneal areas. For example, there may be increase in the hydration in central stromal area of cornea. In addition, the abnormal profile of laser beam also affects the ablation in different areas. For example, exposure to flat ablation beam cause ablation of central hydrated corneal tissue at a slower rate, hence a lesser amount of corneal tissue may be removed from the central zone. Sometimes during procedure discharge of a cloud of gaseous and particulate debris may occur which leads to lesser delivery of laser energy and formation of central islands. Laser beam may have inconsistent energy distribution and undesired optical properties which will cause these islands. Occasionally, non-homogeneous corneal epithelial healing will result in larger epithelial hyperplasia in central area.

  - *Corneal scar:* Any kind of corneal insult will lead to formation of corneal haze or scar. Corneal haze after PRK is specifically more observed in patients who are having high degree myopia (>8 D). During process of epithelial healing there is increase in the amount of activated keratocyte in the corneal tissue. Thus, newly formed collagen and proteoglycans get deposit into the corneal tissue leading to corneal haziness. The corneal haze characteristically appears in the first month of procedure, however, maximum amount of corneal haze is seen typically in first 3 months of post-operative period. The haze gradually decreases over a period of 1–2 years. Clinical grading of the corneal haze is summarized in Table 15.7.

Regular use of topical steroids decreases the corneal haze and improves the refractive status of eye. If corneal haze persists even after six months of surgery, then an excimer laser treatment may be required to improve the visual status of the eye.

Note: Corneal haze until grade 1 is clinically not a major issue and resolves with topical steroids. Corneal haze of more than grade 2 is considered as scar and additional treatment is required to correct the scar.

– *Recurrent erosion syndrome:* After PRK, map dot fingerprint type of changes may take place outside the ablation zone in the surrounding epithelial defect areas. Due to these epithelial changes, recurrent epithelial erosions can occur in the neighboring area of ablation zone or very rarely even in the treatment zone. Excimer laser phototherapeutic keratectomy (PTK) is the treatment of choice to manage this recurrent erosion syndrome.

– *Infectious keratitis:* This may cause corneal scaring and diminished visual acuity. Proper antibiotic coverage is required to treat this condition. Sometimes, excessive use of anti-inflammatory drops without proper coverage of steroids may cause excessive migration of leukocytes as corneal infiltrates. These infiltrates are sterile and usually appear a few days to weeks after the procedure. Treatment of choice is to discontinue the anti-inflammatory drops and start the topical steroids for appropriate time duration.

- **Delayed postoperative complications**
  - *Delayed epithelial healing:* Various factors like dry eye, larger epithelial debridement, excessive topical anti-inflammatory drops or prophylactic topical antibiotics and early withdrawal of steroids may cause delay in epithelial healing of corneal wound.
  - *Visual aberrations:* The visual aberrations like night glare or halos are not very common after PRK, however, a small ablated area of about 3.5–4.0 mm can cause night glare or halos because in dim or scotopic illumination pupil get dilated and the light rays which passes across the mid-peripheral area causes halos of light. In low contrast conditions these glare may persist for longer duration and will cause difficulty in night driving. To solve this problem retreatment with increase ablation zone diameter of 6.0 mm is done because halos are usually not seen with an ablation area of 5.0–6.0 mm.
  - *Corneal ulceration:* Sometimes, patients presenting with delayed wound healing are prescribed bandage contact lens for long periods after surgery. The cornea in these cases may suffer from poor oxygenation which may further delay the process of wound healing. These types of cases have more chances of developing corneal ulcers.

Various advantages and disadvantages of photorefractive keratectomy in comparison to radial keratotomy are summarized in Table 15.8.

Table 15.7: Clinical grading of corneal haze

Grade	Clinical presentation
Grade 0	Transparent cornea
Grade 0.5	Minimally identifiable haze
Grade 1	Mild haze with normal visual acuity
Grade 2	Moderate haze with decreased visual acuity
Grade 3	Marked haze with unclear iris details
Grade 4	Severe haze with no iris details

Table 15.8: Various advantages and disadvantages of photorefractive keratectomy in comparison to radial keratotomy

Advantages	Disadvantages
Eyeball integrity is well maintained as compared to the radial keratotomy	Pain and soreness experienced by patients for several weeks
No diurnal variations in refractive status or night glare as compared to radial keratotomy.	As postoperative epithelial healing is slow, it may delay the regain of good visual acuity.
In moderate myopia (2–8 D) excellent results are seen with a high accuracy of 95% cases achieving ± 0.5 D correction.	Visual acuity may also be affected by residual central corneal haze
	More expensive procedure than radial keratotomy

In cases of significant undercorrection of refractive error, repeat PRK can be carried out with reasonable safety, however, majority of patients do not require a second procedure. PRK retreatment should not be done in the following conditions

- Postoperative refractive status is changing regularly.
- Undercorrection of refractive error is clinically not significant.
- Patient was on steroid therapy till recently.
- First procedure was done before lesser than six months duration.
- Corneal complications like corneal haze or corneal islands are present.

LASIK

LASIK is considered as most popular refractive procedure done for correction of all three refractive errors, i.e. myopia, astigmatism and hypermetropia. Unlike PRK, this procedure keeps the Bowman's capsule as well as corneal epithelium intact and simultaneously also consists of precision of excimer laser ablation. LASIK can correct a high degree of myopia, i.e. up to 12 dioptres and hypermetropia or astigmatism up to 6 dioptres. Though, LASIK has several advantages over PRK or RK, but limitations are that LASIK requires fine surgical skills and very costly pieces of equipment to perform this procedure. Residual refractive errors after PRK, RK or cataract surgery can be corrected by LASIK but variable results are seen.

LASIK Set up

The complete set up of LASIK includes
- Automated microkeratome
- Excimer laser machine

Automated microkeratome: Microkeratomes are the instruments which create a smooth, uniformly planar, precise and desired thickness corneal flap to perform LASIK. All these microkeratomes are motor driven and hence are called automated microkeratome. Various models of microkeratome have been developed since advent of LASIK and are mainly mechanical or laser types. Some microkeratome models are designed for the creation of corneal flaps both for LASIK and epi-LASIK. A few microkeratome are designed to create both types of flaps, i.e. the hinged flaps and free corneal caps. The development of microkeratome was gradual since advent of LASIK and various types and designs of microkeratome have been invented by several manufactures. These microkeratome can be mechanical or non-mechanical in the design and may be disposable or non-disposable in usage. On the basis of their design and usage, microkeratomes can be broadly classified as

- Mechanical microkeratome
- Hydrokeratome
- Epikeratome
- Laser microkeratome

Mechanical microkeratome were developed in early era to create corneal flaps and primarily they had cutting head which was advanced either manually by surgeon or automatically by an electric motor. Initially, to cut the corneal flap diamond blades or metallic (steel) blades were used, however, in advance designs water jet under high pressure (hydro blades) or laser beam is used to create the flap.

Various mechanical microkeratome designs can be grouped as manual, automatic and disposable types. Commonly available mechanical types of microkeratome and their salient features are summarized in Table 15.9.

Hydrokeratome design is based on waterjet principle technique where high pressure fluid beam is used to break the collagen bonds for corneal lamellae. The corneal dissection with this technique produces smoother planar surface with less tissue damage. Under extreme high pressure (more than 15,000 psi) continuous saline beam of very narrow diameter (about 35 micron) is injected at a very high speed (nearly 2000 kph) to cleavage the cornea. This waterjet beam is angled 0° with cornea and a fixed thickness hinged flap is created by this waterjet beam. An image tracking system is present to monitor the position of water pressure and beam of waterjet.

Epikeratome is similar to microkeratome in almost all features, except that it creates an epithelial flap instead of a corneal flap. Epikeratome moves below the epithelial plane (excluding Bowman's membrane) under suction and cut the corneal epithelial layer surface in smooth and homogenous manner. The advantages of epikeratome over alcohol or rotating brush de-epithelization techniques are

– Smoother and linear corneal surface after procedure

Table 15.9: Various mechanical types of microkeratomes	
Manually advanced microkeratome	
Microkeratome types	*Salient features*
Turbokeratome	Fixed head produces 150 m thickness flap, 20° angled with cornea, oscillating speed 10,000 to 24,000 cycles per minute (cpm).
Microlamellar keratome	Corneal flaps from 0 to 450 m thickness, 9° angled with cornea, 20,000 cpm oscillations speed
Lamellar microkeratome	Flap thickness 120,140,160 and 180 m, 21.5° angled with cornea, oscillating speed 15,000 cpm
Automatic advanced microkeratome	
Microkeratome types	*Salient features*
Universal microkeratome	Single unit fixed thickness plate create hinged flap, 0° angled with cornea, oscillating speed 14,000 cpm, pendular movement
Eye-tech microkeratome	Teflon coated steel blades, 26° angled with cornea, oscillating speed 8000 to 14,000 cpm.
Hansatome	Fixed depth 160 and 180 m thickness flaps, disposable metal blade, left and right eye adapters
Disposable microkeratomes	
Microkeratome types	*Salient features*
Automated disposable microkeratome	Moulded plastic, preassembled, single use unit with 130 m and 160 m thickness flaps, metal blade with 10,000 rpm speed
Flipmaker disposable microkeratome	Similar to automated disposable microkeratome with oscillation speed 12,500 cpm.

- Avoids surface toxicity of alcohol
- Epithelial layer can be replaced after surface ablation
- Less postoperative pain because surface nerves are preserved.
- Less postoperative corneal haze because less corneal inflammation

Laser microkeratome are latest version microkeratomes and utilize femtosecond laser beam to create the corneal flap. Femtosecond laser is discussed in detail on page 266. The corneal flaps created by femtosecond laser are of precise thickness, extremely smooth, homogeneous, well centered and significantly stable.

Excimer laser machine: Excimer laser machine is required to ablate the corneal bed as per precalculated data. Basic principle and functioning of various design excimer laser machine have been discussed in detail at page 264.

Preoperative evaluation for LASIK

Ideal patient selection and preoperative evaluation for LASIK includes all points as discussed in detail on page 268. However, there are a few specific points in relation to preprocedure consideration for LASIK.

- Patients with sunken eyeball and narrow palpebral apertures are not ideal candidate for LASIK. In these patients placing of suction ring and passing of microkeratome is difficult because of inadequate eyeball exposure.
- As majority of high myopes is contact lens wearer, they are advised to discontinue the use of contact lens wear before LASIK. Contact lens wearing is discontinued 15 days prior in case of soft contact lens wear and one month prior in case of rigid contact lens wear.
- Central corneal thickness should not be less than 500 μm for LASIK procedure because on an average 100 μm thick corneal flap and nearly 160–180 μm stromal bed is ablated to correct refractive error. To keep the integrity of eyeball and avoid corneal complication

the remaining corneal thickness should be more than 250 μm, hence patients having central corneal thickness less than 550 μm are not ideal candidates for LASIK.

Surgical technique: Surgical technique of LASIK is simple and effective in an ideal surgical atmosphere. It is a day care surgery like other refractive procedures and in an expert hands require less than 15–20 minutes operating time.

Preoperative requisites are meticulous evaluation of refractive status, corneal thickness, corneal topography and IOP measurement on the day of surgery. Patient is advised to use topical preservative free plain antibiotic drops 3–4 times/day for two days prior to procedure. Once everything is set surgeon check the microkeratome and suction unit before commencing the procedure and take up the patient for LASIK. Surgical steps are as follows:

- In majority of cases, topical anesthesia (xylocaine or proparacaine) is used 2–3 times in 15–20 minutes duration prior to start the surgery.
- Careful cleaning of ocular area and proper draping to cover every eyelash is done similar to any other refractive surgery.
- Proper exposure of globe is achieved by use of lid speculum (preferably self-retaining speculum).
- *Corneal marking:* Cornea is marked by using a corneal marker dipped in gentian violet. Several designs of corneal marker for LASIK are available, for example, Hoffer corneal marker, Mendez corneal marker, and Lu corneal marker. For centration of suction ring and precise realignment of corneal flap specially designed corneal marker such as Lu marker (Fig. 15.6A) is used to mark the cornea. This marker has an external circle of 10.5 mm diameter with an internal circle of 3 mm diameter. These two circles are joined by two pararadial lines in an asymmetrical manner as shown in Fig. 15.6B. The inner

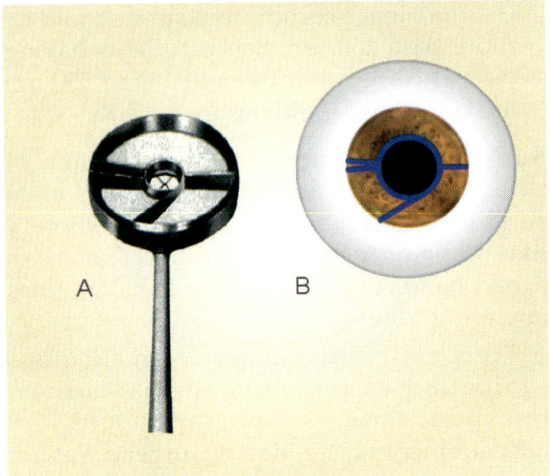

Fig. 15.6: Corneal marking in LASIK. A. Lu corneal marker; B. Markings on cornea

circle is aligned concentrically with the patient's pupil for accurate centration, whereas external circle is aligned to fix the suction ring. In case of an accidental free flap condition, the asymmetrical pararadial lines will help in precise realignment of corneal flap.

- *Suction ring application:* Once the corneal marking is done, suction ring of selected size is placed according to marking with slight decentration towards the hinge. Then the suction is started by attached pump and on an average an IOP of 65 mmHg is achieved. Surgeon instructs the patient that there will be transient blurring but he/she should try to keep the focus on the target light. Proper level of IOP attained can be checked as follows

  – Significant blurring of vision/no vision

  – Dilatation of pupil

  – Barraquer's tonometer measurement

  – Reading in pressure gauge

  It is important to achieve an IOP of about 65 mmHg because it is needed for creation of corneal flap of an accurate thickness and diameter.

Note: An accurate IOP reading by Barraquer tonometer is obtained when both tonometer and corneal surface are dry.

- *Preparation of corneal flap:* After applying the suction ring and increasing the IOP, the cornea is moistened with balanced salt solution (BSS) and microkeratome cutting head is inserted inside the suction ring track.

  Then microkeratome is advanced manually or automatically (depending on design of the microkeratome) to create either superiorly or nasally hinged smooth corneal flap as shown in Fig. 15.7A. Cornea is continuously kept moist with BSS during the movement of microkeratome to prevent any thermal damage to the corneal flap.

Always follow the rule 'wet cutting: dry ablation'

  Care is to be taken to prevent the inadvertent formation of a free flap. Initially superiorly hinged flaps were considered superior against the nasally hinged flaps. Recent studies had shown that superiorly hinged flaps damages the majority of corneal innervations, hence the recent studies recommend the nasally hinged flap creation superior to superiorly hinged flap. Reason being that most of the corneal nerve fibres enter the cornea nasally and a nasally hinged flap saves majority of innervations of the cornea. Only disadvantage of nasally hinged flap is that the flap may be displaced by the movement of upper lid, whereas in a superiorly hinged flap chances of displacement is less.

Note: Majority of LASIK experts recommend releasing of suction pressure immediately after creation of corneal flaps, however, some suggest continuing the pressure until completion of ablation. The explanation is that the amount of damage to optic nerve is the same in both the situations but by keeping pressure, better centration for ablation can be achieved.

To achieve a smooth, linear and precise cut following points must be remembered while creating the corneal flap

- An adequate exposure of eyeball is necessary.
- Continuously maintain IOP between 60 and 65 mmHg during cutting because a lower IOP will make eyeball soft and will produce a flap of variable thickness and diameter.
- Keep cornea well irrigated by using BSS during cutting. This will prevent the damage due to friction produced by microkeratome plate.

- *Corneal stromal ablation:* Lift the corneal flap using micro spatula towards the hinge and then dry the corneal stromal bed using cellulose sponge. Then centration of laser is done and surface corneal ablation is started by excimer laser on the basis of pre-calculated fixed data feed in laser machine by the surgeon as shown in Fig. 15.7B. To achieve better results these points should be followed while doing the ablation

- Apply the rule 'wet cutting and dry ablation', i.e. keep the corneal bed constantly dry during the ablation process.

- Central ablation should be done for better visual outcomes. Latest version LASIK systems have an eye tracker facility which continuously follows the eyeball movements during ablation. Alternately, globe fixation ring can be used to stabilize the eyeball during ablation.
- Do not ablate the hinge of corneal flap, it may cause free flap or poor healing post procedure.
- Complete the ablation process within 30 seconds after flap creation to avoid excessive dehydration of corneal surface.

- *Corneal flap repositioning:* Once ablation is done, the corneal bed and flap are irrigated with BSS to remove any interface debris. Corneal flap is allowed to settle on the corneal bed, and then it is slightly distended and aligned properly using golf club spatula. Excess fluid is dried by wet Weckcell sponge and finally using wet spear sponge or Johnston applanator, the flap is repositioned on the stromal bed. After repositioning the flap it is allowed to get dry for 5 minutes as shown in Fig. 15.7C. This will adhere the flap firmly over the corneal bed. Confirmation of adherence of flap to

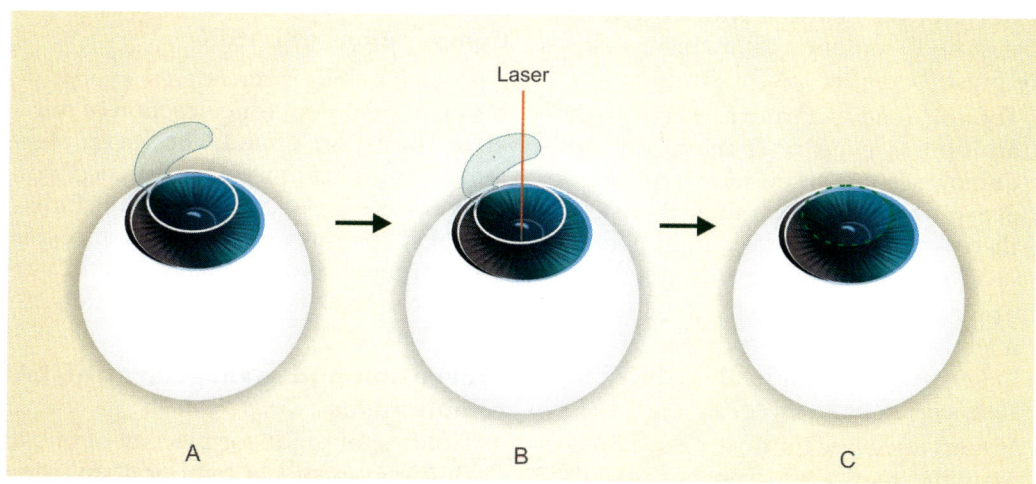

Fig. 15.7: Surgical steps of LASIK procedure

stromal bed is done by performing the **striae test**. Periphery of the cornea is pressed by wet spear sponge to produce striae and these striae can be seen radiating on the flap.

- *Speculum removal:* Removal of lid speculum and drape is the most crucial part of LASIK procedure because a minor negligence can lead to major troubles like epithelial defect or flap displacement. To avoid this gently remove the lid speculum and drape under direct microscopic observation. After removal of lid speculum and drape patient is instructed to blink gently, while the position of flap is observed under microscope. In spite of blinking the flap must remain firmly adhered and properly aligned.

Postoperative treatment

- *Ocular protection:* Majority of surgeons in uncomplicated cases advice goggles after procedure for protection.
- *Systemic medications:* Oral broad spectrum antibiotics (cephalosporins or fluoroquinolones) and long acting analgesics (diclofenac or acelofenac) are prescribed for prevention of infection and pain reduction, respectively for minimum duration of 3–5 days.
- *Topical medications:* To reduce pain, for better wound healing and to decrease foreign body sensation following eye drops are prescribed after LASIK surgery:
  - Topical broad spectrum preservative free antibiotics eye drops usually fluoroquinolones are given in a frequency of every two hours for initial 3 days and then 6–8 times/day for a total period of 2–3 weeks in reducing dosages.
  - Topical steroids usually prednisolone acetate is started 6–8 times/day for 2 days and then gradually reduced for a total period of 3–4 weeks.
  - Preservative free lubricating eye drop or artificial tears eye drop is prescribed 4 hourly for a period of 6 weeks.

- *Preventive measures:* Patient is advised to follow these instruction along with medication for better and faster visual recovery after LASIK
  - Take complete rest for a day or two and then can perform routine daily activities, but still to avoid strenuous work.
  - Avoid rubbing or touching of the eyes and contact with water for 7–10 days period.
  - Avoid direct sunlight exposure and use of eyes for long duration for 2–3 weeks.
  - Do not drive especially, during night time.
  - No sport activities or swimming for 6 weeks duration after LASIK.
  - In case of visual symptoms like pain, excessive redness or diminished vision report immediately to LASIK center.

Follow up: Meticulous corneal examination and measurement of visual acuity is done on following visits

- First postoperative day
- One week after surgery
- One month after surgery
- Six months follow-up
- Yearly follow-up visits

  On every follow up visit check the position and alignment of flap, corneal transparency and anterior chamber status.

Complications of LASIK

Although LASIK is considered a very safe and effective treatment for correction of refractive errors in expert's hands, however, there are several complications which can occur during or after LASIK. Several studies concluded that complication rate of LASIK done by experienced surgeons is less than 0.5–1%. Various complications of LASIK are summarized in Table 15.10.

Prevention and management of LASIK complications

- Holding of globe for placement of suction ring may result in temporal sub-conjunctival hemorrhage which can be easily

Table 15.10: Various complications of LASIK

Related to suction ring fixation	Microkeratome related	Related to photo ablation	Associated with flap handling	Early post-operative	Delayed post-operative	Refraction related
Sub conjunctival hemorrhage	Incomplete flap	Decentered ablation	Flap hydration	Epithelial in growth	Halos and glare	Over and under correction
Conjunctival chemosis	Variable thickness flap	Interrupted ablation	Flap interface debris	Diffuse lamellar keratitis	Interface haze	Induced astigmatism
Ocular hypotony	Free flap	Flap ablation	Flap wrinkling	Flap striae	Recurrent epithelial erosion	Regression of refractive error
	Button hole or flap tear	Central islands	Poor flap adherence	Flap loss	Corneal ectasias	Poor contrast sensitivity
				Infectious keratitis	Dry eye	Diplopia

prevented by using blunt holding forceps. During application of suction ring complication like conjunctival chemosis may occur which can obstruct the pressure of suction ring. Always check the pressure rise and flow before application of suction ring. Rarely, severe ocular hypotony may occur due to sudden vacuum created by the suction ring, hence to prevent this hypotony the pressure in the suction ring should be raised gradually.

- Improper motor functioning, presence of debris in the cutting interface or suction loss during cutting can result in creation of an incomplete flap. Microkeratome components as discussed above should be checked before inserting into the track of suction ring. Always check the IOP before starting the cutting of corneal flap because low IOP can cause variable thickness flap or free flap (especially in small or flat cornea). In addition, the pressure should be checked intermittently to confirm the constant maintenance of IOP during flap cutting. Poor suction mechanism or poor blade quality can cause button hole or tear (especially, in steep cornea) in corneal flap. Always remember the handling instructions

and check the position of blades for proper fit. Maintain the IOP above 65 mmHg during microkeratome movement and use newer blades in every case to prevent these flap complications.

- Photoablation is an important step of LASIK surgery, hence it is important to maintain the centration of ablation and check the program entered in computer data. Decentration of ablation can cause irregular astigmatism and poor visual outcome. To prevent decentration newer machines have an eye tracker system and also patient cooperation is must. Decentration once occurred it is difficult to treat, hence prevention is the only treatment. Sometimes, technical error in laser system can interrupt the ablation process. In this situation, instead of being panic, discontinue the process and reposition the flap after thoroughly irrigating with BSS. Repeat the process on later date once technical problem is solved. Accidental ablation of flap hinge or base of flap can happen because centration for photo ablation and corneal flap are two different points. To avoid flap ablation some surgeons purposely decenter the suction ring about 0.6–0.8 mm, so that photo ablation center and flap center do not coincide. Central islands are mainly related to PRK procedure but they regress with time. However, in LASIK central islands rarely occur but once occur, they hardly regress with time. Latest version scanning laser beams and preprocedure programming data entries have almost abolished the occurrence of central islands nowadays after LASIK.

- Repositioning of flap is a crucial step in LASIK because rough handling of flap can cause damage, dislocation or destruction of corneal flap. Excessive time gap (> 30 seconds) between creation of corneal flap and laser ablation can cause hydration or desiccation of corneal stromal bed. Surgeon must be an expert to reduce this time gap and avoid flap hydration. Intraoperative contamination of corneal surfaces/interface debris can happen due to friction in microkeratome blades. To prevent interface debris during procedure, following steps are advised

  - Appropriate and thorough cleaning of instruments must be done and keep them on plastic surface to avoid the contact with fibres.
  - Powdered surgical gloves should be replaced.
  - Minimize the use of topical anesthetics to prevent epithelial defects.
  - Meticulous corneal flap irrigation with BSS solution should be done.
  - Never touch the posterior surface of corneal flap.

  Repositioning of flap is done properly and golf club spatula is used to remove the wrinkling and striae from flap. Striae test is done as described on page 282. Poor adherence of corneal flap will occur if there is flap hydration or wrinkling.

- In early postoperative period (a few days to week) corneal epithelial cells may proliferate under the corneal flap due to excessive topical anesthesia or flap handling or betadine scrub contact with corneal surface. However, in majority of cases they stabilize without any associated complication. In rare incidences, the epithelial growth is symptomatic and requires treatment in terms of lifting of flap and removal of epithelium using spatula. Repositioning of flap is done with extreme concern to prevent the recurrence of ingrowth.

- Diffuse lamellar keratitis (DLK) is also called *Sands of Sahara syndrome*, due to its appearance similar to sand. It may occur as nonspecific diffuse intrastromal or intralamellar keratitis in early postoperative period. Clinically majority of the patients present with severe pain, photophobia, and diminished visual acuity, usually within 3–5 days after procedure. On slit lamp examination on the basis of location of white granular cells, DLK can be graded as
  - Grade I Peripheral cells
  - Grade II Central cells
  - Grade III Clumps of cells in center with clear periphery
  - Grade IV Stromal melting

  In Grade I and II cases intensive steroids, anti-inflammatory and antibiotic eye drops are prescribed for 5–7 days. If no improvement is seen in infiltrate or if DLK is in Grade III and IV, then it is suggested to lift the flap and irrigate the stromal bed with BSS solution then drying with Merocel sponge should be done to prevent stromal melting.

- Trivial trauma in early postoperative period can lead to flap loss due to poor adherence of flap and the most effective treatment is to prevent trauma by wearing the protective goggles in early postprocedure period. Usually, corneal lamellar grafting is not required in case of flap loss because corneal epithelium will grow over the residual corneal stromal bed and fill the area so that cornea will function normally with minimal haze. Flap striae may be seen in immediate postoperative period. These striae are either macrofolds or microfolds seen in corneal flap.

- Macrofolds are large folds involving entire corneal flap thickness and can be seen easily on slit lamp. Large folds may occur due to the corneal flap slipping from stromal bed and will cause full thickness flap pouching along with diminished visual acuity.
- Microfolds are present within the corneal flap and are occur due to wrinkling in either Bowman's membrane or epithelial membrane. These microfolds occur due to problem in flap adherence.

Flap striae can be managed by lifting the flap and repositioning it carefully to avoid any wrinkling or slipping from stromal bed. Infectious keratitis though very rare but a potentially hazardous condition which necessitate immediate and effective treatment to save useful visual acuity.

- Most common complications of small optical zone, subclinical decentration of ablation and poor repositioning of flap are halos and intolerable glare especially, during night drive. Pupillary dilatation during mesopic conditions, high order aberrations due to decentration and irregular astigmatism due to flap complications are the causes of these halos and glare after LASIK. To prevent the glare and halos, keep the optical zone diameter larger than pupillary size and avoid decentration during ablation.
- Interface haze which can be observed after LASIK surgery is not similar to corneal haze (seen after PRK), relatively a minimal haziness is seen at the interface of corneal flap and stromal bed in LASIK. Generally, the interface haze disappears within 3–6 months duration, leaving a grey circular scar at the edge of corneal flap. There are no symptoms due to interface haze, hence require no treatment. Corneal ectasias is a rare complication and may result if too thin corneal base is left which may result due to formation of a thick corneal flap. It can be managed by penetrating keratoplasty or lamellar keratoplasty. Recurrent epithelial erosions are also uncommon and in these cases bandage contact lenses can be prescribed with variable results. Dry eye remains the most common complication after LASIK especially, in patients having borderline dry eye before surgery. Common hypothesis is that during corneal flap creation superficial corneal nerves are cut as they are coming from nasal side of the cornea. This damage to corneal nerve leads to the decreased corneal sensation and reduced blinking rate which ultimately cause appearance of significant clinical dry eye.

- Improper entry of program in computer is the commonest cause of under or over-correction of refractive error. However, nowadays these errors are very rare because refinement in program and improvised nomogram are available in laser systems. Difference of more than 2 dioptres can be corrected by repeat laser treatment if desired, within a period of 2–4 months because corneal flap can be lifted effortlessly within this duration. Decentration of ablation and improper corneal flap healing can cause astigmatism of regular and irregular types. To prevent astigmatism precise ablation and proper healing of corneal flap is must. Regression in refractive status in early follow up period has also been showed in several studies. These studies reported that initially 0.5–1.0 dioptre hyperopia and then low degree myopia is seen in majority of cases during first 2–4 months period of follow-up however, the refractive status remained stable after six months follow-up in majority of cases. Decreased contrast sensitivity is a troublesome complication seen in many cases. The probable cause of diminished contrast sensitivity is central flattening of cornea in comparison to periphery of cornea.
- In a few selective cases LASIK can lead to the decompensation of latent squint and patient will experience diplopia after surgery. Many a times, in high refractive

error patients the spectacle lenses are fitted with slight decentration to induce the prismatic effect or even sometimes prisms are incorporated in spectacle lenses to compensate for squint. In these cases when LASIK is done this delicate compensation for prismatic effect is lost and patient feels diplopia. To avoid such diplopia it is better to give contact lens trial prior to surgery.

– Recent studies reported a psychological complication after refractive surgeries and termed it *Refractive Surgery Shock Syndrome* (RSSS). Many patients experienced depression, acute stress or anxiety and post-traumatic syndrome features after refractive surgery. Common causes reported for this are improper counseling and surgical consent for disturbing visual symptoms like halos, glare, starburst, and poor contrast sensitivity. These symptoms hampered the routine activities of younger generation, especially at night time. The RSSS condition is still under research process but is a significant complication if occur.

• An unknown origin *GAAP* (Good Acuity Plus Photophobia) *syndrome* is associated with uneventful femtosecond laser treatment. Usually after 4–6 weeks of LASIK procedure a transient increase to light sensitivity is reported, hence it is also called TLS (transient light sensitivity). Short duration topical steroid treatment completely resolves this condition without any remnant long-term effects.

LASIK has several advantages and a few limitations as compared to RK and PRK, which are summarized in Table 15.11.

Sequel of LASIK

• *Imprecise calculation of IOL power:* Post-LASIK the cornea takes an oblate shape, hence the mean keratometry readings used in IOL power calculation formula will give an inaccurate emmetropic IOL power.

• *Imprecise IOP measurement:* Central corneal thickness is decreased after LASIK and hence the IOP measured by applanation

Table 15.11: Various advantages and limitations of LASIK compare to RK and PRK

Advantages	Limitations
Negligible or no pain after surgery	Very expensive
No post procedure residual corneal haze	Not done in patients with inadequate corneal thickness
Minimal or no risk of globe perforation during surgery	Potential risk of corneal flap related complications
No risk of globe rupture due to trauma	Requires commendable surgical skills
Early visual recovery	
Effective in correcting high degree myopia up to 25–30 dioptres	

tonometer gives an erroneous low values. Therefore, to diagnose glaucoma these IOP value needs correction according to the new corneal thickness.

Laser Subepithelial Keratomileusis (LASEK)

In the year 1999, Camellin introduced the technique of LASEK which has combined advantages of both PRK and LASIK. LASEK similar to PRK avoid the corneal flap related complication because in LASEK an epithelial flap is created after loosening the epithelium by using alcohol and like LASIK it offers minimal postoperative pain and faster visual recovery. LASEK can be considered an alternative option in those patients where LASIK is contraindicated like patients having large pupils, thin, steep or flat cornea, deep-set eyes, glaucoma, etc.

Surgical technique (Fig. 15.8): LASEK surgical technique is almost similar to PRK (described on page 472) except the following steps

• **Formation of epithelial flap:** Unlike PRK epithelium is not removed rather a hinged epithelial flap is created by these surgical steps

– *Flap trephination:* Under topical anesthesia using calibrated (70 μm depth) blade an epithelial incison is given with a microtrephine (8 mm in diameter) placed centrally over the cornea. Microtrephines are available in various sizes from 8–10.5 mm diameter and have a blunt 4 mm segment which spares the intact corneal epithelium to provide a flap hinge. Gentle pressure is applied on the microtrephine to cut the corneal epithelium, leaving a 4 mm flap hinge.

– *Chemical de-epithelization:* An alcohol cone of the same diameter as microtrephine is placed centrally over the cornea in marked groove. 20% ethyl alcohol prepared in cold water is then instilled inside the alcohol cone (Fig. 15.8A). After 30 seconds, the alcohol is sucked out of the cone with cellulose sponge. The entire corneal surface and conjunctiva is irrigated generously with BSS. At the time of alcohol application it is recommended to check the light reflex on the alcohol surface regularly, any movement of reflex indicates the leakage of alcohol.

– *Creation of flap:* Wait for another 30–40 seconds so that alcohol treated epithelium get released from Bowman's membrane. Margin of the epithelium is then lifted with the help of a microhoe and epithelial debridement is started. Once epithelium is detached from Bowman's membrane, then epithelial flap is smoothly assembled and slowly rolled towards the hinge with the help of hockey stick spatula (Fig. 15.8B).

- **Surface ablation:** After rolling of epithelial flap, clear Bowman's membrane is seen and then surface ablation is done by excimer laser within precalculated ablation zone to correct the refractive error (Fig. 15.8C).

- **Repositioning of epithelial flap:** Generously irrigate the ablated corneal surface with BSS so that all the debris is removed completely from corneal surface. Then epithelial flap is rolled gently and slowly over the stromal bed using repositioning spatula (Fig. 15.8D).

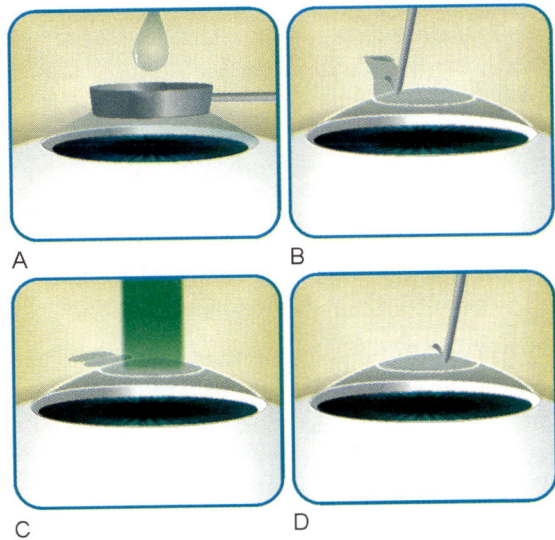

Fig. 15.8: Surgical steps of LASEK. A. Chemical de-epithelization; B. Creation of flap; C. Surface ablation; D. Repositioning of epithelial flap

- Therapeutic soft contact lens is applied over the cornea for a period of 6–7 days.

Postoperative management is similar to PRK or LASIK as described on page 482.

Differential favorable features of LASEK in comparison to PRK and LASIK are summarized in Table 15.12.

Epipolis Laser in Situ Keratomileusis (epi-LASIK)

In the year 2003, Pallikaris commenced a newer technique for correction of refractive errors which had all the advantages of LASEK and also avoided the flap-related complications of LASIK. This recent technique is called epipolis LASIK (epi-LASIK or superficial LASIK), where 'Epipolis' is a Greek word which means 'superficial'. Principle of this technique is that an epithelial flap is prepared by using an epikeratome, rather than using alcohol (as in LASEK). Thus, in epi-LASIK the epithelial cells remain preserved and hence better healing and less postoperative complications occur. Less postoperative pain and corneal haze along with quicker wound healing are some of the advantages of epi-LASIK seen over LASIK.

Table 15.12: Various advantages of LASEK in comparison to PRK and LASIK

Over PRK	Over LASIK
Postoperative pain is less	Lower chances of corneal ectasias
Postoperative corneal haze is less	Absence of corneal flap related complications like free flap, button holing, etc.
Improved epithelial healing, hence an early recovery	Superior option for thin cornea (at 480 μm thickness > 6–7 D myopia can be corrected)
Postoperative complications are limited	Additional 90 μm cornea available for ablation, (additional 5 D myopic correction)
	High order aberrations are excluded
	Postoperative dry eye is less as corneal nerves are preserved
	Large zone treatment is possible

Surgical technique: Preoperative preparations and intraoperative steps of epi-LASIK are similar to that of LASEK (as discussed on page 486) however, the only difference is in the formation of an epithelial flap.

Epithelial flap formation

• For formation of an epithelial flap an advance version of microkeratome called epikeratome is used. This epikeratome create an epithelial flap (similar to corneal flap) of precise thickness.

• Commonly epikeratome consists of a blunt blade or a plastic or stainless steel separator. This epikeratome moves slowly (as compared to microkeratome) over the cornea inside a track controller, while simultaneously it pushes away or slices a much even epithelial flap.

As the epi-LASIK procedure has gained popularity in recent years, various types of automated and disposable types of epikeratomes are available. A few examples of commercially available epikeratome are Morias Epi-K, Centurion Epiedge, Amadeus II, Gebauer Epilift, etc. Epi-LASIK became the procedure of choice in high degree myopes (>10 D) or in patients having thin cornea (<530 μm), because there is an additional corneal thickness of nearly 100 μm which is available for ablation (similar to LASEK).

Custom Laser In situ Keratomileusis (C-LASIK)

Conventional excimer laser surgery is the most common refractive surgery for correction of refractive error, since, the visual outcome after standard LASIK was not satisfactory in terms of high order optical aberrations like contrast sensitivity and glare (specially, in night). Various studies had concluded that a proportionate increase in the spherical aberrations was seen in relation to corneal asphericity after conventional LASIK surgery. In normal conditions anterior surface of cornea gradually becomes flatter from center towards periphery means cornea is prolate in shape normally. After conventional LASIK, the central cornea becomes flatter and peripheral cornea becomes steeper means become oblate shape. This causes an oblate shift, which is directly proportional to the amount of ablation. This change in corneal asphericity causes remarkable inconvenience in the quality of vision, although the visual acuity remains well within normal range. To improve the quality of vision and to maintain the corneal asphericity (i.e. reduction of high order aberrations) the constant search to overcome these problems continued. In the year 1999, Theo Seiler successfully treated one of his patients by customized laser ablation surgery and now C-LASIK is one of the preferred refractive procedures for correction of errors. Various cases having high degree irregular astigmatism due to penetrating injuries, penetrating corneal grafts or extensive peripheral corneal scars cannot be corrected by the conventional laser treatment, hence they are treated by customized LASIK technique.

C-LASIK is also called 'customized ablation' LASIK, named because custom ablation is a pattern of ablation. This ablation pattern includes the patient's requirement and is based on individual eye's optical system and anatomy. This customized pattern of laser ablation utilizes variety of treatment patterns for spherical, cylindrical, aspherical and asymmetrical errors and then the optical system of the eyes are optimized to remove them. For easy understanding we can compare the conventional LASIK procedure with a 'Readymade shirt' present in cloth store as ready to buy stock and customized LASIK with a 'Tailor made shirt' stitched by a tailor on order according to the exact fit for a particular person.

An exact evaluation of an individual eye's optical system is done with corneal topography and aberrometry. Thus, customized ablation selectively corrects all orders of aberrations present in an individual's eyes.

Customized optical ablations can be done by using any one of the following techniques

- Corneal topographic guided ablation
- Wavefront guided ablation

As the name suggests the corneal topography guided ablation is done on those aberrations which are identified during corneal topography. In this the laser treats the corneal irregularities as an integral part of the treatment plan.

Similarly, the wavefront guided ablation works on the aberrations which are produced by the entire human optical system and can be detected by the wavefront measurement devices.

Technique of C-LASIK: As discussed above the C-LASIK is an advancement procedure of standard LASIK, hence majority of steps are same as that of a standard LASIK procedure. However, for customized ablation in C-LASIK technique a few additional steps are required to correct the high order aberrations also.

- *Measurement of optical aberrations:* All the aberrations of the eye are measured using corneal topography and wavefront aberrometry devices. These devices are so accurate and precise that a refractive error of submicron level, i.e. 0.01 D can be measured. This data is utilized to design a customized ablation pattern which is feeded in the laser machine.

- *Linking of data:* All the measured data is combined with the help of software which download this data on a floppy disc. This disc is inserted into laser machine computer to guide and perform ablation pattern.

- *Laser ablation:* Customized ablation is done with a flexible laser delivery system which can deliver small size laser spots (<1–2 mm size). This system is also equipped with an excellent eye tracking system or an eye stabilizing system. To achieve an accurate ablation, registration of wavefront data with laser machine and eye tracking system to eye is a challenging step for surgeons. Any discrepancy in entry of data will give an unfavorable outcome.

Advantages of C-LASIK

- *High quality vision:* As compared to standard LASIK, C-LASIK gives a high quality vision with reduced risk of night glare and halos. Contrast sensitivity is better with C-LASIK.

- *Less invasive:* Comparatively C-LASIK is a less destructive technique than conventional procedure. It ablates a lesser amount of corneal tissue to achieve the desired effect.

- *Correction of irregular astigmatism:* As discussed before, cases following penetrating injuries, penetrating corneal grafts or peripheral corneal scars can be treated by C-LASIK. Nearly 40% of eyes have some degree of corneal irregularities. These eyes can also be treated by customized procedure and shows better results than conventional method.

- *Achievement of super-vision:* As compared to conventional LASIK, the visual acuity up to 6/4 or 6/3 can be achieved. The visual acuity of human retina is usually reduced due to presence of high-order aberrations and diffraction of light. It is seen that chances of high-order aberrations are more with conventional LASIK than custom-LASIK.

Corneal Lenticule Extraction Procedure

The most recent advancement in the correction of myopia is corneal lenticule extraction popularly called SMILE (small incision lenticule extraction) procedure.

Principle: Four photoablative incisions are made in a sequence by femtosecond laser which creates a corneal stromal lenticule and corneal incision. This corneal lenticule is then extracted by either creating a flap (similar to LASIK) or from a corneal incision with the help of a blunt forceps.

Surgical technique

- Procedure is performed under topical anesthesia after cleaning and draping the eye similar to other refractive procedures.
- The positioning of eye is done under a curved contact glass interface and proper positioning of the head of patient is done to avoid nasal contact of the interface. Centration of the eye is done by instructing the patient to look at fixating light.
- Suction is started so that cornea will be held adjacent to the contact glass interface. Now the femtosecond laser is applied to create various photoablative incisions to create intrastromal lenticule and corneal incisions as shown in Fig. 15.9.
  - First incision plane (a) is made from peripheral cornea to central cornea creating the posterior lenticule surface of predetermined diameter depending on the size of optical zone.
  - Vertical 360 degree edge (b) is created along the perimeter of lenticule according to the precalculated depth equivalent to the thickness of lenticule.

  - Third plane (c) is created from central to peripheral cornea about 0.5 mm more than posterior surface of lenticule. This represents the anterior surface of lenticule.
  - Final incision (d) is made at 30–50 degree angle usually superior or superotemporal (to preserve the nasal and temporal corneal nerves and surgical ease) in peripheral cornea from edge of anterior lenticule surface to entire thickness of corneal surface to access the lenticule.

- The entire femtosecond laser procedure takes about 25 seconds and then the suction is switched off automatically. Patient eye is repositioned after releasing the contact glass interface underneath the operating microscope.
- Corneal incision is opened using a sharp tipped delicate instrument and then the anterior surface of lenticule is separated gently and uniformly by using a blunt spatula.
- Using the same sharp tipped instrument the posterior surface of lenticule is opened and

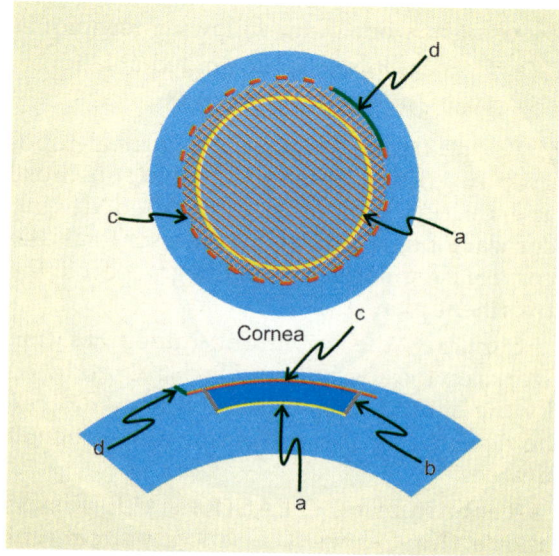

Fig. 15.9: Photoablative incisions of SMILE. a. First incision plane; b. Vertical incisions 360 degrees; c. Third incision for posterior lenticule surface; d. Corneal incision for lenticule extraction

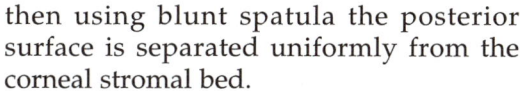
then using blunt spatula the posterior surface is separated uniformly from the corneal stromal bed.

- Once these two planes of lenticule are separated, then using blunt microsurgical forceps the lenticule is manually extracted through the small corneal incision.
- Balanced salt solution is used to flush the corneal pocket with the help of a fine blunt tipped cannula.
- Postoperative treatment is similar to LASIK procedure as described on page 482.

Complications

Intraoperative complications: Rarely, some intraoperative complications can occur during SMILE procedure as follows.

- Sudden loss of suction can occur during femtosecond treatment either due to patient's errors like sneezing or moving head or due to machine faults like gas bubble migration, fluid entry between suction ports. Once the suction is lost, the laser system automatically goes into restart mode. Depending upon the timing of suction loss the procedure can be restarted. For example, suppose if suction is lost at the time of posterior lenticule surface creation (<10%) then restart the SMILE procedure and if suction loss occurs when >10% posterior lenticule creation is done then switch over to LASIK procedure. When suction is lost during side cut stage of either posterior or anterior surface of lenticule, then repeat the side cuts with decreasing the lenticule diameter by 0.2–0.4 mm.
- Microepithelial abrasions at corneal incision site may occur during laser treatment.
- Minute corneal tears at incision site during opening of corneal incision may occur.
- Selection of wrong tissue plane during separation of anterior lenticule surface from overlying corneal plane. Sometimes, the posterior lenticule surface plane is separated instead of anterior surface of lenticule and then it becomes difficult to

remove the lenticule because it gets stuck to overlying cornea.

Postoperative complications: These are very less compared to other corneal refractive procedures. However, following complications can occur in small percentage of cases

- Fine scarring with interface inflammation can occur at the edges of corneal incision site or lenticule, however, it is not in pupillary area, hence no visual symptoms are seen.
- At incision site there may be epithelial in-growth, which is usually self limited and require no additional treatment.
- Occasionally corneal microstriae are seen.
- Complications like dry eye, night glare or decreased contrast sensitivity are seen in lesser magnitude compared to other refractive procedures.

Comparison with Femtosecond LASIK

- Intrastromal lenticule is created within the corneal substance, hence SMILE is independent of treatment factors like corneal hydration, depth of ablation, atmospheric temperature and humidity.
- Total procedure time in SMILE is markedly short because only single laser platform is required unlike femto LASIK where two platforms (one to create corneal flap and second for photoablation) are required.
- SMILE is cost effective in terms of capital investments, maintenance and consumable costs.
- Higher order aberrations, especially spherical are appreciably less in SMILE.
- Amount of corneal tissue requirement per dioptre correction is less compared to excimer LASIK because the peripheral loss of energy fluence is not present with femtosecond laser.
- Corneal nerve arcades are relatively well-preserved during SMILE because no corneal flap is created.
- Postoperative wound healing is faster and better because very small corneal incisions are made during SMILE procedure.

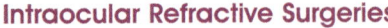

Intraocular Refractive Surgeries

- Refractive lens exchange (RLE)
- Phakic refractive lenses (PRLs)

Refractive Lens Exchange

History: In earlier time even before the invention of IOLs, in the year 1890 extraction of clear crystalline lens was advocated to treat unilateral cases of high myopia of –15 to –20 dioptres, which was commonly called *Fukala's operation*. However, due to high incidence of post procedure retinal detachment, this procedure never gained popularity. In last century the ophthalmic surgery had continuously improvised with invention of better techniques and equipment for extraction of crystalline lens and IOL insertion. These recent innovation encouraged the surgeons to consider the refractive lens exchange (RLE) procedure for correction of high degree myopia or hypermetropia in cases which were not fit for correction by laser surgeries.

Significantly high myopia (25–30 D) is treated by clear lens extraction by phacoemulsification and an appropriate power foldable IOL is implanted. Similarly, in high hypermetrope (+8 to +14 dioptres) phacoemulsification is the procedure of choice with high power foldable IOL implantation. Sometimes in myopes only removal of crystalline lens will achieve emmetrope status means the IOL power requires to achieve emmetropic state is zero but still it is advisable to implant a zero power IOL rather than keeping the patient aphakic, since IOL implantation decreases the chances of retinal complications and posterior capsular opacification.

Refractive lens exchange is an intraocular surgery, hence the complication of the procedure is similar to any other intraocular surgery. Therefore, the surgeon must choose RLE procedure weighing between the surgical complications and expected visual outcome. Various inclusion and exclusion criteria for RLE are summarized in Table 15.13.

As RLE is a refractive procedure and not the routine conventional cataract surgery certain specific preprocedure evaluations along with routine examination are recommended for better visual outcome and patient's satisfaction.

Detailed preoperative evaluation: Majority of patients planned for clear lens extraction are myope, hence the meticulous evaluation of

Table 15.13: Various exclusion and inclusion criteria for refractive lens exchange	
Inclusion criteria	**Exclusion criteria**
High degree myope or hypermetrope in presbyopic age, because complete loss of accommodation occurs after RLE.	Young moderate to high degree myopic patients are better treated with phakic IOLs.
Correction of regular high degree astigmatism not getting corrected by corneal refractive surgeries. Toric IOLs can be successfully implanted in these cases.	Young hyperopic patients are included only when phakic IOL is contraindicated because of shallow anterior chamber, otherwise they are excluded from RLE.
Very high degree refractive error (myopes > 12 D and hyperopes > 7 D) not getting corrected by corneal refractive surgeries or where phakic IOLs are contraindicated.	Patients having retinal conditions like macular degenerations, peripheral degenerations, retinoschisis and retinal tears or holes are not included because the potential visual outcome is unfavorable after RLE.
Borderline presbyope with high degree hypermetropia can be included for multifocal IOL implantation.	Young patients having very high expectations of visual outcome or very apprehensive about RLE.

following retinal lesions are mandatory along with measurement of IOP

- Examination for vitreous degeneration
- Examination for retinal degeneration
- Lattice degeneration with or without hole.

All these lesions should be looked prior to surgery, as high degree myopes are prone for these retinal changes. If these lesions are present they should be treated by photocoagulation or cryotherapy before RLE procedure. Generally, patients having macular degeneration will have poor visual outcome, however, they may get better field of vision after RLE, hence should be informed to patient before procedure.

IOL power calculation: Calculation of IOL power should be perfect to achieve good visual outcome after RLE. IOL power is dependent on axial length of eye, keratometry reading of cornea and formula applied for power calculation so following points are advised

- Immersion technique for measurement of axial length is superior to contact technique.
- Automated keratometry is superior over manual keratometer.
- Optical interferometry based IOL power calculation by use of IOL master gives perfect readings.
- Several studies concluded that most appropriate formula for IOL power calculation in case of myopia is Haigis formula and in case of hypermetropia is any one formula among Hoffer Q, SRK/T, Haigis or Holladay.

Surgical technique

- Phacoemulsification with foldable IOL implantation is the procedure of choice.
- Continuous circular and curvilinear capsulorrhexis is prerequisite. Keep the size of capsulorrhexis a little smaller than optic of IOL for better centration.
- Meticulous flawless phacoemulsification of crystalline lens with minimum surgically induced astigmatism is done because RLE is a refractive surgery.

Postoperative complications: In RLE the immediate or late postoperative surgical complications are similar to any conventional cataract surgery but there may be some additional intraoperative and postoperative complications due to high refractive ocular status.

In high myopes
- Capsular bag is unstable so capsulorrhexis is a little risky and in some cases capsular tension rings are required to perform capsulorrhexis.
- Large axial length is a risk factor for increased percentage of subchoroidal hemorrhage.
- Eyes having axial length >25 mm are at more risk for *capsular bag syndrome*.
- Increased postoperative complications of retinal detachment due to longer axial length, vitreous and retinal degeneration, posterior vitreous detachment and retinal holes.

In high hypermetropes
- Shallow anterior chamber gives poor surgical space for phacoemulsification and IOL insertion.
- Small axial length is a risk factor for increased percentage of choroidal effusion syndrome.

RLE has a high potential to correct even high degree refractive errors but its clinical use is limited in patient's having clear lens, because of these specific complications not seen in routine cataract surgeries. Recently, a huge progress has been done in the field of IOL power calculation, IOL designing and microsurgical instrumentation so gradually RLE is also getting a wider acceptance as refractive surgery.

Phakic Refractive Lenses

Earlier in the year 1954, Strampelli introduced the idea of correction of high degree refractive errors using refractive lenses, but only in last two decades these photorefractive lenses gained popularity as an indispensible tool in refractive surgery. Usually, the refractive power of eye is modified by altering the power of two refracting surfaces, i.e. cornea and lens. The refracting power of cornea and crystalline lens can be altered using laser corneal surgery and refractive lens exchange, respectively. There is another possibility to change the refracting power of eye by introducing third refracting surface without touching cornea or natural crystalline lens, which can be done by using phakic refractive lenses (PRL). High degree refractive errors either myopic or hyperopic can be corrected by PRL with precise predictable surgical outcome. PRL is mainly indicated for correction of high degree refractive errors in young patients having healthy eyes and stable refraction. Patients of more than 50 years age having diabetic retinopathy and/or glaucoma are contraindications for PRL procedure.

Depending on the intraocular position these phakic IOLs can be broadly classified as shown in Table 15.14.

- *Acrysof Cache phakic IOL:* This lens is made up of hydrophobic acrylic material having an optic of 6 mm and four haptics to fit exactly in anterior chamber as shown in Fig. 15.10. Lens is available in sizes 12.5 mm, 13 mm, 13.5 mm or 14 mm with power range from –6 to –16 D.
- *NuVita MA phakic IOL:* Kelman designs IOLs were modified by Baikoff who designed angle fixated anterior chamber IOLs. These original lenses had 25° angulations with 4.5 mm optics. In second modification Baikoff's reduced angle to 20° at the cost of reduced optical diameter. Later on other modifications in the design leads to NuVita MA phakic

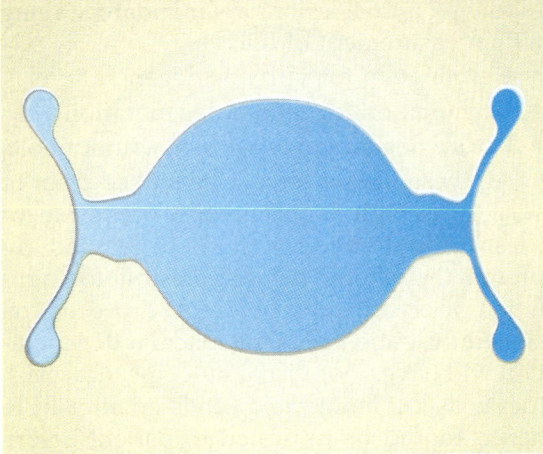

Fig. 15.10: Acrysof Cache phakic intra-ocular lens

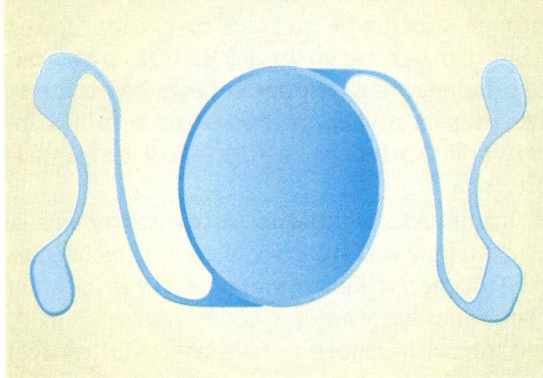

Fig. 15.11: NuVita MA phakic intra-ocular lens

IOL having an optical zone of 4.5 mm and optical diameter of 5 mm. Long legs of this lens engage the angle of eye and optic remains in front of pupillary area as shown in Fig. 15.11. Power range available for myopia correction is –6 D to –20 D. Several modifications are done in past 10 years to decrease the endothelial

Table 15.14: Various designs of phakic IOLs		
Anterior chamber phakic IOLs		Posterior chamber Phakic IOLs
Angle supported	Iris supported	
Acrysof Cache IOL	Artisan	ICL (Implantable contact lens)
Nuvita MA IOL	Artiflex	PRL (Phakic refractive lens)
Kelman duet IOL		
Vivarte IOL		

damage and iris damage by this lens. Glaucoma and intraocular inflammation are main long-term problems with this lens.

- *Artisan:* This lens is made up of PMMA material having an optic of 5 mm/6 mm and two claw-shaped haptics to grasp the iris muscle in mid-periphery as shown in Fig. 15.12. Total size of the lens is 8.5 mm and as this lens is fixed in mid-periphery of iris there is no need of different sizes for various length of patient's eye. 5 mm optic artisan is available in power range of –2 to –23 D, +2 to +12 D and up to 7.5 D for myopic, hypermetropic and astigmatic patients, respectively. However, 6 mm optic artisan is presently available only for myope in power range of –2 to –15.5 D.

- *Artiflex:* This lens has a 6 mm optic, made up of polysiloxane material and two claw shaped haptics made up of PMMA material as shown in Fig. 15.13. Overall diameter is 8.5 mm and is available for

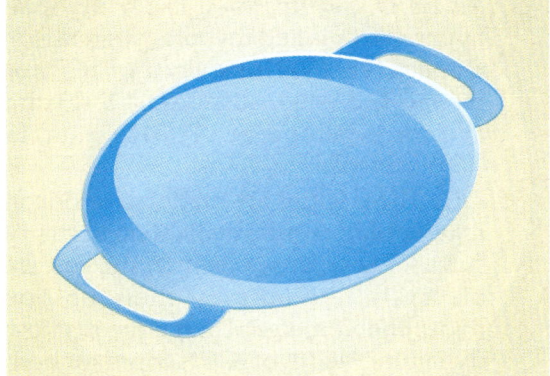

Fig. 15.13: Artiflex IOL phakic intra-ocular lens

myopia in power range of –2 to –14.5 D and myopic astigmatism up to –7.5 D.

- *ICL:* These posterior chamber phakic IOLs (ICL and PRL) are also known as implantable contact lens. ICL is made up of hydrogel collagen co-polymer having a plate design haptic with 4.5 to 5.5 mm size optic. This foldable lens design can be inserted through 2.5 mm incision and its four haptic design plate facilitates proper fixation in the ciliary sulcus. Haptic plate has a forward vault to minimize the IOL crystalline lens touch as shown in Fig. 15.14. Available in power range of –3 to –23 D, + 3.0 to

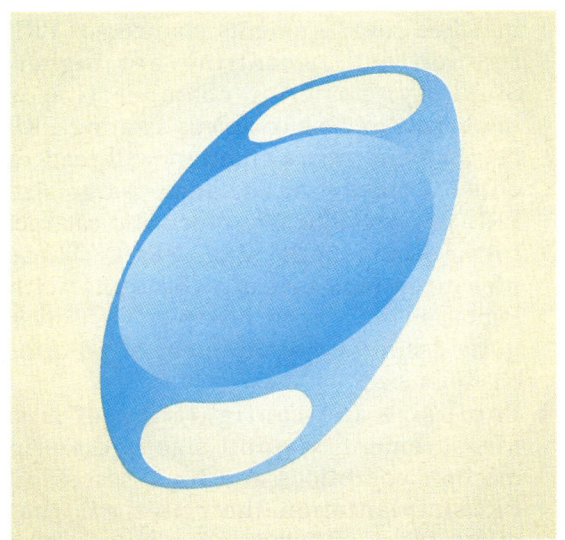

Fig. 15.12: Artisan IOL phakic intra-ocular lens

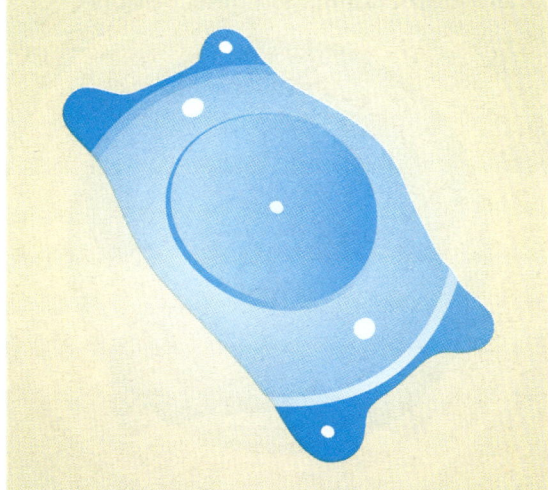

Fig. 15.14: Visian ICL

+ 21.5 D and up to –6 D for myopia, hypermetropia and myopic astigmatism, respectively. Various sizes of ICL for myopia and astigmatism are 11.5 –13 mm and for hyperopia are 11 –12.5 mm, in 0.5 mm steps.

- *PRL:* These lenses are made up of silicon material and require no fixation to ciliary sulcus. These lenses float on the surface of crystalline lens by their unique hydrophobic material and aqueous flow dynamics. Width of ICL is 6 mm for both myopic and hypermetropic patients, however, thickness of lens varies with the dioptric power to a maximum of 0.6 mm as shown in Fig. 15.15. ICL is available in power range of –4 to –22 D and +3 to +16 D for myopia and hyper-metropia, respectively.

Preoperative evaluation: Similar to routine preoperative evaluation as in other intraocular surgery following examinations are done in case of PRL.

- **Vision and refraction:** Uncorrected and best corrected visual acuity should be recorded and meticulous objective, subjective and cycloplegic refraction is done to assess exact refractive status of eye.

- **Anterior segment examination:** Detailed slit lamp examination must be done.

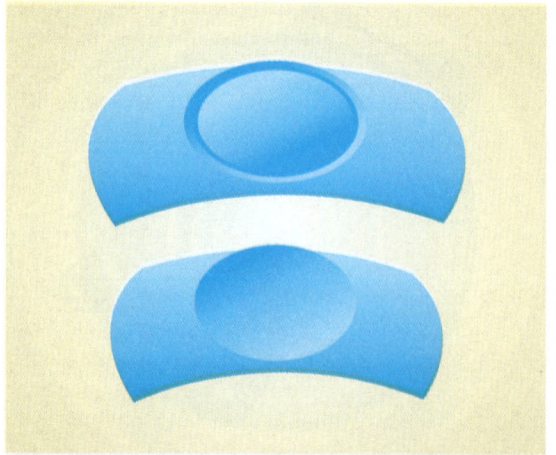

Fig. 15.15: PRL phakic IOL intra-ocular lens

- **Posterior segment examination:** Indirect ophthalmoscopy is done for detail fundus examination with sclera depressor to see the periphery. Any retinal lesions should be recorded and if needed should be treated before surgery.

- **Intraocular pressure** is measured accurately.

Along with these routine examination some important assessments are also done for PRL insertion such as

- **Anterior chamber depth:** This is an important parameter to be measured from corneal endothelium to anterior surface of crystalline lens. Anterior chamber (AC) depth can be measured by use of Orbscan, Pentacam, IOL master or OCT. Although UBM can also measure AC depth but are not preferred because the corneal thickness is also added in the total measurement value. Normal desirable safe AC depth is 3–3.2 mm for PRL insertion, AC depth less than 2.8 mm is considered as unsafe. In shallow AC chances of endothelial cell loss after PRL insertion is very high.

- **Anterior and posterior chamber size:** Measurement of anterior chamber size is prerequisite for implantation of an angle supported PRL because in improperly matched measurements chances of PRL rotation and decentring are higher. Similarly, posterior chamber size is important in case of sulcus fixating PRL because any miscalculation will lead to either occlusion of AC angle (large size PRL) or crystalline lens touch and cataract formation (small size PRL). These measurements can also be done with Pentacam or Orbscan, however, OCT gives quite accurate measurement of anterior chamber size.

- **Pupil size and configuration of iris:** Measurement of pupil size is done in mesopic conditions and for a successful PRL implantation the criteria is that difference of more than 1 mm in pupil size and PRL optic in mesopic conditions is unacceptable. Normal individuals has flat configured iris, whereas high hypermetropes has convex-shaped iris configuration. For implantation of iris fixating PRL the eyes with convex configured iris are not suitable. Accurate evaluation of iris configuration is done by OCT.

- **Endothelium profile:** Normal healthy endothelium having low polymegathism and/or pleomorphism with a cell count of minimum 2400 cells per cubic mm is needed for a successful PRL implantation.

Surgical techniques

- Phakic IOLs can be implanted in topical, peribulbar or general anesthesia depending upon the surgeon's choice and situation. However, for nonfoldable IOLs (for example, NuVita or Artisan), peribulbar or general anesthesia is recommended.

- For anterior chamber IOL (either angle fixated or iris fixated) miosis is required, hence 2% pilocarpine drops are instilled 15–20 minutes prior to surgery. However, posterior chamber IOL insertion requires well dilated pupil so topical tropicamide (1%) with phenylephrine (1%) drop is instilled 2–3 times at an interval of 10 minutes prior to surgery.

- Cleaning and draping of eye is similar to other refractive procedure, however, the following surgical steps are different for various design phakic IOLs.

  - *Angle fixated anterior chamber IOL:* For example, insertion of Acrysof cache IOL is done through clear corneal main incision of 2.8 or 3.2 mm. Side port of 0.8–1 mm is made at 9 o'clock position and main incision is made superiorly, while taking care of anterior lens capsule. Inject viscoelastic preferably of high density in the anterior chamber. IOL is loaded inside the cartridge and then cartridge is inserted through main incision. Now slowly and constantly inject the lens while keep a check on correct unfolding of lens. Blunt dialor can be used through side port to support the correct unfolding of lens. Slowly pull the cartridge outside while trailing IOL haptic is inserted into the eye. Wash the viscoelastic thoroughly using irrigation/aspiration (I/A) cannula manually.

  - *Iris fixated anterior chamber IOL:* For example, Artisan IOL insertion is done through a large corneal or scleral incision of 5.5–6.5 mm length. Two sides are made at 10 o'clock and 2 o'clock positions with a main incision of 5.5–6.5 mm size, superiorly. Inject viscoelastic preferably high density in anterior chamber. Insert the IOL in anterior chamber holding with lens holding forceps and rotate it in horizontal position. Fixate the IOL in midperipheral region of iris by using a blunt needle through side port and pressing the lens optic through main port. Each claw of IOL must be grasping at least 1 mm of iris tissue. Wash the viscoelastic thoroughly using I/A cannula manually.

  - *Posterior chamber phakic IOL:* For example, ICL insertion is done through clear corneal 3.2 mm incision made temporally. Two side ports at 6 and 12 o'clock position with a clear corneal 3.2 mm temporal main incision are made. Inject viscoelastic preferably high density in anterior chamber. Most crucial and important part is proper and precise loading of the ICL in the cartridge. Once loaded cartridge inserted in the anterior chamber and ICL is injected slowly into the anterior chamber while surgeon keeps an eye on the mark on leading and trailing haptic. Leading haptic mark must be on right side and trailing haptic mark on left side of operating surgeon. Once ICL is placed in anterior chamber, slowly press the tip of haptic using a soft tip lens manipulator to posterior chamber. Never press the optic of ICL. Wash the viscoelastic thoroughly using I/A cannula manually.

Note: In case of Acrysof cache IOL, iridectomy is not essential, however, in rest of phakic IOLs iridectomy must be done during surgery or preoperatively using YAG laser.

Postoperative treatment

- Topical antibiotics/steroids eye drops for 6–8 times/day for a period of 2–4 weeks with gradually decreasing the frequency of instillation.
- Topical lubricants 4–6 times/day for a period of 4–6 weeks and later on as and when needed.
- Precautions to be taken as after LASIK surgery described on page 482.
- Follow-up is similar to LASIK as described on page 482.

Complications of phakic IOLs: In a planned and well-executed surgery there are literally no complications seen with phakic IOL insertion, however, a few complications can occur during phakic IOL insertion or post procedure as follows

- Possibility of reverse implantation, i.e. upside down insertion of foldable phakic IOLs is present. This can be avoided by carefully monitoring the mark on IOL while leading haptic is opening inside the eye.
- A few cases of iris bleeding during iridectomy has been reported. This can be prevented by using high density viscoelastic or performing YAG laser iridectomy.

- Occasionally, postoperative decentration of IOL in case of iris fixated phakic IOLs has been reported.
- In small percentage of patients giant granular cell deposits are seen on IOL surface, after Artiflex IOL insertion.
- Variable percentage of cataract formation with ICL lens insertion has been reported by many studies. However, it can be prevented by proper assessment of posterior chamber depth and accurate ICL length calculations.

Several studies have compared the advantages and disadvantages of phakic IOLs in relation to other refractive procedures specially PRK and LASIK. These advantages and disadvantages are summarized in Table 15.15.

Miscellaneous Corneal Refractive Techniques

- Orthokeratology
- Intrastromal corneal ring segments
- Intracorneal lenses
- Gel injection adjustable keratoplasty

Orthokeratology

Orthokeratology means reshaping of the cornea by applying pressure and flattening of the central portion of the cornea. In ancient China, a concept of correction of distance vision was to apply the weight over eyelids

Table 15.15: Advantages and disadvantages of phakic IOLs in comparison to LASIK and PRK

Advantages	Disadvantages
Correct very high degree of refractive errors not suitable for other procedures	Intraocular procedure, possibilities of intraocular infection is higher
Maintain accommodation	Early cataract formation, specially in ICL
Not associated with regression (wound healing)	Endothelial decompensation, specially with anterior chamber phakic IOLs
Reversible procedure with expected outcome	Intraocular hemorrhage due to iridectomy
Maintain prolate shape of cornea hence better vision quality	Iris atrophy and pupil deformation with iris fixated IOLs
Add on procedure can be done to correct residual refractive error	Chronic anterior uveitis with anterior chamber IOLs

during sleeping. Considering this concept first time in the year 1962, George Jessen used PMMA contact lenses of zero power (Plano lenses) flatter base curve than the central corneal curvature for correction of myopia. After introduction of rigid gas permeable contact lenses in year 1980s and a progressive development in the field of corneal topography, a leap change occurred in orthokeratology. In modern days, orthokeratology or Ortho-k fitting has become a valuable non-surgical technique to treat the refractive errors specially myopia (mild to moderate degree) and astigmatism.

Indications: Orthokeratology has been tried to correct all types of refractive error and even presbyopia, however, it is a useful technique to temporarily reshape the cornea in these following conditions

- Progressive myopia in young child
- Low to moderate degree myopia (–2.5 to –6 dioptres) and/or low degree astigmatism (up to 2.5 dioptres) for any age group.
- Younger myopes (< 18 years), who cannot be considered for LASIK.
- Patients having unstable or frequently varying amount of refractive error.
- Sports persons having restrictions in wearing spectacles or contact lenses.
- Early presbyopes (still under evaluation)

Orthokeratology technique

- Cycloplegic refraction is done to record the accurate values of spherical and cylindrical powers. However, spectacle power can also be taken with vertex distance correction without compensating for spherical equivalent.
- Anterior segment examination with slit lamp is done to rule out any corneal pathology or epithelial defects.
- Tear film evaluation by Schirmer's test and tear break up time (TBUT) test is done to rule out dry eye and tear film instability because unstable tear film may cause difficulty in fitting of corrective contact lens.

- Corneal surface mapping is done by corneal topography method with four recordings in each eye.
- Calculate the average apical curvature and eccentricity of cornea from these mappings. Usually patients having steep apical curvature (more than 44 D) and high eccentricity (more than 0.55) are good candidates for orthokeratology because maximum correction is possible with these corneal parameters.
- Measure the horizontal visible iris diameter (HVID) and record the value separately for each eye.
- Once these parameters are calculated then the parameters of corrective contact lens are calculated using these data to correct the desired amount of refractive error.
- Alternately, a trial lens of similar parameters can be tried for one night wear and next day morning the evaluation of trial lens fit can be assessed by recording visual fluorescein pattern, corneal topography mapping and unaided visual acuity.
- Suppose if trial lens fit evaluation is satisfactory then individual corrective (custom ordered) contact lens with specific parameters is ordered to lens manufacturers.
- Therapeutic schedule for majority of custom ordered contact lens designs is that wear the lenses daily for 6–8 hours duration continuously in daytime (awake) and in some specific designs, wear even during nighttime (sleep).
- Usually, custom ordered contact lenses takes 8–10 days to reflect the full effect of correction so patients should keep patience to wait for improvement in unaided visual acuity.
- Once satisfactory visual acuity and expected correction in corneal reshaping has been achieved, then wearing schedule is modified into maintenance schedule.
- Maintenance schedule require wearing of corrective lenses for a few hours in a day during awake usually for 2–3 days a week

or as needed just to maintain the corrected corneal shape and continued to have good unaided visual acuity.

Complications: Orthokeratology is a non-surgical technique hence complications are very less, however, symptoms of foreign body sensation, glare and ocular discomfort had been reported by small percentage of patients. Rarely, potential complications like microbial keratitis can occur due to continuous wear of contact lenses. Regular follow up and early treatment is the only effective method to prevent microbial keratitis.

Various benefits and limitations of ortho-keratology are summarized in Table 15.16.

Intrastromal Corneal Ring Segments

Earlier in the year 1978, Fleming and associates developed synthetic intracorneal implants in the shape of complete ring termed intracorneal rings. They inserted these intracorneal rings in the eye through a peripheral corneal partial thickness incision. However, difficulties occurred during insertion of these rings lead to modification in the shape of rings. The complete rings were later modified and made into two 'C'-shaped segments and renamed intrastromal corneal ring segments.

Principle: Barraquer and Blavatskaya hypothesized that intracorneal rings behave like tissue additives, which when placed will cause the flattening of cornea. Principle of this technique is that a vaulting effect is produced after insertion of intrastromal corneal ring segments in the cornea which shortens the central arc of the cornea. This helps in correction of myopia and astigmatism. The diameter of ring is related in inverse manner to the amount of flattening of cornea, hence smaller the diameter of ring, more will be the flattening and higher degree of myopia gets corrected.

Keratoconus is characterized by increased curvature and thinning of the cornea. In keratoconus, the coefficient of elasticity of cornea is reduced, as a result, the resistance offered by cornea to prevent deformation of cornea is reduced which in turn causes increased stress on the cornea and forward projection of it. Stress is the force applied per unit area means stress is focally more in apical area causing corneal thinning in keratoconus. When the area is large with the same amount of force the stress can be decreased on per unit area. In keratoconus intracorneal rings redistribute the corneal curvature which causes redistribution of stress in apical area and hence break the biomechanical disease progression.

Intrastromal corneal ring segment designs: Currently two types of intrastromal corneal ring segments are available

- Intacs segment
- Ferrara ring segment

Table 15.16: Benefits and limitations of orthokeratology	
Benefits	*Limitations*
Reversible non-surgical alternative correction method for refractive errors	Offers temporary correction of refractive error
Safe and reproducible procedure	Require longer duration to get desired visual outcome
All age group patients can be treated	Repeatedly needs to wear the corrective lenses to maintain the correction
Require no costly equipment or advanced surgical skills, hence cost effective	Only low degree refractive errors mainly myopia and astigmatism can be corrected
Easy acceptance and faster patient adaptation	
Effective and desirable visual results without any visual aids.	

Intacs segment: Intacs segments are available in pair which are made up of PMMA material, each with an arc length of 150° as shown in Fig. 15.16A. External diameter of ring is 8.1 mm and inner diameter is 6.77 mm with a positioning hole diameter of 0.28 mm. Transverse section of ring is hexagonal shape and longitudinal section is conical shape with thickness ranging from 250 µm to 450 µm in 50 µm increments.

Note: Currently new design Intacs segments are introduced for correction of myopia called Intacs SK. This segment has oval shape transverse section and inner diameter is 6 mm.

Nomogram for Intacs: Amount of refractive error correction is dependent on the thickness of Intacs ring selected for surgery and is summarized in Table 15.17.

Ferrara ring segment: In the year 1986, ophthalmologist Ferrara introduced modified PMMA rings for correction of moderate degree of myopia. Subsequently in 1994 he developed a procedure to implant this ring segment in an intrastromal corneal tunnel and then in the year 1996 he substituted the single ring with a pair of ring segments. These rings are popularly called as Keraring and can correct higher degree of myopic error compared to Intacs segments.

Characteristic features of Ferrara ring segments (Keraring, Fig. 15.16B) are
- Rings are made up of PMMA CQ-acrylic material.

- External diameter is 6.6 mm and inner diameter is 5.4 mm as shown in Fig. 15.16B.
- Arc length is 120° and 160°.
- Thickness of segment range available from 150 to 350 µm in 50 µm increments.
- Cross-sectional shape is triangular due to this shape a prismatic effect is created which eliminates the halo phenomenon.

Various indications and contraindications of insertion of intrastromal corneal ring segments are summarized in Table 15.18.

Preoperative evaluation: Depending on the amount and type of correction, the number and thickness of intrastromal corneal ring segments is decided. Routine systemic and ocular examinations are done as in other refractive surgeries. Following evaluations are important to achieve good visual outcome in selected patients.
- Uncorrected visual acuity (UCVA) and best corrected visual acuity (BCVA)
- Spherical and cylindrical power
- Manifest refractive spherical equivalent (MRSE)
- Corneal pachymetry for thickness
- Keratometry (K) value
- Corneal topography
- Examination of anterior segment

Surgical implantation method for rings
- **Anesthesia:** Commonly rings are implanted under topical anesthesia with or without oral sedation.

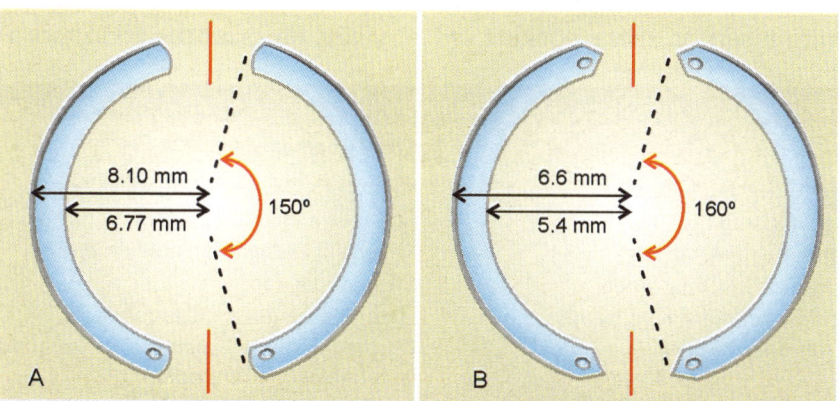

Fig. 15.16: Intracorneal ring segments. A. Intacs segments; B. Keraring segments

Table 15.17: Nomogram for correction of refractive error

Intacs thickness (in µm)	Myopia correction dioptres (D)	Average correction dioptres (D)
250	1.0–1.5	1.3
300	1.6–2.3	2.0
350	2.4–3	2.7
400	3.1–3.9	3.5
450	4.0–4.5	4.2

- **Corneal marking:** For Intacs, marking of geometric center of the cornea is important which can be done by 11 mm zone marker using Sinskey hook. For Keraring, marking of pupillary center is required which can be done preoperatively.
- **Corneal thickness:** Intraoperatively thickness of cornea is measured at incision site and an average of five readings is recorded.
- **Corneal incision:** A 1.8 mm radial corneal incision is made by using a calibrated diamond blade (for nearly 70% of average corneal thickness). Usually incision is made at an axis perpendicular to steepest corneal meridian at inferior position (6 o'clock) and in superior position (at 12 o'clock), about 7 mm away from the optical zone. Incisions are made in such a manner that implants can be placed nasally and temporally.
- **Corneal pockets:** On either side of incisions corneal pockets are made (nearly 70% of corneal depth) using modified microspatula in clockwise and anticlockwise directions. For Keraring insertion these pockets are widened manually using 270° dissection gliders and spatula. Alternately, these corneal pockets can also be made by femtosecond laser.
- For insertion of Intacs segments an instrument is required which generates vacuum in the suction ring and also has lamellar dissector to create stromal channels. Suction ring is applied much similar to LASIK procedure and pressure is checked. At an appropriate pressure the lamellar dissector is placed inside the corneal pockets, which create two semicircular stromal tunnels at 180° apart by dissecting the corneal stroma using rotational movement of dissector.
- Femtosecond laser can be used instead of a lamellar dissector or manual dissector to create stromal channels for insertion of segments. Photodisruptive infrared wavelength femtosecond laser is used to create the tunnels at predetermined stromal depth ranging from 120 to 400 µm. This laser produces smooth walled and of precise depth and diameter tunnels once the required parameters like incision length, width, inner and outer diameter with depth of tunnel had been entered properly in the database.
- **Ring insertion:** Once the appropriate tunnels are created either manually, mechanically or by laser, two ring segments are inserted inside the tunnels, one segment clockwise and another segment anticlockwise. Rings are placed in such a manner that

Table 15.18: Various indications and contraindications of intrastromal corneal ring segments

Indications	Contraindications
Low to moderate degree myopia	High (>45 D) mean K-reading
Progressive keratoconus	Collagen vascular diseases
Pellucid marginal degenerations	Recurrent corneal erosion syndrome
Myopia/astigmatism in thin cornea	Corneal dystrophy
Corneal irregularities after PK or trauma	High degree astigmatism after PK
Corneal ectasias after LASIK	Chronic treatment with drugs like amidarone, isoretinoin or sumatriptan
Postradial keratotomy	Pregnant and lactating women

a gap of about 15–20° nasally and 35–40° temporally is left. Ends of rings are inserted to a length in such a way that about 2 mm and 1.5 mm distance is left from inferior and superior incisions, respectively.

- **Wound closure:** Once rings are placed properly at desired depth and length, the incision wounds are closed by one or two interrupted 10–0 nylon suture. These sutures are usually removed after 12–15 days time to prevent any associated infections.

Postoperative treatment

- Topical antibiotic eye drops are prescribed for 7–10 days in a frequency of 4–6 times/day.
- Steroids eye drops are prescribed for one month period in gradual decreasing frequency starting with 4–6 times/day.
- Lubricating eye drops preferably preservative free drops are given 6–8 times/day for a period of 4–5 weeks.

Complications: In expert hands with proper precautions complications of intracorneal ring segments are negligible, however, following complications can occur in small percentage of cases

- Improper refractive correction
- Deposits in tunnels
- Superficial microbial keratitis
- Migration or expedition of segments.

Note: Femtosecond laser assisted procedures has very less complications specially the microbial keratitis and ring displacement.

- Corneal neovascularization around channels
- Visual symptoms, e.g. glare and halos

Comparative benefits and limitations of intrastromal corneal ring segments over laser ablative refractive procedures are summarized in Table 15.19.

Intracorneal Lenses

Intracorneal hydrogel lenses: In the year 1967, first hydrogel lens was developed for refractive keratoplasty to correct the high myopia, hypermetropia or aphakia. These implants were initially prepared of hydroxy methyl methacrylate (HEMA) having refractive index similar to cornea (1.37). The properties of intracorneal hydrogel lens material are

- Water content is high in range of 70 to 80%
- Lens diameter in the range of 5.0–6.5 mm
- Lens thickness differs as per the type of lens, e.g. for myopia the peripheral thickness is more, whereas for hypermetropia the central thickness is more. Moreover, after implantation the thickness of lens increases because it absorbs the water and permits the nutrients to flow across.

Table 15.19: Advantages and limitations of intracorneal ring segments in comparison to laser ablative refractive procedures

Advantages	Limitations
Better anterior corneal surface is preserved compare to photo ablative procedures	Only mild to moderate degree myopia can be corrected
Central corneal tissue or optical axis remain surgically unaffected	Frequency of over or undercorrection is higher
Natural corneal shape (prolate shape) is maintained	Effect is regressed due to displacement or expedition of segments
Reversible procedure where rings can easily be removed if desired	Complications like tunnel deposits and neovascularization are great hurdles.
Superior visual outcome in mild to moderate degree keratoconus cases.	
Maintains the strength of cornea because no ablation of stroma	

Surgical procedure

- Procedure is performed under topical anesthesia after cleaning and draping the eye similar to other refractive procedures.
- By means of mechanical microkeratome a corneal flap of about 8.5–9.0 mm diameter is created with inferior hinge (about 3.5–4.0 mm). Thickness of corneal flap may vary in range of 180–300 µm depending upon the choice of surgeon.
- Hydrogel lens is implanted underneath the corneal flap over stromal bed in pupillary zone.
- In a few selected cases, corneal suturing is required for stability.
- Postoperative treatment is similar to other refractive procedures, i.e. topical antibiotics (thrice daily × 3 days) and topical steroids (thrice daily with gradual tapering over 15 days).

Note: In this procedure, irrigation of flap interface should not be done after giving cut with microkeratome or implantation of hydrogel lens.

Complications: Limited number of intracorneal hydrogel lens implantation cases and their studies are available to establish the clinical complications related to the procedure, however, following complications after hydrogel lens implantation have been reported in a few studies

- High order corneal aberrations are increased after intracorneal hydrogel lens implantation, especially in cases of high degree hypermetropia or aphakia.
- Intrastromal epithelial cyst and opacification is reported in a few cases.
- Complete regression of refractive error is seen in many cases which require a second corrective surgery to correct the refractive error.
- In some cases formation of membrane around the lens is seen at intrastromal plane.

Note: Many studies reported that predictability of surgical outcome and stability of refractive status is very poor after intracorneal hydrogel lens implantation, hence this procedure is not widely accepted.

Intracorneal polysulfone lenses: Similar to hydrogel lenses, lenses of high refractive index material polysulfone were also tried by several scientists as intracorneal lens implants. However, the initial trials were not successful and results of polysulfone lens implants caused significant clinical problems. Under topical anesthesia, using diamond knife a 5.5–6.0 mm size clear corneal incision was made near limbus. Using blunt spatula a corneal pocket was created and polysulfone lens was implanted and centered. Incision was closed using nylon suture. Postoperative treatment was similar to other refractive surgeries. Severe postoperative complications like stromal melting, wound scarring, anterior chamber perforation, wound dehiscence, irregular astigmatism and neovascularization were reported by several studies conducted on polysulfone intracorneal lens implants. Due to these sight threatening complications this lens never gained any acceptance in clinical practice.

Gel Injection Adjustable Keratoplasty

This is a reversible procedure proposed by Simon G. in the year 1985 for correction of moderate degree of myopia by altering the curvature of cornea. Principle used is that a gel material is injected inside the corneal channel which causes change in the anterior curvature of the cornea and hence correct the refractive error. Several gel materials had been tried for this purpose, however, most commonly experimented gel material is polyethylene oxide.

Surgical technique

- Procedure is performed under topical anesthesia after cleaning and draping the eye similar to other refractive procedures.
- Pachymetry is done at the site of injection and an optical zone 7.0 mm is marked using corneal marker.
- Radial incision of about 1.0 mm size, of nearly 75–80% corneal thickness is made by

using a diamond knife. Blunt spatula is used to separate the stromal lamella and a lamellar plane guide is placed inside the corneal pocket.

- Then a specially designed helicoids spatula is inserted in corneal pocket in lamellar plane and 360° annular dissection is done to create the intrastromal channel.
- Gel material (polyethylene oxide) is injected into intrastromal channel in gradual manner and simultaneously epithelial massage is given to equally distribute the gel inside the channel. An intra-procedural keratometry is done to observe the change in the curvature of cornea happening due to injection of gel. This curvatural change will decide the amount of gel to be injected.
- Once the desired change of corneal curvature had occurred, then stop the gel injection. No sutures are required to close the incision.

Gel injection adjustable keratoplasty is a simple cost effective procedure for correction of myopia and astigmatism. This procedure has an advantage of reversibility without affecting the visual axis and easy adjustability of refractive correction intraoperatively. Postoperatively negligible amount of corneal scar or haze are the additional benefits of this procedure. Limitations of this procedure are quantification of amount of gel require to correct the error and slight opaque nature of gel. To avoid visual symptoms gel is injected in relatively larger optical area.

REFRACTIVE PROCEDURES FOR HYPERMETROPIA

In majority of refractive procedures done for correction of hypermetropia, the principle used is similar to that used in the refractive procedure for myopia correction. However, the major difference is that in myopia the central corneal ablation (thinning) is done, whereas for hypermetropia correction the peripheral corneal ablation (thinning) is done. Various refractive procedures for hyper-

metropia correction can be broadly grouped as

- Incisional refractive surgery
- Laser refractive surgery
- Corneal stromal collagen shrinking procedures: Conductive keratoplasty and thermal keratoplasty

Incisional Refractive Surgery

Hexagonal keratotomy is an incisional refractive procedure which can be performed to correct mild to moderate degree of hypermetropia. In the year 1985, Mendez performed this procedure to correct hypermetropia. This procedure is now obsolete but is discussed because of its historical importance. Originally, in this method, circumferentially connecting peripheral cuts in hexagonal shape were created around 4.5–6 mm clear optical zone as shown in Fig. 15.17A. This causes the buldging of central cornea and hence correction of hypermetropia occurred. Later on, Jensen and Mendez improvised the technique by creating shorter, non-connecting incisions in hexagonal shape as shown in Fig. 15.17B. In spite of this modification, the complications like higher amount of aberrations, corneal scarring, irregular astigmatism, corneal perforation on trivial trauma, and keratitis were observed in high percentage of cases. Hence, due to high risk of complications over advantages this procedure is not preferred.

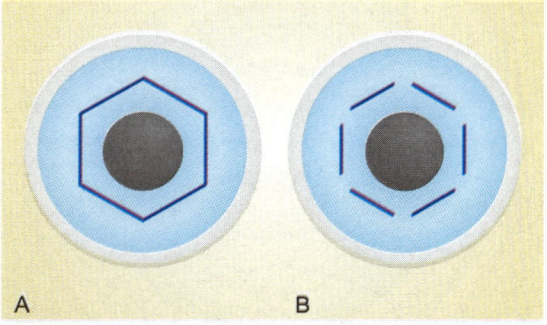

Fig. 15.17: Hexagonal keratotomy. A. Original method; B. Modified method

Laser Refractive Surgeries

Similar to myopia the laser systems can also be used to correct hypermetropia and various laser refractive surgeries for correction of hypermetropia are

- Hypermetropic photorefractive keratectomy (PRK)
- Hypermetropic LASIK
- Hypermetropic epi-LASIK
- Hypermetropic LASEK
- Hypermetropic customized LASIK

Hypermetropic PRK: Prerequisite and initial surgical steps of hypermetropic PRK technique are same as that of myopic PRK. Under topical anesthesia excimer laser is applied to correct the hypermetropic refractive error, however, the preparation of stromal bed and pattern of laser delivery is entirely different from myopic pattern.

- In hypermetropic PRK a large diameter (about 9 to 9.5 mm) optical zone is prepared by removing corneal epithelium, against smaller area in myopic PRK.
- Then large dough-nut shaped laser photoablation is done as shown in Fig. 15.18, whereas in myopic PRK the central optical zone photoablation is done. This peripheral

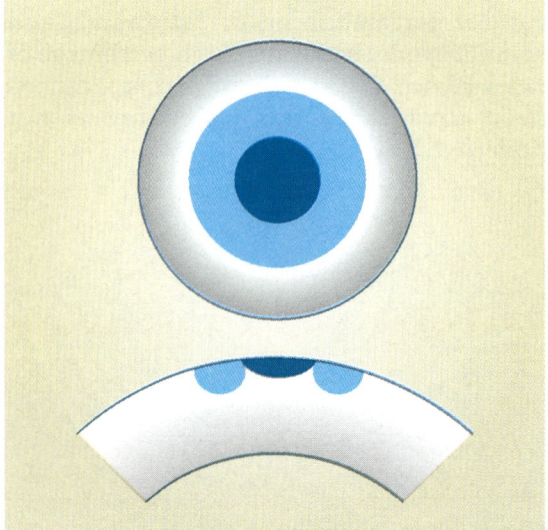

Fig. 15.18: Hypermetropic photorefractive keratectomy

zone photoablation produces corneal thinning in peripheral area and hence buldging of central cornea occurs.

- Nearly three times of laser energy is required in hyperopic PRK to ablate the equivalent amount of corneal stroma as compared to myopic PRK. For example, to correct 2 D hypermetropic error amount of laser spots require to ablate cornea are equivalent to the spot require to correct 6 D myopic error.
- Increased amount of laser ablation increase the chances of corneal dehydration and centration.

Centration of optical zone is an important step in hypermetropic PRK, hence proper patient alignment and target fixation is must. In hypermetropic PRK the epithelial healing is also delayed because of

- Large size epithelial defect is created.
- Longer duration of photoablation is required
- More amount of laser energy is delivered

Postoperative treatment and complications of hypermetropic PRK are similar as that of myopic PRK (discussed on page 474–477).

Hypermetropic LASIK: Principles and surgical technique of hypermetropic LASIK is same as that of described for myopic LASIK on page no 479–482. A refractive error of +1 to +8 D can be corrected by this method.

Hypermetropic epi-LASIK: Prerequisite and surgical steps of this technique are same as that of described in myopic epi-LASIK on page 487–488. Epi-LASIK for correction of hypermetropia (especially, moderate to high degree error) is preferred to PRK or LASIK due to several advantages as described in myopic epi-LASIK on page 488.

Hypermetropic LASEK: This procedure has its specific advantages over LASIK and can correct high degree of refractive error. Basic principle and surgical steps of hyperopic LASEK are same as that of myopic LASEK (described on page 486–488).

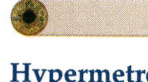

Hypermetropic C-LASIK: Most recent procedure to correct moderate to high degree of hypermetropia is customized LASIK. It has an edge over conventional LASIK in terms of visual outcome and postoperative comfort to patient. Basic principle and surgical steps of hyperopic C-LASIK are same as that of myopic C-LASIK (described on page 488–489).

Corneal Stromal Collagen Shrinking Procedures

Principle: Anterior curvature of cornea can be altered using various energies like thermal (heat) energy, radiofrequency energy or laser energy which cause shrinkage of the corneal stromal collagen structure. This change in the anterior corneal curvature will cause the correction of refractive error.

Correction of hypermetropia or presbyopia can be done by various procedures based on this principle and can be grouped as

- Thermal keratoplasty
- Conductive keratoplasty

Thermal Keratoplasty (TK)

In the year 1898, Lans applied thermal energy on the cornea through heat or thermal cautery for correction of astigmatism. The exposure to heat caused change in the curvature of anterior cornea due to the shrinkage of corneal stromal collagen, which corrected the refractive error. Later on, thermal energy was delivered using a radiofrequency probe instead of heat cautery. This procedure is termed thermal keratoplasty, however, with use of simple heat cautery or probe the control of thermal energy delivery was difficult, hence this original nonlaser thermal keratoplasty procedure was widely abandoned because of these reasons

- Poor predictability of refractive outcome
- Corneal scarring
- Delayed epithelial healing
- Stromal necrosis
- Corneal vascularization

After the invention of lasers this procedure again gained some attention because of better control over the delivery of thermal energy to cornea by use of laser energy. A wide range of anterior corneal curvature changes can be brought by using several treatment parameters like laser wavelength, pulse duration, pulse energy, number of laser spots, pattern of spots, and size of laser spots. Originally, Holmium: YAG laser was used to deliver the thermal energy and this procedure is termed laser thermal keratoplasty (LTK). Ho: YAG laser penetrates cornea up to depth of about 480–520 µm which is considered perfect depth range to provide heat to stroma without causing damage to adjoining tissue. In addition, Thermal footprint produced by laser is conical shape (whereas, a hot needle produces cylindrical thermal profile). As compared to cylindrical thermal profile, these conical shape profiles or footprints produces shrinkage of stromal collagen more in the anterior stroma than posterior stroma, hence better correction in refractive error is achieved with long lasting results.

Mainly two types of laser delivery systems are studied widely

- Contact probe LTK
- Non-contact type LTK

These two types of system delivers different amount of temperature, spot size, space distribution and time of laser delivery.

Contact laser thermal keratoplasty: In this type of delivery system a sapphire probe is used to deliver the thermal energy at an angle of 120°. The solid state infrared range laser of 2060 nm wavelength at 0.3 millisec pulse rate is emitted as electromagnetic radiations by this probe to treat about 700 µm diameter spot size corneal area at 450 µm depth.

Surgical technique

- Procedure is performed under topical anesthesia after cleaning and draping the eye similar to other refractive procedures.
- Under topical anesthesia along with 1% pilocarpine the cornea is marked with a

specifically designed marker to denote the probe placement.

- Then probe is placed perpendicular to corneal surface and typically eight to sixteen spots are applied in peripheral cornea either in single ring or double ring pattern. After procedure, remove the coagulated epithelium with a cotton tip applicator.
- Postoperative management is similar to other refractive procedures.

Non-contact thermal keratoplasty: In this type of delivery system the slit-lamp is used to deliver the laser energy to cornea. Ho: YAG laser of 2130 nm wavelength at 0.25 millisec pulse rate is emitted by a slit-lamp laser delivery system to create a spot size of 600 µm having nearly 90% of energy per spot.

Surgical technique

- Before starting the procedure topical anesthesia is administered 4–5 times in each eye at 5 minutes intervals and then patient is made to sit on laser delivery slit-lamp system.
- Patient is instructed to focus the fixation red light source and a self-retaining lid speculum is applied to keep the eyes wide open.
- Corneal surface is dried either by waiting for 5–10 minutes or using a moist cellulose sponge because corneal hydration plays an

important role in Ho: YAG laser tissue interaction effects.

- Once the corneal surface is ready for laser then either 8 or 16 treatment spots are applied in single or double ring patterns as shown in Fig. 15.19. Diameter of treatment spot ring can be in the range of 4–8 mm depending upon the type and amount of refractive error correction required. Double ring pattern can be either staggered or radial as shown in Fig. 15.19B, C.
- Postoperative treatment includes topical antibiotics and anti-inflammatory drops 4–6 times a day for one to two weeks duration.

In both these methods the laser treatment causes the thermal contraction of stromal collagen matrix, which in turn creates a constriction band in peripheral cornea. This peripheral constrictive band causes the steepening of central cornea and hence the correction of hypermetropia.

Several studies on laser thermal keratoplasty have been done for correction of hypermetropia and astigmatism. Majority of these studies concluded that LTK is useful in correction of low to moderate degree (range of 1–4 D) of hypermetropia and is an effective alternative in conditions like monovision induction or to improvise the overcorrected LASIK/PRK patients. LTK is very economical and has low maintenance cost, hence it is an

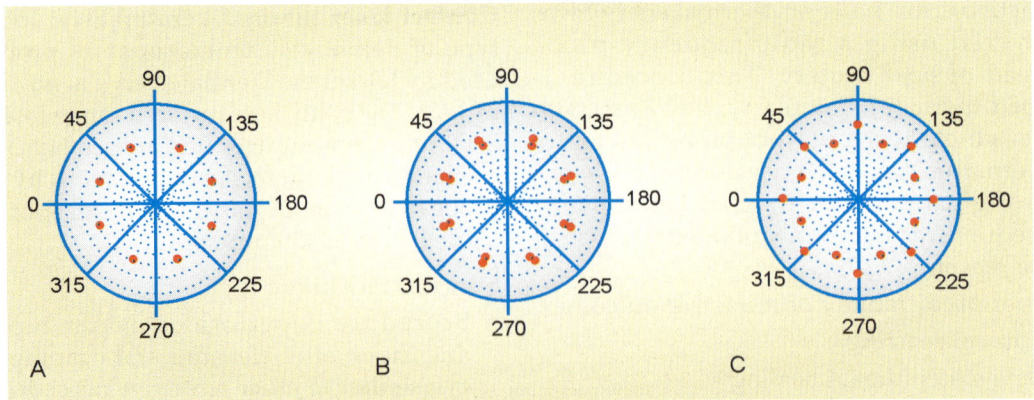

Fig. 15.19: Laser thermal keratoplasty ablation patterns. A. Single ring pattern; B. Double ring radial pattern; C. Double ring staggered pattern

effective way to treat hypermetropia. Several studies also concluded that nearly one-third of the total patients in presbyopic age group corrected by LTK retained functional near vision with hyperopic correction. No significant postoperative complications have been reported after LTK.

Conductive Keratoplasty

In an approach to develop a procedure having combined advantages of theromkeratoplasty and uniform heat application to corneal stroma with better predictable outcome, Mendez and colleagues introduced a non-laser refractive procedure for correction of hypermetropia and presbyopia, called conductive keratoplasty (CK). In place of laser, radiofrequency energy is used to reshape and steepen the cornea in conductive keratoplasty. In CK, current of low energy and high frequency (350 kHz) is given to heat the corneal collagen tissue in the periphery which results in shrinking of peripheral and paracentral stromal collagen. This shrinking results in flattening of cornea in the periphery and steepening in the central part. Thus hypermetropia and/or presbyopia is corrected by this method.

Indications: CK is preferred in patients of hypermetropia with age more than 40 years with a stable refractive error as more benefits are seen with CK in this age group than younger patients.

- Hypermetropia of +1 D to +3.5 D, with or without astigmatism of up to +1 D.
- Presbyopia

CK equipment: Primarily CK system consists of following components

- CK console: This is a radiofrequency energy generating device.
- CK Hand piece (probe) this is a pen shaped reusable part which is attached to console system with a removable cable and connector.
- Keratoplast tip this is a disposable stainless steel needle attached to probe. Needle length is 450 μm and diameter is 90 μm. It delivers radiofrequency energy directly to cornea and has a cuff, which ensures the correct depth of delivery.
- Foot pedal to control the release of radio-frequency energy.

Preoperative assessment
- Near and distance vision
- Refraction for far and near
- Keratometry
- Corneal topography to rule out keratoconus or other irregularities
- Pachymetry
- Anterior segment examination by slit lamp
- Monovision tolerance assessment using contact lenses

Procedure of CK: CK is done under operating microscope as following steps
- Topical anesthesia using xylocaine or proparacaine drops.
- Self-retaining lid speculum is applied for adequate corneal exposure and also to serve as ground electrode.
- Corneal marking is done using a corneal marker dipped in gentian violet ink. Marker is placed exactly in center of cornea to avoid any postprocedure astigmatism.
- Delivery of radiofrequency energy is done by keratoplasty tip insertion at defined spots in a ring pattern marked over cornea as per nomogram as shown in Fig. 15.20.

Nomogram in CK: Important points to be remembered during delivery of radiofre-quency energy are
- Keep keratoplast tip exactly perpendicular to corneal surface to get full depth penetra-tion of energy.
- Avoid high touch, i.e. more pressure on cornea during procedure, use light touch technique, i.e. minimum pressure while delivering the energy to form a spot size of 0.5–1 mm.
- Smooth and even size spots are applied using 350 kHz with 60% power.
- 0.6 seconds treatment time is required per spot.

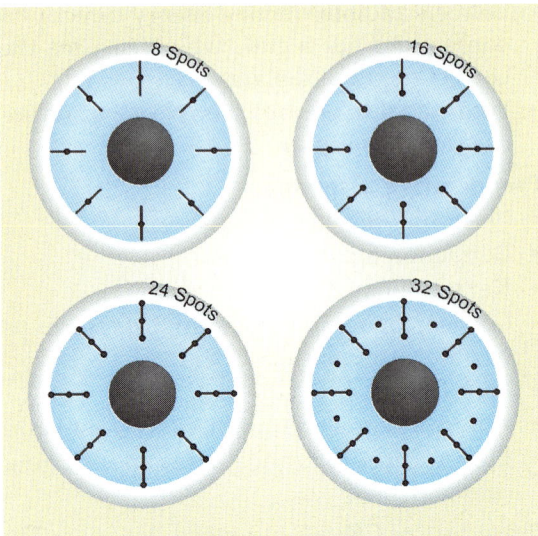

Fig. 15.20: Nomogram for conductive keratoplasty

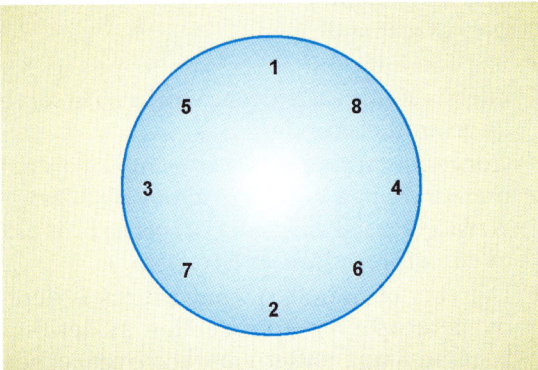

Fig. 15.21: Spots placement order in conductive keratoplasty

- Start treatment from 12 o'clock position and move as per sequence shown in Fig. 15. 21.
- Second and third ring treatment spots are applied in relation to first ring in such a pattern that they do not touch each other.
- Number of treatment spots is dependent on the amount of error needed to be corrected. Number and placement of treatment spots

Note: Shape of CK footprint is cylindrical, whereas after LTK it is conical. Footprint is nearly up to 80% depth of cornea because corneal tissue receives same temperature from surface till bottom. Visual recovery is seen after one week time.

require with respective spherical correction is summarized in Table 15.20.

Postoperative management
- Topical antibiotic/anti-inflammatory eye drops 3–4 times per day for one week.
- Lubricating eye drops 4–6 times per day for 4–6 weeks.
- Follow up is done after CK on
  - One day
  - One week
  - Three weeks
  - Six weeks
  - Three months

Various advantages and disadvantages of CK are summarized in Table 15.21.

REFRACTIVE PROCEDURE FOR ASTIGMATISM

Various surgical techniques have been developed for correction of simple astigmatic error or compound astigmatic error in association with spherical refractive errors or high degree astigmatic error associated with post-penetrating keratoplasty. These astigmatic corneal refractive procedures can be grouped as shown in Table 15.22.

Relaxing Incisions

Astigmatic refractive error is quite common and is usually treated with spherical refractive error through various laser based or lens based corrective procedures. Astigmatism correction based on corneal relaxation principle is performed with limbal relaxing incisions and astigmatic keratotomy. Basic principle of correction in both the procedure is same. According to the depth of cornea two or more peripheral corneal incisions (transverse or arcuate shape) are created perpendicular to the steepest meridian. Once these incisions heal due to biomechanical characteristic of cornea the steeper meridian becomes flat and the flatter meridian becomes steep, hence the astigmatic error gets corrected. The effect of incision is directly related to the position (distance from the central cornea), length and depth of incision.

Table 15.20: Number of treatment spots required in relation to spherical equivalent correction of error

Spherical equivalent (D) correction	Number of treatment spots			
	First ring (6 mm)	Second ring (7 mm)	Third ring (8 mm)	Total spots
0.75–0.875	–	8	–	8
1.0–1.625	8	8	–	16
1.75–2.25	8	8	8	24
2.375–3.0	8	16	8	32

Table 15.21: Advantages and disadvantages of conductive keratoplasty

Advantages	Disadvantages
Safe and effective in hypermetropia and presbyopia	Ineffective in high degree (>4 D hyperopia and 1 D astigmatism) refractive error
Minimal invasive technique	Not reversible
Stereopsis or depth perception remains maintained	Regression can occur at rate of 1 D per 2–3 years duration. Hence repetition of procedure may be required every 2–3 years time period
BCVA is improved after procedure	Complications rarely seen are
	• Corneal perforation
Contrast sensitivity remains maintained	• Corneal erosions
	• Iritis
	• Decreased BCVA

Table 15.22: Various refractive surgeries for correction of astigmatism

Simple and compound astigmatic errors		Post-penetrating keratoplasty induced astigmatism
Relaxing incisions	**Laser based surgery**	Suture removal
Limbal relaxing incision	Astigmatic PRK	Relaxing incisions
Corneal relaxing incisions (Astigmatic keratotomy)	Astigmatic epi-LASIK	Relaxing incisions with compressing sutures
	Astigmatic LASIK	Corneal wedge resection
	Astigmatic C-LASIK	Ruiz procedure
		Astigmatic LASIK

Limbal relaxing incision: Astigmatic error of more than 0.5 dioptre can be appreciated by sensitive patients and may influence optical quality of vision in these patients. Low degree residual astigmatism (0.5–2.5 dioptre) after cataract surgery or refractive lens exchange or phakic IOLs (without toric lenses) can be corrected by limbal relaxing incisions (LRI). This procedure can be performed along with cataract surgery for an effective correction. As these incisions are peripherally placed and heals very fast their influence on the visual acuity and optical quality of cornea is minimal. Thus, LRI is the primary indications for low degree astigmatic error correction.

Corneal relaxing incisions (astigmatic keratotomy): The concept of astigmatic keratotomy (AK) was introduced by Lans in 1898. This procedure is similar to limbal relaxing incision, however, it is used to correct high degree astigmatic errors (3–8 dioptres) which may appear following penetrating keratoplasty or post-cataract. In this method to correct high degree astigmatism the incisions are given on the cornea. Basic principle of this procedure is same as described above.

In AK two or more transverse or arcuate shape incisions of predetermined depth and length are given on corneal mid-periphery region perpendicular to the steepest meridian as shown in Fig. 15.22. The incision on the steep meridian will lead to flattening of that meridian while steepening of unincised (flat) meridian 90 degree away (called coupling effect). Incisions short in length cause more flattening of steeper meridian than steepening of unincised meridian (coupling ratio >1). Generally the transverse incisions of 3–5 mm and arcuate incisions of 30–90° causes coupling ratio of one. Too deep or too long incisions must be avoided as there are increased chances of globe perforation, induction of irregular astigmatic error and overcorrection of astigmatic error in post-surgical period.

Surgical method: Corneal incisions are made depending on the amount and type (with the rule, against the rule or oblique) of astigmatism using a diamond knife, as per the existing nomogram for relaxing incision. Alternately, laser can be used to make incisions in more précised way with accurate length and depth of incisions. On an average in case of 'with the rule' type astigmatic error (up to 2 dioptre) two incisions are given, whereas for same amount of error only one incision is given in the case of 'against the rule' or oblique astigmatism. These incisions are ideally made in 2.5–3.5 mm radius around the pupillary center or the center of cornea as shown in Fig. 15.22.

Two types of incisions can be given in AK

- Transverse (T-cut) incisions: Usually, two incisions of 3 mm length are given as a pair on the steepest meridian on mid-peripheral cornea as shown in Fig. 15.23A. In specific cases to increase the effect of incisions, sometimes another pair of incision is added in the same meridian adjacent to previous incisions as shown in Fig. 15.23B. As the length of these transverse incisions increased their flattening effect decreases because these transverse incisions are made tangentially to optical zone of cornea. Incisions which are deeper, longer and more centrally located will produce greater effect.

- Arcuate incisions: Usually these incisions are made at a fixed distance from pupil center at any length in an arcuate shape in pair as shown in Fig. 15.24. For any length or any given optical zone size these arcuate

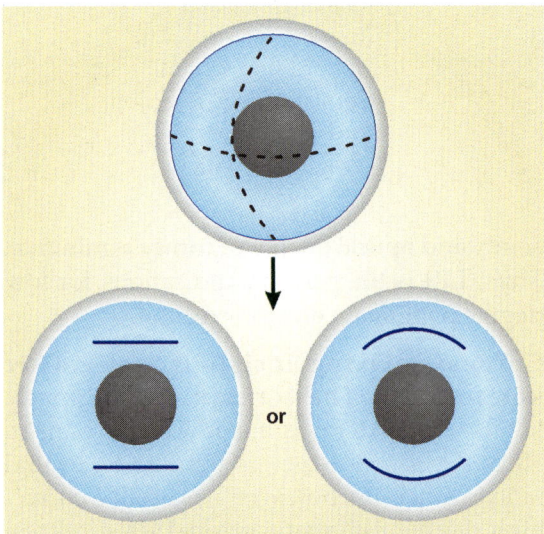

Fig. 15.22: Incisions made in astigmatic keratectomy procedure

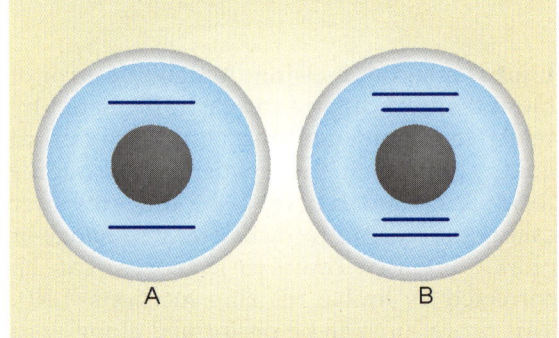

Fig. 15.23: Transverse (T-cut) incisions in astigmatic keratectomy. A. Single pair incisions; B. Double pair incisions

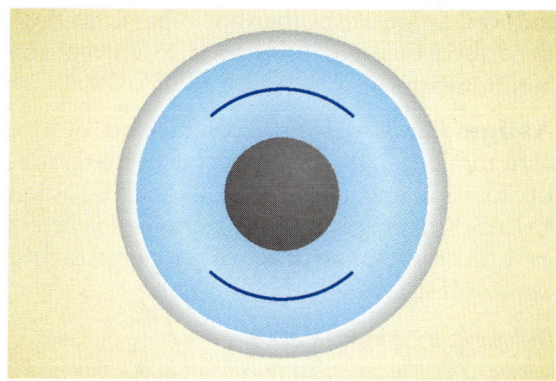

Fig. 15.24: Arcuate incisions in astigmatic keratectomy

incisions are more effective as compared to transverse incisions. The reason is that with increasing the length of incision (maximum up to 90°), flattening effect of arcuate incision increases.

Laser-based Surgery

Astigmatic PRK: Astigmatic photorefractive keratotomy (PRK) is similar to photoablation procedure (describe on page 472–474) done for correction of spherical errors like myopia or hyperopia except that the ablation pattern created by laser in astigmatic PRK is cylindrical, not spherical as done in myopia as shown in Fig. 15.25. If patient has combined

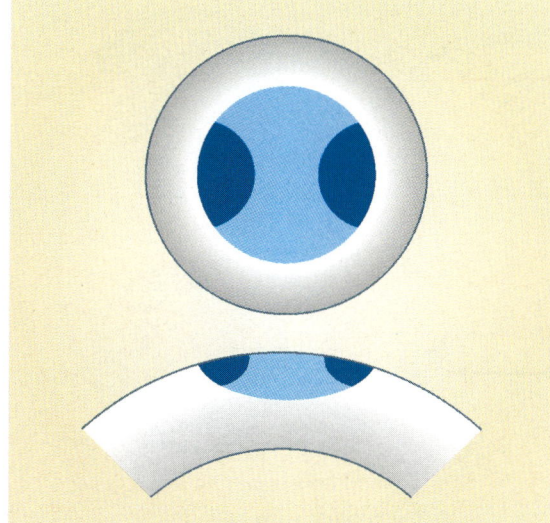

Fig. 15.25: Photoastigmatic refractive keratectomy

refractive error of myopia and astigmatism, then an elliptical ablation pattern is used to correct both these errors together. Marking of astigmatic axis on patient's cornea must be done while patient is in sitting position because in lying down position the axis mark will shift from the original position.

Astigmatic epi-LASIK: Astigmatic epi-LASIK procedure is similar to the epi-LASIK procedure described in detail on page 487–488. This procedure is a better choice for correction of moderate to high degree astigmatism as compare to PRK because of the advantages as described on page 488.

Astigmatic LASIK: Astigmatic LASIK is a similar procedure to conventional LASIK as described on page 477–480 , except in terms of laser ablation pattern. Astigmatic LASIK can effectively correct an astigmatic error in the range of 2–10 D with minimal complications. This procedure has an edge over PRK in terms of visual outcome and safety.

Astigmatic C-LASIK: Currently, astigmatic C-LASIK especially, wavefront guided is considered as first choice refractive procedure for correction of moderate to high degree astigmatism with negligible complications and satisfactory visual results. Technique of C-LASIK is same as described on page 488–489.

Postpenetrating Keratoplasty (PK)-induced Astigmatism

High degree of astigmatism (5–30 D) may be induced after penetrating keratoplasty. Various methods advocated to manage this astigmatism are:

Suture Removal

Suture removal is the most effective, easiest and fastest way to correct the astigmatism induced due to penetrating keratoplasty. This can be done as follows

• Examination of central and peripheral portion of the corneal graft and measurement of central corneal graft curvature is done by using keratoscope and keratometer, respectively. These parameters will help the examiner to decide exactly which suture should be removed to correct the astigmatism. Keratoscopic mires become closer and exhibit a 'V' pattern indentation near a tight suture as shown in Fig. 15.26A. Alternately, in case having no induced astigmatism, no such indentation pattern will be seen on keratoscopy as shown in Fig. 15.26B.

- Once the indentation pattern is seen and suture is identified by the examiner, removal of selected sutures present in most steep meridian will correct both the regular and the irregular type of astigmatism.
- Depending on the degree of induced astigmatism usually in case of interrupted sutures surgeon can remove the selected suture after 3 months duration of surgery. Whereas, in case of continuous sutures, the selected sutures are ideally removed after one year duration of surgery.

Penetrating keratoplasty induced astigmatism is initially corrected by suture removal technique only. However, once all the sutures are removed and patient has a stable refractive status with a significant amount of residual-induced astigmatism, then any other procedure described below can be tried to correct the astigmatism.

Astigmatic LASIK: As discussed before astigmatic LASIK can correct astigmatism of up to 10 D and currently wavefront guided C-LASIK is the procedure of choice to correct astigmatism produced after penetrating keratoplasty.

Relaxing Incisions Post PK

- As described earlier the arcuate relaxing incisions are given on the steepest meridian to correct the astigmatism. Normally, a pair of arcuate incision about half millimeter inside the donor graft junction is given on the donor cornea. These relaxing incisions can correct astigmatism in the range of 2.5 to 8 dioptres.
- Under topical anesthesia these arcuate incisions are created with a diamond knife or femtosecond laser beam as described on page 466. Pair of arcuate incision (180° apart) are made deep up to 70–75% of corneal thickness. Length of incisions can be extended in a range of 60° to 100° according to the degree of astigmatism.

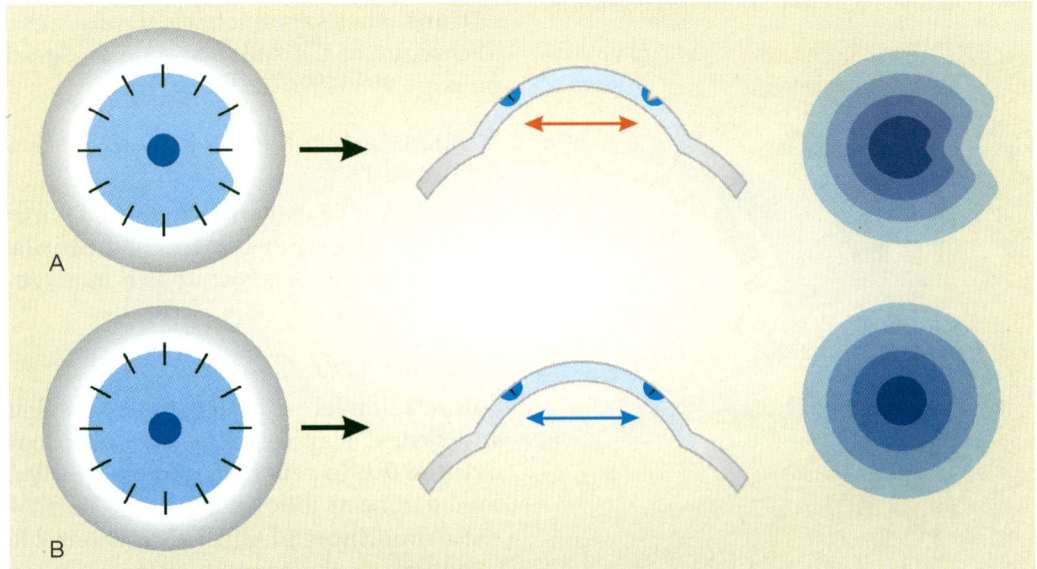

Fig. 15.26: Post-penetrating keratoplasty astigmatism

Relaxing incisions with compression sutures

- High degree astigmatism (6 to 15 dioptres) can be corrected by applying compression sutures along with relaxing incisions.
- Relaxing incisions are given on the cornea at desired angle in a manner explained above. Two or three interrupted suture by 10–0 nylon suture are given on each side at graft-host junction, perpendicular to the steepest meridian as shown in Fig. 15.27.

Corneal Wedge Resection

For very high degree astigmatism (16 to 25 D) before attempting a repeat penetrating keratoplasty, corneal wedge resection or Ruiz procedure can be tried to correct the residual astigmatism.

- Retrobulbar or peribulbar anesthesia is given and under complete aseptic precautions corneal wedge is removed from the recipient cornea.
- Usually a 1–1.5 mm wide base and approximately 90° in extent from the flattest meridian of recipient cornea is selected near host graft junction as shown in Fig. 15.28A.
- Using fine microsurgical blade the selected corneal wedge is removed from the donor cornea as shown in Fig. 15.28B.

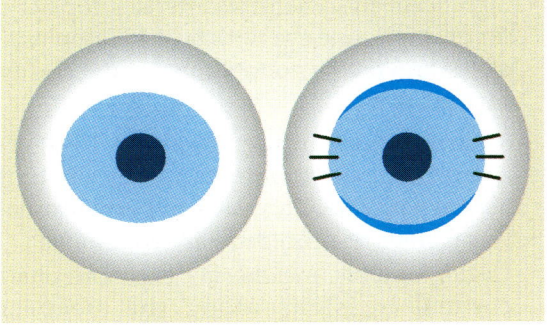

Fig. 15.27: Relaxing incisions with compressing sutures

- Then about six to seven interrupted compressing sutures by 10–0 nylon or prolene are applied to close the gap as shown in Fig. 15.28C.
- These compression sutures should be applied tight enough to attain an over correction by nearly 1/3 amount of the present astigmatism.

Ruiz Procedure (Trapezoidal Keratotomy)

Ruiz procedure is performed in the following cases such as

- Failure of wedge resection
- Highly equivalent spherical myopic refractive error

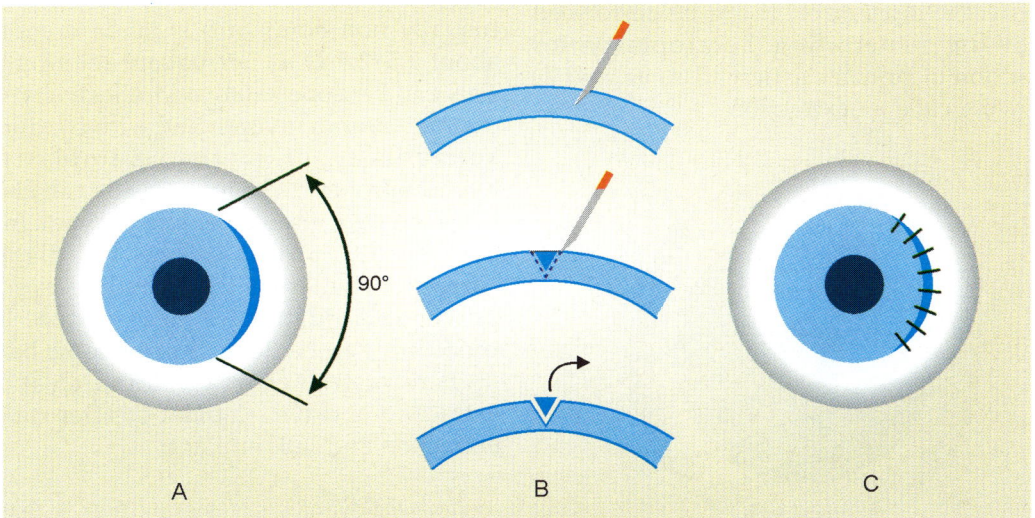

Fig. 15.28: Corneal wedge resection. A. Corneal wedge selection; B. Removal of corneal wedge; C. Interrupted compressing sutures

- Significant anisometropia after keratoplasty, for example, one eye with post-keratoplasty status and fellow nonoperated eye is highly myopic eye.

Ruiz procedure can correct about 10–12 D astigmatism with simultaneous shift in spherical equivalent towards hypermetropia. Surgical steps of procedure are as follows

- Under suitable anesthesia deep horizontal corneal incisions along the steepest meridian are made by using a guarded diamond knife, in a step ladder manner as shown in Fig. 15.29.
- Two sets of horizontal (transverse) corneal incisions (keratotomy) are performed opposite to each other. The depth of incisions must be 80% of corneal thickness.
- Each set of horizontal keratotomy are bordered by two radial incisions in such a manner that they do not cross with the horizontal incisions.
- Cross connection of horizontal and radial incisions can result in wound gaping, delayed wound healing, and epithelial microcystic dystrophy.

Results of Ruiz procedure are significantly variable though it can correct penetrating keratoplasty induced astigmatism along with spherical myopic error. It can be performed following penetrating keratoplasty for correction of primary astigmatism as well as following cataract extraction.

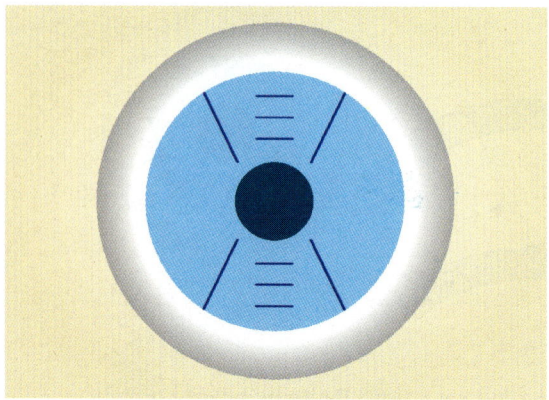

Fig. 15.29: Ruiz procedure

Note: After penetrating keratoplasty when corneal wedge resection and/or Ruiz procedure get fail to correct the residual induced astigmatism, a repeat penetrating keratoplasty should be performed.

Modified Ruiz procedure (rectangular incision pattern) has also been described where the radial incisions are made perpendicular to the horizontal incisions. This modification helped to obtain full correction of astigmatism band in the periphery.

REFRACTIVE PROCEDURE FOR PRESBYOPIA

Presbyopia is not a refractive error rather it is an ageing process which ultimately affects every individual. Presbyopia usually happen around 40–42 years of age and many people consider it a sign of old age, hence resist wearing of bifocal or progressive spectacles. A large number of people do not want to wear glasses or due to professional reasons wants correction of presbyopia by surgical procedures. Various procedures to correct presbyopia by surgical means are summarized in Table 15.23.

Corneal Procedures

Monovision procedure: Monovision simply means one eye (usually dominant) is fully corrected (made emmetropic) and fellow eye (usually non-dominant) is made myopic of about 1.5–2.5 D as per patient requirement. This can be done safely and effectively with excimer laser in myopes and with conductive keratoplasty or thermokeratoplasty in hypermetropes. Even monovision can also be achieved with intraocular lens implant. In one eye the IOL power is kept for distance correction, whereas in the fellow eye IOL power is adjusted for near vision. This procedure can be done in presbyopic having high refractive error by doing clear lens extraction and IOL implant or after cataract extraction and IOL implant.

Note: Disadvantage of monovision is that an intermediate distance vision usually remains uncorrected.

Table 15.23: Classification of various presbyopia corrective surgeries		
Corneal procedure	*Lens-based procedures*	*Sclera-based procedures*
Monovision procedure	Multifocal Intraocular Lenses	Anterior ciliary sclerotomy
Laser procedures	Accommodative IOLs	Sclera spacing procedures
Corneal implants	Refractive lens exchange	Sclera expansion with laser

Laser procedures: Excimer laser can also be used for correction of presbyopia similar to refractive errors.

- Laser thermal keratoplasty can be done but CK is more preferred than laser thermal keratoplasty.
- Monovision LASIK can be performed. In this method, one eye is corrected for distance vision and the other eye for near vision with the help of epi-LASIK or C-LASIK.
- Presbyopic bifocal LASIK this is also called as LASIK-PARM (presbyopia by Avalos Rozakis Method). In this method, instead of one zone as created with routine LASIK two concentric ablation zones are created on the cornea. This changes the shape of cornea at two places, which enable the patient to have distance vision from one zone and near vision from another zone. Surgical steps of this laser are as follows

  – Cornea is anesthetized using topical anesthesia.
  – Under aseptic precautions hinged corneal flap of size 8.5 to 9.5 mm is made.
  – Hyperopic ablation of cornea is performed to make it steeper centrally (prolate shape) which will facilitate for near vision.
  – Myopic ablation of cornea is performed over central 4 mm zone to make cornea flatter centrally (oblate shape) which will facilitate the distance vision.
  – At the end of laser, cornea is of oblate shape or flatter in center for distance vision and a surrounding ring of prolate shape or steeper periphery for near vision.
  – Repositioning of corneal flap is done as described on page 481.

- Multifocal excimer laser: Most recent and effective treatment to correct presbyopic myopes, hypermetropes, or emmetropes is multifocal LASIK. In this method a multifocal cornea is created by giving multistep, independently calculated, ablation zones using flying spot excimer laser. Surgical steps are as follows

  – Cornea is anesthetized by topical anesthesia.
  – Under aseptic precautions hinged corneal flap of size 8.5 to 9.5 mm is made.
  – In next step, central multifocal LASIK is performed where central ablation of cornea for correction of distance refractive errors is done.
  – Peripheral multifocal LASIK is the last step where multiple paracentral ablations in several optical zones of cornea are done to correct the near and intermediate vision defects.

Corneal implants or inlay: Various implants to correct presbyopia were tried in past but failed due to several disadvantages. Recently after the development of microkeratomes, femtosecond laser and better biosynthetic material this idea of presbyopic implants has revived. A few examples are

- **Kamra inlay (AcuFocus):** This implant is a polyvinylidene fluoride material ring which has an outer diameter (3.8 mm) and inner or central opening of 1.6 mm, with a thickness of 10 μm. This is implanted uniocularly (non-dominant eye) under a corneal flap as created in LASIK. The central opening of inlay is positioned in such a way that it remains in front of the pupil of eye and produces a 'pinhole camera' effect, thus increases depth of focus. It is first corneal inlay which has been approved by FDA in 2015.

- **PresbyLens (raindrop near vision inlay):** This is a hydrogel material implant having 1.5 mm diameter with an edge thickness of 10 μm, which progressively increases up to 24–40 μm towards center. This implant is similarly placed in non-dominant eye after creating a corneal flap by LASIK. This implant alters the curvature of cornea. It was approved by FDA in 2016 for presbyopia.

- **SDICL:** Recently, an intracorneal inlay lens of small diameter has been produced for correction of presbyopia. This lens is inserted in a intrastromal pocket created via a 3–4 mm circumferential corneal incision made in periphery as shown in Fig. 15.30. No suture is required to close the incision.

Main advantage of these implants is that they can be removed if not tolerated or if a cataract surgery has to be done in later stage.

Lens-based Procedures

Multifocal intraocular lenses: These lenses can be implanted either after cataract surgery or refractive lens exchange procedure. Mainly two types of lenses are present: Refractive and diffractive multifocal lenses.

- **Refractive multifocal IOLs:** These IOLs have two or more ring-shaped spherical zones of different refractive powers as shown in Fig. 15.31. Near power zone is usually situated in the central portion of

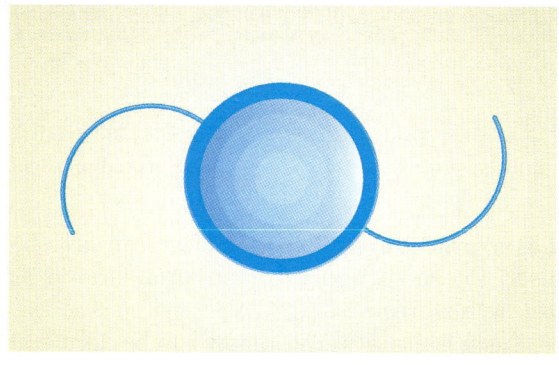

Fig. 15.31: Refractive multifocal intraocular lens

lens optic. The effectiveness of these IOLs depends on the surgical centration of lens and size of patient's pupil.

- **Diffractive IOLs:** These IOLs have two focus points, one point for near and another for distance vision. There are diffractive concentric rings on anterior and posterior surface of IOL optic to diffract the incoming light rays and focus them either to near or distance focal point of IOL as shown in Fig. 15.32. The effectiveness of this type of IOL is independent to surgical centration and patient's pupil size.

Accommodative IOLs: These IOLs are designed in such a way that movement of ciliary muscle is transformed into an ocular dynamic change in terms of dioptric power.

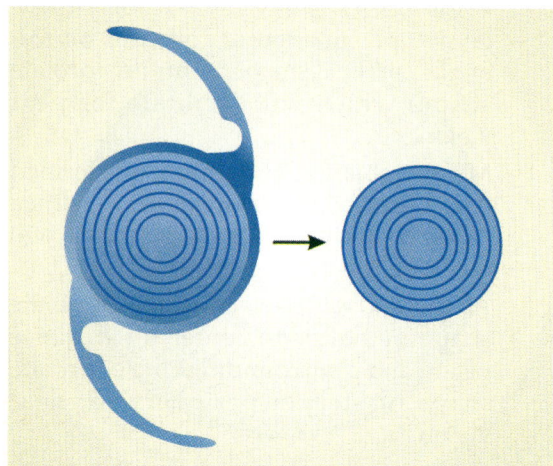

Fig. 15.32: Diffractive intraocular lens

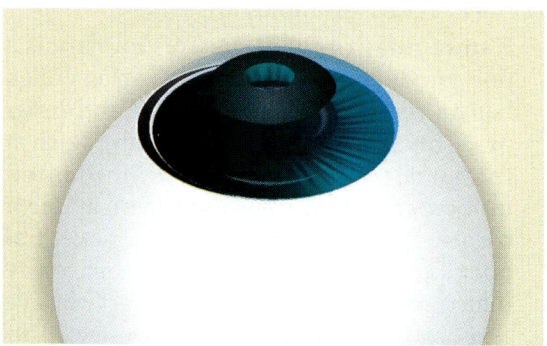

Fig. 15.30: Small diameter intracorneal implant

Presently available accommodative IOL designs are

- *Humanoptic 1CU:* It is a single piece IOL made up of hydrophilic acrylate material and has four wide haptics with a flexible haptic-optic junction as shown in Fig. 15.33. Optic is 5.5 mm in diameter and haptics is 9.8 mm in width. These haptics are so designed that they get compressed by capsular bag with accommodation and move the optic forwards.

- *AT-45 Crysta lens:* This IOL has an optic of high refractive silicon material with a modified plate haptic design. Optic is of 5.0 mm diameter with a groove at optic haptic junction. There is a pair of arch-shaped stabilizing polymide haptic at the end of each plate haptic as shown in Fig. 15.34. This mechanism helps in moving the lens forward when a pressure gradient is generated between vitreous cavity and anterior segment during accommodation due to ciliary muscle movement.

- *Visogen synchrony:* This IOL design has two optics, i.e. the anterior is convex with 32 D power and other with posterior concave optic. These two optics are connected by a spring mechanism. During accommodation process the anterior optic moves inside the capsular bag and posterior optic remains constant.

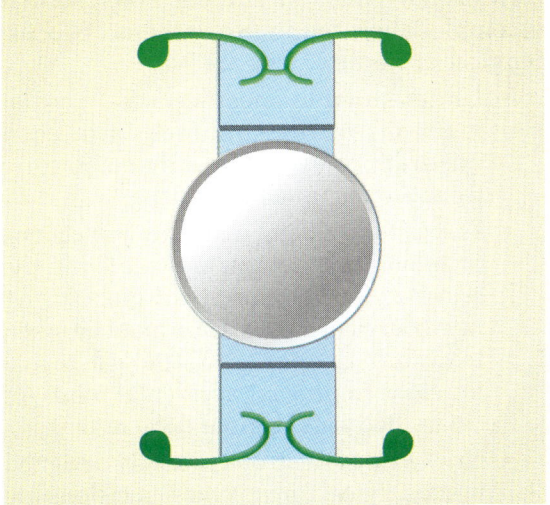

Fig. 15.34: AT-45 intraocular lens

Refractive lens exchange: Rarely, to correct presbyopia in emmetropes the clear lens extraction with IOL implantation is done. However, in cases having high degree refractive errors clear crystalline extraction with multifocal IOL implantation can be done at presbyopic age. Detailed surgical procedure with associated complication is explained on page 492–493.

Scleral Based Procedures

Anterior ciliary sclerotomy: Various accommodation theories assumes that

- Outward movement of equator of crystalline lens during near accommodation causes increase in the diameter of lens.
- In ageing process due to natural lenticular growth, the equatorial diameter of crystalline lens increases.
- Decreased space between lens equator and ciliary body resists the outward movement of crystalline lens during near accommodation, hence causes presbyopia.

Aim is to increase the space between lens equator and ciliary body, hence an anterior ciliary sclerotomy has been tried to stretch and enlarge the eyeball with variable results. This procedure is performed to facilitate extra space for ciliary muscle to contract and force

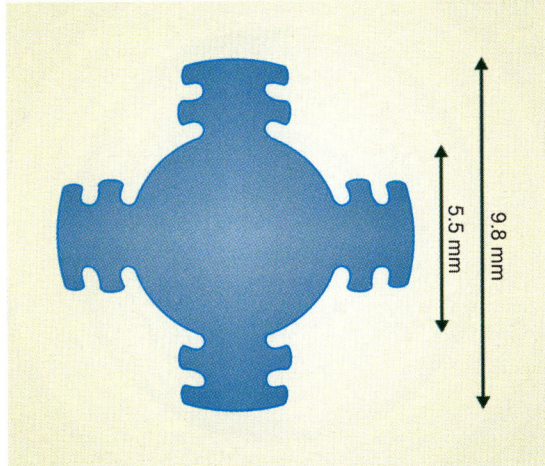

Fig. 15.33: Humanoptic 1CU intraocular lens

forward movement of vitreous body, so that accommodation can improve the near focus. Surgical procedure steps are

- Under suitable anesthesia four radial incisions in the conjunctiva in each quadrant of eyeball are made starting from limbus up to pars plana.
- Then about 600 μm deep radial incisions of about 3 mm length are created in the sclera in four quadrants of globe using microsurgical blades. Care must be taken to avoid deeper and too posterior incisions to prevent accidental injury of ciliary body and retinal detachment.
- Now with the help of a specially designed microsurgical forceps these incisions are separated very minimally to create desired scleral space. Be careful about globe perforation or ciliary body injury.
- No sutures applied for scleral incision but conjunctiva is cauterized to avoid ocular infections.

In spite of good initial surgical outcome in majority of cases the incisional wound regress and space gets decreased. So to maintain the space, silicon expander plugs are used to be placed in incision wounds. Normally, silicon expander of 0.6 mm width and 2.5 mm length are used based on the estimated dimensions of incisional wound and expected circumferential expansion of globe.

Majority of studies reported that presbyopic correction of moderate degree can be achieved by anterior ciliary sclerotomy. Postoperative complications include subconjunctival hemorrhage, photophobia, and ocular irritation.

Sclera spacing procedures: As discussed above to correct presbyopia various scleral implants have been tried to increase the circumferential space of globe. PMMA segments scleral implants commonly available as PresView implants are used to increase the scleral space. Posterior scleral tunnels are made in four scleral quadrants. PMMA segments are implanted over ciliary body in these sclera tunnels in four quadrants by using an automatic microsurgical instrument. Results of this procedure are yet to be expected.

Scleral expansion with laser: This is an advancement of anterior ciliary sclerotomy where partial thickness radial incisions are made on sclera over ciliary body region to increase the circumferential space by using Erbium: YAG laser instead of a routine microsurgical blade. This facilitates the outward movement of crystalline lens to provide increased focal power and focal depth during accommodation. This procedure is in experimental stages with variable outcome.

Low Vision

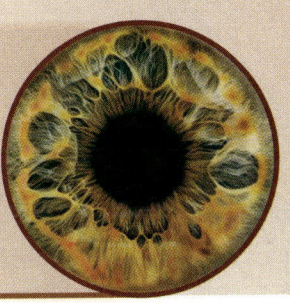

LOW VISION EVALUATION

Introduction

Low vision can simply be considered as the poor utilization of eyes or visual system. Various similar terms like visual impairment, visual disability or visual handicap are explained in relation to low vision, however, low vision never implies visual blindness. Low vision person can present with functional ocular defects like poor distance and/or near visual acuity, suppressed visual fields, decreased contrast sensitivity and excessive glare. Low vision symptoms also include distortion of image, diplopia or difficulty in visual perceptions. Visual impairment can cause significant visual disability which in turn restricts the daily routine activity of an individual and also hampers his/her ability to carry out any work independently.

Thus, low vision or visual handicap condition confines the personal, economical and social independence of an individual. The person suffering from visual impairment is unable to independently perform several personal and social activities like reading, writing, moving in public transport, identify people or attend social gatherings moreover, these people are economically dependent on relatives or others.

Young children having visual impairment since birth or soon after birth will develop delayed physical and mental milestones, especially in the area of coarse and/or fine motor abilities. Similarly, students suffering from low vision are unable to read books with standard sized font, unable to see blackboard or screen projection or computer. Hence, these students face a huge loss of their educational development. In these cases parents and teachers should be aware about visual abilities of student and they must apply various possible techniques to make best use of the remaining useful functional vision of student.

Visual impairment fundamentally means that the concern person is not blind, although the vision is markedly less as compared to the normal individual and cannot be corrected by regular optical devices, medical or surgical methods. Hence, these patients are best corrected by low vision devices such as large print, image magnifiers and increased illumination.

Several ophthalmological and/or neuro-logical disorders can also lead to a wide range of visual impairment starting from moderate visual loss to total blindness. It means that visual loss is not all of a sudden rather it occurs over a range from poor visual acuity to complete blindness.

Definition and Classification of Low Vision

World Health Organization, International Classification of Impairment, Disabilities, and Handicaps (ICIDH) system, define and classify various vision related conditions as follows

- Visual disorder means an ocular condition regardless of its origin (such as trauma, disease or any anomaly) which can cause a considerable damage to visual structures.
- Visual impairment is any loss or anomaly in an ocular structure causing reduction of physiological or psychological ocular functions such as vision, visual field, contrast sensitivity or color.
- Visual disability means any restriction or inability (due to visual impairment) to perform routine ocular functions. For example, reading, writing, moving around independently or recognize familiar faces.
- Visual handicap is a condition which shows that a person is having an unfavorable status in society resulted from visual impairment and/or visual disabilities.

Visual impairment or low vision can be considered as the functional restriction of visual system caused by visual disorder that can lead to visual disability or visual handicap. For better understanding consider the example of age-related macular degeneration (ARMD). In an individual, ARMD (visual disorder) will lead to decrease visual acuity (visual impairment); which in turn causes inability to read small size font (visual disability), hence, finally a limitation of personal, social and economical independence (visual handicap) will occur.

Note: In a nutshell, low vision is referred as an insufficient amount of vision unable to fulfill the routine requirements of a person.

Worldwide, low vision or visual impairment is classified in different manner, but here we are considering the classification and definitions given by World Health Organization (WHO), International Classification of

Diseases (ICD) categories and Indian National Programme Control of Blindness (NPCB). Various low vision conditions as defined by WHO are summarized in Table 16.1.

- Advantage of these functional definitions is that patients who have vision < 3/60 are included for low vision services, which help these patients to utilize their remaining useful vision to its maximum prospective.
- Functional visual impairment may result in the following conditions such as
  - Inadequate visual resolution
  - Insufficient field of vision
  - Decreased peak contrast sensitivity

Inadequate visual resolution and/or peak contrast sensitivity in high or low illumination causes difficulty in performing routine daily activities.

For several health management purposes and clinical uses ICD is the international standard diagnostic classification body. Diseases and other health-related problems recorded on various types of health and vital records such as death certificates and other health records are mainly classified by ICD. Classification of low vision as per ICD-10 (International

Note: Clinical significance of legal blindness is mainly for legal benefits.

Classification of Diseases) is summarized in Table 16.2.

In India, according to National Programme Control of Blindness (NPCB), definition of visual impairment is as follows

- Low vision refers to a state when an individual has the following conditions
  - Visual acuity not more than 6/18 (20/60) and less than 6/60 or 20/200 in better eye (with best refractive correction).
  - Limitation of visual field ≥ 20° and up to 40°.
- Low vision means an individual having poor visual function in spite of receiving standard treatment or full refractive error correction; however, still is able to utilize the remaining vision for planning and/or performing an assignment with suitable supportive instruments.
- Blindness refers to a state of complete absence of visual perception or visual acuity ≤ 6/60 (20/200) in better eye (with best refractive correction) and/or visual field of ≤ 20°.

Table 16.1: Various low vision conditions with their definition (WHO)	
Visual conditions	*WHO definition*
Visual impairment	A condition which range from partial sight to total blindness
Low vision	Visual acuity in range of 3/60 to <6/18 (after best possible correction) and visual field < 20° from the point of fixation in the better eye
Functional visual impairment	Significant reduction of visual capability resulting from some pathological conditions which cannot be corrected or treated
Functional low vision	A person with low vision having an impairment of visual functioning even after treatment, has a visual acuity in range of <6/18 to light perception and /or a visual field of <10° from point of fixation but who is potentially able to use his /her vision for planning and/or execution of a task
Blindness	Visual acuity <3/60 (after best possible correction) and visual field <10° in better eye from the point of fixation. This can also be simplified as no usable vision with exception of light perception
Legal blindness	Visual acuity 6/60 or 20/200 (after best correction including contact lenses) with a visual field of 20° (in the widest meridian) in better eye

Table 16.2: Classification of low vision according to ICD

Type	Visual acuity	
	Maximum	Minimum
Low Vision		
1	6/18 (20/60)	6/ 60 (20/ 200)
2	6/60 (20/200)	3/ 60 (20/ 400)/Finger count at 3 meters
Blindness		
3	3/60 (20/400)/ Finger count at 3 meters	1/ 60 (20/ 1200)/Finger count at 1 meter
4	1/60 (20/1200)/ Finger count at 1 meter	Light perception (PL)
5	No perception of light (NPL)	
9	Undecided or unspecified	

Epidemiology of Low Vision

Incidence: An accurate estimation of people having low vision or visual impairment is difficult to assess because the study outcome will differ according to the norms used to calculate the population affected. Prevalence of low vision increases with rise of ageing population; hence when an increasing population and an ageing population are grouped together they result in a considerable rise in total number of people suffering from low vision.

People more than 50 years age: About 20% of world's population is in the age group 50 years or above, whereas nearly 65% people out of total low vision sufferers belong to this age group. In many developed countries prevalence of low vision is increasing because of a rising percentage of population falling in this age group of 50 years and above.

Children less than 17 years of age: Worldwide, children below 17 years of age suffering from low vision are estimated to be about 2 crores in number. Out of these children nearly 1.2 crore children have uncorrected refractive errors causing low vision. These refractive errors can easily be screened and corrected by routine evaluation methods. Approximately, 15 lakh children are suffering from irretrievable blindness, because of various congenital pathologies for their remaining life. Exact analytic records of visual impairment prevalence in school going children and very young adults is insufficient, however, this is an important population which needs timely visual rehabilitation related care and services.

Risk factors: Various factors can increase the risk of visual impairment in a person, which includes various ocular pathologies along with trauma and systemic illnesses. Most common risk factors for low vision in adults are

- Cataract
- Diabetic retinopathy
- Glaucoma
- Age-related macular degeneration

Etiological Factors for Low Vision

Several congenital or inherent, acquired, ocular or systemic conditions can lead to low vision however, conditions causing irreversible damage to ocular structures or visual pathway remain the major cause of low vision. Most common conditions causing low vision in various age groups is summarized in Table 16.3.

MANAGEMENT OF LOW VISION

Visually impaired patients present a big challenge to practitioners in terms of diagnosis and treatment, although management of low vision in these patients is complicated and require a thorough knowledge of science but an accurate diagnosis will lead to a satisfactory treatment. In most of the cases both patient and doctor feel that nothing can be done for improvement in vision but a positive

Table 16.3: Etiological factors for low vision in various age groups

Age group	Etiological factors
Children	Nystagmus (congenital), cortical visual impairment, congenital cataract, albinism, Leber's optic atrophy, retinitis pigmentosa, optic atrophy, retinoschisis (juvenile)
Younger	Malignant myopia, traumatic brain injury, keratoconus, histoplasmosis, toxoplasmosis, solar retinopathy
Elder or older	Age-related maculopathies, cataract, diabetic retinopathy, glaucoma (primary open angle), cerebrovascular accident, central retinal vein occlusion, macular hole, central retinal artery occlusion, angioid streaks

approach should be kept by the practitioner. An accurate diagnosis and several treatment strategies will definitely help the visually impaired patients in performing the routine activities of their life.

Management of low vision can be broadly grouped as

- Diagnosis of low vision
- Treatment strategies for low vision

Diagnosis of Low Vision

Diagnosis of etiology of low vision is very challenging and sometimes may require other procedures or steps in addition to following steps mentioned below

Guidelines for diagnosis of a low vision case:
Following components are important to diagnose a case of low vision
- Detailed history
- Ocular examination
- Structural ocular examination
- Functional ocular examination
  - Visual status
  - Refractive status
  - Visual field
  - Binocular vision

- Supportive evaluations
  - Contrast sensitivity testing
  - Color vision testing
  - Glare testing
  - Electroretinogram (ERG)
  - Visually evoked potential (VEP)
  - Electro-oculogram (EOG).

Detailed History

Most important aspect in diagnosis of a case of visual impairment is to obtain an elaborative and precise history of illness from the patient. When detailed history cannot be elicited from the patient then we can ask for help from family members. Sometimes, history can also be obtained from health care personnel, therapists or supportive personnel. History should include
- Chief complaint regarding visual and professional activities.
- Character and extent of chief complain.
- Visual problems in terms of more for distance or near vision.
- Systemic illness history including previous diagnosis and treatment
- Related ocular problem history in family members
- Medication usage and medication allergies
- Social history and psychological framework of patient.
- Vocational, educational and professional visual requirements of patient
- Related medical history of family member in support to patient's visual difficulties.

Ocular Examination

Detailed evaluation of ocular system is a prerequisite to achieve an accurate diagnosis especially in cases of low vision patients. Ocular examination includes
- Structural examination by using slit lamp
- Functional ocular examination which includes
  - Visual acuity
  - Refractive status
  - Visual field
  - Binocular vision

Ocular structural examination: Gross ocular asymmetry or periorbital structural anomalies like ptosis, lid lesions or significant orbital lesions should be looked for and are recorded in examination sheet. Detailed anterior and posterior segment examination is done using slit lamp biomicroscopy.

Any corneal, lenticualr or anterior segment pathology should be examined by using slit lamp. Similarly, examination of fundus is done using indirect ophthalmoscope to rule out any posterior segment pathology.

Functional Ocular Examination

Visual Status

Estimation of amount of visual acuity (VA) is an important part of low vision evaluation and is used to calculate the degree of high contrast visual losses. For practitioners visual acuity measurement helps to correlate the chief complaint of patient and actual visual impairment status, hence this VA assessment is utilized in

- Monitoring the steadiness or progression of visual detoriation
- Monitor the changes in visual performance with the advancement of rehabilitation
- Evaluate typical head positions due to eccentric viewing
- Judge the amount of motivation in patient
- Demonstrating the basic approach and techniques related to rehabilitation process.

In low vision patients visual assessment is done after placing best correction (spectacle or contact lenses) in trial frame using various techniques. Initially check Snellen's visual acuity after putting the best corrective appliance, but to confirm the accuracy of best corrected vision pinhole test is performed.

Pinhole test: Primarily this test is performed to assess whether visual acuity can be further improved by refraction or changing the existing best correction or not. After placing full optical correction lenses in trial frame, pinhole glasses or a multi pinhole occluder as shown in **Fig. 16.1** is placed over this

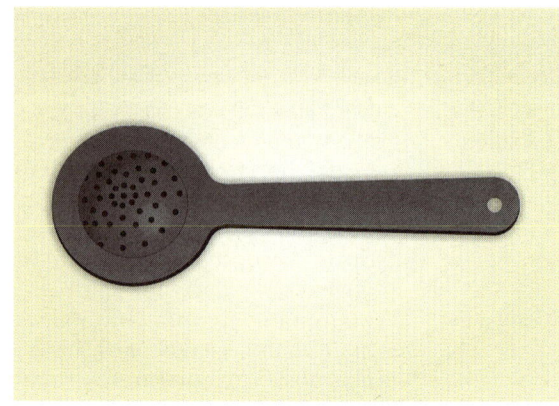

Fig. 16.1: Multi pinhole occluder

correction. Suppose an improvement in visual acuity occurs, it means this patient VA can be improved by further correction of the refractive power, however, if no improvement in visual acuity is seen it means refractive power prescribed is best correction.

Distance and near visual acuity is checked by using either of these following specially designed charts.

Distance vision charts: Distance vision assessment in low vision patients is done with specially designed charts which are portable, having large numbers of optotypes, high contrast and wide range (100–800 foot size) of optotypes size. Along with these features low vision charts poses variable ambient illumination to evaluate minimum lighting conditions that can cause glare and also to decide about the requirement of filter to reduce photophobia and glare.

Various distance vision charts (Fig. 16.2) commonly used to record visual acuity in patient's having low vision are

- Sloan's chart
- Feinbloom charts
- Bailey-Lovie Log MAR chart

Note: Most of these low vision charts are designed to test visual acuity at non-standard testing distances of 10 feet, 2 meters, 1 meter or closer, against standard 20 feet or 6 meters distance for Snellen's distance visual acuity chart.

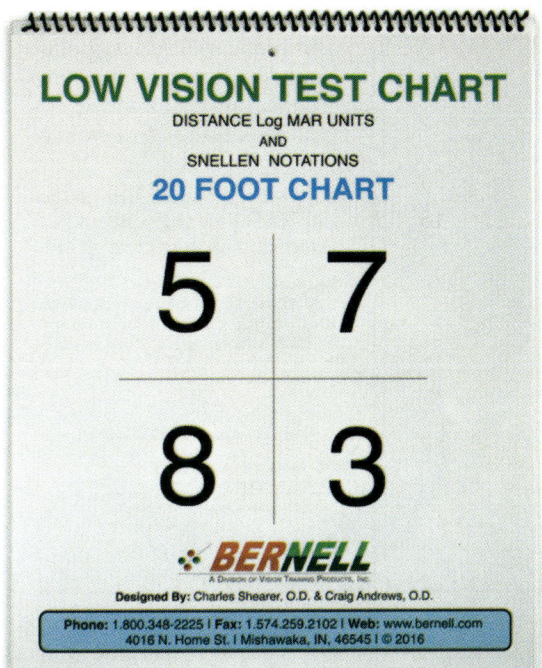

Fig. 16.2: Distance vision chart for low vision (*courtesy:* Bernell Corporation)

Fig. 16.3: Near vision chart for low vision (*courtesy:* Bernell Corporation)

- Modified ETDRS (Early Treatment Diabetic Retinopathy Study) chart
- SOHS (Student Optometric Services to Humanity) charts.

Near vision charts: Similar to distance vision charts various near vision charts are designed to record not only the near vision but also the amount of magnification require to see the near letters clearly. For measurement of near visual acuity different types of acuity charts have been designed especially for visually impaired patients. Commonly used near vision charts (Fig. 16.3) in low vision patients are

- Sloan's M charts
- Feinbloom charts
- Modified ETDRS charts
- Lee charts

Note: These low vision charts are designed with special features such as single letters, isolated words or short sentences.

Feinbloom charts: William Feinbloom designed both distance and near vision charts for partially sighted patients popularly called Feinbloom's low vision charts (Fig. 16.4). Distance vision chart originally designed by Feinbloom is a thirteen page spiral bound book consisting of number optotypes (based on Snellen's optotypes and Sloan's letters). This chart was designed to be tested from 10 feet distance and covers 10/10 to 10/700 visions, although it can be tested from any distance but conversion for distance is done. For example, suppose if a patient read 100 size letter from 2 feet distance clearly then vision is recorded as 2/100 (equivalent to 20/1000 or 6/300).

Feinbloom near vision test cards are different from distance vision charts because on one side they contain numbers optotypes with seven levels (3.2 M to 0.5 M size), whereas other side of test card provides continuous reading lines in five levels (3.2 M to 0.8 M size). Graded continuous text lines provide more

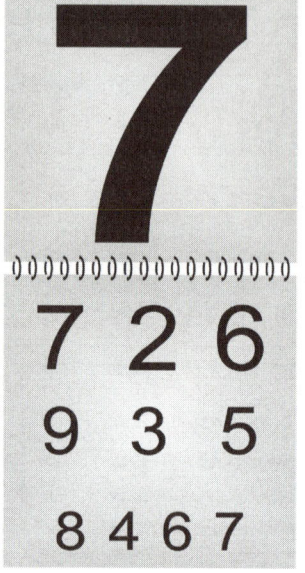

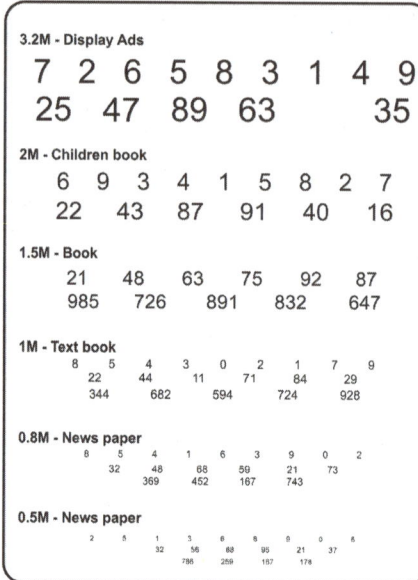

Fig. 16.4: Feinbloom distance and near vision charts for low vision

accurate measurement of reading ability as compared to a number optotypes measurement.

Main advantages of these charts are large optotypes size, easy portability and can be measured at any examination test distance, however, disadvantages are inconsistent width to height ratio and irregular progression of optotypes sizes.

Sloan's M chart: In low vision patients visual assessment using Sloan's M system is widely used because it gives equivalent Snellen's values which can be compared with distance visual acuities of normal person. For example, letter sizes present at 1 M or 2 M in Sloan's chart indicate the distance similar to Snellen's chart print for angular size of 6/6 optotype. Here an angle of 5 minutes of arc is subtended by 1 M print optotypes at 1 meter distance, hence visual acuity can be calculated by this simple formula as

Test distance in meters/M size letter read by patient

Suppose a patient read 8 M size letter clearly from 40 cm distance, then

$$VA = 0.4/8$$
$$= 20/400$$

Similarly, it also helps in assessment of the amount of magnification required to improve the near vision by simply multiplying the size of letter clearly read by patients.

Suppose if, a patient read 8 M size letter clearly at 40 cm distance, then to read 1 M size letter from same distance he/she will require 8 times magnification of letters.

Refractive Status

As discussed above uncorrected or under corrected refractive errors remains major cause of diminished visual acuity all around the world, thus full correction of refractive error is mandatory in low vision cases because it is the deciding factor for further addition of low visual aids. Although pinhole test remains the standard in decision of performing refraction, however, in cases of low vision (less than 6/18 after correction) cycloplegic refraction is done irrespective of pinhole test results.

Objective and subjective refraction is performed in a routine manner as discussed in Chapter 11, when pupil size is normal and clear media is present, however, when retinal reflex is dull, small size pupil or media opacity are present, then radical retinoscopy is performed to assess the refractive status of the eye.

Radical retinoscopy simply means performing a retinoscopy from a closer distance than usual distance (50 or 66 cm). This may be helpful to detect high refractive errors like pathological myopia, high hypermetropia, or astigmatism.

Just noticeable difference (JND) simply means a minimum amount of change in lens power, appreciated by the patient which is expressed in denomination Snellen's acuity equivalent of 20 foot distance. For example, just noticeable distance of 2 dioptres is nearly equivalent to a visual acuity of 10/100 or 20/200 in a retinoscopy range of +1 D. This simply means that examiner needs to starts his/her subjective refraction by placing +1 D power lens, over existing retinoscopy lenses or patient's present spectacle prescription.

Effects produced by various ocular pathologies like irregularities of cornea, irregular astigmatism or lenticular changes on quality of retinal images can be determined with the help of a stenopic slit or pinhole as discussed above.

Visual Field Evaluation

Many studies had confirmed that visual field evaluation, especially in cases of low vision is equally essential like the assessment of visual acuity or reading ability. Visual fields play vital role when a patient's independent travelling is concern. Central, peripheral, or both visual field assessments is done to evaluate the existence and position of the relative or absolute field losses. These field assessment findings are then interrelated with visual functioning of the low vision patient. Following tests are used to evaluate visual fields in low vision patients

- Confrontation test
- Amsler grid test
- Automated static perimetry
- Goldmann kinetic perimetry
- Tangent screen testing

Central visual field evaluation using low vision field charts (Fig. 16.5) or kinetic perimetry is done to look for the presence of relative or absolute scotoma in all the cases of low vision. In these patients having poor visual acuity or visual function the supportive assessment with Amsler grid test and static perimetry is done to rule out the presence of metamorphopsia and decreased sensitivity. This evaluation will help in determining that whether a patient having low vision can be improved with low visual aids or not, because

- Size and position of an absolute scotoma will have an effect on near vision specially in reading capability in spite of an improvement in the image magnification and visual acuity of patient with the help of visual aids.

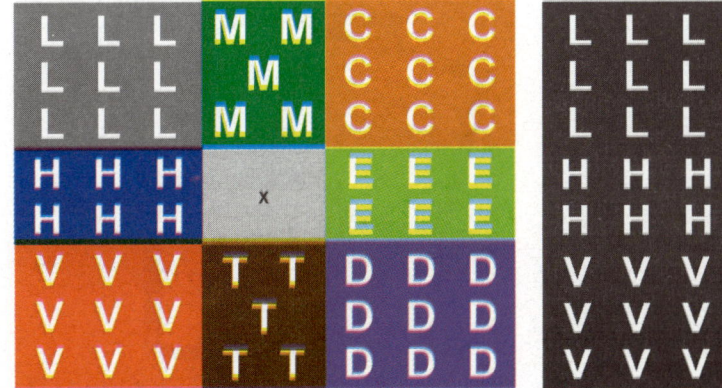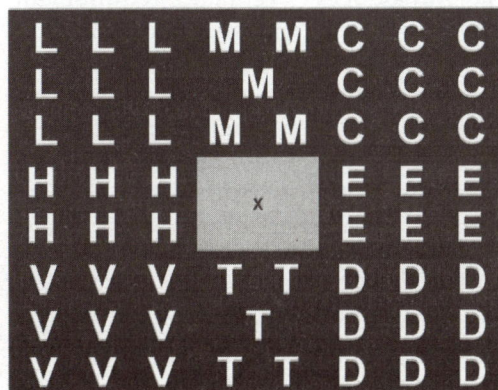

Fig. 16.5: Central visual field charts for low vision (*courtesy:* Bernell Corporation)

- Significant image distortion (if present) will require nearly twice more magnification as compared to an estimate done only on the basis of visual acuity measurement.
- In patients having field losses in peripheral areas the amount of field loss in terms of area and depth and amount of presence of vision specially in peripheral islands is assessed to decide whether patient having low vision is a good contender for visual field expander devices or not.

Binocular Vision Assessment

Treatment options or visual performance in low vision patients are greatly affected by visual deficiencies such as nystagmus, squint, ocular motility defects, imperfect binocular vision, or diplopia. To assess binocular function following procedures can be done

- Hirschberg corneal reflex test for coarse judgment of ocular alignment
- Worth four dot, stereo fly test, etc. for testing of sensor-motor function
- Amsler grid test
- Contrast sensitivity assessment tests

Note: Both Amsler test and contrast sensitivity tests are done monocularly versus binocularly to identify the dominant eye and hence the requirement of occlusion therapy.

Mostly low vision patients have one eye as their favorite or better eye, hence requirement for a binocular prescription is insignificant. However, following possibilities for improvement in binocular vision must be considered

- possible utilization of binocularity or binocular use of low vision optical devices
- possibility of an improved ocular function by occluding the non-preferred eye

Supportive Evaluation

Various supplementary tests may be required, especially in unsatisfied patients, insufficient improvement in magnification, education or work-related necessities, occurrence of particular disease, or other unexplained findings. These supplementary tests are as follows

- Contrast sensitivity
- Color vision
- Glare
- Electroretinogram (ERG)
- Electro-oculogram (EOG)
- Visually evoked potential (VEP)

Contrast sensitivity: Newer studies had concluded that to correct the same amount of visual acuity, patients having low contrast sensitivity require nearly thrice the lens power as compared to patients having normal contrast sensitivity. Hence, contrast sensitivity appears to be an important parameter of visual function especially, in low vision patients.

Contrast sensitivity in low vision patients can be measured by specially designed contrast sensitivity charts **(Fig. 16.6)**, which helps in detection of certain range of spatial frequency losses. Because

- Mid-frequency range loss of contrast sensitivity affects the independent mobility of person.
- High frequency range loss produce difficulty in reading and identification of familiar faces.

Color vision: Presence of color vision abnormalities many a times helps in the diagnosis

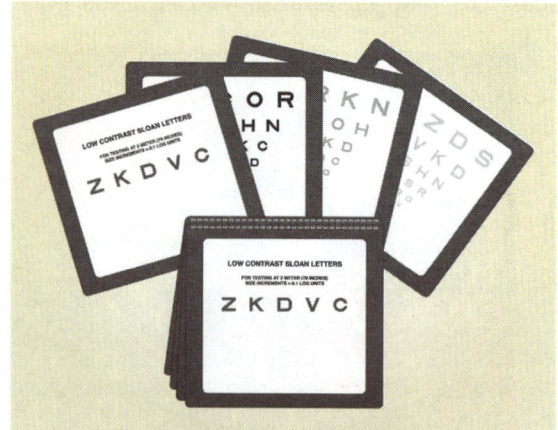

Fig. 16.6: Contrast sensitivity charts for low vision

of specific conditions and may considerably influence the professional, educational, day-to-day activities and independent movement of an individual. In patients having low vision, tests like Holmgren wool test and Farnsworth dichotomous test are commonly used to evaluate the practical inferences for loss of color vision. For example,

- Hereditary or congenital retinal dystrophies such as Best vitellifrom disease, Stargardt disease, central areolar choroidal dystrophy, they all cause red green color deficiency,
- Acquired conditions like ARMD, diabetic retinopathy and hypertensive retinopathy, usually causes blue–yellow color deficiency.

Glare sensitivity: Glare can disable the low vision patients because it may cause increased risk for slipping and difficult movements while walking independently. Glare sensitivity of an individual may be evaluated by environmental stress testing procedures or specific devices available in market. Evaluation of glare sensitivity of low vision patient helps in quantifying the amount of problem and gives a clue for the requirement of special glare filters.

Various conditions such as cataract, posterior capsular opacification, corneal edema or macular edema can cause variation in glare sensitivity. These conditions are treatable, hence low vision can be improved in these cases by proper surgical treatment. Several special filters such as ultraviolet light blockers, contrast enhancers or low intensity filters can be incorporated in glasses to protect from glare.

Supportive exhaustive and specific electro diagnostic tests such as ERG, EOG and VEP are important to establish diagnosis, especially when clinical information and routine tests are insufficient or incompatible to produce results. Moreover, if the patients having low vision are very young and/or handicapped, these tests are useful to establish the diagnosis.

TREATMENT APPROACH FOR LOW VISION

Every patient of low vision requires an individualized treatment approach. Based on the following factors clinician can plan various strategies for low vision therapy.

- Chronological age and mental development of patient
- General, physical and ocular health condition of patient
- Primary cause of low vision and its final outcome
- Extent of visual loss or visual disability or visual handicap
- Visual necessities, aim and objectives of the treatment
- Patient's hopes and amount of inspiration
- Mental aptitude of the patient to take part in the process of visual rehabilitation
- Associated physical handicap which can obstruct visual rehabilitation
- Existing optical systems or low vision aids
- Accessible supportive treatment modalities

These treatment strategies are planned presuming that patient's refractive error has been fully corrected before evaluating the expected amount and type of magnification or else refractive status is not contributing in to the optics of correcting visual aids. Devices used to improve various elements of low vision are called low visual aids.

Low visual aids are the devices which make objects to appear larger, brighter or clearer, even an improvement in contrast sensitivity with reduction in glare also happens. These low visual aids work on the following strategies

- Object enlargement
- Optical magnification
- Contrast improvement
- Electronic magnification

Broadly, we can group these low vision devices as

- Optical devices
- Non-optical devices

Both types of optical and non-optical low vision devices use abovementioned strategies to provide improvement in low vision elements. Magnification or enlargement of the objects remains the key approach among all, whether an optical or non-optical low vision device is used to improve the vision.

An increase in angulations of objects relative to eye's optical system provides the desired magnification for patients having low vision. Most commonly used magnification methods are

- Relative size magnification
- Relative distance magnification
- Angular magnification
- Projection magnification

Relative size magnification: Relative size magnification (RSM) is simply the magnification in the size of the object at same position as shown in Fig. 16.7. For example, outsized print books, magazines and newspapers use this principle of magnification.

Relative size magnification is calculated by keeping the fixation distance (*d*) similar for both object sizes. For example, an object of height *H* (say 1 mm) kept at 25 cm distance has been magnified to height *H′* (say 3 mm) at same distance (25 cm), then

$$RSM = \frac{3}{1} = 3 \text{ times magnification.}$$

Relative distance magnification: Relative distance magnification (RDM) refers to the amount of magnification produced by altering the distance between an object and the observer's eye as shown in Fig. 16.8. To denote the amount of RDM, it is essential to use an

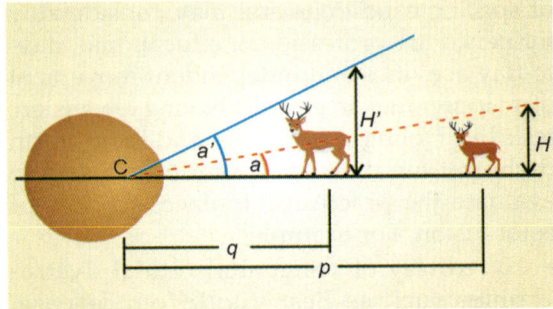

Fig. 16.8: Relative distance magnification by an optical system

original standard or reference distance (typically 40 cm or 25 cm) and RDM is expressed as

$$RDM = \frac{\tan a}{\tan a'}$$

$$= \frac{p}{q}$$

For example, if an object of the same size is moved from 25 cm (*p*) distance to 5 cm (*q*) distance, then

$$RDM = \frac{25}{5} = 5 \text{ times magnification.}$$

Angular magnification: Angular magnification (AM) of an optical system refers to the ratio between angle formed by an object image when viewed via optical system and the angle formed by the object when viewed directly as shown in Fig. 16.9. Here, both these angles are measured presuming that both these angles are formed at pupillary center of eye (C).

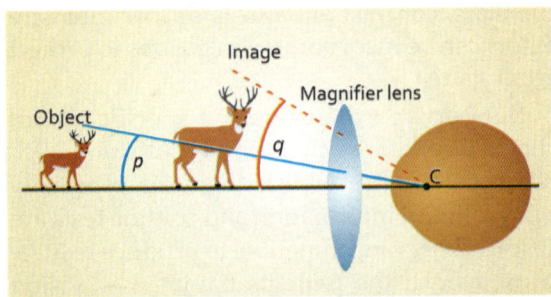

Fig. 16.9: Angular magnifications by an optical system

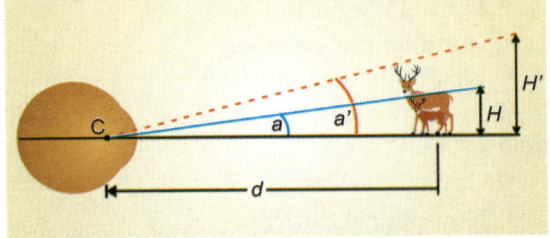

Fig. 16.7: Relative size magnification by an optical system

Angular magnification (AM) = angle formed by image of an object/angle formed by same object when viewed directly.

$$AM = \frac{q}{p}$$

Hence in an angular magnification the comparison of an apparent increase in the object size is done with optical system and without optical system in place.

Projection magnification: Projection magnification simply means formation of an enlarged image of an opaque or transparent object on a screen. Projection magnification system can be optical magnification system or electronic magnification system such as a closed circuit television (CCTV) system. A high amount of magnification at the observer's suitable distance is possible, by using projection magnification. This system has an additional advantage that, it can be used in combination with relative distance magnification for high amount of magnification as shown in Fig. 16.10.

Optical and Non-optical Low Visual Aids

Low vision optical devices: For easy understanding of low vision treatment, various management approach using low vision optical devices are

• Improvement of diminished visual acuity
• Enhancement in contrast sensitivity and glare
• Management of central visual field defects
• Management of peripheral visual field defects

Improvement of Diminished Visual Acuity

Initially it is important to identify the most suitable magnification system for low vision patient having diminished best corrected visual acuity with routine refractive correction. Improvement in the distance and near visual acuity is done on the basis of specific requirements of the patient. Mostly this required level of magnification for either distance or near vision is characteristically work oriented, means it is distinctively different for various activities.

Magnification for Distance

Determination of the expected amount of magnification for improvement in distance visual acuity is simply calculated by taking a ratio of denominators of both the existing best corrected visual acuity (BCVA) and the desired visual acuity level.

For example, suppose existing BCVA is 10/240 and desired visual acuity is 10/60, then simply the magnification required is 240/60 = 4 times.

Devices commonly used for enhancement of distance magnification are telescopes or head mounted electronic devices, however, it is important to consider these following factors before prescribing a distance magnification system

• Visual requirements for specific work
• Need of variation in amount of magnification
• Extent of visual field required for specific task

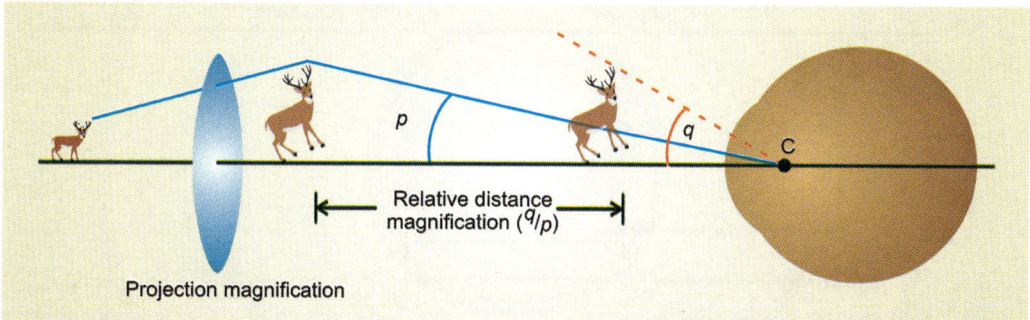

Fig. 16.10: Relative distance magnification combined with projection magnification by an optical system

- Amount of brilliance/contrast at work place
- Use of binocularity

Telescopes

Optical system: An optical system which offers an angular magnification without causing alteration in vergence is termed afocal telescope. These afocal telescopes have two basic optical elements, i.e. an objective and an eyepiece. In all types of telescopes the objective lens is of plus power to obtain an angular magnification and is kept facing the object, whereas an eyepiece is either a plus or minus power lens (significantly larger in power as compared to objective) and is kept nearer to the observer's eye.

Principle: Basic optical principle in all types of afocal telescope is that the secondary focal plane of objective lens and primary focal plane of eyepiece lens coincides with each other. The parallel rays falling on objective lens will form an image at the secondary focal plane of this objective lens and this image now acts as an object for the eyepiece lens. Since the object image is situated at the primary focal plane of eyepiece lens, the emerging rays from this optical system are again parallel in nature. However, these emerging rays form a larger angle with the optical axis of the system as compared to the angle produced by the incident rays.

Telescope designs: Most commonly used telescopes as low vision devices are classical afocal telescope designs such as

- Galilean telescope
- Keplerian telescope

Galilean or terrestrial telescope

Optics: In Galilean telescope objective lens (O) is of convex (plus power) and eyepiece (E) lens is of concave (minus power). Incident rays when falls on convex objective lens then a virtual image of height (H) is produced and the central light ray after passing through the optical center of objective lens subtend an angle (A) with optical axis of system as shown in Fig. 16.11. Another light ray passes via optical center of the eyepiece lens which forms the tip of virtual image and emerges out from eyepiece lens without any deviation, forming an angle A' with the optical axis of system. Hence, in this optical system bundle of parallel rays enters an objective lens at an angle A, whereas a similar bundle of parallel rays emerges out from the eyepiece lens at an angle A'.

D = distance between the objective and eyepiece lens; Fo = secondary focal length of objective lens, Fe = primary focal length of eyepiece lens.

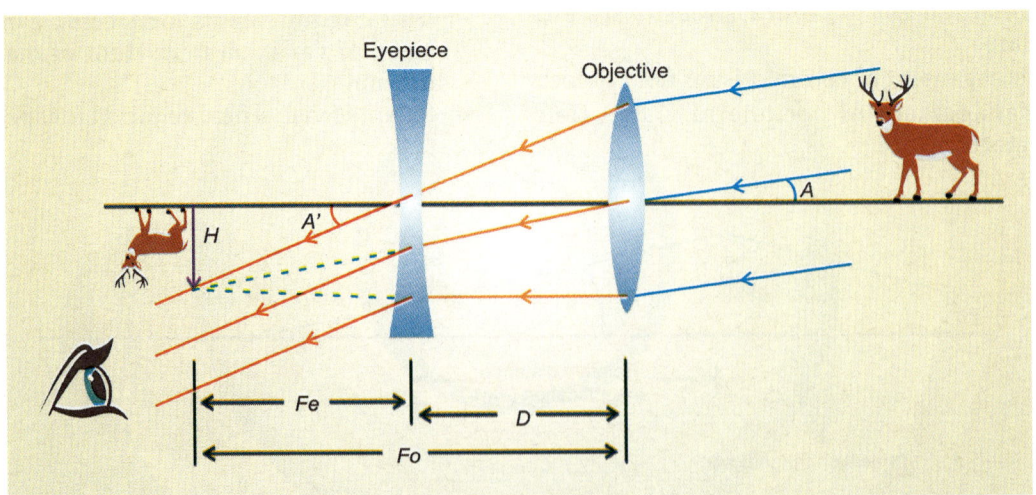

Fig. 16.11: Optics of Galilean telescope

Here, the ratio of angle A'/A represents an angular magnification, which can also be expressed as

$$M = \frac{\tan A'}{\tan A}$$

$$= \frac{Fo}{Fe}$$

Consider that Po is power of objective lens and Pe is power of eyepiece lens, then by simple calculation

$$\text{Magnification} = \frac{-Pe}{Po}$$

In a nutshell since for a Galilean telescope Po is always a positive lens and Pe is always a negative lens hence, magnification formula, ($M = -Pe/Po$) will have a positive sign which means that image formed will be always erect.

Keplerian or astronomical telescopes is combination of two convex lenses means a plus power (convex) objective (O) lens and a stronger plus power (convex) eyepiece (E) lens as shown in Fig. 16.12. When parallel rays falls on the objective lens at an angle A passing through the optical axis of system, it will produce a real image of height (H) at the secondary focal plane of the objective lens. As

per principle, the primary focal plane of eyepiece lens coincides with secondary focal plane of objective lens, thus the emerging rays from eyepiece lens are parallel, forming an angle A' at optical axis of system.

Magnification provided by this telescope system is also

$M = -Pe/Po$ here Po is power of objective lens and Pe is power of eyepiece lens

Since secondary focal length of the objective lens is positive and primary focal length of eyepiece lens is negative, sum (D) of them is equal to total length of telescope.

In a nutshell since for a Keplerian telescope both Po and Pe are always a positive lens, hence magnification formula, ($M = -Pe/Po$) will have a negative sign which means that image formed will be always inverted.

Galilean versus Keplerian telescope: Various features of Galilean telescope and Keplerian telescope are compared in Table 16.4 and the image formed in a standard telescope is shown in Fig. 16.13.

Types of telescopes: Telescopes for low vision patients are available as hand-held or head-borne (spectacle mounted) telescopes, either in monocular form (as shown in Fig. 16.14) or

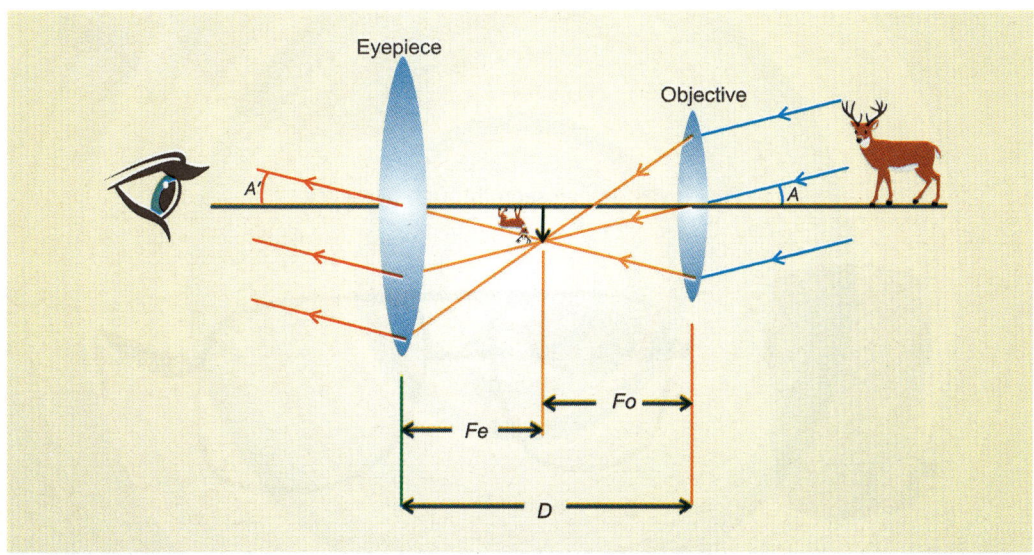

Fig. 16.12: Keplerian telescope

Table 16.4: Galilean telescope versus Keplerian telescope

Telescope features	Galilean telescope	Keplerian telescope
Telescope design	Simpler	Complex
Telescope weight	Lighter	Moderately heavy
Telescope length for a given amount of magnification	Shorter	Longer
Image formed	Erect	Inverted (hence needs an additional erecting system, to be used as a low vision device).
Quality of image and brightness of view field	Lower	Better
Image magnification	Lesser usually up to 4X	Higher usually up to 20 X
Observer's fields of view	Smaller	Larger
Exit pupil	Virtual, falls inside the telescope (between objective and eyepiece lens), present usually at some distance in front of entrance pupil of eye	Real, situated at short distance behind the eyepiece very close to entrance pupil of eye

Position and size of exit pupil are two important factors which determine the degree of field of view in a telescope.

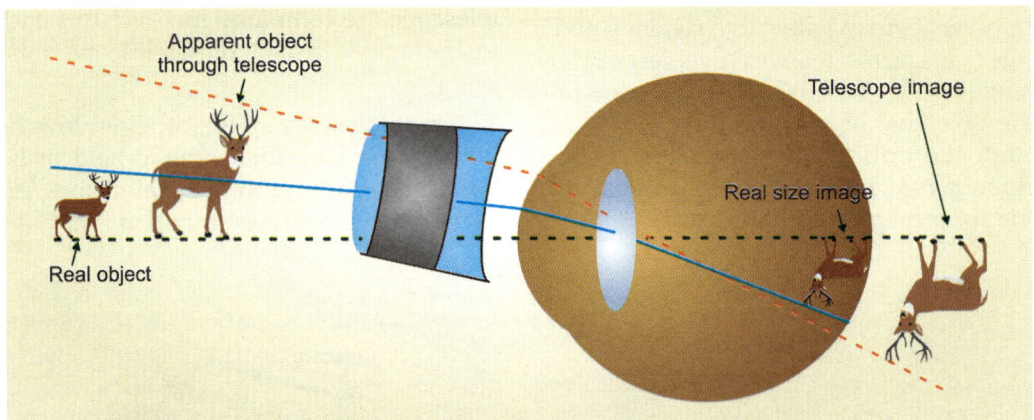

Fig. 16.13: Image seen through telescope

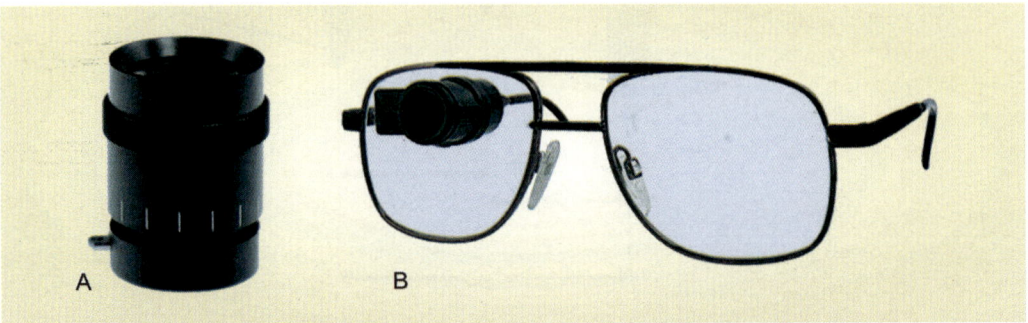

Fig. 16.14: Monocular telescopes: A—Hand held, B—Spectacle mounted (uniocular)

binocular form (as shown in Fig. 16.15). Spectacle mounted telescopes can be either center mounted (full diameter) devices or off center mounted (bioptic, or reading/surgical) devices. Among off centered devices bioptic are superiorly off centered to view the distance objects, whereas reading/surgical devices are inferiorly off centered.

Headborne telescopes (fixed in spectacle frames) are available as full diameter telescopes and the telescope engages the total aperture of the spectacle lens. Similarly, bioptic telescopes are small diameter telescopic unit, mounted in the upper portion of carrier lens fitted in the spectacle frame as shown in Fig. 16.15.

Various design telescopes are available for low vision patients. These telescope designs and their power range is summarized in Table 16.5.

Indications of telescope

- Hand held telescopes are very useful for purpose of viewing for short period such as to read the bus numbers or street signs, can also be used to view blackboard work in classroom or wall mounting.

Table 16.5: Various telescope designs and their power range

Telescope type	Design	Power range (X)
Galilean telescope	Full diameter telescope	1.3–2.2
	Bioptic telescopes	2.2–4
Keplerian telescopes		2–8

Clinically most useful Galilean Bioptic telescopes are 2.2X power and Keplerian telescopes is 3X or 4X power.

- Headborne telescope (spectacle mounted) systems are indicated where viewing is desired for long duration such as watching television or sports event.
- Spectacle mounted telescopes are prescribed depending on the need of patient, mobility and head posture. For example, a bioptic version is preferred when patient mainly needs telescope for distance or mobility, however, a full diameter version is advised when patient needs telescope mainly for watching television or computer work.

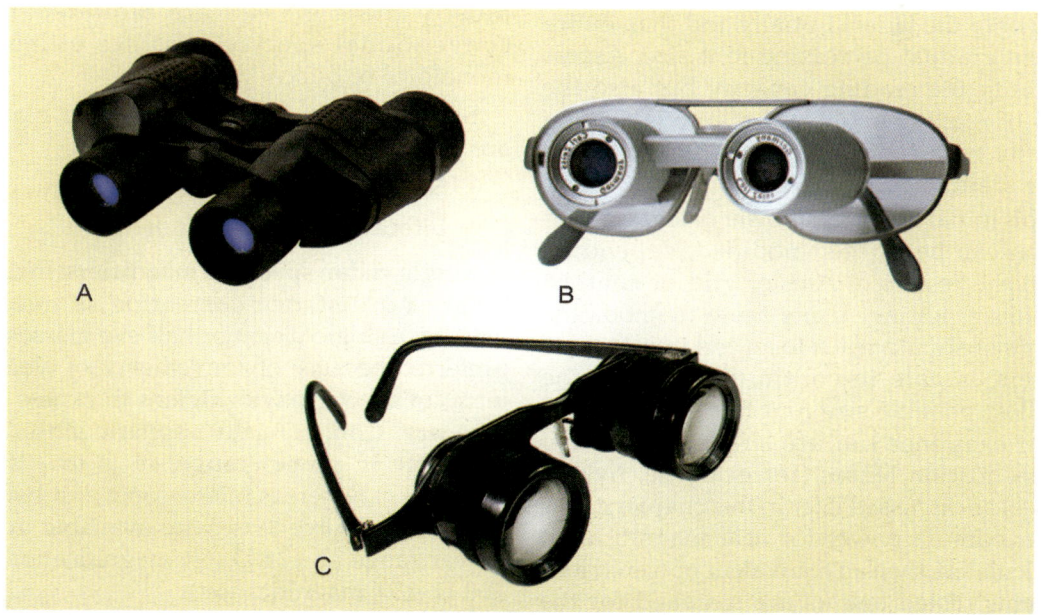

Fig. 16.15: Binocular telescopes: A. Hand held; B. Spectacle mounted (bioptic); C. Spectacle mounted (full diameter)

Head mounted electronic devices: Recently, various head mounted video devices or electronic magnification systems have been developed, having features such as changeable autofocus magnification, and/or contrast enhancement. Although electronic devices can be used for correction of both near and distance low vision but still are not suggested for mobility tasks such as driving or ambulation.

Magnification for Near

Unlike distance magnification no simple formula is present for near magnification hence, various calculation processes were employed in the past to determine the minimum addition power, required for near magnification in low vision cases. Most of these calculation processes required an assessment of best corrected distance visual acuity using maximum lens power and then estimation of additional near power to visualize the smallest object clearly. To evaluate the amount of near magnification required, this calculated near power is placed in the trial frame and the patient is asked to read only the letters initially and then entire line in gradual decreasing font size. Assess not only the reading capacity but also the flow of reading because continuous reading usually requires higher magnification than mere identification of words.

This initial calculated power of lens for near vision can be further modified, depending upon the results of Amsler grid or contrast sensitivity testing. Using these methods the examiner should reach to an end point where patient is able to continuously read the smallest possible size font text. For this end point examiner can use singlet or doublet magnification lenses (for example, hybrid lenses) as discussed later in this chapter. Once the maximum power for near magnification is calculated, then an equivalent powered lens systems (listed below) are searched for the correction of near vision in visually impaired patients.

Most commonly used low vision optical devices to correct near vision are

- Microscopic lenses or spectacle mounted reading glasses
- Telemicroscopes
- Image magnifiers
- Electronic magnifier appliances

Microscopic lenses or spectacle mounted reading lenses: Microscopic lenses are most commonly used low vision devices in majority of patients for improvement of near vision. Visual outcome and comfort of wear is very satisfactory in most of the wearers because these devices are suitable for both near and intermediate distance vision.

Optical system: Simple magnification system is present, where object magnification is achieved by bringing the object (O) within the focal length (f) of high powered convex lens. Hence, a virtual, erect and magnified image (I) is formed behind the object. Object forms an angle 'a' at point C, whereas image forms a larger angle 'b' at the same point C (Fig. 16.16).

Types of spectacle magnification glasses: Mostly these glasses are mounted in a conventional spectacle frames either as monofocal or bifocal glasses.

Broadly, these spectacle mounted glasses are grouped as

- Single vision spectacle magnifiers
- Bifocal spectacle magnifiers

Single vision spectacle magnifiers: In cases where no distance correction is needed usually, a single vision or half eye glasses are preferred because of convenience of wear in terms of spectacle weight, lens thickness and lens size. Commercially aspheric lenses are available in power range +4 D to +20 D. (Fig. 16.17), whereas microscopic and hybrid diffractive double lenses are available in the power range of +24 D (6X magnification) to +60 D (15X magnification).

Hybrid diffractive lenses or double lenses: Hybrid diffractive spectacle lenses or double

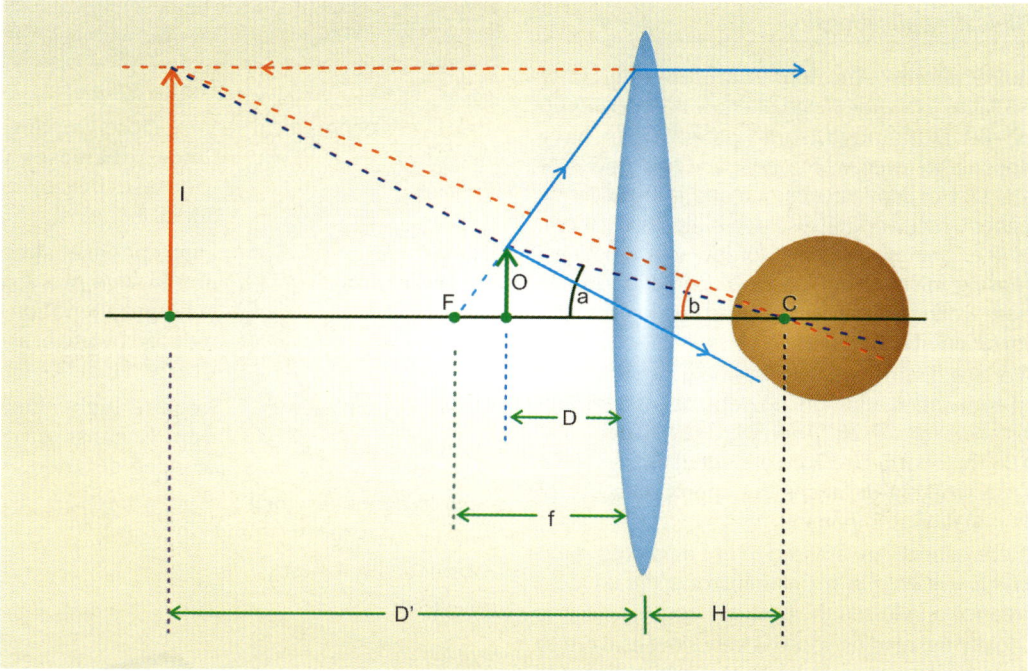

Fig. 16.16: Microscopic lenses produces image magnification, here D' = distance between image and magnifying lens and H = distance between eye and magnifying lens.

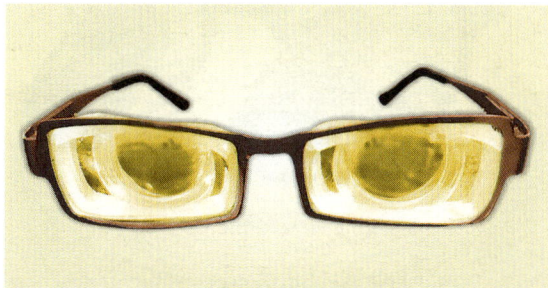

Fig. 16.17: Spectacle magnifier with aspheric lenses (*see* text)

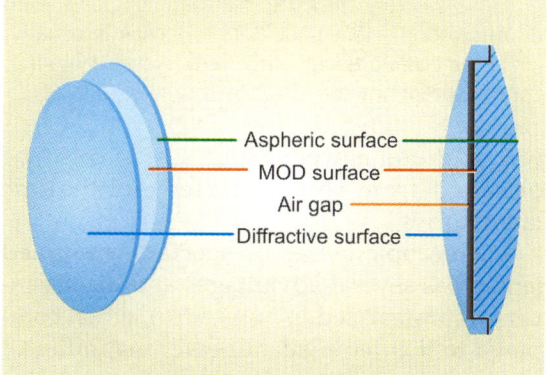

Fig. 16.18: Hybrid diffractive lens

lenses consist of two elements, one in front and another in the back portion of lens. Front element consists of an aspheric curve front surface and multi-order diffractive (MOD) back surface. Similarly, back element also has a first order refractive front surface and a plano back surface.

These two elements are separated by an air interface and are assembled in such a manner that diffractive surfaces of each element faces each other as shown in Fig. 16.18.

Bifocal spectacle magnifiers: To work as an effective low vision aid, power of additional microscopic lens must be extremely high. Semi finished bifocals usually present in ready stock by many ophthalmic laboratories, rarely have an addition power more than +4 D, even on special order addition available for fused bifocals are usually just up to +4.5 D. However, on special order single piece bifocals

Clinical Applications

- These microscopic lenses are commercially available in a wide range of equivalent power up to +80 D although, some patients can have binocularity even with a near addition power of +10 D, but convergence demand is significantly higher when working distance is less than 16 cm. Hence, greatest challenge for low vision patients in using microscopic lenses is adaptation to this close working distance produced due to very high power additional lenses.

- Working distance (meters) is simply the reciprocal of equivalent addition power, means working distance for a +20 D lens is 1/20 meters, i.e. 0.05 meter or 5 cm. To work optimally in such a close working distances the appropriate use of illumination is important.

- These patients are advised to use a reading stand which will help in maintaining of accurate focal distance and lessen the postural fatigue.

- Usually the reading speed is very slow as word to word reading because of close working distance and illumination. Patients are advised to keep patience and slowly learn to read at this close distance. Once patients are accustomed to this close working distance, the reading speed with microscopic lenses or double lenses is usually faster compared to other lens systems having equivalent power.

with addition power as high as +20 D can be obtained from some selected ophthalmic laboratories.

Microscopic lenses or spectacle mounted lenses has several advantages and disadvantages (summarized in Table 16.6), when compared to their equivalent power magnifiers.

Telemicroscopes: These are popularly called reading telescopes which are particularly designed for near work by using afocal telescopes (also used for distance magnification) and modified reading caps. In these telescopic systems usually a reading cap is fitted in the front portion of an afocal telescope which can easily be removed and carried separately by the patient as shown in Fig. 16.19. This reading cap can easily be worn when patient needed to perform near work. Near

Table 16.6: Various advantages and disadvantages of spectacle mounted lenses

Advantages	Disadvantages
Relatively economical	Very close working distance (decreases with increase in power of additional lens)
Hands free magnification	High spherical aberration in high plus lenses, although aberrations are reduced by use of aspherical or diffractive lenses.
Wider field of view	Require high illumination, because of close working distance
Simultaneous distance and near vision	
Cosmetically better accepted	

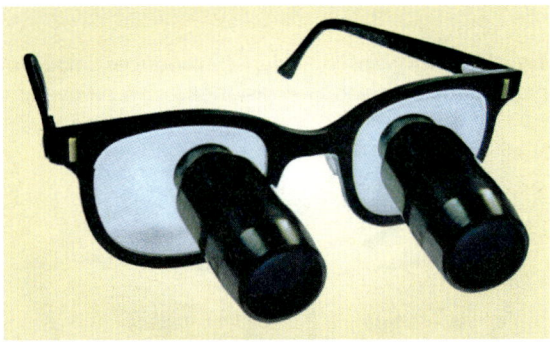

Fig 16.19: Telemicroscope

Note: In nutshell, combination of an afocal telescope and a reading cap is called as a telemicroscope.

working distance is predetermined by the power of reading cap added above the telescope. For example, reading cap of +2.5 D power will produce a 40 cm working distance, similarly for 10 cm working distance, reading cap must have +10 D power.

Optical system: As discussed above a telemicroscope has two elements, i.e. an afocal microscope and reading cap, hence the total amount of magnification by a telemicroscopic system is represented by multiplying the angular magnification of afocal telescope with

Clinical Applications

This simple relationship that equivalent power of a telemicroscope is equal to the product of reading cap power and angular magnification of afocal telescope is very useful in selecting various combinations of reading cap and afocal telescope for a predetermined magnification with desired working distance.

For example, consider following three telemicroscopes, each of them providing the same amount of equivalent power, say 24 D with same magnification as shown in Fig. 16.20.

- Telemicroscope A has 4X telescope with a +6 D reading cap
- Telemicroscope B has 8X telescope with a +3 D reading cap
- Telemicroscope C has 12X telescope with a +2 D reading cap

However, working distance for these three telemicroscope is different depending upon the power of reading cap, i.e. 16.7 cm (1/6 meter) for A, 33.34 cm (1/3 meter) for B and 50 cm (1/2 meter) for C telemicroscope with variable field of view. Whereas, an equivalent microscopic lens of the same power (+24 D) will have only 4.17 cm (1/24 meter) working distance as summarized in Fig. 16.20.

relative distance magnification of the reading cap. This total magnification is in turn can be equated with the amount of relative distance magnification produced by the equivalent single plus power lens. This simply means that different telemicroscopes having same equivalent power will produce same amount of magnification for wearer but working distances will be different in different telemicroscopes depending upon the power of reading cap.

Advantages

- Provides magnification of similar amount at a greater working distance when compared to microscopic lens of an equal power.
- Can be useful for those patients, who are incapable (because of specific working distance requirements) or unwilling to regulate closer working distance of microscopic lenses, although desires a hands free magnification.

Disadvantages

- Size of field of view is reduced because an increased working distance is achieved at the cost of decreased field of view, this can cause a reduced reading speed.

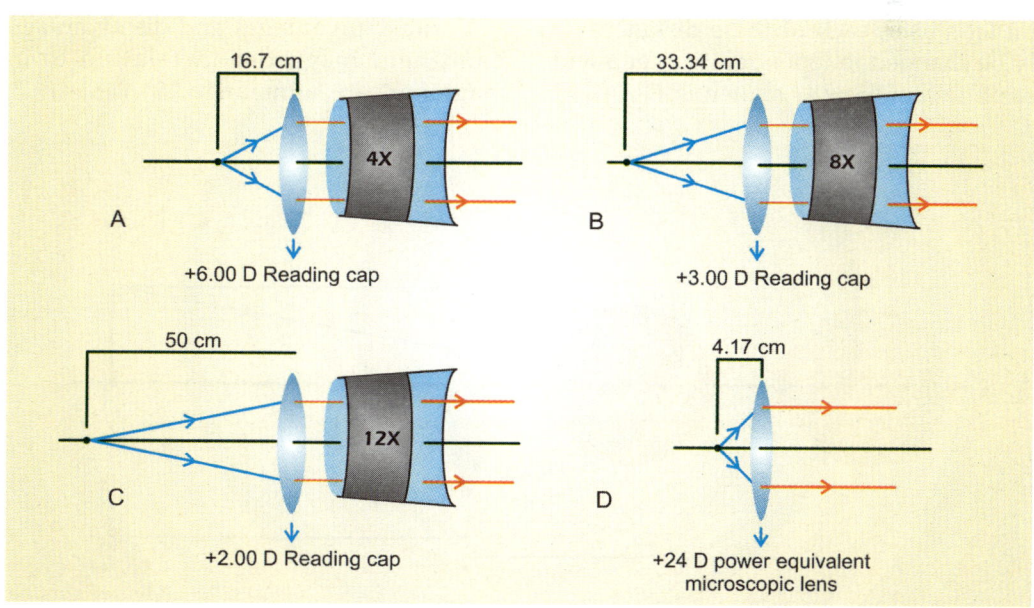

Fig. 16.20A to C: Various power telescopes, having equivalent power of +24 D, showing different working distances. D: Equivalent power microscopic lens showing very less working distance

Image magnifiers: Various image magnifiers used to improve near vision in a low vision patient can be grouped as

- Hand-held magnifiers
- Stand magnifiers
- Paper weight magnifiers

Hand-held magnifiers: Hand-held magnifier are common in use as they provide magnification at variable working distances, hence are especially useful in seeing objects within reading distance or during spotting tasks such as seeing the expiry date on medicine package. By use of this type of device a larger field of view is achieved due to shorter distance between the lens and eye.

Optical system: Hand-held magnifier is comparatively a simple device although optical principles used in this device are relatively complex because magnification is not in terms of a specific number. Magnification depends on two factors, i.e. equivalent power of the device and position of the magnifier, hence both distances, i.e. from lens to the observer's eye (either d1 or d2) and distance from the object to magnifier lens (D) affects the amount of magnification. According to desire of magnifier's user, each of these distances can easily be changed independently over a wide range of field of view as shown in Fig. 16.21.

The amount of magnification for a particular hand-held magnifier can be denoted by using the formula mentioned below which is based on two assumptions, i.e. the standard reference distance for an unaided vision is 25 cm and another is that an object is situated at primary focal point of the magnifier lens.

Magnification = Primary focal point of magnifier lens/4

Hence the emerging light rays from the object will be parallel from magnifier lens (Fig. 16.21) and these parallel rays will fall on the observer's eye irrespective of the distance between magnifier and observer's eye.

Types and designs: Various types of hand-held magnifiers are shown in Fig. 16.22

- Conventional hand-held magnifiers
- Pocket or foldable hand-held magnifiers
- Self-illuminating hand-held magnifiers

These magnifiers are available in the power range of +4 D to +60 D with variable range of magnification; because field of view varies with distance between the position of object and focal length of magnifier lens. These magnifiers are selected according to individualized need of patient and their working distance.

Various advantages and disadvantages of hand-held magnifier in relation to other magnifiers are summarized in Table 16.7.

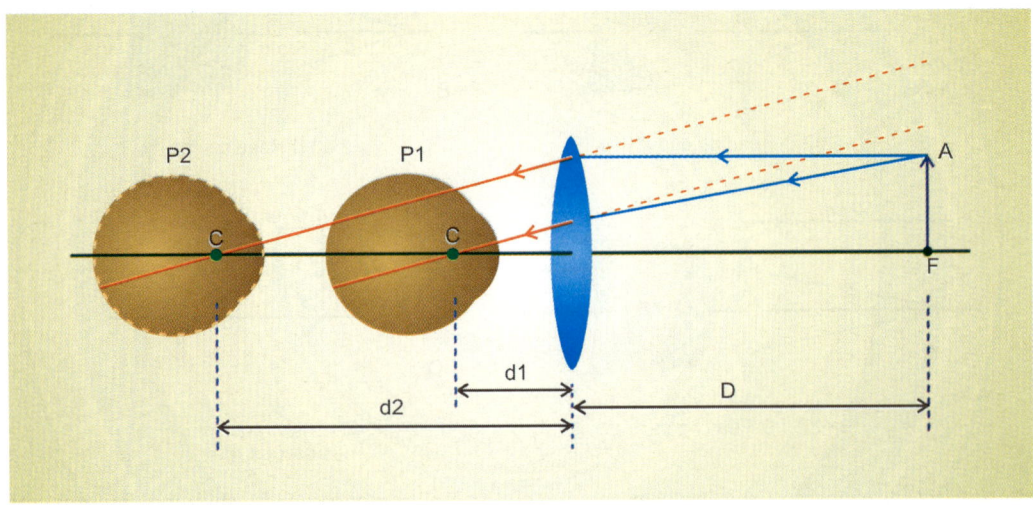

Fig. 16.21: Optics of hand-held magnifier

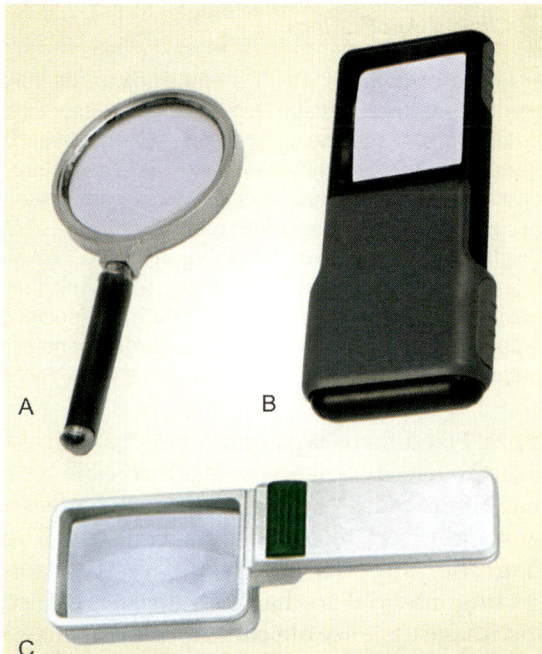

Fig.16.22: Various types of hand-held magnifiers. A. Conventional; B. Foldable; C. Self-illuminated

Clinical Applications

Suppose patient's already wearing bifocal spectacles require the magnifier along with their spectacles, then they should be guided by practitioner about the maintenance of distance between eye and magnifier lens. These patients must be guided that from which portion of bifocal glass the maximum magnification will be achieved at desired object distance.

- Suppose patient holds the object at focal distance of magnifier lens, where magnifier lens to eye distance is greater than focal length of magnifier lens, then patient is instructed to view through distance portion of his/her bifocal glasses. Because viewing through the reading power of bifocal glasses would actually reduce overall equivalent power to less than magnifier power alone.
- Suppose patient held the object at focal distance of magnifier lens (as shown in Fig. 16.21), where magnifier lens to eye distance is less than focal length of magnifier lens, then patient is instructed to view through reading portion of bifocal

glasses. Because equivalent power is greater with bifocal than without it, hence bifocal can be used for maximum magnification.

- Where magnifier lens to object distance is less than focal distance of magnifier lens, divergent light rays emerge from the system, hence an addition power lens or patient's accommodation or both in combination are used.

Table 16.7: Various advantages and disadvantages of hand-held magnifier

Advantages	Disadvantages
Simple and economical device	Users require great practice to maintain proper lens to object distance.
More working distance compared to micro-scopic lenses	Field of view is reduced compared to micro-scopic lenses.
Eccentric viewing is easy	Hands are engaged
During reading no accommodation is needed	Tiring and cumbersome to hold the lens at fixed position from object
	Difficult to use by patients suffering from systemic illness like Parkinsonism, or neurological deficiency.

Stand magnifiers: Stand magnifiers provides a larger working distance compared to spectacle magnifier glasses having equivalent power; however, the relative field of view becomes smaller than spectacle glasses.

Optical system: Stand magnifier forms an image at infinity when plane of reading matter overlaps with primary focal plane of magnifier lens. Normally for magnification reading matter is placed a little inside the focal plane of magnifier lens, so that image is formed at a position between infinity and plane of reading matter. This object image is virtual, larger and erect in nature and is located behind the magnifier lens as shown in Fig. 16.23A.

While prescribing the stand magnifiers for a visually impaired person, practitioner must be in a position to locate the image plane of

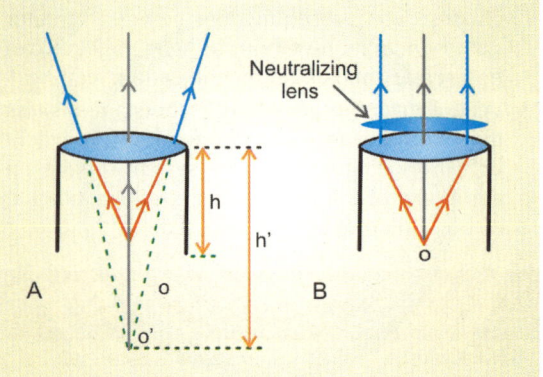

Fig. 16.23: Optical system of stand magnifier. A. Image plane shown in a stand magnifier; B. Optical power of neutralizing lens determines the position of image plane by making emergent light rays parallel

that particular stand magnifier because instructions can be given to the patient regarding proper viewing distance, and also practitioner can estimate the amount of accommodation or power of near addition needed by the patient to observe the object image clearly. Location of image plane is determined by calculations done after neutralizing the emerging divergent rays with an appropriate power plus lens. This plus lens will make the emerging rays parallel and image will form at infinity as shown in Fig. 16.23B.

Types and design: Stand magnifier as shown in Fig. 16.24 are available both as fixed focus (common) and focusable (less common)

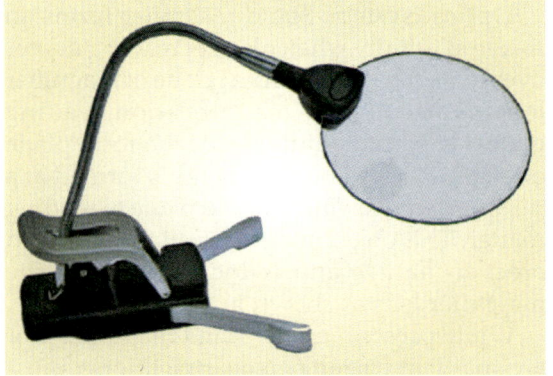

Fig. 16.24: Stand magnifier design

Clinical Applications

Majority of patients prefer a stand magnifier for reading purposes, because lens to object distance is predetermined and fixed. In addition, self illuminated stand magnifiers are useful in situations where lighting control is difficult. Usually, the optical parameters provided by the magnifier manufacturers' are insufficient for clinical uses, hence practitioner needs to evaluate equivalent power of magnifier with the position of object image and prescribe the specific type of stand magnifier to match the requirements of patient.

types. Fixed focus type magnifiers has a fixed object to lens distance, whereas focusable type magnifiers require fixing of distance between lens and object to see the image clearly. The magnifier support is placed directly upon reading material so that both object distance and image distance are constant. Several fixed focused designs are fitted with self-illumination which has an additional advantage of glare free light source. Power range of these magnifiers is +4 D to +80 D.

Various advantages and disadvantages of stand magnifier in relation to other magnifiers are summarized in Table 16.8.

Paperweight magnifiers: Paperweight magnifiers are very popular low vision aids, because of convenience and availability. These aids can be used in very old people who have tremors

Table 16.8: Various advantages and disadvantages of stand magnifiers

Advantages	Disadvantages
Simpler to use, because object distance is pre-determined and magnifier lens is mounted on a stand	Field of view is smaller as compared to spectacle magnifying glasses
Can easily be used by patients suffering from systemic illness and who are unable to use hand-held magnifiers	Cannot be used for non-planar object surface, because lenses will not focus equally at different levels of planes.

or are unable to hold objects for longer durations. These are thick planoconvex lenses kept directly on the reading matter and person slowly slides this magnifier across the page while reading the printing matter. Hence, paperweight magnifiers can be considered as modified version of stand magnifiers.

Optical system: Magnification power of a paperweight magnifier can be calculated by locating the image position and applying a simple linear magnification formula usually, used for a single spherical refracting surface.

$$\text{Magnification} = \eta' h' / \eta h$$

Where, η = refractive index of air, η' = refractive index of magnifier lens material, h = central thickness of paperweight magnifier and h' = object distance from top of magnifier. This can further be simplified as

$$\text{Magnification} = \eta' h' / h \text{ (because refractive index of air is 1)}$$

Here, in Fig. 16.25, A = object location, A' = image location, h = central thickness of paperweight magnifier and h' = object distance from top of magnifier, R = radius of curvature of sphere, C = center of curvature

Similarly, if a paperweight magnifier has equal amount of radius of curvature (R) and central thickness (T) means it is in the form of a hemisphere, then magnification will be equal to refractive index of lens material, i.e. η' as shown in Fig. 16.26, because here $h = h'$ and image will be located at object plane.

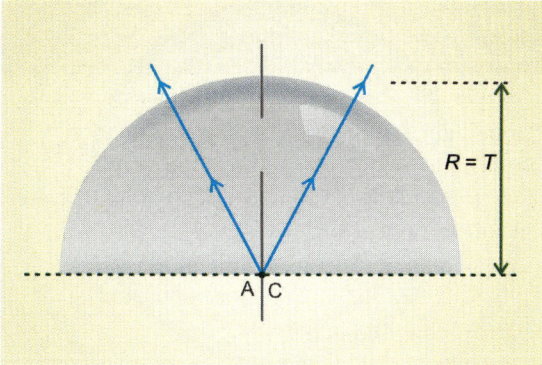

Fig. 16.26: Magnification through paperweight magnifier where R = T

Types and designs: Various types of paperweight magnifiers are commercially available, but most commonly used paperweight design are bar, dome shaped and LED illuminated as shown in Fig. 16.27.

Various advantages and disadvantages of paperweight magnifier in comparison to other commercially available magnifiers are summarized in Table 16.9.

Electronic magnifying appliances: Several electronic magnifying appliances like closed circuit television systems (CCTV), head-mounted devices (HMD) and computer-based adoptive softwares are available for visually

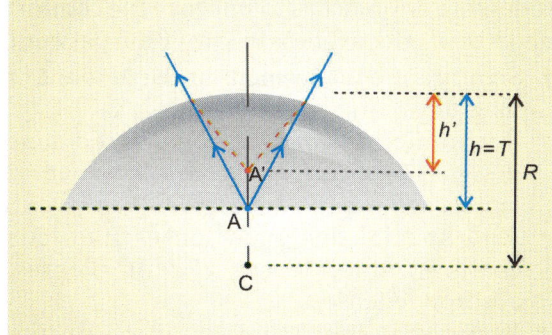

Fig. 16.25: Magnification through paperweight where T < R

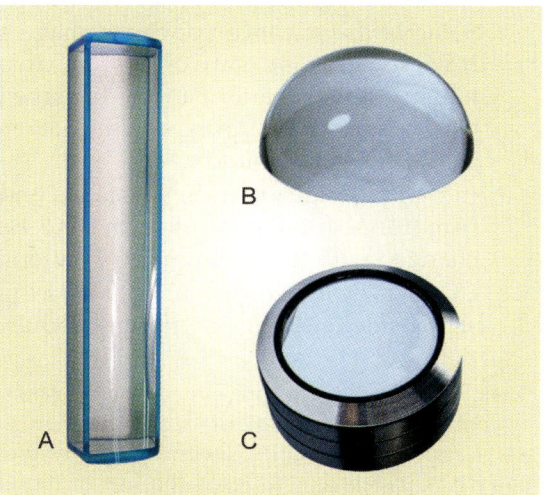

Fig.16.27: Various types of paperweight magnifiers. A. Bar design; B. Dome shaped; C. LED illuminated

Table 16.9: Various advantages and disadvantages of paperweight magnifiers	
Advantages	*Disadvantages*
Good light gathering power	Low magnification power
Easy to handle and maintain	Restricted field of view
Very economical	Difficult to read continuous text
Can also be used in old age patients, with unsteady hands	

impaired persons. Unlike abovementioned magnifiers majority of these appliances are bulky and non-movable, hence recently compact designs of electronic magnifying appliance like HMD devices are manufactured so that they can be easily carried to different places by the patient.

Salient features of various electronic magnifiers are

- These electronic magnifying appliances magnify the object image and also provide binocular presentation with a contrast enhancing system.
- Patients using these appliances can control the image size magnification and amount of contrast.
- Some of the advance appliances have a reverse contrast control system also where printed matter can be displayed in reverse contrast, means as white letters on a black background.
- In many designs working distance and functional field of view can also be changed with the willingness of patient.
- CCTV is designed for patients desiring an extended reading or writing schedule.

Note: The choice of an appropriate magnification system for improvement of near vision in a particular person require several visits by the patient as patient has to learn the use of these complicated lens system according to their required working distance and posture.

These devices are explained in detail later in this chapter in non-optical devices.

In a nutshell final selection of a distance or near magnification system to correct low vision is based on the following factors

- Comfort in utilization of magnifier especially in relation to the field of view, scanning or focusing the object.
- Patient's need of mobilization or driving vehicle after wearing low vision aids.
- Contrast or image brightness required by the patient especially for reading.
- Lightness of magnifier.
- Social acceptance or cosmetic appearance with device.
- Expenditure for purchase and maintenance of low vision device.

Enhancement in Contrast Sensitivity and Reduction of Glare

Change in contrast and glare sensitivity are two important associated factors along with amount of visual acuity which influences the various routine works especially in a low vision patient. The routine activities such as reading, writing, moving around and other day-to-day living activities are adversely affected due to reduced contrast sensitivity, whereas excessive sensitivity to glare will cause the defective functional abilities in visually impaired patients. In cases of low contrast sensitivity or altered glare sensitivity the practitioner should concentrate on the following approaches to improve the comfort and visual effectiveness in low vision patients.

- Significant enhancement in the amount of magnification.
- Recommendations of specialized lens designs like biconvex aspheric lens, hybrid lenses, achromatic doublets.
- Add special designed lenses like lens coatings, tinted lenses, UV filter lenses, absorptive lenses.
- Best possible lighting condition during routine activities by using illuminated appliances.

- Advice to use the non-optical supportive articles like eye shades, sunscreen, peak hats, signature guides, typoscopes.

Several studies had concluded that low vision patients show higher degree of sensitivity to alteration in lighting conditions, hence to achieve comfort at work and maximum visual performance these visually impaired patients need particular amount of illumination. In general to improve visual performance, modifications in lighting conditions at house or at job place are strongly recommended. In visually impaired patients reduced near visual acuity is commonly associated with reduced contrast sensitivity, hence image magnification alone is not sufficient to improve the reading capability, rather special illumination adjustments should be searched during reading or performing other near activities for better visual functioning.

Best suitable illumination for house or job place can be decided by simply comparing the illumination between various light sources like LED bulbs, fluorescent lamps, halogen bulbs, gas tube lights, or assemblage of these light sources. Distance of the light source from the target and angle of the light rays on the object are also essential parameters. Visibility comfort is assessed with the alteration of illumination because an excessive illumination will produce intolerable glare (sensitivity to glare is reduced in low vision patient).

In critical lighting situations illuminated, optical appliances play a major role in enhancement of contrast, however, some of these appliances are incapable to produce uniform illumination, hence may require an additional supplementary light source.

Low vision patients suffering from mild to moderate amount of decreased contrast sensitivity require specialized type of reading glasses fitted with lens designs having hybrid doublets, or aspheric lenses with antireflective coatings. These lenses transmit an increased amount of light and hence produce sharper object images, so they are useful in poor contrast sensitivity conditions. Low vision patients suffering from significantly decreased contrast sensitivity require only increased amount of magnification over and above the estimated visual acuity. Visibility of low contrast print materials can be improved by using tinted lenses or acetate superimpose. A variety of regulatory filters and lens tints are available to increase contrast in surroundings or decrease glare sensitivity. Some studies concluded that yellow and orange tints increased contrast sensitivity in patients having age related macular degeneration similarly, dark red tints has conventionally being used in patients having albinism and retinitis pigmentosa.

Altered sensitivity to glare can be evaluated inside the house or outdoor at public places in different problematic lighting atmosphere such as LED bulb lighting in job place or shopping mall. Non-optical aids like peak hats and shades either used single-handedly or in combination with sun filter glasses reduces significant amount of annoying glare.

Reflected glare from printed matter produced due to additional illumination done for contrast enhancement can be markedly decreased by using typoscope, because it cuts down the surrounding light area during reading.

In low vision patients having decreased contrast sensitivity electronic devices (e.g. CCTV or head mounted devices) remain a better option because they help in handling of contrast, brightness, and magnification especially when illuminated magnifiers are increasing the amount of glare.

Approach for Central Visual Field Defects

Visual field defects in terms of either relative or absolute scotomas which are located centrally produce significant amount of deterioration in basic visual task such as reading or writing. Moreover, the size, position and the depth of these central field defects influence the outcome of near magnification, hence in several cases in spite of a suitable near magnification various factors like size of printed matter, understanding of material, reading speed and duration gets compromised.

In patients having macular scotoma the positive stimulus to focus the object on fovea may be present, hence with duration and proper training these patients will learn to observe the target eccentrically. However, eccentric viewing of the target needs to build up a new preferred retinal location (preferably near to macular scotoma) to which the patient's eye treat as a new fovea.

In spite of a relatively superior visual acuity and magnification response, scotoma situated right side of fixation will make continuous reading of text matter very difficult. Similarly, scotoma situated left side of the fixation will make judgment of the text matter in subsequent line difficult.

Learning of an eccentric viewing (EV) becomes difficult in scotoma (situated in the surrounding area of an absolute scotoma) having areas of relative sensitivity loss and/or distortion. Many patients learn EV with their own efforts, but proper training is more advantageous for an improvised reading skill. Training of EV is usually done for improvement of reading by using suitable magnification devices. Eccentric viewing (EV) training comprises these approach

- Patient is taught to become responsive for scotoma.
- Develop improvised reading techniques like moving of the reading matter (not the head), read single letter, read large print matter in lower magnification.
- Learn to adjust the image relocation happened due to the use of prisms.

Once patient develops responsiveness to scotoma then they can learn to locate this scotoma with ocular movements. Control of head and eye movements can be achieved in a gradual guided practice manner, using above threshold objectives like large printed matter or television screen. Various types of printed matter have been developed both for supplemented magnification and non-complimented reading conditions. Prism relocation technique is very useful in shifting the image closer to new preferred retinal location.

Patients can be explained the advantages of these approaches, however, success with reading systems can hamper the growth of this vital ability of eccentric viewing. Patient's motivation play a major role in final result of eccentric viewing training, although size and site of scotoma greatly affects and poses difficulty in controlling eccentric viewing and reading speed even after good training in a highly motivated patient.

Approach for Peripheral Visual Field Defects

Patients having peripheral visual field defects face more difficulty in moving around independently compared to persons having only decreased visual acuity. Various training methods like scanning approach or organized searching technique will improve understanding of surrounding and independent travelling ability, especially in patients having incapacitating peripheral visual field defects.

After completion of an estimation of visual field loss, both factors, i.e. patient's appreciation about field loss and his/her capability to cover the defect are investigated by proper questioning and observing the functional abilities. Following devices are used as field expander to enhance visual fields in low vision patients

- Reverse telescopes
- Concave lens
- Prisms
- Mirrors
- Field expanders
- Honey Bee lens systems

Reverse telescopes: Reverse telescopes are nothing but reversely fitted telescopes, which shorten or diminish (in place of magnify) the whole visual field either in one meridian or all meridians. As a result of diminution of visual field, more objects can condense in a smaller area but at the cost of decreased visual acuity. In these telescopes the objective lens is kept near the eye, hence image formed is minified. Similar to distance magnification telescopes, these reverse telescope designs are also commonly available as hand-held or spectacle mounted design as shown in Fig. 16.28. Good visual acuity is a prerequisite to use these reverse telescopes, because minification effect occurs at cost of visual acuity.

Concave lenses or minus lenses: Minus lenses are placed a little away from the eyes and they will also minify the entire field of view, hence can be used as field expanders in cases of low vision patients. These minus lenses help in direction purposes, especially to find objects or locate people or view a large print matter.

Prisms: Prisms are basically used to reallocate an image toward its apex and to produce this prismatic effect prisms are incorporated segmentally in the desired section. For example, prisms are fixed on spectacle lens in such a manner that the prism base remain toward the field defect. Usually this prism segment is fixed away from the central portion of the lens (like in temporal side to right or left eye, or in upper part as shown in Fig. 16.29) so that prism does not obstruct the view of patient when he/she is looking straight ahead.

When patient look through these prisms, the objects can be detected in non-seeing area of the eye with very less ocular movement as compared to the movement required without

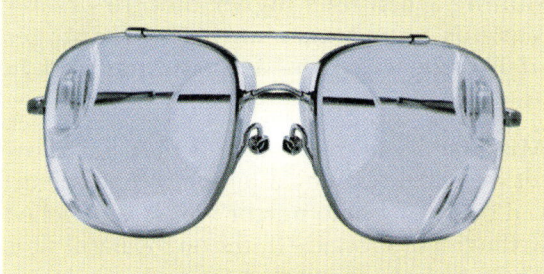

Fig. 16.29: Prism segments fitted in spectacle frame

the prism. Prisms are very useful in cases of constrained visual field conditions like hemianopia or generalized field constriction.

Various designs of prisms are available as
- Fresnel prisms also called press on prisms
- Simple prisms grounded or cemented segmentally into any part of lens.

Fresnel prisms: Fresnel prisms are used to move an image from non-seeing area to seeing or functional retinal area. Majority of the patients suffering from homonymous hemianopia will be benefited by use of these prisms.

Fresnel prisms are press on spectacle lenses (Fig. 16.30) in direction of field loss in a position in front of the eye, these prisms bends light at nearly half dioptric value. Stronger dioptric prisms form larger blind spot which creates image jump, hence patient feel more image

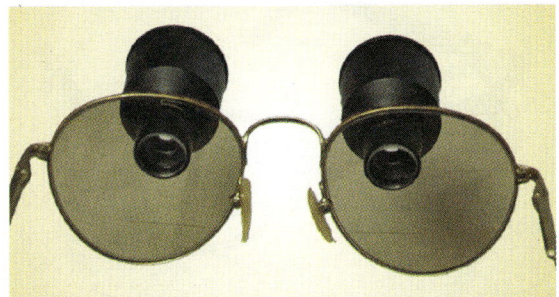

Fig 16.28: Spectacle mounted reverse telescope

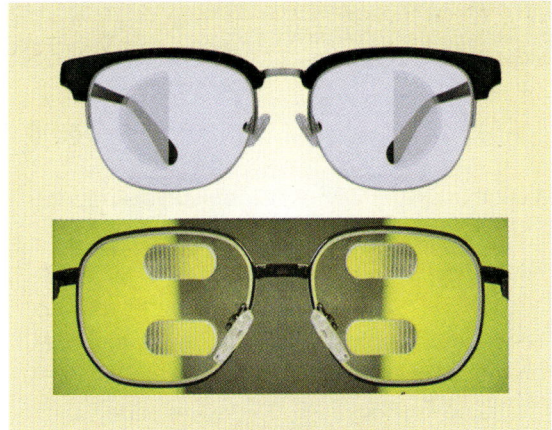

Fig. 16.30: Fresnel prism

shifting when uses higher dioptre prisms. Various advantages and disadvantages of Fresnel's prisms are summarized in Table 16.10.

Mirrors: To improve visual field in a low vision patient having a temporal field defect can be given plano mirror which is attached in the rim of spectacle frame on the nasal side. These mirrors are angled toward non-seeing area in such a manner that by looking into this mirror (just like the review mirror of a jeep) the patient can easily detect the targets or objects lying within the field defect.

As discussed before the image formed in a plane mirror is reversed, hence the patient should learn and understand left to right reversal of the object image seen in the mirrors. These mirrors are available in two designs, i.e. a removable hook-on form or a permanently fixed form, however, both the types has their merits and demerits. Mainly these mirrors are recommended for right or left hemianopic field defects.

Field expanders: Although the field expanders are similar to prisms but contain high powered lenses fused in the temporal aspect of a spectacle lens which helps in improving the field of view. For example, Gottlieb field expanders (Fig. 16.31) are easily available in various power ranges.

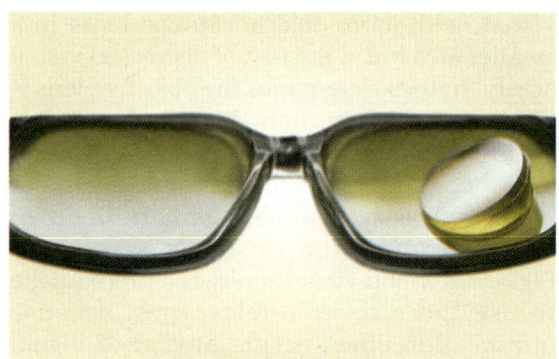

Fig. 16.31: Gottlieb field expanders

Honey Bee lens system: These are nothing but spectacle mounted triple telescopic systems, like a honeycomb, hence the name of system. This type of visual system offers largest visual field to low vision patients in their present respective powers.

Three telescopes of similar power are optically aligned in one housing, which is fitted on a spectacle frame as shown in Fig. 16.32. Special wedge designed prisms are placed over the outer telescopes, angling in a manner such that visual fields of outer telescopes direct towards middle telescope. This mechanism results in filling the blind spots of both the eyes, hence this system provides a larger continuous horizontal field of view.

In a nutshell proper training to utilize these visual field enhancement aids is very important before deciding the actual outcome of their success. Usually low vision patients

Table 16.10: Various advantages and disadvantages of Fresnel's prisms	
Advantages	Disadvantages
Light weight	Creates significant image distortion
Very thin	Chromatic aberrations are increased
Economical	Not stable on glasses, fall off easily
Easy to use, simply press on spectacle glasses	Increases photophobia
Available in wide range 20–60 Δ	Decreases acuity and contrast sensitivity

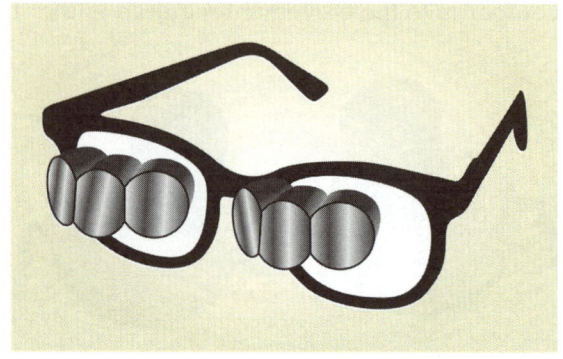

Fig. 16.32: Honey Bee lens system

are not familiar to these complex lens systems and their optical features, hence for an effective utilization of these lens systems patient must have a basic knowledge of optics involved in these systems. So the low vision patients must develop these basic visual proficiencies in

- Object spotting especially for using reverse telescopes and minus lenses.
- Scanning the surroundings for using the prisms and/or mirrors.
- Development of techniques to utilize these complex lens systems.

Non-optical Visual Aids

Visual aids which do not utilize the lenses for improvement in amount and quality of the vision, especially in visually impaired persons are called as non-optical visual aids. Various types of non-optical visual aids have been developed on the basis of magnification of object's size, improvement in the contrast sensitivity or providing the sensory clues like touch or hearing. Aim of these non-optical visual aids is to discover the possibility to assist low vision persons so that they can use their residual vision more efficiently or perform some specific jobs non-visually.

Following are non-optical aids used in specific situations in a low vision patient

- Reading aids
- Script aids
- Auditory aids
- Object magnification aids
- Orientation and mobility aids
- Sight substitution aids

Reading aids: Low vision patient can be benefited by the use of either highly illuminated reading surface or contrast enhanced reading area. This can be achieved by use of reading stands or typoscopes.

Reading stands: Maximum illumination (avoiding eyes) on reading material is helpful in majority of low vision patients. This purpose is served by use of a reading stand with lighting facility. Many patients feel uncomfortable in high intensity fluorescence

lights, rather patients suffering from albinism, cataract or maculopathies feel relaxed in low intensity yellow lights.

Typoscopes: It is a reading tool, which helps in fluent reading through a small rectangular box; shows only 2–3 lines at a time as shown in Fig. 16.33. Surrounding dark background cuts the glare from page and facilitates an easier reading of selective text, hence also considered as contrast enhancer.

Script aids: Many script aids (writing aids) are available for visually impaired persons such as felt tip pens, signature guides, envelope guides, witting templates as shown in Fig. 16.34. These aids help the visually impaired person to write routine important matter inside a guided box like signing the bank cheques or writing the postal address. Even Braille or Moon method of writing is also an example of writing aid.

Auditory aids: Several auditory aids like talking watches or clocks, large print auditory calculators, speech synchronized computers, help enormously in severely poor visual acuity patients.

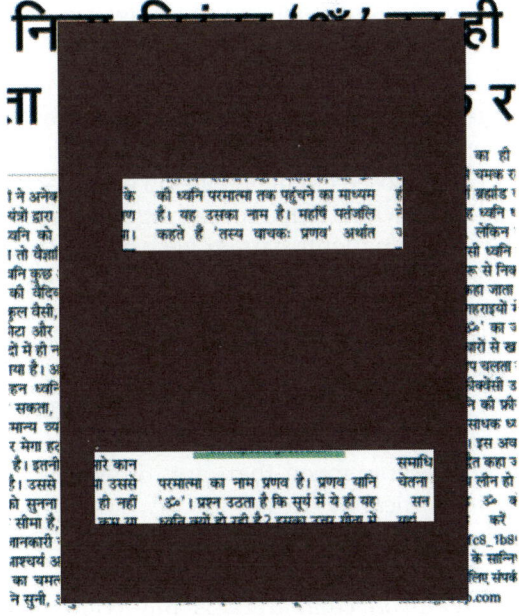

Fig. 16.33: Typoscope

Fig. 16.34: Writing aids

Object magnifications aids: Increase in the size of object helps low vision patients to identify various things. For example, large print books or playing cards, high contrast clock dials or telephone dials. Similarly, various electronic devices are also available for magnification of object size.

Electronic devices: Electronic devices magnifies the objects for easier visibility in low vision patients and are available as follows

- CCTV
- Large print computers
- Electronic head mounted magnification devices

CCTV: Closed circuit television is an electronic device, which helps in reading and writing activities in patients having very poor vision. In these devices a camera pick the picture of concern object and project it on a TV screen which is several times magnified (up to 40 times) as shown in Fig. 16.35.

CCTV provides more comfortable reading/writing posture, increased work duration and faster reading speed than any other similar type of optical devices.

Various benefits and limitations of CCTV are summarized in Table 16.11.

Large print computers: A few computers are available with specially designed software

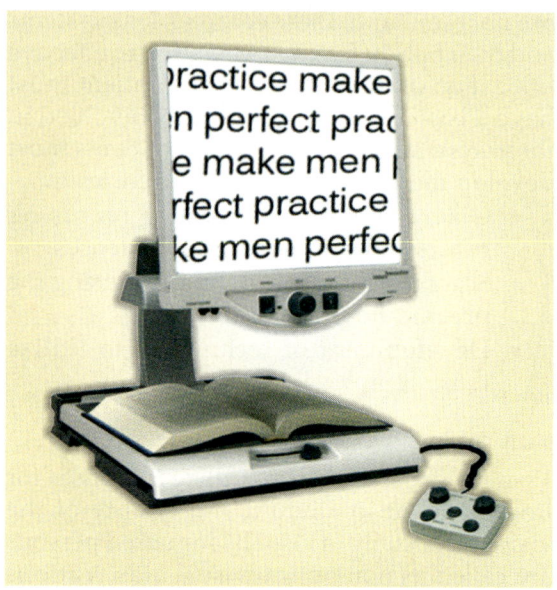

Fig. 16.35: Closed circuit television

Table 16.11: Various benefits and limitations of closed circuit television

Benefits	Limitations
Instantly convert any material into large print	Very expensive
Only device which provides binocularity at very high magnification.	Not easily available
Provides larger field of view with distortion free, highly magnified image.	Non-portable
Provides high illumination and contrast enhancement	Long learning curve
Make reading of continuous text easier at high magnification	
Enable the patient to perform writing tasks such as writing cheques	

which provides large size prints with movement of objects towards viewer's eyes. Sometimes this software is also incorporated with an auditory facility which provides speech along with the printed text. Although

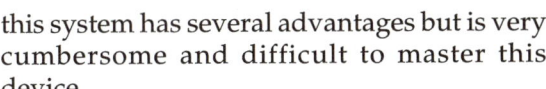

this system has several advantages but is very cumbersome and difficult to master this device.

Electronic head mounted magnification devices: In the year 1992, scientists from John Hopkins Wilmer Eye Institute introduced a unique low vision system aid, called low vision enhancement system (LVES) which was later on marketed as low vision imaging system (LVIS).

Examples of various commercially available head mounted electronic devices are

- LVIS
- V-max
- Jordy system
- MaxPort
- NuVision

In LVIS, a video camera (monocular) is mounted on a binocular head-mounted display system which provides enhanced contrast with changeable degree of magnification. This head mounted system is connected with a control device. Maximum magnification is about 10 times with field of view about 50° horizontally and 40° vertically.

V-max is next generation LVIS which has a color video camera and magnification up to about 20 times, however, field of view reduced to half than previous generation LVIS, i.e. about 25° horizontally and 20° vertically. Its control device is more simple compared to LVIS.

Jordy system came with more advanced features than V-max, like zooming magnification of objects as high as 30 times and variable viewing options such as color view, black and white view, high contrast images, positive and negative contrast images and reverse contrast imaging systems.

Although several advantages are present in these devices but main disadvantages are

- Very expensive
- Field of view is reduced
- Not easily available
- Complex operating system
- Difficult mobility

- Not suitable for patients having head tremors
- Difficult to navigate

Orientation and mobility aids: Various non-optical devices are designed to support a visually impaired person for better orientation of objects and mobility. A sighted person holding hand of a visually impaired person and guiding the path was a traditional method employed for many centuries. Gradually, devices were developed to aid the mobility of low vision patients.

Mainly following methods are used to guide slightly impaired persons

- Guide dogs
- White sticks and canes
- Electronic devices

Guide dogs: Very small percentage of visually impaired persons uses guide dogs for mobility, however, they can be referred by health workers, clinicians or ophthalmologists to rehabilitation centers for proper training. Dog owner must be in a physical health status to direct the dog for a desired route of walk.

White sticks and canes: To guide impaired sighted persons these white sticks or canes are available

- *Symbol cane:* This is specially designed to symbolize that consumers of this cane are visually impaired persons and need special attention usually in a crowded place such as market, shops or roads. This cane is made up of multiple sections of foldable hollow light weighted tubes. Some amount of training is required to use this kind of cane.

- *White walking stick:* Visually impaired patient use this cane as a symbol cane rather using it for mobility or finding the directions. It is primarily used by low vision patient to take support while walking. Occupational counselor and physiotherapist commonly recommend these types of canes for visually impaired patients.

- *Guide cane:* Mainly used by people who have some useful vision to identify various routine objects such as footsteps and staircase, doors or furniture. It is a longer and sturdier cane compared to symbol cane.
- *Long cane:* Primarily used by virtually blind people to scan the ground in front of them for the recognisation of the obstructions or some risks ahead of them. It is a long light weighted cane having a rubber grip with a roller ball tip on one end.

Electronic devices: Several electronic devices are available for orientation and mobility aid for visually impaired persons. These devices can be used in addition to canes, for localization of various obstructions in routine surroundings such as ceilings, corridors, turning roads, small bushes.

Commonly available electronic devices for visually impaired patients are

- *Sonic aids:* These devices use sound waves to detect the presence or absence of an object similar to Radar. Hence, when an obstacle comes across, the user receives an auditory warning or vibratory signal so that person can move away from hazard.
- *Global positioning system:* Commonly called GPS and are similar devices used in automobiles or mobiles for finding the directions of desired destination. These devices give a voice command to visually impaired person once the patient specifically feed the desired route in GPS device.

Sight substitution aids: As we know that sight is the most important sense in individuals because nearly two-thirds of information around us is received by sight. A significantly visually impaired or practically blind person uses his other sense of hearing or touch more efficiently than better sighted people. Although person may be literally blind but many still like to use their visual sense in a mixture with other senses. For example, use of a magnifier for reading newspaper and using an auditory device for novel or storybook.

Mainly two senses, i.e. hearing and touch, substitute the sight; hence various devices are designed for sight substitution is as follows

- *Hearing substitutes:* These devices are based on the principle that when a desired work is complete, an indicating sound like beep or siren will blow so that a visually impaired person can notice that desired work is complete. For example, fluid or water level devices which beep when water or fluid has reached the desired level in a coffee mug. Similarly, several popular movies or videos are available with audio described narrations. Talking microwaves, talking books, clocks, watches are also available so that the visually impaired person can perform routine activities. At some places annual subscription of talking newspaper, magazine and books are also available.
- *Touch substitute:* These are touch-based reading and writing methods and are popularly called Braille or Moon. Braille is considered as most popular and most widely accepted method of touch related reading in writing by blind people whole over the world. Specific combination of six raised dots are arranged like numbers on various surfaces such as charts, dice or board; which produces each of 63 symbols of letters as shown in Fig. 16.36. Mostly people use this technique to tag short text matter or read small paragraphs. Reading and writing using Braille require a significant amount of training, by professionals. Moon is simpler than Braille both in terms of practice and learning because shapes of symbols resemble the routine letters, however this method is not used widely because limited trainers and books are available on Moon technique.

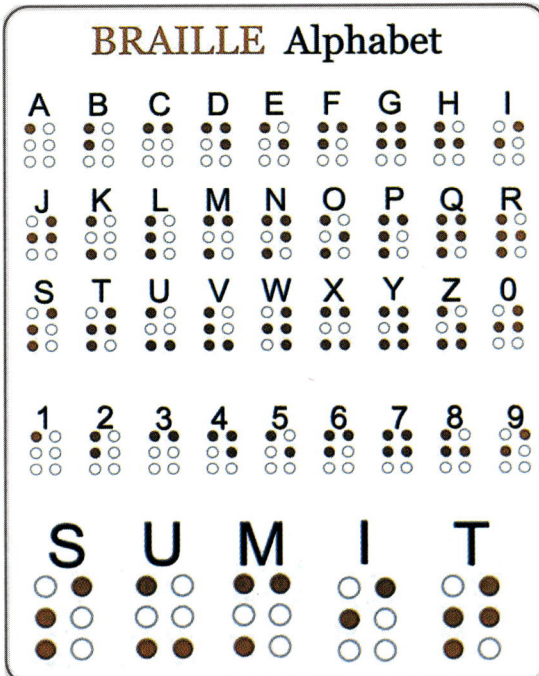

Fig. 16.36: Braille

PRESCRIPTION OF LOW VISION DEVICES

Introduction

As discussed an accurate diagnosis and magnitude of visual problem is assessed. Once the visual status of patient is evaluated, then the appropriate low vision aid is prescribed which fulfill the objectives of prescription of low visual aids.

Objectives in Prescribing a Low Vision Device

While prescribing a low vision device clinician should consider following objectives

- Primary objective of prescription is to give maximum visual acuity, contrast and visual field with minimal influence on the movements of the patient.
- Keep an appropriate balance between amount of magnification, field of view and working distance.
- Individualize the requirement of low vision devices in different persons because motivation and mental status varies from person to person even if their visual status may be similar.
- Prescribe simpler, portable, economical and light weighted devices because complex devices are not very user friendly.
- Before finalizing the prescription, attempt similar types of low vision aids having comparable designs and /or magnification.
- Always try to prescribe binocularly, where magnification difference is not significant. However, in cases where complex electronic devices are required or patient is single eyed, it is better to prescribe the best low vision device (telescopes or hybrid double glasses) for better seeing eye.
- Avoid prescribing low vision devices for very young children or very old people mainly because both are not competent enough for accepting a low vision device.

For better understanding of the patient's requirement and before prescribing the low visual aids which satisfy the objectives of our prescription, following elements are determined

- Distance vision correction requirement
- Near vision correction requirement
- Peripheral visual field enhancement requirement

Distance vision correction requirement

- For improvement of distance vision in a visually impaired person primarily we need to magnify the distance object so that person can see the object clearly. Amount of object magnification required by a particular patient is simply calculated by dividing the denominator of their present visual acuity with the denominator of the desired visual acuity, considering that the numerators of both the acuity are the same. For example, suppose if present visual acuity is 10/120 and desired visual acuity is 10/20, then
  Amount of magnification required for distance correction = 120/20 = 6 times.
- Spectacle mounted magnifiers or head mounted electronic magnifiers are selected

on the basis of expected amount of magnification and contrast enhancement requirements.

- Appropriate telescopic system either Galilean or Keplerian is decided on the basis of desired amount of magnification, extent of field of view, contrast in image quality, and position of exit pupil.

Near vision correction requirements

Near vision correction requirements in low vision patients is not as simple as distance requirements, where simply the magnification of object is sufficient to improve the distance vision. For near vision we need to assess

- Starting addition with distance correction
- Refine the starting correction
- Equivalent power calculation

Starting addition is the power of lens requires to be added initially with the calculated distance power. This starting addition is assessed using single letter charts and can be calculated by using any one of following methods

- Starting addition calculation depending on starting near visual acuity with proper accommodation: The M system is used to measure near visual acuity and stated as a fraction (means testing distance/M letters read). Suppose if the expected target for near visual acuity is 1 M, then simply equating it in fraction representation with the present near acuity will give the amount of near correction.

  For example, suppose 6 M size letter is read at 30 cm (0.3 meter) distance. This can be represented in a fraction as 0.3/6 M.

  When equate this

  $$0.3/6\ M = X/1\ M,$$
  $$X = 0.3/6\ M\ \text{or}\ 0.05,$$

  Which means this patient require 100/5 (+20 D) dioptre addition power to read 1 M size letter, from 30 cm distance.

- Another method to calculate the starting addition power is that Snellen's distance

visual acuity is measured at 6 meters distance and then desired near visual acuity is converted into Snellen's equivalent at 40 cm. Now denominator of distance visual acuity is divided with denominator of desired near visual acuity (Snellen's equivalent at 40 cm) and the product is multiplied by 2.5 (for near distance).

For example, suppose distance visual acuity is 20/240 and desired visual acuity is 20/40, then starting addition is 240/40 multiplied by (2.5)

$$= 6 \times 2.5 = 15$$

Means +15 D power lens is required as starting addition.

- Kestenbaum's rule: It is very simple where the distance visual acuity represented in Snellen's fraction is reversed. Final product of this reversed value represents the starting addition in dioptres.

  For example, suppose distance visual acuity is 20/240, and then the reverse representation is 240/20 = 12

  Hence + 12 D starting addition is required in this case.

Refining the starting correction is done by using near vision charts having continuous reading text matter. As discussed above the starting addition power for near vision is calculated by different methods using single letter charts, however, refinement in near power is done with considering the contrast sensitivity and Amsler grid results along with near acuity require to read the text matter (newspaper, textbook, etc.) effortlessly and uninterruptedly from the desired distance. The refined power required for near correction is usually greater than the starting addition power because continuous reading of text matter require more magnification and better contrast.

Equivalent power is nothing but the power of a single lens which is equating the power of entire optical system required for magnification. Formula used to calculate the equivalent power has the power of low vision device (say P_1) and power of accommodation or addition (say P_2) and the distance between P_1 and P_2 (say d).

For spectacle magnifiers, equivalent power (say P_e) is simply the addition of two powers, i.e. P_1 and P_2. It means for spectacle magnification the equivalent power is

$$P_e = P_1 + P_2$$

For hand-held magnifiers, the distance (say d) between the low vision device and patient's eye also come into calculation, hence equivalent power for hand-held magnifier is calculated by formula

$$P_e = P_1 + P_2 - d\,(P_1 P_2)$$

Formula required in calculating the equivalent power for electronic magnifiers or CCTV is complex but this is also based on the above mentioned parameters.

Peripheral visual field enhancement requirement: Majority of low vision patients has an associated reduced peripheral visual field, hence while calculating the distance and near vision requirement we should also consider the requirements to enhance the peripheral visual field in these cases. To increase the peripheral visual field an appropriate optical system is selected and then patient is trained to use this system. To enhance the peripheral visual field in a low vision patient, various optical systems can be used as follows

- *Prisms:* As discussed above prisms can be incorporated in spectacles by keeping the base towards the visual field defects, so that when patient sees through prism the object image will shift towards the apex of prism and will be seen by the patient.
- *Mirrors:* Use of mirrors is another method of shifting the object image from non-seeing area to seeing area by placing the mirror angle towards the field defects.
- *Reverse telescopes and minus lenses:* Both of these optical systems enhance the field of view in low vision patients by minifying the image so that more information is seen in a particular visual field.

In a nutshell, prescription of a low visual aid is done in the following sequence

- First of all try a spherical convex lens in spectacle frame to correct distance vision then add an appropriate power of near addition as calculated by various methods (as discussed above), either in the form of monocular or binocular glasses.
- Suppose field of view is not adequate then add a converging prism in the above prescription.
- If no improvement with spectacle glasses is seen then advice hand-held magnifier with an appropriate magnification, whereas no improvement with hand-held magnifiers will be followed by the prescription of a stand magnifier.
- Telescopes, and electronic devices are complex to use and expensive hence are kept as reserved and are rarely prescribed in some cases showing no improvement with conventional devices.

Supportive Services in Low Vision Management

Visual rehabilitation is an important and integral part in the management of low vision patients. It consists of education, training, assistance and support or provides means which may benefit a visually impaired person. In addition to low vision, many patients especially in older age group may develop depression due to hazardous effects of visual impairment. Following supportive services and their recommendations can be done with the help of several governmental and non-governmental organizations

- Medical condition related counseling (psychiatric or psychological)
- Nutritional counseling (especially, for diabetics)
- Genetic counseling
- Employment related training
- Supportive medical/ocular services
- Procurement of supportive devices such as talking books or computer softwares from public library

Training/Instructions to Patient

Training of the patients about the uses and drawbacks of prescribed optical system is an important part while dispensing the visual aid device. Individually patients must be taught about the best way of utilization and maintenance of that particular low vision aid. Optical systems which are complex in nature will need harder and longer training for optimal usage of device, however, in majority of cases regular practice, improves the handling and usage of even a complex optical devices. Regular practice and proper training of low vision aid has shown good reading speed and even longer duration wear of complex devices in majority of cases.

Following instructions and training about the prescribed low vision device are given to the patients at the time of dispensing or during successive meetings for better outcome

- Type of low vision aid.
- Functioning of low vision device.
- Coordinating usage of prescribed low vision aid such as distance maintenance, proper lighting and proper timing of usage.
- Timely maintenance, i.e. changing the battery or recharging the device and proper care of device.
- Avoid any hazardous situation by using the device at improper timing like during driving or coming down from staircase with head mounted devices.

Apart from abovementioned routine and general instruction, many visually impaired patients also need some additional training to utilize their remaining vision more proficiently.

Various specialized training procedures are advised on individualized pattern based on remaining visual acuity, category of prescribed low vision appliance, size and position of scotoma (if present), and specific objectives.

Specialized training requires to use remaining vision include the following strategies

- Eccentric viewing
- Recognition of the sentence from words

- Interpretation of blur images
- Target scanning and identification
- Fixating the eyes during saccadic eye movements
- Identify the pursuit movements
- Memorize the target and recognize it on reappearance

Patient Education

Patient education is equally important as that of an effective treatment, hence after the completion of clinical evaluation all practitioner must analyze and should discuss about their examination findings with the patients and their concern relatives. This discussion with patient and their family members give a comprehensive understanding of the eye disease, natural course and prognosis of present ocular disease with various functional limitations. This healthy discussion and patient education will help in a successful management and rehabilitation of visually impaired person.

For successful treatment these following factors evaluated during examination should be discussed with patients and their family members, while dispensing the visual aids

- Amount of motivation evaluated in the patient.
- Benefits and limitations of the treatment offered.
- Description of treatment strategies with probable prognosis for success of offered treatment.
- Expected time required for training of use of device and desire of compliance for successful rehabilitation.

Patient counseling and education elements include these strategies

- Establish the relationship between patient's visual status and visual signs/symptoms evaluated during examination.
- Select the best possible rehabilitation strategy with its decisive factors and expected outcomes in terms of achievement of treatment objectives.

- Prepare the evaluation facts and/or directives for patient in detailed written document.
- Discuss in detail about importance of the regular follow-up and patient obedience in relation to the prescribed low vision management.
- Time framing for re-evaluation and follow-up advices.

Prognosis and Follow-up Visits

Overall prognosis and visual outcome in low vision therapy depends on several factors such as

- Primary cause of poor visual acuity
- Category and amount of visual impairment
- Physical and mental status of patients
- Aims and objectives of rehabilitation
- Patient's approach, enthusiasm and hopes towards low visual aids
- Practitioner's mindset and impulse towards visual outcome

Frequency and duration of follow-up visits will be decided by these aspects

- How well the patient is reacting to the prescribed low vision treatment
- Whether the ocular status of patient is stable or deteriorating

When desired aims and objectives of therapy are achieved then follow-up visits to assess various aspects related to treatment should be done on a regular basis. The follow-up visit schedule can be decided by both the practitioner and the patient. These routine follow-up visits should be done to evaluate the patient's

- ocular health status
- visual condition
- visual performance
- low vision aid adaptation

Although patient's requirements and visual condition may change over time period, but it is essential for a visually impaired patient to realize the necessity of re-evaluation. Patients should know that there will be a gradual change in visual condition, however, they should not presume that sudden drop in vision is normal for their ocular condition. Similarly, practitioner should also be aware that if there is a sudden change in the patient's requirements, re-evaluation is necessary to resolve their recently developed visual status.

Problem-based Learning

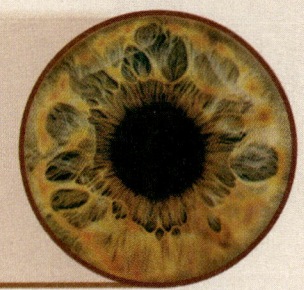

CHAPTER 17

Problems Related to Refractive Errors and Presbyopia

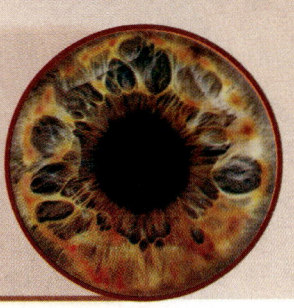

MYOPIA

Problem 1: A young person aged 17 years, having mild asthenopic symptoms was presented to clinic. On examination, distance visual acuity was found relatively normal, however, on performing a subjective refraction patient is accepting minus spherical power of reasonable degree.

1. Why patient is accepting minus power?
2. How do you manage such cases?

Solution:

1. While performing a subjective refraction it is very important to keep in mind that the patient should not be corrected with too much minus power. Many a times, young patients use accommodation during subjective refraction, hence they accept minus power lenses. Usually young patients prefer extra minus power because when compensated by accommodation, letters on acuity chart look smaller and darker which patient think as better vision.

2. For managing such situation following methods can be used during refraction

   - Patient must be trained to compare only the clarity of letters on vision chart. Inform the patient that if letters become smaller and darker, then they should be considered as same choice, not as better choice.
   - Fogging or astigmatic dial technique (Chapter 11 Page 290) should be performed where patient begins with a choice from plus power lenses.

   - Duo-chrome test (Chapter 11 Page 292) should be done to know if more minus power is given or not.
   - Finally, if we are not satisfied with above mentioned methods then cycloplegic refraction or wet retinoscopy (Chapter 11) can be done to relax the accommodation. This gives us the accurate refractive status of this young patient who is accepting the significant degree of minus power.

Note: In young asymptomatic patients accepting minus power spheres for distance vision, always perform cycloplegic refraction specifically with atropine to know the correct refractive status.

Problem 2: A 60 years old lady presented with complain of fluctuation in distance vision since 3–4 years. She had a history of radial keratectomy done about 40 years back and since then she had problem of glare and poor contrast sensitivity. Recently, since 15 years her power of glasses for distance and near had increased regularly and abruptly.

1. What are the causes of symptoms and fluctuation in refractive error?
2. How would you manage this case?

Solution:

1. Most probable cause of symptoms like glare and poor contrast sensitivity may be

   - Radial keratectomy (RK) especially, with smaller treatment zone and deeper incisions to correct higher degree myopia. Size of pupil plays an important role for manifestation of glare because if

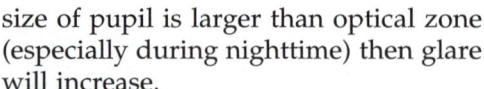

size of pupil is larger than optical zone (especially during nighttime) then glare will increase.

- Formation of cataract is another possibility for increased glare at nighttime at the age of 60 years.
- Fluctuation in refractive error may also be due to change in refractive status post-radial keratectomy because contraction of incisional wound usually causes refractive shift mostly towards hypermetropia.
- Similarly, the corneal irregularities, scarring and smaller optical zone are causes for fluctuation in refractive errors. Moreover, formation of cataract especially nuclear sclerosis will also contribute to the change in refractive status.

2. Management of this case includes detail evaluation of
   - Pupil size in daylight and dim light
   - Status of cornea in terms of optical zone, scarring and keratometry
   - Cycloplegic refraction twice in daytime and evening
   - Assessment of cataract if present
   - Detailed fundus evaluation
   - Suppose the size of pupil is large, then advice the pharmacological treatment using pilocarpine to induce miosis which will reduce the glare, especially during nighttime. Perform meticulous cycloplegic refraction to know the amount and type of refractive error and prescribe glasses accordingly. Majority of these post-RK patients will have irregular type of astigmatic refractive errors, hence they may require refractive surgical procedures for correction of refractive error.
   - Hypermetropic refractive shift (due to radial keratectomy) and presbyopia (due to progressive age) will cause difficulty in near vision, hence she may require higher additional power than usual to see the near objects.
   - Suppose cataract is present, then decide according to the best corrected visual

acuity with glasses, if BCVA is satisfactory, prescribe glasses and if not, then advice for cataract surgery with possible visual outcome.

Problem 3: An elderly person of age about 68 years presented to clinic with diminished distance vision with existing spectacles (fitted with two years old prescription). On examination, an additional –1.5 D change was found in each eye.

1. What are the probable causes for this acquired myopia?
2. How you will prescribe a new spectacle power in this case and what all possibilities you will consider in management of this case?

Solution:

1. Probable causes for acquired myopia at an age of 68 years may be
   - Cataract (most probably nuclear sclerotic type)
   - Diabetes mellitus of recent onset or with poor glycemic control
   - Recent retinal detachment surgery (scleral buckling)
   - Medications (e.g. chloroquine, anti-depressants, sulfa drugs, chlorthalidone, etc.)

2. Prescription of new spectacle power requires consideration of following possibilities
   - Suppose cause of acquired myopia is cataract, then patient must be described in details that change in power in spectacles will improve the vision but will not solve the problem of cataract.
   - New prescription power should be placed in trial frame and shown to the patient binocularly to check the distance and near vision. Suppose there is an improvement in the distance visual acuity with new prescription power but the near vision get more adverse due to increased myopic shift, then more add power should be prescribed.

- Consult with the patient whether the change in prescription will allow them to carry out their daily activities adequately or not. Suppose outcome is that they can perform their daily activities comfortably with glasses, then offer new prescription. However, if they feel difficulty in performing daily activities with new prescription, then advice cataract surgery for vision improvement. When patient is unclear about outcome, then prescribe the new glasses and wait for the outcome in follow-up visits.

- If cause of acquired myopia is uncontrolled diabetes, then first it is necessary to stabilize the blood sugar level. Once the sugar level is stabilized, then do cycloplegic refraction again and prescribe new glasses.

- If cause of acquired myopia is exposure to medications, then first of all discontinuation of medications is required. In addition, also discuss with patient about the duration of exposure to medications which will decide whether patient requires change in prescription or not.

- Myopia secondary to retinal detachment surgery is usually astigmatic error and will improve when scleral buckle is removed after some time, however, until that period appropriate power glasses with prisms should be prescribed to maintain the visual acuity and avoid monocular diplopia.

Problem 4: An adult aged 38 years having moderate degree myopia appeared for routine eye checkup to the clinic. This patient was habitual of wearing contact lenses in office and outdoor activities. On examination, a small increase in the myopic correction was found.

1. What should be further course of management in prescribing new refractive power?
2. How will you reduce the accommodative demand and also increase the retinal image size in this 38 years old patient?

Solution:
1. An ideal way to manage this case is that show the amount of change in vision quality to the patient, first by placing the older prescription and then the newer prescription. Now ask the patient whether he/she would like to wear a new pair of glasses (contact lenses) or not depending on the improvement in vision noticed by him/her during examination. This methodology (i.e. let the patient decide about the change) should be followed in every case presenting for any probable change in prescription.

2. To reduce the accommodative demand we will advice use of spectacles for correction of myopia because in myopes spectacle glasses not only increase the retinal image size but also reduce the efforts of accommodation, which is very useful in person approaching the age of presbyopia (Chapter 13, Page 367).

Note: As this patient is approaching the age of presbyopia any amount of increase in minus power will affect the near vision significantly, hence it is advisable to evaluate the patient both for distance and near vision if we are correcting the myopic error at this age.

Problem 5: 40 years old male presented with diminished distance vision with monocular diplopia from left eye since one month. He had undergone an encirclage band buckle surgery in left eye for large retinal tear about one month back. The retinal tear was located in the periphery and was not involving the macular area. After scleral buckle surgery the unaided visual acuity was 6/6 in the right eye and 6/60 in the left eye, however, with pinhole the visual acuity in left eye improved to 6/9. On further evaluation left eye showed 12Δ exotropia with 4Δ hypertropia.

1. What are the causes for his symptoms?
2. Outline the effects of lenses on tropia.
3. How would you mange this case?

Solution:
1. Scleral buckling causes myopic shift due to elongation of posterior segment of eye. This

myopic shift leads to diminution of distance vision in this case. Simultaneously, the pressure effects and changes in corneal curvature after scleral buckling lead to irregular astigmatic error which causes monocular diplopia in some cases. These symptoms are more pronounced in those cases where encirclage buckle is applied compared to partial buckle.

2. As per the rule the minus lenses show more deviation than plus lenses, hence with minus lenses the tropia appears more and with plus lenses the tropia appears less. Simple formula 'percentage difference = 2.5 × deviation' can be used to calculate the prismatic effect of lenses on tropia.

3. As significant amount of increase in visual acuity is seen with pinhole test, the diminished distance vision and also the diplopia can be managed by correction of refractive error alone. Cycloplegic refraction is done to estimate the complete amount of refractive error and glasses are prescribed. To correct exotropia prisms (base in) are added, this will also eliminate the monocular double vision.

Note: If diplopia is not improved with correction of refractive error with glasses and prisms, then the cause of diplopia is probably muscular misalignment. This needs correction in scleral buckle or removal of buckle once retina is settled.

Problem 6: A 46 years aged person is reading book comfortably without using reading glasses or bifocals or progressive glasses at routine reading distance.

1. What are possible reasons for clear near vision at this age in this patient (normally we expect symptoms of presbyopia at this age)?

2. What sort of management is needed in this case?

Solution:

1. Various possibilities of this patient reading comfortably without using glasses are
   - Patient may be having low degree myopia and not using glasses for distance vision.

- Another possibility is that patient is wearing glasses for myopia, but almost certainly his/her myopic refractive error is not fully corrected.

- Sometimes, a myopic person might be reading after taking off their spectacles, a condition called natural near sightedness.

2. Various possible modes of management in this patient are
   - Suppose patient is low degree myope and is satisfied with his/her distance and near vision, then there is no need to prescribe glasses either for distance or near vision.

   - In the situation where patient is wearing myopic glasses but is undercorrected, then the best way is not to prescribe an additional minus power to fully correct the distance refractive error because patient is not complaining about distance vision and also is comfortably seeing the near objects. Moreover, keeping them under-corrected allows them not to move for a bifocal or progressive addition lens immediately. However, correction of myopic prescription may be required along with addition of a bifocal or progressive addition lens if patient performance for distance is not satisfactory.

   - In case of natural near sightedness where patient is comfortable, then there is no need to prescribe for a bifocal or progressive glasses because these patients are used to read from a nearer distance than normal reading distance and prescription of bifocals or progressive lenses will disturb their routine reading distance.

Problem 7: An elderly person aged 52 years having high degree myopia, wearing progressive glasses regularly arrived to clinic for eye check up with desire to remove heavy progressive glasses. Ocular examination reveals that spectacle power is accurate, needs no correction and eyes are also in good health.

1. What kind of advice we should give to this patient considering that he/she has no systemic illness?
2. What other alternatives we can offer to this patient to get rid of heavy glasses?

Solution:

1. Considering the age of patient and high degree of myopia following advices can be given to this patient:
   - Usually high degree myopes have increased chances of development of posterior segment complications like lattice degenerations, retinal holes or tears and macular degenerations. In this patient a detailed fundus examination should be done to rule out any posterior segment lesion and the patient should be informed about potential complications of high degree myopia.
   - We must advice the patient to report immediately if he/she develops symptoms of retinal damage in the form of change in temporal vision, floaters or flashes.
   - On every regular follow-up visit including present visit a detail dilated fundus examination is done to rule out any pathological myopic changes. If changes are present an immediate treatment should be done to prevent any devastating outcome like retinal detachment.
2. Various alternatives to high power myopic glasses can be offered to this patient after performing the corneal keratometry and corneal topography
   - Suppose patient is fit for refractive surgery, then the best possible alternative to glasses is laser correction of myopic error. Considering the age of patient and degree of myopia, the best possible laser treatment is with Femtosecond Lasik surgery (Chapter 15, page 477).
   - If the patient is not fit for refractive surgery, then other optical alternatives such as contact lenses of suitable designs (rotational non-spherical contact lenses) and aspherical high index lenses (reduces the weight and thickness of glasses) can be offered to this patient.

Problem 8: An adult aged 36 years having moderate degree myopia, presented with complaint of difficulty in reading while using existing glasses. However, the reading fluency is increased when glasses slides down on the patient's nose.

1. Can we consider this as presbyopia and what is the possible diagnosis for near vision problem?
2. How will you manage this case?

Solution:

1. For an individual of 36 years of age, presbyopia is very unlikely diagnosis for difficulty in near vision. Most strong possibility is that patient was over corrected for myopic error with minus lenses for distance vision since starting of glasses wear. This is further confirmed by the fact that reading ability improves with sliding down the glasses on nose, because with increase in vertex distance the minus power decreases. At a younger age, the patient's accommodation power was able to compensate for this extra minus power prescribed in glasses. However, with advancing age (at 36 years) the accommodative ability is decreased gradually which is now not sufficient to overcome the excessive minus power in the present glasses. So this myopic patient is not left with enough accommodation to be use for reading purposes and developed symptoms of near vision.
2. Best method to mange this patient is to perform a cycloplegic refraction (preferably using atropine) and estimate the accurate degree of myopia. Once the exact amount of myopic error is determined, then the patient may be prescribed with the new prescription, which most likely will have less minus power.

Problem 9: A 38 years old asymptomatic patient walked in clinic for routine eye check-up. He had never used spectacles for either distance or near vision and presently working comfortably on computers. However, after ocular examination and post-cycloplegic refraction, a small degree of myopia is revealed.

1. What should be our course of management in this case?

Solution:

1. On discussion and examination, following advices can be given to this patient
   - If patient feels that his/her distance vision is adequate and on examination only a slight myopic correction is needed, then it is better for the patient to continue his/her routine work without distance glasses.
   - At the age of 38 years avoid any kind of near correction, especially when we found a small degree of myopia.
   - Manage this patient just by Counseling and advice of regular follow-up.

Problem 10: A 48 years old –2 DS myopic patient presented to clinic with the complain that he has to remove the distance vision glasses off and on to read the books or newspaper. Presently patient's near vision without glasses is satisfactory at routine reading distance, however, the patient desires to prescribe new glasses so that he needs not to remove the glasses either to see the distance or near targets.

1. Describe the problem with possible solutions.
2. Explain the various prismatic effects associated with bifocal or multifocal glasses.

Solution:

1. The patient is presbyopic at the age of 48 years and his accommodation is completely exhausted. Hence he is unable to compensate for 2 dioptre myopia while reading a book so he needs to remove the myopic glasses to read the book comfortably. As patient does not want to remove his glasses to read, then the best option for him is to use either bifocal or multifocal glasses so that he can see both the distance and near targets without removing the glasses. Suppose patient works on computer, then options are trifocals, computer glasses or progressive glasses.

2. In case of bifocal lenses the common prismatic effects (discussed in Chapter 12, page 348) are
   - Differential displacement at segment top (image jump): This image jump occurs due to near segment in bifocal lens and is more problematic than other prismatic effects of bifocal lens. When person sees suddenly from distance portion to near portion the image of the object appears as if jumped from its place, which take some time for adjustment.
   - Differential displacement at reading level (image displacement): This occurs due to the relative reading position in near segment and is minimum with straight top D bifocal lenses design.
   - Total displacement is the sum of both these prismatic effects and is dependent on the refractive power of distance and near addition portion.

Problem 11: A 40 years old office executive having moderate degree (–3.5 DS) myopia presented to clinic with a desire of corrective refractive surgery for myopia. There is history of wearing contact lenses during family functions or gatherings. No history of medical illness is present.

1. What advice would you give to this patient?
2. Compare refractive surgery and progressive glasses in relation to this case.

Solution:

1. As this patient is approaching the presbyopic age and might not have been aware about the fact that refractive surgery will correct only distance refractive error in his case, our prime duty is to counsel this patient about the pros and cons of myopic corrective refractive surgery. Patient should be well informed that after surgery the distance vision will be alright and there is no need to wear optical correction for distance vision ever, however, as the person is nearing presbyopic age there will be requirement of reading glasses in coming years. The patient will also loose the advantages of natural near sightedness after laser surgery. Moreover, complications related to laser surgery should be explained in detail before performing the surgery.

2. Considering the age of patient and work profile, progressive glasses are also very good alternative for his problem because the patient can have quality vision with less accommodative demand in progressive glasses. For cosmetic reasons patient can occasionally use contact lenses of bifocal or multifocal design (Chapter 14, page 428). Post-LASIK surgery patient needs to wear glasses for near vision and moreover there are chances that intermediate vision may also get affected after LASIK, hence progressive glasses are very good choice at age of 40 years.

Note: Many moderate degree myopes feel comfort in reading without glasses during presbyopic age and do not want to lose this natural nearsightedness at presbyopic age.

■ **Problem 12:** 56 years old moderate degree (–2.75 DS) myopic patient presented to clinic with a desire of myopic corrective refractive surgery. Patient is already wearing progressive glasses since 14 years and having a vision of 6/6 and N6 in each eye with glasses. There is no history of medical illness or symptoms of cataract, however, grade one peripheral cortical lenticular changes are seen on dilated fundus examination.

1. How will you counsel the patient?
2. What is line of management in this case?

Solution:

1. Before counseling the patient clinician must confirm about
   - Status of anterior segment specially cataract.
   - Posterior segment status
   - Corneal surface status and related problems like dry eye or scars.
   - Pupillary assessment in bright and dim light conditions

   Once these evaluations are recorded and found to be within normal limits, then explain the patient regarding their refractive status, stating that the patient needs refractive correction both for distance and near vision and counsel the patient with these options.
   - Suppose distance vision is corrected fully in both the eyes by refractive surgery, then he/she will need to wear glasses for near vision.
   - There is no option that only near vision gets corrected by refractive surgery.
   - Rate of progression of cataract or any other ocular condition will not be affected by refractive surgery and patient will eventually require cataract surgery when it will mature.
   - With gradual maturity of cataractous changes there will be slight changes in refractive status specifically for distance vision.

2. Management of this particular case is slightly on different line compared to routine refractive surgery case because practitioner needs to correct both the distance and near vision in an elderly patient by corneal refractive surgery. Following treatment options can be given to the patient
   - Monovision LASIK can be done which means one eye is corrected fully for distance vision and fellow eye will be

fully corrected for near vision, so that no spectacles are required for both distance and near vision.

- Multifocal LASIK is another good option to correct both distance and near vision simultaneously in both the eyes.
- Alternately multifocal intraocular lenses can be advised in both the eyes one after the other.
- Monovision with IOL, where in one eye the IOL of distance power correction and in fellow eye IOL of near power correction can also be done to correct both the distance and near vision.

Note: In adult patients having 6/6 and N6 vision in each eye, the multifocal LASIK is good option for correction of refractive error.

HYPERMETROPIA

Problem 1: An elderly person aged 47 years presented in clinic with difficulty in distance vision, although there was no such complaint in the past. The patient is wearing half eye reading glasses for near work comfortably without a prescription since 10 years. Recently the power of half eye glasses was increased by the optician.
1. Describe the probable cause of difficulty in distance vision?
2. How will you manage the case?

Solution:
1. The most probable cause of difficulty in distance vision at this age is uncorrected latent hypermetropia. The latent hypermetropia usually remains uncorrected because young healthy person does not experience any difficulty in distance vision since they have sufficient reserve of accommodation and can use his/her accommodative power to overcome the defect in distance vision. However, as the age advances, the ability of person to accommodate get deteriorate and no enough accommodation is left to overcome the latent hypermetropia, which ultimately

will appear as manifest hypermetropia. In this case also prior to age of 47, the person used accommodation to correct distance vision and as the age increased his/her latent hypermetropia has now turn into manifest hypermetropia.

2. This patient requires correction for both the near and distance vision after performing the cycloplegic refraction. The correction can be given in the form of bifocal or progressive addition lenses or if the patient is comfortable with two pairs of glasses (used separately for distance and near), then it is another economical option. Moreover, over the counter available reading glasses can also be used if patient is having low and binocularly equal degree of hypermetropia without astigmatism. For example, +1 D pair for distance and +2.75 D pair for near.

Note: In these types of cases it is mandatory to perform a cycloplegic refraction preferably using atropine drops to evaluate the exact degree of latent and manifest hypermetropia.

Problem 2: A 21 years old college student presented to clinic with history of ocular strain, frontal headache and brow ache since 2 years. His symptoms are exaggerated with continuous reading or studying in classroom. Past history revealed that he had been prescribed spectacles for distance and reading purposes about 3 years back, which he used off and on to relieve the symptoms of headache. Patient has no history of medical illness.
1. What all additional evaluation you would like to perform to reach the diagnosis in this case?
2. On cycloplegic refraction of this patient, the error found in right eye is +0.75 DS (6/6) and left eye is +0.25 DS (6/6), and orthoptic examination showed orthophoria for distance and 4Δ exophoria in near. Discuss the differential diagnosis of this case.
3. Outline the management strategies for this case.

Solution:

1. To establish diagnosis in this case we should perform cycloplegic refraction, orthoptic assessments and measure the range and amplitude of accommodation. This additional information will help us to confirm the diagnosis like hypermetropia, and/or muscular imbalance in this young patient.

2. Various possible diagnoses in this patient are hypermetropia, convergence insufficiency or accommodation insufficiency. As for distance there was orthophoria and exophoria for near and the range and amplitude of accommodation was also normal, thus this case may be of low degree hypermetropia with convergence insufficiency.

3. Management of this patient is mainly done by advising orthoptic treatment of convergence insufficiency (discussed in Chapter 8, page 177). Optical correction of low degree hypermetropia should not be recommended because it may worsen the asthenopic symptoms in case of convergence insufficiency. As the amount of exophoria is small there is no need of additional prism therapy in this case, however, sometimes for rapid and effective results base in prisms can be added. Surgical treatment of convergence insufficiency will not be required in this particular case.

▌ Problem 3: Young adult male, aged 36 years wearing hypermetropic correction was having no problems with distance and near vision with prescribed glasses since last 12 years. Now this patient is presented to clinic with difficulty in near vision with his present glasses, however the distance vision with these glasses is comfortable and clear.

1. Whether this patient became presbyopic and if not, what is the likely diagnosis?

2. What sort of management is required to correct near vision problem?

Solution:

1. As we have discussed on page 567 that appearance of presbyopia at the age of 36 years is very unlikely. Most possible diagnosis is that the hypermetropia of this patient was not corrected completely with the glasses prescribed to him, i.e. latent hypermetropia persisted in spite of correction for hypermetropia. This latent hypermetropia was getting compensated by the excessive accommodation efforts of the patient till age of 36 years. As the age advanced the accommodation ability decreased gradually, as a result an inadequate amount of accommodation is left for reading so this patient experienced difficulty in near vision. Most likely diagnosis in this case is under corrected hypermetropia, where only the manifest part was corrected and latent part was not corrected by glasses.

2. Management strategies for this under-corrected hypermetropic patient are

   • The latent hypermetropia can be revealed by doing cycloplegic refraction or retinoscopy, i.e. testing refraction after abolishing the tone of ciliary muscle so that hypermetropia cannot be overcome by accommodation of patient. If latent hypermetropia of high degree is detected on refraction with cycloplegia, then it is recommended to do post-cycloplegic refraction to confirm that the additional plus power prescribed to patient during cycloplegic refraction is adequate for patient without cycloplegia also, because as the accommodation tone of the eye returns to normal, the visual acuity may alter.

   • On the other hand, a push plus technique can be performed during non-cycloplegic refraction to know the maximum plus power which the patient can tolerate. During testing, the plus spherical power is added progressively until the patient notices slight blurring or discomfort. This plus power indicates full hypermetropic correction to be given and it should be corrected in stages to avoid intolerance because tone of ciliary

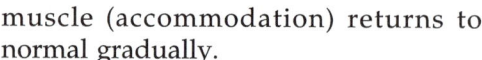

muscle (accommodation) returns to normal gradually.

- Alternately, contact lenses can be prescribed to this patient, because the mechanism of relaxation of accommodation is much gradual and also the tolerance to high plus power is better.

Note: Many a times patients of younger age group having quite well distance and near vision without any glass may also complain the problem in near vision when they approaches the presbyopic age because of latent hypermetropia.

Problem 4: A 5 years old child having history of occasional mild deviation of eyes was brought by parents to the clinic for detailed evaluation. There is no past history of any systemic illness. On examination no manifest squint was seen, however, cycloplegic refraction has revealed a refractive error of +1.75D in both the eyes.

1. Explain the probable cause of deviation of eyes.
2. What should be the course of management?

Solution:

1. Most probable causes of occasional deviation of the eyes in young child are mild degree of hypermetropia or muscular imbalance due to systemic illness. As there is no history of systemic illness in this child then the most probable diagnosis for deviation of eyes is hypermetropia.

2. There is no need of any optical correction in this case. Usually, young children presenting with low to moderate degree of hypermetropia, with no strabismus and no visual difficulty do not require any correction for refractive error because child has enough amount of accommodation to overcome the hypermetropia which is elicited without any conscious effort by the child, i.e. without any symptoms of eye strain. However, if hypermetropia is more than 3 D and child also having symptoms of eye strain then optical correction should be prescribed. If there is associated strabismus or amblyopia, then other therapies like occlusion therapy, etc. are also required with optical correction.

Problem 5: An elderly male aged 70 years wearing bifocals since 28 years is presented to clinic with recent onset of diminution of vision for distance and near. On examination, a change in refractive power suggestive of recent onset hypermetropic shift was found.

1. What are the possible causes for this recent onset hypermetropic shift?
2. How would you mange this case?

Solution:

1. Diminution of both distance and near vision along with refractive shift towards hypermetropia in this age may probably occur due to

- Diabetes mellitus: Recent onset diabetic mellitus having poor glycemic control or fluctuations in glucose levels due to long standing diabetes mellitus may cause hypermetropic shift.

- Cortical cataract in some cases may cause mild hyperopic shift in older age patients, however, majority of cortical cataract causes an associated astigmatic error which can lead to the difficulty in distance and near vision.

- Anterior shifting of retina due to retinal edema or central serous chorioretinopathy will lead to hyperopic shift because of the defective focusing of light rays on the retina.

2. The management of this patient includes detailed posterior segment evaluation and sometimes even assistance of advance diagnostic instruments like optical coherence topography, fundus angiography to establish the cause of hyperopic shift.

- If poorly controlled diabetes mellitus is the cause of change in refractive status, then the patient should be referred to physician for better control of blood sugar.

- In case of cataract if change in glasses gives satisfactory vision, then we can prescribe new power of glasses and if vision is not satisfactory with glasses then patient should be advised to undergo the cataract surgery.

- If posterior segment lesions are the cause of hyperopic shift, then treatment of the lesions is advised.

Problem 6: Parents of a 3½ years old child brought him with complaint of deviation of eyes and inattentiveness of surroundings while playing with toys. Parents noticed deviations of eyes when child tries to focus the near objects, however, the deviation was less marked when child watches the television. The birth history is normal and child is showing normal developmental milestones.

1. What is the probable diagnosis?
2. If on refraction moderate degree of hypermetropia found in the child, how will you manage the case?

Solution:

1. Most probable cause of deviation of the eyes in young child having no other ocular abnormalities is uncorrected refractive error specially hypermetropia. To confirm the diagnosis cycloplegic refraction should be done using atropine ointment. Suppose the refractive error found in this case was moderate degree hypermetropia (say +6.5 DS in each eye). Thus, the diagnosis of this case is accommodative squint due to high degree hypermetropia with high AC/A ratio.

2. Management of the case includes correction of hypermetropia by plus power glasses. In this case the full correction is given in spectacle power and parents are advised to make sure that the child must wear the glasses regularly. Due to defective accommodation and high AC/A ratio the child may show deviation in near vision in spite of using hyperopic glasses. Suppose after full correction this child shows deviation of eyes (esotropia) in near vision, then the bifocal glasses are advised, where an add is given to compensate for high

AC/A ratio (discussed in Chapter 9, page 197). The power of bifocal lenses is gradually adjusted as the age of child advances, where add power is gradually decreased because accommodation efforts are slowly compensated with plus lenses. Follow-up of child should be done strictly at 6 months interval to evaluate the amount of visual acuity and deviation of eyes.

Note: Accommodative esotropia with high AC/A ratio remain the only ophthalmic condition where bifocal glasses are advised for very young child (2–8 years age group).

Problem 7: An asymptomatic young adult aged 24 years presented to clinic for routine ocular examination. On cycloplegic refraction and examination a diagnosis of latent hypermetropia was made for which plus power glasses were prescribed to the patient. After a few days the patient again came to the clinic with complaints of intolerance to newly prescribed glasses to him.

1. What could be the causes of these symptoms?
2. How we should manage this case?

Solution:

1. In this case the most probable causes of intolerance to the prescribed glasses may be

- Imperfect cycloplegic refraction
- Post-mydriatic test (PMT) was not performed

Most probably the refraction performed was not correct (*see* the guidelines in Chapter 11 for refraction techniques) and either an overcorrection or undercorrection of hypermetropia has been done. In both these situations accommodation ability of patient will affect which lead to asthenopic symptoms or intolerance to glasses. Moreover, a post-mydriatic test was also not performed to assess the tolerance of the plus power lenses, because this patient was going to wear the plus power spectacles first time in his life. In these patients the ciliary muscle tone had been used to overcome the latent hypermetropia since long duration and this increased ciliary tone is difficult to get relaxed all of a sudden by use of plus power lenses.

2. To manage the condition of intolerance this patient should be advised to come for a repeat cycloplegic refraction to check the accuracy of prescription.

   • If cycloplegic refraction is found accurate and significant amount of plus sphere power is detected then advice the patient to come again for a post-mydriatic test. Post-cycloplegic refraction gives an accurate assessment of patient's tolerance of new plus power prescribed to him so it is mandatory to perform this test before writing the final prescription. In first prescription it is recommended to prescribe less plus power lenses than the total power required to correct the entire hypermetropic error. Gradually, in subsequent follow up visits the plus power can be increased as the tolerance of patient increases to plus power spectacles.

   • Suppose the refraction was incorrect and an undercorrection or overcorrection had been done, then simply perform a PMT and write a new prescription with accurate power of lenses.

> **Note:** Once the plus power lenses are started to be used by the patient then this increased ciliary muscle tone will gradually decline. Now gradually the power of plus lenses can be stepped up to correct the entire degree of hypermetropic error.

Problem 8: A 21 years old high hyperopic (+7 DS in each eye) female patient presented to the clinic with dissatisfaction of wearing thick lenses and she wants to get rid of her spectacles.

1. What all possible options are available for her to get rid of her glasses?
2. What best advice you will give to this patient?

Solution:

1. The various possible options for this high hyperopic patient to get rid of glasses are

   • Contact lens wear: As the power of glasses is only spherical, she can comfortably wear contact lenses and get rid of glasses. Advantages of contact lenses are better cosmetic appearance and lesser spherical aberrations compared to the spectacles. Efforts on accommodation are also reduced due to decreased vertex distance in the contact lenses (Chapter 13, page 367).

   • Refractive surgery: Her hyperopia can be permanently corrected by refractive procedures specially C-LASIK or Femtosecond LASIK (discussed in Chapter 15, on page 489). Advantages of refractive surgery are lifetime correction of refractive error, however, a few disadvantages are dry eye, glare and decreased contrast sensitivity (discussed in Chapter 15).

2. Considering her age and amount of the refractive error the best possible advice for this young lady is to undergo the refractive procedure for correction of high degree hypermetropia. Using contact lenses for long period are very cumbersome and also not complication free, hence refractive surgery is a better choice in this case.

Problem 9: Young college student aged 25 years presented with difficulty in reading for some duration continuously. There is no history of wearing glasses and previous ocular examination. This student tries to read in installments and get relief when take rest in between reading.

1. Discuss the possible diagnosis in this case.
2. How will you manage the problem?

Solution:

1. At 25 years of age presbyopia is not a diagnosis so reading difficulty might be due to these following situations

   • Latent hypermetropia: A large amount of latent hypermetropia may cause difficulty in near vision in young adult because at this age, the accommodation ability of person is unable to compensate the hypermetropic error and the hidden refractive error will manifest.

- Convergence insufficiency: Patients having convergence insufficiency face difficulty in reading for longer duration and develops asthenopic symptoms. Normal near point of convergence should not be farther than 8 cm, however, a receding in NPA will cause reading difficulty.

- Drugs: Several pharmacological agents used to treat condition like common cold, migraine, motion sickness or some central nervous system disorders may affect pupillary sphincters. This causes faulty accommodation and leads to difficulty in reading. A detailed treatment history is must before concluding the cause of reading difficulty in a young adult.

2. Management of this case depends on the cause of near vision problem

- Suppose the latent hypermetropia is the cause, then perform cycloplegic refraction and prescribe the full correction in first sitting.

- Suppose convergence insufficiency is the cause of problem, then the convergence exercises (discussed in Chapter 8) are very effective in relieving the symptoms.

- Suppose the patient is on any drug causing difficulty in near vision then the best option is refer the case to physician and ask the opinion about discontinuing the drug.

ASTIGMATISM

Problem 1: Young adult of age 20 years, having mixed myopic error came for routine follow-up visit. The patient is presently wearing a small cylindrical power lenses, whereas now on subjective refraction suddenly the patient was found to be accepting a larger degree of cylindrical power.

1. What could be the possible reasons for this change in cylindrical power?
2. How would you prescribe new power?

Solution:

1. Various possible reasons for sudden acceptance of large cylindrical power in this case are

- Firstly, the reason of increase cylindrical power may be increase in the astigmatic power of the patient. Though it is very unlikely that there is only increase in the astigmatic error of patient's present prescription; thus it becomes necessary to recheck for inaccuracy of earlier prescription.

- Another possibility is that the patient is using too much minus spherical power which will ultimately lead to increase in cylindrical power. In this case chances of over minusing are high, because for every half dioptre of over-minused prescription, the cylinder plus power needs an increase by one dioptre to maintain the spherical equivalent.

For example, suppose the exact refractive error of patient is: $-2 \times +1.0 \times 90°$; means the spherical equivalent is -1.5 D.

- If spherical power of this patient gets wrongly overcorrected by -0.50 dioptre sphere, then to maintain a spherical equivalent of -1.5 D an additional $+1.0$ D cylinder power is needed to equalize this spherical overcorrection. So the resultant final prescription will become $-2.5 \times +2.0 \times 90°$.

- Suppose this patient is overcorrected by -0.75 D spherical power then to maintain a spherical equivalent of -1.5 D, an additional $+1.5$ D cylinder power is needed to equalize this spherical overcorrection. So the resultant final prescription will become $-2.75 \times + 2.5 \times 90°$.

2. In this patient repeat cycloplegic refraction is done to know the exact power of spherical

and cylindrical errors. Post-mydriatic test (PMT) is done to know the minimum power of minus sphere and maximum power of plus cylinders acceptance by the patient. After PMT the power must be prescribed for spectacle lenses.

Problem 2: Middle-aged patient having a mixed astigmatic refractive error was presented to clinic for routine follow-up. Previous prescription of glasses was –5.5 DS × + 1.5 DC × 90° in both the eyes. After cycloplegic refraction the new glasses prescription came out to be –5.25 DS × + 2 DC × 95° for right eye and –6 DS × + 2.75 DC × 85° for left eye.

After wearing this new prescription for 2–3 days, this patient came back with a complaint of severe asthenopic symptoms like sloping of computer screen, and rising of ground on walking with nausea.

1. What could be the cause of these asthenopic symptoms?
2. How does the corneal topography will appear in this case?
3. How would you manage this case?

Solution:

1. The strongest possibility of these asthenopic symptoms is the modification done in new prescription for improvement in refractive error. Among all types of refractive errors the most sensitive part of a prescription is corrections in the astigmatic portion of entire prescription. Usually a change in > 0.5 D power and >5 degree of axis in astigmatic error can cause asthenopic symptoms, especially in patients who are already wearing the astigmatic glasses with different power and axis of cylindrical lenses.

2. In this case the corneal topography will show a typical bow and tie appearance in vertical orientation. This patient has the regular with the rule type of astigmatism, where topography shows a plus astigmatic power in vertical direction.

3. This case can be managed by performing a trial screening of prescription before prescribing the final total correction in cylindrical power and axis. Initially place trial lenses of changed cylindrical power and axis in a trial frame and ask the patient to look around in the clinic or walk around wearing this trial frame. Suppose patient feels discomfort, then immediately remove the trial frame. Suppose the visual acuity is showing significant improvement with new prescription, then the change in cylindrical power is first prescribed. Once patient is adjusted to new power of cylinder, then gradually change in axis of cylinder is prescribed till the total power and axis of cylinder gets corrected.

Problem 3: In our routine village camp 26 years old person presented with complain of gradual diminution of vision for distance and associated frontal headache, since few years. This patient has no medical illness and also no history of wearing glasses in the past. In our camp set up there is no facility for retinoscopy or autorefraction.

1. What are the methods to determine an accurate astigmatic error (if present), without these facilities?

Solution:

1. When a young adult presents with gradual diminution of vision for distance and we do not have facility of autorefraction or retinoscopy; perform accurate subjective refraction as per guidelines described in Chapter 11. Many a times young adults have uncorrected astigmatic errors of mild to moderate degree. As the accommodation gradually diminishes with age, these astigmatic errors produce symptoms of diminution of vision and asthenopia. After subjective refraction patient can be prescribed the glasses to be used constantly for distance and near work.

Problem 4: A young female aged 19 years undergraduate student of college presented with complain of difficulty in seeing the letters on whiteboard in classroom and also reading book for long duration, since a few months. There is history of associated frontal headache and brow ache off and on with occasional blurring of letters in book. She has no history of medical illness or wearing of glasses in the past.

1. Outline the evaluation method to reach the proper diagnosis.
2. How will you manage the case?

Solution:

1. Complete anterior segment examination on slit lamp with unaided visual acuity is recorded. Fundus examination with optic disc evaluation is done to rule out retinal pathology and glaucoma. Cycloplegic refraction is done to assess the refractive status of the patient. Blood tests to rule out systemic conditions like anemia, thyroid disease or microelement deficiency (e.g. calcium) are ordered.

2. Suppose all the medical investigations and ocular examination came out to be normal; then probably the cause is refractive error. Cycloplegic refraction in these sorts of cases usually show a simple or mixed astigmatic error of mild to moderate degree. To manage the case complete amount of astigmatic error is recorded and initially glasses are prescribed after performing PMT, so that patient can tolerate the new prescription. Once the patient is comfortable with glasses, then complete amount of astigmatic error can be advised. After a few months of comfortable wear of glasses she can be advised to go for toric contact lenses. Once the refractive error becomes stable she can go for astigmatic refractive surgery to get rid of glasses or contact lenses.

Problem 5: An adult aged 44 years was presented with complaint of difficulty in reading small fonts since a few months. On examination along with signs of presbyopia he also had a plano-astigmatic error of −0.75 DC × 180° for distance vision in each eye. There is no history of using distance vision glasses in the past and also the patient is asymptomatic till recently. On subjective refraction this patient is well accepting a +1.5 DS × −0.5 DC + 180° for near correction.

1. What is the probable diagnosis of this case?
2. What should be our prescription?

Solution:

1. The most probable diagnosis of this case is recent onset presbyopia, because the small degree with the rule astigmatism is very common and produces no clinical symptoms. Usually these small degrees with the rule astigmatism require no correction for distance vision.

2. As per the past history patient was comfortably seeing at distance till now and would simply require correction for reading. A prescription of +1.25 D sphere is advised depending on the spherical equivalent calculated from the subjective refraction of +1.5 DS × −0.5 DC × 180°. In this particular patient there is no need to prescribe an additional astigmatism correction; however, astigmatic addition can be prescribed if patient feels an improvement in either reading or distance acuity with the addition of cylindrical power, or patient prefers to use bifocal or progressive additional glasses.

Problem 6: A 11 years old class 6th student was brought by the parents with complaint of difficulty in seeing the letters properly on blackboard. History revealed that child usually sits in front row in the class and never worn glasses; also there is no previous history of refraction done. Subjective refraction of this child is OD −1.75 DS (6/12), OS − 1.5 DS × + 0.75 DC × 70° (6/6).

On detail examination no ocular pathology was found, and VA in right eye was improving to 6/6 with pinhole.

1. What is the cause of low visual acuity in right eye?
2. How it should be managed?

Solution:

1. Most probable cause of low visual acuity in right eye is improper refraction, because

young children may have different degree of ciliary tone in each eye and hence subjective refraction may not give accurate amount of refractive error. Secondly, in majority of patients astigmatic correction is symmetrical, so it is better to search for this possibility.

2. To manage this case we need to perform a cycloplegic refraction with atropine eye drops. On PMT a complete symmetry in astigmatic error would have been indicated when refractive error for the right eye is $-1.5\,DS \times +0.75 \times 110°$, so a repeat subjective refraction for the right eye can be done considering this symmetrical prescription.

Note: When there is significant improvement is seen in visual acuity with pinhole and no ocular pathology is found on examination; then the most common cause of low visual acuity is inaccurate refraction.

▌ Problem 7: A middle aged 52 years old patient presented with complain of diplopia since few days. Ophthalmic history revealed that the patient was wearing a sphero-cylindrical correction of moderate degree in each eye since many years. On clinical evaluation monocular diplopia was discovered in right eye; however there was no deviation of eyes and extraocular movements were free and full. There is no history of medical illness like diabetes mellitus, hypertension or thyroid disease.

1. Whether refractive error can cause this recent onset diplopia?
2. How will you investigate this case?
3. Outline the management of this problem.

Solution:

1. Few selective refractive errors especially irregular astigmatism of moderate to high degree can cause severe blurring of vision with distortion of images; which occasionally can manifest as monocular diplopia. In this particular case the moderate degree astigmatic error was wrongly corrected either in terms of spherical power, cylindrical power or axis; hence the symptom of monocular double vision was appearing.

2. Any case of diplopia should be thoroughly investigated in terms of blood parameters (complete blood count, blood sugar, thyroid profile, lipid profile, etc.), MRI brain and ocular B-scan. Clinically a detail posterior segment evaluation is also necessary to rule out any intraocular lesion.

3. For the management of this case perform a meticulous cycloplegic refraction to determine the exact refractive power and cylindrical axis.
   • Suppose new prescription eliminates the symptoms of diplopia, then the cause was established and patient will be alright in a few days after wearing the new glasses.
   • However, if symptoms of monocular diplopia are still present and investigation data shows some deviations from normal, then search for other causes of monocular diplopia. Then the line of management is either medical or surgical.

Note: In cases of monocular double vision suppose pinhole test abolishes the diplopia, then the cause is either refractive error or cataract.

PRESBYOPIA

▌ Problem 1: A 44 years old office employee started facing difficulty in performing the routine desk work. He has no difficulty in distance vision and was not wearing any glasses. On his own he purchased an over the counter reading glasses for near vision, but after advise from colleagues he presented to clinic for ocular evaluation. This patient asks following question during examination

1. Whether using over the counter reading glasses are correct for my eyes?
2. What are the advantages and disadvantages of over the counter reading glasses?
3. What is the problem with my vision and using over the counter glasses will affect my vision?
4. How would you treat me?

Solution:

1. Usually when the patient of 44 years age are asymptomatic and have good distance vision without glasses, the near vision

problem is due to presbyopia. For this usual presbyopic condition over the counter (OTC) glasses are good alternative, when given by trained ophthalmic personnel. In this particular case the OTC glasses were purchased by patient under no supervision, so chances of overcorrection or under-correction are high.

2. Most common advantages of OTC glasses are economical, easily accessible and immediately available to use.

Disadvantages of OTC glasses are

- These glasses have equal power on both sides, however, majority of person have some amount of difference in refractive status of both the eyes.

- OTC glasses are available in common size small frames, whereas facial anatomy of people are quite different; hence the optical center and reading center may not properly align in OTC glasses.

- Quality of lenses used in OTC glasses is usually poor because of mass production; hence proper refractive correction is not possible.

Note: Indirect disadvantage of OTC glasses is that patient does not feel like visiting an ophthalmologist at presbyopic age; hence the chances of missing potentially blinding conditions like glaucoma and cataract increase.

3. Problem in this case is simple presbyopia due to decreased accommodation ability at 44 years of age. Using OTC glasses prescribed by ophthalmic personnel will not weaken the eyes, however, in this case the patient had purchased OTC glasses without any prescription so these glasses may not be correct for him. Many a times due to unproven concern of weakening of eyes, occasionally patients report that despite of having difficulty in reading they avoided using the recommended reading glasses; to keep their eyes strong.

4. To manage this case we will perform dry retinoscopy to evaluate any refractive error

for distance and then check the near vision monocularly then binocularly. Suppose distance vision retinoscopy is normal, then near vision is corrected using plus power spherical lenses monocularly and then binocular balancing is done as discussed in Chapter 11, page 297.

▎**Problem 2:** A 50 years old presbyope using over the counter reading glasses since 8 years presented with difficulty in seeing the fine near objects. On examination it was found that patient needs an increase in the strength of the existing over the counter reading glasses. On declaring that patient needs to increase the power of their existing reading glasses the patient asked these routine questions:

1. Can I still use my old reading glasses which are less strong?
2. Will the old glasses harm my eyes?
3. Write an appropriate solution with explanation.

Solution:

1. The patient can continue to use his/her old reading glasses as long as patient feels that the glasses are providing satisfactory vision for reading.

2. Suppose these old reading glasses are not causing any eyestrain; means they are also not doing any harm to patient's eyes, by using them. However if there is difficulty in seeing small objects or performing fine work, then change of glasses is recommended.

3. Best option for this patient is to perform a cycloplegic refraction to record the exact amount of refractive error. Suppose there is no refractive error for distance vision, then the power of near vision is determined and balancing is done as discussed in Chapter 11, page 297. It is always better to wear the glasses of exact power rather than OTC reading glasses for the reasons explained in the above solution. Suppose patient is an office employee and do computer work, then it is better to use the progressive glasses rather than OTC reading glasses.

Problem 3: A 55 years old moderately high myope successfully using progressive addition lenses for normal reading recently discovered that now she is facing difficulty in threading a needle. There is no history of medical illness and the power of her present glasses is nearly one and a half year old.
1. What might be the cause of her problem?
2. How will you solve the situation?

Solution:
1. The most probable cause of her difficulty are
   • Change in refractive power.
   • Beginning of cataractous changes.
   • Power of addition used since beginning was less (means just sufficient to read).
2. Various possible solution for her problem are dependent on the cause
   • In case of change in refractive power it is better to perform retinoscopy and prescribe new glasses having sufficient near add to see very small objects like needle hole or thread margin.
   • Perform a dilated examination to see the lenticular changes and if the cataract is only in grade one or two and patient is achieving N5 with near add then prescribe glasses and if the vision is not improving up to the patient's satisfaction, then perform cataract surgery.
   • Alternately in moderate degree myopes the simplest solution to this problem is just take off the present glasses and thread the needle; because by doing so they are using their natural nearsightedness to see close, hence no accommodation or additional plus power is needed.

Note: This strategy will also be useful when patient try to read very small print, or when it is necessary to read while at the same time patients require distance vision. However the reading material needed to be held closer than the normal reading distance.

Problem 4: A 42 years old asymptomatic emmetrope presented with the complaint of difficulty in focusing the distance objects after reading book for some time. Patient is not wearing glasses for distance or near and has no medical illness. Presently patient feels that it takes a few seconds for his vision to become clear when he looks across the room after reading for some duration. He also feels that words overlap when he read the book continuously for some duration.
1. Explain the etiology of this off and on blurring of vision both in distance and near?
2. How you will manage this case?

Solution:
1. This symptom is classical presentation of presbyopia, especially in an emmetrope. The remaining accommodation at 42 years of age is functioning very strongly so that this patient can read for some duration; however due to this extra efforts of accommodation patient's eye takes a few seconds for the accommodation to relax when patient look distance objects. Similarly while reading for some duration the small amount of accommodation gets exhausted and patient feels that words are getting overlapped.
2. To manage this case the options are dependent on the amount and severity of symptoms
   • If these symptoms of blurring off and on are accidental findings by the patient and are not causing any major inconvenience or difficulty; reading glasses can be deferred for some more period of time.
   • However, suppose patient has also noticed some difficulty with small print or would like to eliminate this problem; then reading glasses are recommended.
   • Suppose patient has to perform work on computers and also desire to have crisp intermediate vision then progressive glasses are recommended as the first choice.

Problem 5: A 44 years old emmetrope not wearing any glasses for near presented to the clinic with complaints of difficulty in reading newspaper inside the room especially during early morning or evening time; however, he is able to read the newspaper in balcony in daylight without any glasses. This patient also feels that he faces difficulty in reading the magazine in bed during nighttime; however, the same magazine he can read easily while sitting on table in daylight.

1. Explain the causes of this problem along with the diagnosis.
2. How would you manage this patient?

Solution:

1. The most probable cause of these symptoms is weakening of accommodative power of eyes, due to onset of presbyopia at the age of 44 years. These symptoms are occurring because

   • Normally when accommodation power decreases the pinhole effect helps in the ability to read clearly by producing miosis of eyes. Hence this patient was able to read newspaper in daylight. On contrary, normally pupils dilate when surrounding illumination decreases, which cause loss of the pinhole effect; hence this patient was unable to read inside the room.

   • In normal circumstances accommodation is achieved by contraction of the ciliary muscle, which in turn relaxes the zonules and allows the crystalline lens to become more convex. During early morning period the ciliary muscles are mildly slower and until late night the muscle gets fatigued; so this patient has difficulty in reading the newspaper especially during early morning and late nighttime.

   • Usually inside the bed person holds the magazine closer as compared to sitting position during daytime; this decrease in reading distance demands more accommodation power, which this 44 years old patient do not have. Hence this patient faces difficulty in reading the magazine in bed during nighttime.

2. As this patient is having an early onset presbyopia and has on official work we can manage this patient by prescribing the reading glasses. For an emmetrope at 44 years of age, usually a +1.25 DS power half eye reading glasses will work very

satisfactorily. Patient can wear these glasses during reading work by keeping them slightly in front over the nose, so that he can see the distance objects above the glasses.

Note: In bright sunlight reading is much easier for an emmetropic early onset presbyope because of the pinhole effect. The pinhole effect can be produced either by stimulating the eye with bright light or squinting the eyes.

Problem 6: A 52 years old emmetropic presbyope was using half eye reading glasses since 8 years for reading purposes. He has no history of medical illness or any other ocular problem. This patient walked into the clinic overwhelmed saying that he is capable of reading magazines without his reading glasses on tour, especially when he lay down on seashore.

1. Write an appropriate explanation of improvement in near vision.
2. Is this problem require any additional treatment?

Solution:

1. When this elderly emmetropic presbyope is on a tour and lay down on seashore in bright sunlight his eyes get the pinhole effect as discussed in the above problem. Normally on seashore the bright sunlight causes miosis of pupil to produce a significant pinhole effect and this pinhole permits only the central rays (coming from an object) to enter the eye. This effect neutralizes the refractive error and also compensate for the demand of accommodation. Hence this patient is able to read the magazine without wearing his reading glasses.

2. As this pinhole effect is a normal phenomenon and causes no harm to the eyes of patient, no additional treatment is recommended in this case. However, patient can continue to wear his reading glasses in all other situation while reading. Patient must be counseled and explained about the phenomenon of pinhole effect for improvement of his near vision in sunlight.

CHAPTER 18

Problems Related to Refraction, Post-refractive Corrections and Low Vision

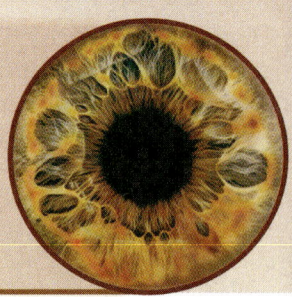

REFRACTION

Problem 1: A 65 years old patient having pesudophakia in both eyes came for routine follow-up without any significant complaints. A meticulous cycloplegic refraction was performed on this patient and glasses were prescribed. After a week this patient again came to the clinic with complaint that new glasses prescription given to him are not good and he is facing a lot of difficulties in seeing with new spectacles compare to his old spectacles. This patient has no history of systemic medical illness.

1. What could be the possible cause of non-acceptance of new prescription?
2. How will you manage this case?

Solution:

1. To find out the cause of discomfort and non-acceptance of glasses ask the following leading questions to this patient
   - Whether problem of seeing is in one eye or both the eyes?
   - Is their difficulty in seeing at distance, near or both with new glasses?
   - Is there any associated symptoms like ocular strain, tilting of edges of plane object, nausea, sudden blurring?
   - From where these new spectacles were made?

   Suppose the patient answers that he is having difficulty in seeing both at distance and near and has no associated symptoms of eye strains then re-evaluate the patient

with the old glasses. During re-evaluation examine these points
   - Check the power of old glasses.
   - Compare the visual acuity with both the old and new spectacles and note down the difference and comfort level (sometimes patient may have better visual acuity and comfortable feel with new glasses).
   - Perform a repeat refraction (preferably with cycloplegic drug, e.g. cyclopentolate)

2. Manage the patient according to outcome of examination as follows
   - Suppose a change in prescription of glasses is must, then advice the patient for new glasses (give complimentary consultation) and also explain him the cause of his difficulty in vision.
   - Suppose the glasses power prescribed were correct but there was an error in making of glasses by optician; handle the situation gently and consult with optician for arrangement of new complimentary spectacles.
   - Suppose the power of new prescription is accurate and also the glasses made are correct then counsel the patient that sometime a change in power requires adjustment period of one to two weeks, hence do not panic and continue to wear the new prescription.

Problem 2: Two 75 years old patients came together to clinic with complaint of gradual painless diminution of distance visual acuity since few months. A meticulous cycloplegic refraction is done and on subjective refraction best corrected visual acuity with glasses was recorded for both the patients as follows

- Patient A: Distance visual acuity 6/24 and near visual acuity of N12 in each eye.
- Patient B: Distance visual acuity 6/24 and near visual acuity of N6 in each eye.

Considering these abovementioned visual status, explain

1. What is the possible diagnosis of each patient?
2. How will you manage them?

Solution:

1. Considering the disparity between distance and near visual acuity
   - Patient A is more likely to have age-related macular degeneration, because in case of age-related macular degeneration, distance and near acuity are comparable. After correction with glasses both the distance and near visual acuity rarely get fully corrected in case of ARMD.
   - Patient B is more likely to have a cataract, because in an early to moderate grade cataract usually a disparity between distance and near acuity is seen where near acuity is always better than distance acuity. After correction with glasses the near acuity is usually corrected in normal range, however, the distance acuity is rarely get fully corrected in case of cataract.
2. Management of these patients include
   - In case of patient A having ARMD the treatment of choice is best correction with glasses and also by low visual aids (discussed in Chapter 16).

Note: Suppose a patient present with gradual painless diminution of vision and has both cataract and macular degeneration; then the discrepancy in improvement of distance and near visual acuity can be helpful in deciding which condition is more responsible for the reduced visual acuity.

- As patient B having cataract is not satisfied with distance vision with glasses then cataract extraction with IOL implantation is the treatment of choice.

Problem 3: A young patient having mixed refractive error came for follow-up after a period of two years with complain of slight difficulty in distance vision with existing glasses. Two years back an excellent refraction was performed by you and patient is wearing the same power glasses since then.

1. What type of refraction should be performed to resolve the present problem?
2. Describe the management in this case.

Solution:

1. As this patient is having a mixed refractive error and was comfortably wearing the previously prescribed glasses since two years, it means the cylindrical power and axis determined during previous cycloplegic refraction was accurate. This time as the patient is having slight problem in distance vision with existing glasses, means there is no need of changing the cylindrical power or axis in this patient and simple over refraction for correction of spherical power is required to correct the distance vision problem. In over refraction the patient is asked to wear the present glasses and a dry retinoscopy is performed to neutralize the reflexes. New power is recorded and difference in power is considered for prescription.
2. New prescription is dependent on the visual outcome after over refraction. Suppose over refraction produces an excellent vision in distance, then only a change in the sphere is prescribed along with the existing cylindrical power and axis. Thumb rule of prescription is that do not change the astigmatic error frequently. Difficulty in adjusting to the new prescription will be less in cases where astigmatic power was kept same as compared to the cases where cylinder power (especially cylindrical axis) was changed in new prescription.

Note: Additional advantage of performing an over-refraction is that there is no need to adjust vertex distance (distance between the lens and cornea) in new glasses. Since the new glasses will be fitted in same plane as existing and adjustment of new glasses will be easier for patient. Remember that larger the prescription power, the vertex distance becomes more relevant.

Problem 4: An elderly patient of 85 years age presented to clinic with low distance vision (6/60 in each eye). He is a diagnosed case of age-related macular degeneration (ARMD) and is on medical management. There is no history of medical illness; however, both eye cataract extractions with IOL implantation was done about two years back in right eye and one year back in left eye.

1. Whether routine type of refraction technique will help in improving the visual acuity in this case?
2. Describe an appropriate type of refraction method to improve the visual acuity in this case.

Solution:

1. Routine type of dry or wet retinoscopy will not help in this particular case, because the reflexes seen are not very bright and also the patient is not able to appreciate the small changes during subjective refraction. Hence we need to modify the refraction method to improve the visual acuity.
2. Most appropriate refraction technique is to perform the objective refraction under cycloplegia (specifically homatropine) and selecting large steps of lens power correction in ARMD patients having low vision. Once the objective refraction is done and estimated amount of refractive error is recorded then the subjective refraction power measurement and comparison of spherical and cylindrical powers are done in larger steps like 0.75 to 1 dioptre; not in routine smaller steps of 0.25 D. After changing the power of lenses at every step the patient is asked to compare the visual acuity and then proceed accordingly. Even

Note: There is no role of auto-refractor in these kinds of cases.

the axis of cylindrical lens is shifted in steps of 15–20 degrees, not as 2–5 degrees as done in routine refraction method.

Problem 5: An elderly 86 years old patient came to the clinic with complaint of having a lot of confusion about spectacles he needs during daily activities. He has no history of medical illness; however, both eyes cataract extraction with IOL implantation was done about 10 years back. On further investigation four pairs of spectacles were found in a carry bag, which he is wearing for various daily activities.

1. How will you proceed in this case?
2. How will you solve the problem of multiple spectacles?

Solution:

1. Primary aim of consultation is to reduce the number of spectacles in this patient which are being used for various activities and simplify the things. Following questions are asked to the patient to understand the real requirement in his daily activities
   • Which pair of spectacle he wishes to wear most of the time?
   • For what kind of activities he requires other pair of glasses?
   • How long he wear other pairs of spectacles?
   • Since how long he is using these four pairs of spectacles?

   Answers to these questions will help the practitioner to understand the real requirement of multiple pair of glasses. Based on the answers clinician can decide and accordingly reduce the spectacles which are not really needed by this old man.

2. Management of this problem depends upon the outcome of evaluation of patient and all four pairs of glasses
   • Suppose prescription of all glasses is very old and patient wear most of these

spectacles for very short duration then it is better to perform a cycloplegic refraction and prescribe new pair of glasses preferably separate spectacles for distance and near vision. This will reduce the number of glasses to only two pairs from four pairs. Alternately a pair of bifocal glasses having distance and intermediate power and second pair of glasses having only near power can be prescribed.

- Suppose patient is using these four pairs of glasses regularly and comfortably during various daily activities, then it is advisable to continue all pairs of spectacles as before, because change in pattern may create newer visual problems.

Problem 6: A 65 years old male patient presented to clinic overwhelmed that since a few months he does not require near vision glasses to read newspaper, although he was using half eye reading glasses since 22 years for reading purpose. He has not undergone any medical check up since 6–8 years and also has no symptoms of illness.

1. What are the possible etiologies for improvement in near vision at such an elderly age?
2. How will you manage this case?

Solution:

1. Most common phenomenon causing an improvement in reading ability in elderly age group patients is due to acquired myopia. As discussed before the common causes for acquired myopia are
   - Nuclear sclerosis of crystalline lens
   - High blood sugar levels in a diabetic (recent onset) patient.
   - Retinal detachment surgery (recent)
   - Chronic use of medications.

   As this particular patient has no history of recent ocular surgery (specially retinal detachment with scleral buckling), drug intake for longer duration or high blood sugar levels; the probable cause of improvement in near vision is nuclear sclerosis of crystalline lens. Cataract especially of nuclear sclerosis type causes a condition commonly called second sight of nearness because the patient again starts seeing the near objects without reading glasses after wearing the near vision glasses for 20–25 years.

2. To manage this case first evaluate the distance vision with best optical correction and following options are available for this elderly patient
   - Suppose the distance vision improves significantly by optical correction and patient is also satisfied with the amount of vision, then it is better to recommend the progressive glasses for some more year with regular six monthly follow up.
   - Suppose there is not significant improvement in distance vision or patient is not satisfied with the amount of distance vision with glasses, then it is better to recommend the cataract surgery.

Problem 7: An elderly 85 years old patient presented to clinic with visual symptoms due to excessive scratches on present spectacle lenses. On examination the refractive power of present glasses was accurate and a new prescription of same glass power was prescribed.

After a few days patient came with complain of intolerance to new glasses and exaggeration of visual symptoms.

1. How will you evaluate the case?
2. What will be the next step of management?

Solution:

1. First we check the power of old glasses on lensometer and also compare the new prescription with the old power of glasses. Once the power of both the old and new prescriptions are checked then
   - Suppose the power of old and new glasses are different, then ask the optician to correct the power of new glasses.
   - Suppose both the power of glasses are the same, then the most likely cause for

this problem of intolerance is that the new lenses have a different base curve than that of the old lenses. Change in base curve will affect the accommodation efforts of eye and refractive power of lens, hence will cause intolerance to the patient.

2. Most preferred method to solve this problem is to ask the patient to carry the old lenses to the optician along with new prescription of glasses with specially mentioned note for optician. In this note request the optician to simply duplicate the old prescription including the base curve of lenses.

Note: Suppose patient is wearing prisms in old prescription then simply write a note to the optician to duplicate the existing prisms in new lenses.

█ **Problem 8:** A 41 years old moderate degree myope recently developed presbyopia presented to clinic with a desire of monovision contact lens fitting. He has no medical illness and contraindications to contact lens fitting.

1. How will you evaluate the case for monovision?
2. What will be your recommendations in this case?

Solution:

1. All the basic evaluations for fitting of contact lens are done as discussed in Chapter 14, page 430. In case of monovision contact lens fitting we need to establish which eye of patient is dominant for a successful prescription. Easiest clinical method to determine the dominant eye of patient is as follows
   • Instruct the patient to outstretch both the arms keeping hands one on top of other. Tell the patient to create a small gap between two thumbs of outstretched arms.
   • Then patient is asked to look at a fine object like quotation on wall through this small gap between the thumbs (keeping both the eyes open).

• Examiner then alternately occludes one eye by an occluder while patient is still looking to the distance object.
• Patient must be able to see the distance object clearly with one among two eyes. The eye which sees the distance object clearly is termed dominant eye.

2. For a successful monovision contact lens fitting, the recommendations are
   • Determine the dominant eye and prescribe the distance correction contact lens for this dominant eye. A monofocal contact lens of near power is prescribed in fellow eye (non-dominant eye).
   • Alternately bifocal contact lens can be prescribed in both the eyes.

POST-REFRACTIVE CORRECTION

█ **Problem 1:** A 70 years old presbyope was comfortably wearing flat top bifocal glasses since 26 years. He developed difficulty in visualizing the TV caption from an intermediate distance with his present glasses. After cycloplegic refraction his glasses were changed from flat top bifocal to progressive type of glasses elsewhere. Now this patient is presented to our clinic with discomfort in vision both at distance and near.

1. How will you evaluate this case?
2. What will be the solution to this problem?

Solution:

1. For evaluation of problem
   • First inquire when the patient has been changed from a standard bifocal to progressive glasses or since how long patient is wearing these new progressive glasses. Usually there is an adjustment period for progressive glasses; some individuals may take approximately 2–3 weeks time period for adjustment of progressive glasses.
   • Following problems are asked to decide the cause of patient's difficulty in using progressive glasses:
     – Troublesome inbuilt blur at the sides of progressive glasses

- Necessity of any abnormal head posture for seeing the distance or near objects

- However, if there is a significant need for the correction of intermediate distance, for example, to see the television; it was reasonable to make the change in glasses from bifocal to progressive.

2. To solve the problem

  - Suppose the patient feels inbuilt blur or require abnormal head posture to see clearly, then check the proper pantoscopic tilt (described in Chapter 12, page 345).

  - Check the power of new progressive lenses by automatic lensometer (to be sure about the fitting of correct prescription).

  - Counsel the patient that usually progressive lenses require some amount of training in viewing the target and also viewing through progressive lenses takes some time for adjustment.

  - Suppose no problem is identified or it is confirmed that patient is unable to tolerate progressive glasses, best option is to change back to standard bifocal flat top glasses.

Note: Generally when patient is doing perfectly well with standard bifocal and has no complaints, it is better to continue the same type of glasses in new prescriptions.

■ **Problem 2:** A 55 years old patient was refracted and prescribed new glasses for both distance and near vision. This patient was previously wearing the D-bifocal glasses and hence made the new prescription in same lens design. After 2–3 days the patient came back with the complaint of having difficulty in reading with the recent prescription received from us; although the distance vision is fine with the new prescription.

1. What are the probable causes for difficult near vision with new prescription?

2. What should be the line of management?

Solution:

1. Various situations can cause the reading difficulty in this case.

  - To reach a proper diagnosis some more information is required in this case. Ask the patient whether changing the reading distance (means either keeping the book a little away from eyes or bringing the book a little closer to eye), affects the clarity of reading. Suppose the answer to any one of these situations is yes, means the reading addition given was improper. Always keep in mind that in the making of bifocal lenses, near power is always added with the distance prescription. Suppose the distance prescription is incorrect, then the reading segment prescription will automatically be wrong and patient will have difficulty in reading.

  - Classically position of the upper line for D-bifocal segment is fitted at the level of lower lid margin as described in Chapter 12, page 350. Suppose on inspection the reading segment is found to be fitted too low or too high, then the problem is not in addition power rather the cause is improper fitting of lens in the spectacle frame.

  - Spectacles are verified whether the lower portions of the lenses are fitted with an inwardly angled position (pantoscopic tilt) or not. Proper pantoscopic tilt is mandatory to read comfortably as described in Chapter 12, page 346.

2. Management of problem

  - Suppose if an improper addition was given in new prescription, then re-examine the patient and give proper addition power.

  - Suppose patient feel more comfortable in reading by pushing the glasses up or lifting the chin up, then reading difficulty is because of improper fitting of glasses in spectacle frame. In these cases the opticians are advised to fit the bifocal segment properly in spectacle frame as described in Chapter 12.

Note: In some individuals spectacle frame slides down from nose while person lowers the head to read a book; so the working position of bifocal near segment is fitted slightly lower than the usual position (i.e. at lower lid margin) in these cases.

- Suppose improper pantoscopic tilt was noticed in this case then correction of the pantoscopic tilt will enhance the comfortable reading ability of this patient.

Problem 3: A 47 years old emmetrope was presented to clinic with the complaint of recently developed problem in viewing the labels of medicines with his near vision half eye glasses. He was using +1.75 D power half eye reading glasses without any prescription very successfully since one year. He used to purchase the reading glasses from the opticians without any prescription. He has no history of medical illness and also presently has no complaint for distance vision.

1. What are the possible causes for this difficulty in near vision with reading glasses?
2. Outline the solutions to this problem?

Solution:

1. Possible causes for difficulty in reading the labels of medicine with present near vision half eye glasses are
    - Whether patient is attempting to see the medicine labels in bright sunlight. If yes, then the probable reason is that significant miosis in sunlight will cause difficulty in near vision with reading glasses because pinhole effect increases the near vision.
    - Is there any history of purchase of different reading glasses for fine near work, because fine near work requires higher addition power at nearer working distance.
2. Best possible solutions for this problem are
    - Advice the patient to purchase different half eye glasses with stronger power for this kind of fine near work.
    - Suppose patient requires seeing of medicine labels regularly and have multiple half eye reading glasses; then he/she can wear two glasses one above the other for this kind of fine near work.

Problem 4: A 48 years old an office executive who was wearing D-bifocal glasses since many years comfortably is now presented with difficulty in performing the excel work on his computer wearing glasses. The prescription of his bifocal glasses was recently changed about 3 months before and he is having crisp distance and near vision with the D-bifocal glasses.

1. What could be the probable cause for this problem in computer work?
2. Write down the possible solutions for this difficulty in intermediate vision.
3. Describe the tips to remember while prescribing a computer glasses.

Solution:

1. Most common cause for difficulty in viewing computer screen clearly is the distance of monitor. The desktop computer monitor is usually situated at a further distance than the normal reading distance. This distance is referred as the intermediate distance of vision; where person is unable to visualize the objects clearly either from the distance portion or near portion of his/her standard bifocal glasses.
2. To correct this problem possible solutions are
    - Prescribe a trifocal lens as discussed in Chapter 12, page 336. Patient is able to view the computer screen clearly and perform excel work comfortably when see through the intermediate segment of trifocal lens. However a small amount of chin lift is required to position the intermediate segment of trifocal lens in visual line of eyes.
    - Alternately progressive lenses can be prescribed, where multiple power will take care of intermediate distance; however a slight chin lift is recommended even for a progressive addition glasses.

- When patient is not agreeing for either of the above two solutions, then prescribe a separate computer glasses having intermediate correction in top portion and near correction in bottom portion of lenses. For distance vision patient is advised to use a separate spectacle. Patient will see the computer monitor while looking straight ahead, because the intermediate power is fitted in top portion. These computer glasses also eliminate the necessity of chin lift to see the computer screen, hence are useful in patients having neck problems.

3. Remember these points while prescribing the computer glasses
   - Never prescribe single vision glasses having intermediate power, because patient also needs to see near fonts while trying in computer key board.
   - Always prefer progressive glasses as computer glasses, because jumping of images is negligible in progressive glasses.
   - When only computer bifocal glasses are advised, then the near addition look very unusual, because nearly half of near power is required to be fitted in top portion of glasses as intermediate power and only remaining half power will be fitted in near segment.
   - To avoid this unusual looking situation a convenient method to calculate the intermediate power is by use of a near vision test card and slit lamp. Fix the near vision test card in chin rest position of slit lamp; this test card will serve as computer screen. Now gradually change the power of lenses in trial frame until patient comfortably read the smallest line on near test card. This will give the desired intermediate vision with minimum lens power.

Note: Suppose patient is suffering from a significant neck problem and feels difficulty in maintaining a chin lift position then both trifocals and progressive glasses are not suitable as computer glasses.

Problem 5: A 62 years old professor is presented with the complaint of difficulty in reading book during taking a class standing against the classroom dice; although professor is wearing the D-bifocal glasses since many years and has clear distance and near vision with glasses. Professor has no history of medical illness or not on any drugs.

1. What could be the possible cause for this problem?
2. How would you manage this problem?

Solution:

1. Strongest possibility is that the height of reading dice is such that professor need to read the book at an intermediate distance, which is beyond the reading distance and nearer than distance vision. So professor is unable to read either from distance segment or near segment of his/her present D-bifocal glasses.
2. This problem can be solved by following methods
   - Prescribe the progressive additional glasses or trifocal glasses and replace present D-bifocal glasses.
   - Prescribe a separate pair of glasses (on patient desire) with full distance correction in the upper portion and add of intermediate correction in the lower portion of D-bifocal glasses; so that professor can see the classroom students from upper portion of spectacles and book with the near segment simultaneously, while taking the class.

Note: Similar management is useful for various professions where person needs distance vision clarity with intermediate correction to read the subject matter kept on the dice.

Problem 6: Patient of age about 45 years working as vegetable vendor presented to clinic with problem in near vision. This patient requires glasses which he can wear continuously during the work. Explain which

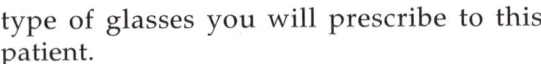

type of glasses you will prescribe to this patient.

1. Whether a bifocal glass that is fitted with too weak power of addition and why?
2. Whether a bifocal glass that is fitted with too strong power of addition and why?

Solution:

1. To this presbyopic patient working as vegetable vendor we will prescribe either the half eye reading glasses or bifocal glasses fitted with weak addition power. Because weaker addition glasses will produce a wider and longer range of reading. This patient does not require reading of book or fine matter, hence weaker addition will work better.
2. Usually bifocal glasses fitted with too strong power are not prescribed because they will create more problems than a too weak fitted bifocal glass. A closer and narrower range of reading produced by too strong bifocals is less tolerated as compared to longer and wider range of reading produced by weaker bifocal glasses.

Note: Suppose half eye glasses are prescribed then patient needs to advise to keep these glasses slightly lower on the nose so that he can see the distance objects from top of glasses.

▌**Problem 7:** A 55 years old golf player presented with the complaint of difficulty in seeing the score card, since few months. However, the player is comfortably wearing flat top D-bifocal glasses since 12 years.

1. What could be the cause for difficulty in viewing the score card?
2. How will you mange this case?

Solution:

1. Cause of problem in this case is that usually bifocal addition power is fused in lower segment of glasses and near segment is placed in bottom nasal portion of lens during fitting of spectacles. So normally people read from nasally fitted lower near segment of glasses, because while reading the eyes converge and hence the reading segment lie in front of pupillary center in normal circumstances. In case of golfers they view the score card from temporal side and hence they face difficulty because near segment is fitted nasally.

2. Management of the problem in special cases like golfers near add is required on opposite side of corner of glasses, i.e. temporarily, so that they can read score card while aiming for golf ball straight down. The golfers are fitted with special type of golfer's lenses in one eye and normal fitting in fellow eye as per requirement of golfer (described in Chapter 12, page 335).

Note: Similarly several other professionals like electricians, musicians specially French horn players and watch makers, require near add in top portions of glasses. These bifocal glasses are commonly called occupational bifocals (discussed in Chapter 12 on page no 334).

UNCOMMON REFRACTIVE CONDITIONS

Study these following clinical refractive scenarios which are not so common in routine clinical practice. Plan the strategies to manage these uncommon clinical refractive problems.

▌**Problem 1:** A 22-year-old boy came to the clinic for consultation regarding maintenance of his eyes. Presently the boy has no ocular complaints. He had past history of ocular trauma and on examination had no perception of light (PL) in right eye and left eye was emmetropic.

1. What advice you will give to this patient?

Solution:

1. It is most important to protect the left eye as this patient is having only one visually useful eye. Following advice can be given to look after the eyes
   - Wear protective goggles while playing contact games like football, cricket or badminton.
   - Wear Plano power anti-reflex coated glasses specifically made from polycarbonate

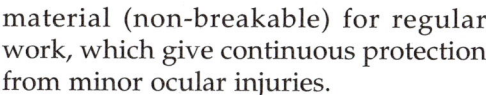

material (non-breakable) for regular work, which give continuous protection from minor ocular injuries.

- Use preservative free lubricants, because this boy is working on computers for more than 7–8 hours per day.
- Regular six monthly ocular examinations.

Problem 2: 28 years old patient working on computers for 5–6 hours daily came for an ocular examination to the clinic. Apparently patient is having no visual symptoms, however he occasionally feel foreign body sensation in both the eyes. On detailed examination and after cycloplegic refraction the patient had 6/6 visual acuity in each eye with –1.75 DS power in right eye and plano power in left eye. He also has mild dry eye in both the eyes.

1. How will you prescribe this patient?
2. Will there be any clinical symptoms if we prescribe glasses for this patient?

Solution:

1. As we can see that there is significant difference in amount of refractive status of both the eyes in this patient, so it is better to leave the decision on patient whether he wants to wear glasses or not. Prescription of glasses can be done as follows
   - Normally patient is asymptomatic and seeing the distance objects clearly with both the eyes open, because left eye is emmetropic. At the age of 28 years with one eye having moderate degree myopia the patient is comfortable in reading from any distance. Some of patients feel that correcting one eye will not produce any significant improvement in distance vision and hence refuses to use the glasses.
   - On contrary some patient may feel that correction of refractive error in one eye will improve the quality of vision by depth perception and also will not hamper the vision of better eye, so they agree to wear the glasses.
2. As discussed in Chapter 6, page 125 when the difference in refractive error between

two eyes (anisometropia) of less than 2.5 dioptres is present, it will not produce clinical significant difference in image size (aniseikonia). Hence in this particular case we can prescribe the glasses without producing any new clinical symptoms.

Problem 3: A 50 years old asymptomatic patient walked into the clinic for consultation. On examination when left eye was occluded the distance vision was affected and vice versa when right eye is occluded the near vision gets affected. However, patient is comfortably seeing both the distance and near targets without any glasses binocularly. On performing the refraction patient had –2.25 DS refractive error in right eye and plano power in left eye for distance. Also patient is accepting + 4 DS in right eye and +2 DS power in left eye for near vision.

1. What is the diagnosis of this condition?
2. What kind of consultation you will give to this patient?

Solution:

1. This particular patient is asymptomatic because of phenomenon called natural monovision, where patient is comfortably seeing distance objects clearly with one eye (left eye in our example) and vice versa near objects with fellow eye (right eye or myopic eye in our example).
2. Depending on the requirement of patient we can give following advise to this patient having natural monovision
   - Suppose patient require full correction of distance as well as near vision in each eye then we need to advice either bifocal or progressive glasses for this patient, where right eye glasses will have both distance and near powers, whereas left eye glasses will have only near correction power.
   - Suppose patient is happy with present visual status and desire not to wear

Note: In natural monovision cases it is always better not to prescribe any glasses.

glasses, then patient will do extremely well even without glasses for some more years.

Problem 4: An elderly 60 years patient presented to clinic with difficulty in seeing the distance and near objects since last few months. Patient is wearing glasses for distance since few years and has no history of medical illness. On examination right eye has a refractive error of $-2.5\,DS \times -1.5\,DC \times 90°$ with a near add of $+3\,DS$, whereas left eye has only perception of light.

1. What type of advice you will give to this patient?
2. Does this patient require some special type of prescription for making of glasses?

Solution:

1. As discussed above on page 590 protection of eyes specially the right eye having useful visual acuity is most important in this kind of patients. So we will advice the patient in similar manner as discussed.
2. As the distance refractive power is significant in right eye and left eye has no useful vision, we will prescribe the patient with the prescription having fully corrected power for refractive error on right side column and a balance written in left side column. The optician will understand the meaning of balance and fix an almost matching power of glass in front of left eye also, so that cosmetically both the glasses appear equal and more acceptable. This left eye lens is commonly called balance lens which appear almost equal in thickness and style to its fellow lens. This patient can manage the near vision by simply removing the glasses and keeping the object a little nearer than usual reading distance. Suppose the patient is not comfortable in removing the glasses too often and require near addition, then he can be prescribed bifocal glasses with $+3\,D$ addition in both eyes.

Problem 5: An elderly 85 years old patient presented with complaint of reading difficulty with the present bifocal glasses. On examination the distance visual acuity was 6/18 in right eye and 6/12 partial in left eye with present glasses. Patient is wearing an addition of $+2.75\,DS$ in both eyes and is having a near vision of N36 with present bifocal glasses. Patient is a diagnosed case of dry age related macular degeneration (ARMD) and is on medical treatment.

1. Describe the management outline in this case.
2. What will be your prescription for this patient?

Solution:

1. Normally in emmetrope at this age the maximum near addition given is in the range of $+2.5$ to $+3.0\,DS$. As this patient is having ARMD we can consider managing this case on the guidelines of low vision rehabilitation (discussed in Chapter 16). This patient can be managed by using various low vision optical aids at this stage of disease.
2. Prescription for this elderly ARMD patient include
   - A higher addition of $+3.5$ to $+4.0\,DS$ can be prescribed when patient is getting a significant improvement in near vision and also is mentally prepared to keep the reading objects little nearer than usual reading distance.
   - Suppose a higher addition more than $+4.0\,DS$ is required in this case to improve the near visual acuity then we can prescribe separate near vision glasses having high plus power.

Note: Suppose near vision further deteriorates, then consider magnification for near objects by using low vision optical aids as described in Chapter 16.

Problem 6: 17 years old young college student presented with complain of difficulty in seeing letters on blackboard, especially when he/she sit on last bench in classroom.

There is no history of wearing glasses or any eye examination in past. On examination after cycloplegic refraction the right eye has –5.5 DS refractive error and left eye has –0.5 DS refractive error.

1. Describe this condition in detail.
2. Outline the management strategy for this patient.
3. Write the management of this patient in follow-up visits.

Solution:

1. The difference between refractive status of both the eyes is considerably high; hence this condition is called anisometropia (described in Chapter 9). The difference in degree of refractive error is of 5 dioptres, hence when right eye is fully corrected there will be significant amount of aniseikonia (described in Chapter 9), where patient will see the significantly smaller size images from right eye after full correction of refractive error.

2. To manage this patient initially we need to prescribe trial corrective lenses, means correct the right eye refractive error partially by giving lesser power (say –2.25 DS) lenses than total power (–5.5 DS in our example). Patient is instructed to wear these trial lenses and report after some time about the quality of vision and associated symptoms (if any).

3. In follow-up visit this patient can be managed as follows
   - Suppose patient remains asymptomatic with trial run lenses, we can gradually increase the power of right side lenses (until tolerated by patient) to improve the visual acuity in right eye.
   - Suppose patient shows symptoms of aniseikonia, then we can prescribe contact lens for right eye which will improve the visual acuity and also eliminate the aniseikonia symptoms by abolishing the vertex distance factor.
   - Later on when refractive status of right eye becomes stable and visual acuity has

Note: Unlike monovision cases always correct the young anisometric patients to prevent amblyopia and other vision related symptoms.

also improved after correction, refractive surgery on right eye is done to correct the anisometropia in this case.

Problem 7: An elderly couple, husband of 65 years age and wife 63 years of age presented to clinic with recent onset difficulty in seeing the distance objects from their present glasses. On examination husband had a large chalazion in right upper eyelid and wife had ptosis of left eye. Both of them had no significant history of systemic medical illness. On performing the refraction a change in spherical power and cylindrical axis was found in respective eyes of both the patients.

1. Explain the cause of change in refractive status on one eye.
2. Describe the course of management in both the cases.

Solution:

1. Explanation for change of refractive status in one eye having ocular pathology are
   - In both these cases pressure changes on cornea due to mechanical push of lesion will be seen.
   - In case of husband the large upper eyelid chalazion is mechanically pushing the cornea due to its weight on eyelid and hence a refractive error especially astigmatic type will occur.
   - Similarly in case of wife the left eye ptosis will cause the change in corneal curvature. These changes in cornea can produce astigmatic error (usually irregular astigmatism) due to distortion of cornea.
   - Hence in both the cases these conditions are responsible for recent onset change in refractive status of one eye.
2. Management of problem
   - Surgical removal of chalazion is the treatment of choice, to relieve the mechanical

pressure on cornea in case of husband. This will automatically correct the refractive status of right eye; because once the chalazion is removed the cornea will come back to its original shape within a short period of time.

- Similarly in case of wife correction of ptosis will eliminate the indentation of cornea by left upper eyelid and hence will correct the refractive status of left eye gradually over period of time.

Note: In these cases correction of refractive error by glasses or other optical means is not helpful.

LOW VISION

Study these following low vision cases very carefully and explain the low vision evaluation methods along with management strategies in each specific condition.

Problem 1: An 85 years old patient walked into the low vision clinic with the support of his grandson. He was teacher by profession and presently is unable to read or write since a few months. Nearly 6 months ago patient was examined by retina specialist for gradual painless diminution of vision and was diagnosed as a case of dry ARMD both eyes where right eye is affected more than left eye. Presently patient is unable to move around alone and facing difficulty in performing daily activities.

Past history revealed that in both eyes cataract extraction with intraocular lens implantation was done, about 12 years back in right eye and 11 years back in left eye. Since post cataract surgery patient is wearing bifocal glasses and his present power of glasses is nearly two years older. Patient has no medical illness and no surgical history in the past.

In this case of dry ARMD

1. Outline how you will evaluate the low vision status of this patient.
2. Write down in detail about the management for this ARMD patient having significant visual impairment.

Solution:

1. Low vision evaluation: Low vision evaluation is done according to following headings as discussed in Chapter 16
   - Detailed patient history
   - Visual acuity assessment
   - Refractive status
   - Visual field assessment
   - Color vision
   - Contrast sensitivity and glare

Detailed history in terms of various target related activities is taken from the patient and his keen (relative accompanying the patient). He is unable to move alone in known or unknown places or identify the people meeting him in surroundings. With existing glasses he is unable to read the bus numbers or read a sign board on railway stations or roads, hence is not able to move in the common crowd without any support.

This elderly patient had difficulty in reading, writing and also watching television. He is also not able to sign on cheques or documents and also faces great difficulty in identifying the labels of his routine medicines. However, he is able to eat from his plate, wear clothes, identify the currency notes and take bath on his own.

- Visual acuity assessment is done both for distance and near vision using low vision distance and near charts with best possible optical corrections. Visual acuity in right eye (OD) is 3/60, in left eye (OS) 4/60 and OU 5/60
- Near visual acuity OD is 8 M, OS is 6 M and OU 5 M
- Refractive status OD $-2.25 \times +1.75 \times 90°$ and OS $-3.5 \times -1.5 \times 160°$
- Acceptance OD is $-2.5 \times +1.5 \times 90°$ (5/60) and OS is $-3.5 \times -1.5 \times 160°$ (6/60)
- Low vision device trial for near vision done and near visual acuity improved to 1.6 M with +10 D half eye spectacle magnifier at 8 centimetres distance in normal illumination, whereas with

+12 D hand-held magnifier the binocular near visual acuity improved to 1.2 M.

- Color vision testing done with color plates and was found to be within normal limits. Visual field assessment with low vision visual charts showed OD moderate superior suppression and OS mild temporal field suppression.

- Contrast sensitivity showed diffuse reduction in both eyes where right eye was more affected than left eye. Glare was markedly reduced with the usage of photochromic glasses.

2. Rehabilitation and management

- Complete distance vision correction was prescribed. Patient was advised to get these glasses in photochromic lenses and wear the spectacles regularly for daily activities.

- +10 D half eye magnifying near spectacles in white lenses were prescribe for near work.

- Use of signature guide and envelop guide to sign the cheques and write letters are advised along with usage of magnifying near glasses. However, to search near objects hand-held magnifier of +12 D power can be used occasionally by the patient.

- Use of peak cap and dark goggles was advised while patient goes out in sunlight and advised to avoid going out alone in nighttime.

- To watch TV patient was counselled the role of approach magnification.

- Regular monthly visits till three months and then every three months were recommended for follow-up.

Problem 2: A 70 years old female came with her husband to the clinic for low vision evaluation. She was referred by her family physician and is a diagnosed case of bilateral diabetic retinopathy with left eye affected more than right eye. She also had history of associated hypothyroidism for which she is taking oral medications since 15 years. She also had history of osteoarthritis for which she takes oral anti-inflammatory medications off and on as per her requirements. Treatment history revealed that twice she had received retinal laser treatment in both the eyes in last 3–4 years.

Presently she complains of gross diminution of distance and near vision in spite of wearing progressive multifocal glasses. The prescription of present progressive glasses is about 8–10 months old and she is using separate near glasses for reading books. Her history of diabetes is about 40 years old, initially she was only on oral hypoglycaemic and gradually she came to the present status of insulin with oral hypoglycaemic usage since 10 years. With insulin she is maintaining her blood sugar levels well in control and rarely have fluctuation in blood sugar levels. Presently she is not using any low vision aids or any other supportive visual aid.

1. Outline how you will evaluate the low vision status of this patient.

2. Write down in detail about the management for this diabetic retinopathy patient having significant visual impairment.

Solution:

1. Low vision evaluation: Elaborated history in terms of various target related activities is taken from the patient and her husband. She is facing difficulty in identifying the numbers of channel on television and also in reading books with present glasses. She feels very uneasiness while coming down from the staircase especially during nighttime. She has great difficulty in writing notes or any letter and also found continuous reading of novel very tiresome. However she is able to do her routine activities like bathing, prayers, walking in house and eating food, etc. independently.

- Visual acuity assessment is done both for distance and near vision using low vision distance and near chart (Feinbloom's chart) with best possible optical corrections. Best corrected visual acuity

(BCVA) in right eye (OD) is 6/60, in left eye (OS) 5/60 and OU 6/24

- Refractive status of respective eyes were OD $-1 \times -2.5 \times 90°$ and OS $- 2.5 \times -2 \times 90°$
- Near visual acuity with present near vision glasses OD is 3.2 M, OS is 2 M and OU 1.5 M
- Low vision device trial for near vision done and near visual acuity improved to 0.8 M with +6 D half eye spectacle magnifier at 30 cm distance in normal illumination, whereas with +8 D hand-held magnifier binocular near acuity was 0.5 M.
- Color vision testing done with color plates and was found that she is able to identify the normal colors within normal limits.
- Visual field assessment with low vision visual charts showed no suppression of visual fields either in right eye or left eye.
- Contrast sensitivity showed mild diffuse reduction in both eyes where left eye was more affected than right eye. Glare was marked reduced with the usage of antireflex coated polarized glasses.

2. Rehabilitation and management
- Complete distance vision correction was prescribed and patient was advised to get these glasses in antireflection coated polarized lenses. She was instructed to wear these spectacles regularly for her routine household activities.
- +6 D half eye magnifying near spectacles either in high index aspheric lenses or in hybrid lenses were also prescribe for near work. She was instructed to remove the distance glasses and wear these near spectacles for reading writing purpose only.
- Use of signature guide and envelop guide to sign the cheques and write letters are advised along with usage of magnifying near glasses. However, to search near objects hand-held magnifier of +8 D power can be used occasionally by the patient.

- She was advised to avoid going out in sunlight, however, if required she was advised to wear peak cap with dark goggles or take umbrella while goes out in sunlight. However, she was advised to avoid going out alone in nighttime.
- To watch TV patient was counselled to use distance glasses with the application of the approach magnification by reducing the viewing distance of television and also enlarging the screen size of TV.
- Regular monthly visits are must till initial three months and then every three months to observe the adjustment of low vision devices and then a regular follow-up is recommended to watch for any deterioration in visual acuity.

Problem 3: A 57 years old patient walked into the clinic with holding the hand of his wife and straightway sat on the examination chair when asked to take a seat for evaluation. He is a diagnosed case of open angle glaucoma since 28 years and using anti-glaucoma medication since then. Treatment history revealed that right eye trabeculectomy was done about 8 years back and left eye trabeculectomy was done 5 years back. Both eyes cataract extraction with IOL implantation was done one after the other in last 3 years. No associated history of medical illness is present.

Presently patient is wearing progressive glasses and having satisfactory visual acuity for distance and near, however, his visual fields done one month back is showing significant peripheral scotoma with ring scotoma in both the eyes. He is using anti-glaucoma medications latanoprost with brinzolamide and brimonidine combination eye drops regularly in both the eyes.

At present patient is unable to identify large furniture in room and need to move the head to see the various objects present in room. He is unable to watch the entire TV screen in one view and also not able to perform continuous reading in computer screen or textbook. However, patient is able to perform routine daily activities independently and can walk alone in garden.

1. Outline how you will evaluate the low vision status of this patient.
2. Write down in detail about the management for this advance glaucoma patient having significant visual impairment.

Solution:

1. Low vision evaluation: Detailed history in relation to various task related activities are taken from the patient and his wife. Patient is able to identify the distant objects very clearly, however, is unable to see the entire object in a single view, hence is facing difficulty in identifying the numbers of channel on television and also in reading books. He feels difficulty and uneasiness in crowded places because he often bumps up with people walking around him. He is unable to enjoy any tour or scenery places because of limited view of visual field. However he is able to perform daily activities like bathing, clothing and eating independently. He is also able to sign the documents and read the letters.

- Visual acuity assessment is done both for distance and near vision using Snellen's distance and near chart with best possible optical corrections. Best corrected visual acuity (BCVA) in right eye (OD) is 6/9, in left eye (OS) 6/6 and OU 6/6

- Refractive status of respective eyes were OD – 1 DS and OS – 0.75 × –0.5 DC × 90°

- Near visual acuity with +3DS power near vision glasses, OD is 0.8 M, OS is 0.8 M and OU is 0.5 M

- Color vision testing done with color plates and was found that he is able to identify the normal colors within normal limits.

- Visual field assessment with low vision visual charts showed significant suppression of visual fields in both the eyes, where right eye was affected more than left eye. Right eye showed ring scotoma with presence of only 8 degrees central visual field and left eye has inferior and superior arcuate field defects with presence of only 12 degree central field.

- Contrast sensitivity showed marked diffuse reduction in both eyes where right eye was more affected than left eye. Glare sensitivity was not much affected.

2. Rehabilitation and management

- Complete distance and near vision correction was prescribed and patient was advised to get these glasses in progressive lenses. He was instructed to wear these spectacles regularly during his routine activities.

- Central visual field expanders as discussed in Chapter 16 are prescribed to improve the visual field. Patient was instructed to wear these field expanders during daily activities or reading, however, try to avoid them wearing in public places.

- He was advised to avoid going out alone in crowded places and if absolute necessary then he has to take support of a sighted person.

- To watch TV patient was counselled to use distance glasses with the application of the field expanders specially the reverse telescopes or minus lenses, so that larger field of view is seen.

- Patient and relatives are explained the prognosis of advanced glaucoma disease and patient is encouraged to learn some additional skills like Braille or Moon for future survival as there are chances of further deterioration in visual field.

- Regular follow-up at two months interval is advised to observe the adjustment of low vision visual field expanders and assessment of visual fields.

Problem 4: Retina specialist referred a 36 years old patient having the diagnosis of retinitis pigmentosa (RP) with optic atrophy, for low vision evaluation and management. This patient came to the clinic with holding the hand of his brother and was searching the examination chair when asked to take a seat for evaluation. Present and past history was explained by his brother because patient was not very comprehensive and also was not precise in answering the leading questions. He had no significant contributory birth or past history related to the present illness. About at the age of 19 years he was diagnosed as a case of RP and since then the patient is on irregular follow up due to social and financial constrains. Patient is third child among five children and two of his siblings had similar kind of problem. One of his paternal uncle and grandfather also had problem of poor night vision. He has no associated systemic illness and there is no history of consanguineous marriage in his family. His present complaint is diminution of distance and near vision since 7–8 years and was unable to go around in the night time since past 22 years. Patient is a vegetable seller and now he is unable to identify the currency or weight of vegetables at night time, so he closes down his vegetable sale in the evening time only. He is presently not using spectacles for either distance or near, although elsewhere he had been prescribed distance glasses about 4–5 years before which he hardly worn in past few years. There is no history of any previous low vision evaluation or prescription of any kind of low vision devices.

Solution:

1. Low vision evaluation: Detailed history in terms of various target related activities is taken from the patient and his brother. He is facing difficulty in identifying the currency and weight of vegetable sale especially during nighttime. Patient is unable to search the road for home or move around independently in market place especially during nighttime. He is not much educated but has great difficulty in signing the bank cheques or any other documents. However, still he is able to perform his day-to-day activities like bathing, clothing, identifying house furniture and eating food, etc. independently in bright daylight.

- Visual acuity assessment is done both for distance and near vision using low vision distance and near chart (Feinbloom's chart) with best possible optical corrections. Visual acuity in right eye (OD) is 4/60, in left eye (OS) 4/60 and OU 5/60.
- Near visual acuity OD, OS is 6 M and OU 5 M
- Refractive status of respective eyes were OD $-2.5 \times -0.75 \times 110°$ (5/60) and OS $-1.5 \times -0.5 \times 70°$ (5/60) and OU with glasses 5/60.
- Low vision device trial for near vision done and near visual acuity improved to 1.8 M with +8 D half eye spectacle magnifier at 30 centimetres distance in normal illumination, whereas with +10 D hand-held magnifier binocular near acuity was 1 M.
- Color vision testing done with color plates and was found that he is able to identify basic colors, however, he fails to identify the specific design color plates.
- Visual field assessment with central low vision visual field charts showed that only 15 degrees central vision in both the eyes is present.
- Contrast sensitivity showed moderate degree of reduction in both eyes where left eye was slightly more affected than right eye. Glare was marked reduced with the usage of amber tint glasses.

2. Rehabilitation and management
- Complete distance vision correction was prescribed and patient was advised to get these glasses in amber tint lenses for better visibility in daylight. He was instructed to wear these spectacles

regularly during his routine vegetable business timings.

- +8 D half eye magnifying near spectacles preferably in high index aspheric lenses were also prescribe for near work. He was instructed to remove the distance glasses and wear these near spectacles for identifying the currency and reading the weight of vegetables on weighting machine.

- Use of signature guide to sign the cheques and documents was advised along with usage of magnifying near glasses. However, to search any specific vegetable items or small coin hand-held magnifier of +10 D power can be used occasionally during business hours.

- He was advised to avoid going out alone in nighttime and if absolute necessary, then he has to take support of a sighted person.

- To watch TV patient was counselled to use distance glasses with the application of the field expanders specially the reverse telescopes or minus lenses, so that larger field of view is seen.

- Genetic counselling and examination of other family members for visual status and disease identification is advised.

- Patient and relatives are explained the prognosis of disease RP and patient is encouraged to learn some additional skills like Braille or Moon for future survival as there are chances of further deterioration in distance and near vision.

- Regular follow-up at three months interval is advised to observe the adjustment of low vision devices and assessment of visual fields.

Problem 5: A 22 years old young male was diagnosed as a case of Leber's hereditary optic neuropathy (LHON) in both the eyes by retina specialist recently. This patient was presented to our clinic with his parents for low vision evaluation and management. Birth history was normal and he is younger among two sons. He had almost normal developmental milestones except that since 2–3 months he started difficulty in identifying the faces, reading the books and also started watching the television from very closer distance. Presently he is a college graduate student in a regular college and sits in second row of classroom, however, his professors complains that he is very restless in classroom and is not doing well in studies.

Presently the chief complaint is that he is unable to see the distant objects clearly and is not able to read the book from normal reading distance. This diminution in distance and near vision has occurred since 2–3 months and visual acuity markedly decreased in right eye and then after 3–4 weeks into the left eye. There is no history of consanguineous marriage in his family and his elder brother is absolutely normal with no such complains, however, one of his paternal uncle had similar kind of ocular problem. No systemic or other ocular complains are present. Patient is not on any chronic use of drugs and also there is no previous history of ocular examination or usage of glasses or any other optical aids for poor visual acuity.

Solution:

1. Low vision evaluation: Detailed history in terms of various target related activities is taken from the parents. Patient is facing difficulty in reading/writing and also was unable to see the distance objects clearly. His behaviour and eye contact was normal on gross evaluation and has no difficulty in moving around in market places, however, was uncomfortable in bright sunlight in daytime and with vehicle headlights in nighttime. He faces difficulty in identifying the friends and relative faces from some distances and also is unable to read the school bus number or road sign-boards. He is also unable to read the book continuously in fluency even if he changes the reading distance frequently. Patient is

able to perform daily activities like bathing, clothing and dining independently.

- Visual acuity assessment is done both for distance and near vision using low vision distance and near charts. Distance visual acuity in right eye (OD) is 3/60, in left eye (OS) 4/60 and OU 5/60.
- Near visual acuity OD, OS is 4M and OU 3 at 20 cm distance.
- Refractive status of respective eyes were OD + 1.75 Ds and OS + 1.5 × + 0.5 × 90°
- Acceptance OD and OS + 1.75 DS, 5/60. Near visual acuity 2.6 M at 18 cm.
- Color vision testing done with Munsell 100 hue test and was found that he is not able to identify basic colors; especially had difficulty in identifying red color.
- Visual field assessment with peripheral and central low vision visual field charts was attempted but patient is unable to complete the test accurately, because he is not fixing the central visual target of charts. His visual field charts showed centrocecal scotoma in both the eyes and in right eye the scotoma was extending on both sides of vertical meridian.
- Contrast sensitivity testing showed 15% moderate degree of diffuse reduction in both eyes where left eye was slightly more affected than right eye.
- Distance low vision aids 8X telescope (monocular type) was tried with latest distance correction glasses. He was able to read 6/36 size letters comfortably from 6 meters distance fluently. Overall response for distance and near vision improved and both the parents and patient were accepting the final visual acuity when telescope was added with spectacle lenses.

2. Rehabilitation and management
- Complete distance vision correction was prescribed and parents were advised to get these glasses in photochromic grey lenses for better visibility in daylight. He

was instructed to wear these spectacles regularly throughout the day.

- 8X telescope (monocular type) is fitted with his distance spectacle power and he is trained to read the text on blackboard wearing these telescopic lenses. Specific instructions were given to the professor to cooperate in terms of seating arrangements and training of patient to see with telescopic spectacles. Once patient is accustomed to these telescopic spectacles, then he is advised to wear them regularly.
- To watch TV patient was counselled to use approach magnification by reducing the viewing distance of television and also enlarging the screen size of TV.
- Parents are explained about the prognosis of Leber's hereditary optic neuropathy condition and are instructed to promote the patient to adjust the low vision device and to learn some additional skills where vision is not much hurdle.
- Regular follow-up at two months interval is advised to observe the adjustment of low vision devices and assessment of retinal status with visual fields.

Problem 6: A 9 years old female child presented to clinic with her father for low vision evaluation and management. She is an established case of Oculo-cutaneous albinism with rotatory nystagmus having very poor visual acuity. History was presented by the father because child was unable to focus on questions and was not able to maintain the eye contact. Birth history reveal normal hospital delivery and she is the elder among two daughters.

She had almost normal developmental milestones except that since early childhood she used to keep the things very close to her face and watches television from very near distance. She also was not able to maintain the gaze and had constantly moving eyes especially in rotatory movements. Her skin color is also very fair, whereas her parents and sister are having normal brownish colored skin. Presently she is a class third student and sits in front rows of classroom, however, her teacher complains that she is very less attentive in class and do not copy the subject matter correctly from the blackboard.

Presently she is unable to see the distant objects clearly and is not able to fix her eyes on any target. She also read and writes from very close distance. No systemic or other ocular complains are present. There is no history of consanguineous marriage and her younger sister is absolutely normal with no such complains.

Solution:

1. Low vision evaluation: Detailed history in terms of various target related activities is taken from her father. She is facing difficulty in reading/writing and also unable to see the distant objects clearly. She needs support to move in crowded places and also feels irritation in bright sunlight. She has right-sided head tilt while try to focus the distance objects or speak to some person. This head tilt is more significant when she focuses on specific tasks like watching television, or sees the blackboard in classroom. She is able to move around in the house independently and also is able to perform her daily activities like bathing, clothing, eating and moving around without any support.
   - Visual acuity assessment is done both for distance and near vision using low vision distance and near chart (Feinbloom's chart) with best possible optical corrections. Distance visual acuity in right eye (OD) is 3/60, in left eye (OS) 2/60 and OU 3/60.
   - Near visual acuity OD, OS is 3.2 M and OU 3 M at 8 cm distance.
   - Refractive status of respective eyes were OD – 6.5 × – 0.75 × 90° and OS – 7.5 × – 0.5 × 90°
   - Acceptance OD –6.× –0.75 × 90° (6/18) OS –6.5 × –1.0× × 90° (6/24), with head tilt towards right. Near visual acuity 2 M at 15 cm.

- Color vision testing done with HRR color plates and was found that she is able to identify basic colors, however, she fails to identify the specific design color plates.
- Visual field assessment with central low vision visual field charts was attempted but child is unable to complete the test because of her rotatory nystagmus.
- Contrast sensitivity testing done with chart showed moderate degree of diffuse reduction in both eyes where left eye was slightly more affected than right eye. Glare was markedly reduced with the usage of photochromic glasses and shades.
- Nystagmus evaluation shows the presence of rotatory nystagmus with null zone in primary gaze and exaggeration in lateral gazes.
- Cover uncover test revealed left exophoria with nystagmus.
- Low vision aids tried for distance vision with use of 6X telescopes over distance correction glasses. She was able to read 6/9 size letters comfortably from 6 meters distance fluently. She was also able to identify the near objects and locate various objects in the examination room.

2. Rehabilitation and management
   - Complete distance vision correction was prescribed and parents were advised to get these glasses in photochromic brown tint lenses for better visibility in daylight. She was instructed to wear these spectacles regularly during her routine activities.
   - 6X telescope (monocular type) is especially designed with her spectacle power and she is trained to see the blackboard wearing telescope lenses. Specific written instructions were given for school teacher to arrange the front row seat for child and cooperate in training the child to see with telescopic spectacles. Gradually once she is accustomed in

using telescope mounted spectacles, then she should wear these telescopic spectacles regularly.

- She was advised to avoid going out in sunlight and if absolute necessary then she has to cover the body with proper clothing and wear dark shade spectacles with peak cap. For additional protection from sunlight she can use UV protection sunscreen lotions (SPF > 12).

- To watch TV patient was counselled to use approach magnification by reducing the viewing distance of television and also enlarging the screen size of TV.

- Genetic counselling and examination of other family members for visual status and systemic disease identification is advised.

- Patient and relatives are explained the prognosis of oculo-cutaneous albinism disease and parents are instructed to promote the child to learn some additional skills where vision is not much hurdle.

- Regular follow-up at three months interval is advised to observe the adjustment of low vision devices and assessment of visual fields.

Bibliography

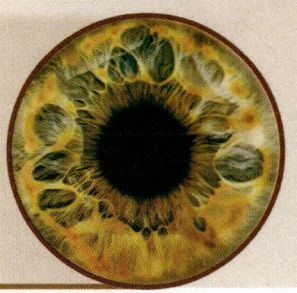

1. AK Khurana. Theory and Practice of Optics and Refraction. Elsevier (A division of Reed Elsevier India Private Limited); 2008.

2. David Abrams. Duke-Elder's Practice of refraction. Elsevier (A division of Reed Elsevier India Private Limited); 1983.

3. George L. Spaeth, Helen V. Danesh-Meyer, Ivan Goldberg, Anselm Kampik. Ophthalmic Surgery Principles and Practice. Elsevier; 2012.

4. Gholam A. Peyman, Donald R. Sanders, Morton F. Goldberg. Principles and Practice of Ophthalmology. Jaypee Brothers; 1987.

5. Gunter K. von Noorden, Emilio C. Campos. Binocular Vision and Ocular Motility. Mosby inc.; 2002.

6. John M. Corboy, David J. Norath, Richard Reffiner, Ron Stone. The Retinoscopy Book. *An Introductory Manual for Eye Care Professionals*. SLACK incorporated; 2003.

7. Myron Yanoff, Jay S Duker. Ophthalmology. Mosby international ltd; 1999.

8. Norman S. Jaffe, Mark S. Jaffe, Gary F. Jaffe. Cataract Surgery and its complications. Harcourt Asia PTE. Ltd;1999.

9. Paul L. Kaufman, Albert Alm. Adler's Physiology of The Eye, Clinical Application. Mosby Inc; 2003.

10. Troy E. Fannin, Theodore P. Grosvenor. Clinical Optics. Butterworth-Heinemann; 1996.

Index